CASES IN DIAGNOSTIC REASONING

ACUTE & CRITICAL CARE

NURSE PRACTITIONER

Notice

Medicine is an ever-changing science. As new research and clinical experience broaden our knowledge, changes in treatment and drug therapy are required. The authors and the publisher of this work have checked with sources believed to be reliable in their efforts to provide information that is complete and generally in accord with the standards accepted at the time of publication. However, in view of the possibility of human error or changes in medical sciences, neither the authors nor the publisher nor any other party who has been involved in the preparation or publication of this work warrants that the information contained herein is in every respect accurate or complete, and they disclaim all responsibility for any errors or omissions or for the results obtained from use of the information contained in this work. Readers are encouraged to confirm the information contained herein with other sources. For example and in particular, readers are advised to check the product information sheet included in the package of each drug they plan to administer to be certain that the information contained in this work is accurate and that changes have not been made in the recommended dose or in the contraindications for administration. This recommendation is of particular importance in connection with new or infrequently used drugs.

ACUTE & CRITICAL CARE

NURSE PRACTITIONER

SUZANNE M. BURNS,
MSN, RN, ACNP-BC, CCRN, RRT,
FAAN, FCCM, FAANP
Professor Emerita
School of Nursing
University of Virginia
Consultant
Critical and Progressive Care
and Clinical Nursing Research
Charlottesville, Virginia

SARAH A. DELGADO,
MSN, RN, ACNP-BC
Clinical Practice Specialist
American Association of
Critical-Care Nurses
Aliso Viejo, California

Mc
Graw
Hill
Education

New York Chicago San Francisco Athens London Madrid
Mexico City Milan New Delhi Singapore Sydney Toronto

Cases in Diagnostic Reasoning: Acute & Critical Care Nurse Practitioner

4 5 6 7 8 9 0 LCR 22 21

ISBN 978-0-07-184954-8
MHID 0-07-184954-8

This book was set in 10/12 Chaparral Pro by MPS Limited.
The editors were Andrew Moyer and Susan Barnes.
The production supervisor was Catherine Saggese.
Project management was provided by Poonam Bisht, MPS Limited.
The text designer was Eve Siegel.
RR Donnelley was printer and binder.

This book is printed on acid-free paper.

Library of Congress Cataloging-in-Publication Data

Burns, Suzanne M., author.
  Cases in diagnostic reasoning : acute and critical care nurse practitioner / Suzanne M. Burns, Sarah A. Delgado.
    p. ; cm.
  Includes bibliographical references and index.
  ISBN 978-0-07-184954-8 (pbk. : alk. paper) — ISBN 0-07-184954-8
  I. Delgado, Sarah A., author. II. American Association of Critical-Care Nurses, sponsoring body. III. Title.
  [DNLM: 1. Critical Care Nursing—methods—Case Reports. 2. Nursing Diagnosis—methods—Case Reports. 3. Acute Disease—nursing—Case Reports. 4. Decision Making—Case Reports. 5. Nurse Practitioners—Case Reports. WY 154]
  RT48
  616.07'5—dc23
                                                                                    2015026232

Dedication

To our fellow nursing faculty who work tirelessly to assist nurses with the transition to advanced practice. And to acute and critical care nurse practitioners everywhere who manage this vulnerable population with knowledge and care.

Sincerely,
Suzi and Sarah

CONTENTS

CONTRIBUTORS

Kwame Asante Akuamoah-Boateng MSN, RN, ACNP-BC
Division of Trauma, Critical Care, and
 Emergency Surgery
Virginia Commonwealth University
Richmond, Virginia

Rachel Anderson MSN, ACNP-BC, CCRN, CMC, CSC
Lung Transplant Program
University of Virginia Health System
Charlottesville, Virginia

Julie K. Armatas MSN, RN, ACNP-BC
Vascular and Endovascular Service
University of Virginia Health System
Charlottesville, Virginia

Caroline Austin-Mattison FNP-BC
Cardiac Telemetry and Cardiac
 Catheterization Units
Mount Sinai Hospital
New York, New York

Michelle Beard MSN, RN, ACNP-BC, AOCNP
University of Virginia's Cancer Care
 Clinics in Farmville and Charlottesville
University of Virginia Health System
Charlottesville, Virginia

Carolyn Brady MSN, RN, ACNP-BC
Heart Failure Clinic
University of Virginia Health System
Charlottesville, Virginia

Steven W. Branham PhD, RN, ACNP-BC, FNP-BC, FAANP, CCRN
Acute Care Nurse Practitioner Program
Texas Tech University Health Sciences
 Center
Lubbock, Texas
Texas Woman's University
Denton, Texas

Mary M. Brennan DNP, RN, AGACNP-BC, ANP
Adult Acute Care Nurse Practitioner
 Program
New York University, New York
Cardiology Inpatient Service
New York, New York

Helen F. Brown MS, RN, ACNP-BC, FNP-BC
Emergency Department
Anne Arundel Medical Center
Annapolis, Maryland
Acute Care Nurse Practitioner
 Program
Georgetown University
Washington, District of Columbia

Denise Buonocore MSN, RN, ACNP-C, CCRN, CHFN,
Heart Failure Service-St. Vincent's
 Multispecialty Group
St. Vincent's Medical Center
Bridgeport, Connecticut

Suzanne M. Burns MSN, RN, ACNP-BC, CCRN, RRT, FAAN, FCCM, FAANP
Professor Emerita, School of Nursing
University of Virginia
Consultant, Critical and Progressive
 Care and Clinical Nursing Research
Charlottesville, Virginia

Donna Charlebois MSN, RN, ACNP-BC, CCDS
Heart and Vascular Center-
 Outpatient Interventional
 Cardiology Service
University of Virginia Health
 System
Charlottesville, Virginia

Jie Chen MSN, RN, ACNP-BC, CMSRN
Transplant Service
University of Virginia Health System
Charlottesville, Virginia

Sarah A. Delgado RN, MSN, ACNP-BC
Clinical Practice Specialist
American Association of Critical-Care Nurses
Aliso Viejo, California

Charles Fisher MSN, RN, ACNP-BC
Medical Intensive Care Unit
University of Virginia Health System
Charlottesville, Virginia

Shawn Floyd MSN, RN, ACNP-BC, CCRN, CCTC
Cardiopulmonary Transplant Team
University of Virginia Health System
Charlottesville, Virginia

Elizabeth S. Gochenour MSN, RN, ACNP-BC, CWON
Inpatient Wound Care Team
University of Virginia Health System
Charlottesville, Virginia

Kelly Godsey MSN, RN, ACNP
Advanced Heart Failure and Cardiac Transplant Outpatient Clinic
University of Virginia Health System
Charlottesville, Virginia

Elizabeth W. Good MSN, RN, ACNS-BC, ACNP-BC
Hepato-Pancreato-Biliary Surgical Oncology Service-Department of Surgery
University of Virginia Health System
Charlottesville, Virginia

Eliza Ajero Granflor MSN, RN, APRN-BC, ACNP-BC, CNS, CCRN
Surgical Intensive Care Unit
The Queens Medical Center
Honolulu, Hawaii

Julie A. Grishaw MSN, RN, ACNP-C, CCRN
McGraw-Hill Education
New York, New York
Medical Intensive Care Unit
University of Virginia Health System
Charlottesville, Virginia

Tonja M. Hartjes DNP, RN, ACNP-BC, CCRN, CSC
Adult Gerontology Acute Care Program
University of Florida College of Nursing
Gainesville, Florida

Janie Heath PhD, RN, ACNP-BC, FAAN
University of Kentucky College of Nursing
Lexington, Kentucky

Tara C. Hilliard MSN, RN, ACNP-BC
Acute Care Nurse Practitioner Program
Texas Tech University Health Sciences Center
Lubbock, Texas

Sheryl Hollyday MSN, RN, FNP-BC
Cancer Center-Palliative Care Inpatient and Outpatient Program
St. Vincent's Medical Center
Bridgeport, Connecticut

Theresa R. (Roxie) Huyett MSN, RN, ACNP-BC, CCRN
Cardiothoracic Postoperative Intensive Care Unit
University of Virginia Health System
Charlottesville, Virginia

Janet H. Johnson DNP, RN, MA, ANP-BC, ACNP-BC, FAANP
Cardiology Telemetry Service
Mount Sinai Hospital
New York, New York

April J. Kastner MS, RN, ACNP-AG-BC
Neurocritical Care Service
Ohio State University Wexner Medical Center
Columbus, Ohio

Lynn A. Kelso MSN, RN, ACNP-BC, FCCM, FAANP
Department of Pulmonary, Critical Care, and Sleep Medicine
Acute Care Nurse Practitioner Program
University of Kentucky
Lexington, Kentucky

Joan E. King PhD, RN, ACNP-BC, ANP-BCG
Acute Care Nurse Practitioner Program
Vanderbilt University School of Nursing
Pre-anesthesia Evaluation Clinic
Nashville, Tennessee

Karen L. Kopan DNP, RN, ACNP-BC, CCRN
Critical Care Consult Team-Surgical Intensive Care Unit
North Shore University Health System
Evanston, Illinois
Department of Adult Health and Gerontological Nursing
Rush University College of Nursing
Chicago, Illinois

Donna W. Markey MSN, RN, ACNP-BC
University of Virginia's Cancer Care Clinics in Farmville and Charlottesville
University of Virginia Health System
Charlottesville, Virginia

Sheila Melander PhD, RN, ACNP-BC, FCCM, FAANP
Acute Care Nurse Practitioner Program-College of Nursing
University of Kentucky
Lexington, Kentucky

Helen-Marie Molnar MSN, RN, ACNP-BC, FNP-BC
Outpatient Cardiology Practice
University of Virginia Health System
Charlottesville, Virginia

Nancy Munro MN, RN, CCRN, ACNP-BC, FAANP
Critical Care Medicine Department and Pulmonary Consult Service
National Institutes of Health
Bethesda, Maryland
University of Maryland School of Nursing
College Park, Maryland

Angela Nelson MSN, RN, ACNP-BC, CCRN, FCCM, FAANP
Department of Neurosurgery
New York University Langone Medical Center
New York, New York

Nicolle L. Schraeder MSN, RN, ACNP-AG-BC, CCRN, CNRN
Neuroscience Department
Littleton Adventist Hospital
Littleton, Colorado

Megan M. Shifrin DNP (C), MSN, RN, ACNP-BC
Adult Gerontology Acute Care Nurse Practitioner Program
Vanderbilt School of Nursing
Nashville, Tennessee

Joshua Squiers PhD, RN, ACNP-BC, ACNP-AG-BC, FCCM
School of Nursing-Acute Care Nurse Practitioner Program
Division of Cardiac and Surgical Subspecialty Critical Care
Department of Anesthesiology and Perioperative Medicine
Oregon Health and Science University
Portland, Oregon

David V. Strider, Jr. DNP, RN, ACNP, CCRN
Vascular and Endovascular Service
  Surgery Service
University of Virginia Health System
Charlottesville, Virginia

Carol K. Thompson PhD, DNP, RN, ACNP-BC, CCRN, FCCM, FAANP, FAAN
College of Nursing
University of Kentucky
Lexington, Kentucky

Bonnie Tong DNP, RN, ACNP-BC
Cardiology Service
Mount Sinai Hospital
Acute Care Nurse Practitioner Program
New York University
New York, New York

Allison Walton MSN, RN, FNP-BC, ACNP-BC, CNRN
Neurovascular-Neurosurgery
  Department
University of Virginia Health System
Charlottesville, Virginia

Michelle A. Weber MSN, RN, ACNP-BC
General Surgery
Milwaukee, Wisconsin

Mary Ann Whelan-Gales DNP, RN, ANP-BC, CCRN
Inpatient Cardiology Service
Mount Sinai Hospital
New York, New York

Brian Widmar PhD, RN, ACNP-BC, CCRN, CSC, CMC
Adult Gerontology Intensivist
  Subspecialty Program
Vanderbilt University School of
  Nursing
Cardiovascular Intensive Care Unit
Nashville, Tennessee

Briana Witherspoon DNP, RN, ACNP-BC
Department of Anesthesiology
Division of Critical Care
Vanderbilt University School of
  Medicine
Nashville, Tennessee

Cynthia Wolfe MSN, RN, ACNP-BC
Step-down Cardiac Surgical Unit
University of Virginia Health System
Charlottesville, Virginia

Kelly Wozneak MSN, RN, ACNP-BC
Medical Intensive Care Unit
University of Virginia Health System
Charlottesville, Virginia

Susan Yeager MS, RN, ACNP-BC, CCRN, FNCS
Neurocritical-Care Service
Ohio State University Wexner Medical
  Center
Columbus, Ohio

ACKNOWLEDGEMENTS

Suzi and Sarah thank the authors for their hard work and dedication to making the cases "come alive" for readers by "thinking out loud" as they work through the process of diagnostic reasoning in acute and critical care patients. Their knowledge, expertise, and ability to guide others in diagnostic reasoning and evidence-based management of the patients will benefit nurse practitioners, faculty, students and most importantly our patients!

PREFACE AND HOW TO USE THE BOOK

This book on diagnostic reasoning is for faculty who teach in ACNP programs, ACNP students, graduate ACNPs who will be taking the ACNP certification exams, and practicing ACNPs who want to test and expand their diagnostic skills. The book is sponsored by AACN and covers blueprint topics in AACN's ACNP certification examination.

When we were teaching acute care nurse practitioner students at the University of Virginia, we found that teaching diagnostic reasoning was best accomplished by using a case-based approach that guided the students in thinking systematically to rule in, or out, specific diagnoses on their differential. The approach is reminiscent of Eliza Doolittle's request to Henry Higgins when he was describing how to be a lady. She sang to him: "don't tell me, show me!" We developed a teaching method using a case format to do just that, to "show" the students how to evaluate data to support or refute a diagnosis.

The first step in diagnostic reasoning is to develop a list of potential diagnoses that may cause the patient's presenting symptom(s) or condition(s). Because our ACNP students were all nurses with extensive experience, we recognized the tendency to "jump to a diagnosis" based on patterns they recognized as representing a specific condition (ie, inductive reasoning). To ensure that the students did not "jump to a diagnosis," but instead methodically deduced the cause of the presenting symptom(s), we asked them to analyze case history and physical examination (H & P) findings bit by bit, identifying key information as pertinent positives and significant negatives. Stopping at regular intervals as we progressed through the H & P data, we asked them to "think out loud" about how each pertinent positive or significant negative supported or refuted the items on their differential diagnoses. In addition, the students were asked to consider what additional information was needed (diagnostics or other information from different sources), and in what order they would proceed, to further refine their differential. The students loved these sessions and found the process of "thinking out loud" very helpful. Subsequently, some of our past students have stated that they wished a book existed that would walk them through this process, for a variety of diagnoses, so they might reinforce their own skills, as well as those of the clinicians they teach and/or work with in their practice.

To that end, we designed this book to teach nurse practitioners, including students, clinicians, and clinical faculty, how to use deductive reasoning to systematically and comprehensively evaluate data to confirm or refute a potential diagnosis. We accomplish this with cases written by expert nurse practitioners practicing in a variety of acute, critical, and specialty care areas around the country. Each author presents a case by "thinking out loud" as they systematically evaluate the data acquired in the H & P to hone their differential. They start by first noting the diagnoses that are critical, move quickly to rule these in or out, then consider other diagnoses that may be causing the patient's problem or condition. Readers may note that the cases move more slowly than in actual clinical practice. One of our authors summed this up when she stated in the margin of one of her case drafts to us: "Yikes … my patient is going to die before I state the actual diagnosis." The idea is to allow the reader to "hear" what is happening in the mind of an expert diagnostician. Thorough diagnostic reasoning is essential to avoid the error of "satisfaction of search" where the diagnostician settles for a specific cause and does not consider other diagnoses.[1] Our goal is to assure a thoughtful, comprehensive, and reasoned approach.

Many of the authors struggled with this, which we did not find surprising, as we were asking them to explain thinking that has long since become so fast and so integrated into their diagnostic process that they are unaware of how they do it. This speed is essential especially if the patient's condition is critical. Assuredly, working through the cases in this book may seem a laborious task at times, but doing so forces the reader to consider diagnoses that otherwise might be missed. As noted by Lucien Leape, safe practice happens when we acknowledge the potential for error and build-in error reduction skills at each stage of clinical practice.[2] We believe that two of the first steps in error reduction related to diagnosis generation are to ensure accurate H & P skills, and then to develop solid diagnostic reasoning skills. This book attempts to make this process logical, systematic, and fun to accomplish.

How to use the book

1. We start with a chapter on diagnostic reasoning. The chapter discusses inductive and deductive reasoning and a stepwise approach to diagnosing disease as we move through a traditional H & P.

2. The cases begin with a chief complaint and the actual diagnosis is not revealed until the case presenter determines it in the course of moving through the case. In addition, the case diagnosis does not appear at the top of the cases so that it is not revealed prematurely to those who do not want to know the diagnosis a priori. This is useful if one wishes to work through the cases as in real life and is especially helpful for use with students and new NPs. For faculty, or preceptors, they can access specific conditions for their students by using the case listings at the front of the book.

3. The cases are formatted similarly throughout the book. The information provided is called "case information." At different points in the case the reader is cued to stop and evaluate the "case information" provided to that point. Questions are posed that prompt the reader to list the pertinent positives and significant negatives, then to consider whether these findings help rule in, or out, the diagnoses in their differential. The authors of the cases then provide their analyses using the same data. These sections are highlighted as "case analysis" and represent the author "thinking out loud." There are also sections that ask the reader to consider "what additional information or diagnostics are needed, and in what order," to encourage the reader to carefully consider the necessary information required to further hone the potential causes of the patient's symptoms. Last, the author discusses the management of the disease or condition diagnosed in the case.

4. The cases are listed in the two front "Case Listings" as follows:

a) By diagnosis: Seventy-one case diagnoses are listed alphabetically and numbered consecutively. The page number where you can find the case is next to the diagnosis. We have not put the diagnosis at the top of each case in the book so if you wish to work through the case without knowing the diagnosis, you can do so.

b) By symptom: The symptoms found in the cases are listed under a system heading such as "cardiovascular" or "pulmonary" or by a specific topic. The category listings include: "cases managed in the ICU," "postsurgical cases," and "end-of-life cases." The presenting symptom is listed alphabetically under each heading. The secondary symptoms, as they appear in the chief complaint, follow. We have put many of the presenting symptoms under more than one heading. For example, since "chest pain" may be due to a cardiac event or perhaps musculoskeletal cause, we list the symptom under both "cardiovascular" and "musculoskeletal" headings.

We hope you enjoy the cases in the book as much as we have and that you find the book helpful in honing your diagnostic skills. Our patients will benefit!

Suzi Burns and Sarah Delgado

References

1. Fleck MA, Samei E, Mitroff SR. Generalized "satisfaction of search": adverse influences on dual-target search accuracy. *J Exp Psychol Appl*. March 2010;16(1):10.1037/a0018629. doi: 10.1037/a0018629.
2. Leape L. Error in medicine. *JAMA*. 1994;272(23):1851-1857. doi:10.1001/jama.1994.03520230061039.

CASE LISTING BY DIAGNOSIS

CASE LISTING BY SYMPTOM

Symptoms Listed by System (as in H & P)

Constitutional:

Cardiovascular:

Pulmonary:

Neurological:

Altered mental state (Case 49), *541*

Altered mental state: post-operative neurosurgery, coma with unilateral weakness and eye deviation (Case 67), *751*

Altered mental state, confusion (Case 17, 71), *195, 789*

Altered mental state, confusion, fatigue, abdominal pain, weakness: post lung cancer surgery (Case 4), *45*

Altered mental state, confusion, hypertension- (Case 35), *387*

Altered mental state, decreased responsiveness (Case 1), *9*

Altered mental state, dementia (Case 56), *625*

Altered mental state, hyperglycemia (Case 25), *273*

Altered mental state, somnolence, confusion, abdominal pain (Case 41), *447*

Altered mental state: post-trans-spenoidal pituitary surgery, increased thirst, increased urine output (Case 24), *263*

Altered mental state, unresponsive (Case 70), *779*

Fever: post-operative cancer surgery, confusion, agitation (Case 47), *517*

Headache (Case 12), *141*

Headache, arm weakness, nausea and vomiting (Case 42), *459*

Headache, dysarthria, left sided weakness- (Case 68), *759*

Headache, subarchanoid hemorrhage (Case 69), *771*

Hypoxemia, altered mental state (Case 2), *21*

Seizures, progressing to status epilecticus (Case 40), *437*

Seizures (refractory), acute psychosis (Case 27), *297*

Syncope- (Case 9, 18, 63), *99, 205, 705*

Hematologic/Oncologic/Lymphatic:

Abdominal mass: post-transplant surgery (Case 13), *151*

Back Pain (Case 43), *471*

Bloody stools, leg, abdominal and scrotal swelling, anemia (Case 30), *331*

Bruising, thrombocytopenia (Case 36), *399*

Erythema, tenderness, swelling: post-operative colorectal surgery (Case 22), *245*

Fatigue (Case 6), *69*

Fatigue, hypotension after dialysis (Case 5), *57*

Fatigue, pancytopenia (Case 38), *417*

Headache (Case 12), *141*

Jaundice, fatigue, nausea, diarrhea, weight loss (Case 50), *551*

Endocrine:

Altered mental state, confusion, fatigue, abdominal pain, weakness (Case 4), *45*

Altered mental state, hyperglycemia (Case 25), *273*

Altered mental state: post-trans-spenoidal pituitary surgery, increased thirst, increased urine output (Case 24), *263*

Failure to wean, weakness (Case 46), *503*

SYMPTOMS LISTED BY SELECTED TOPIC OR MANAGEMENT SETTING

DIAGNOSTIC REASONING: AN OVERVIEW

A key element in the scope of practice for all nurse practitioners is the ability to diagnose medical conditions. This sets nurse practitioners apart from other licensed nurses who, consciously or unconsciously, apply nursing diagnoses to their patients but are not expected to establish medical diagnoses. A nursing diagnosis addresses a patient's response to a disease state, while a medical diagnosis identifies the disease. Developing the skill set to accurately and efficiently establish a medical diagnosis as the cause of a patient's illness is essential in the transition from nurse to nurse practitioner.

Experienced nurses are aware of how certain disease states typically present; a patient having a myocardial infarction complains of crushing chest pain, a patient with appendicitis reports intermittent, sharp right lower quadrant pain. This knowledge is applicable in diagnostic reasoning; however, the process of forming a diagnosis involves approaching the patient from the other side of the lens. Rather than connecting a disease with a specific symptom, the diagnostician must work from the symptom back to the disease state. This requires considering all possible causes of a particular complaint, and using a stepwise approach, narrowing the list to establish a theory regarding the specific cause of the patient's complaint. The nurse practitioner relies on past clinical experiences, recommendations from evidence-based practice resources, and the clinical information from the history, physical examination, and diagnostic testing to arrive at a medical diagnosis.

Inductive and Deductive Reasoning

The process of reasoning generally takes two forms: inductive and deductive. Inductive reasoning involves noting particular details about a phenomenon, recognizing a pattern in what is observed, and developing a theory about the cause of that phenomenon. Applying deductive reasoning means that the theory is established first and observations and information are collected to confirm or refute the theory. Consider the following example:

INDUCTIVE REASONING: I work on a general medical unit on the third floor and there is a similar unit on the fourth floor. I have noticed that nurses on the other unit leave for other jobs more often than the nurses on my unit do. When I ride the elevator with nurses from the other unit, I notice they complain a lot. A friend of mine briefly worked on the other unit and said she had a bad experience. Therefore, the work environment on my unit is better than the work environment on the other floor.

DEDUCTIVE REASONING: The work environment on my unit is better than the work environment on the fourth floor. To test this, I e-mailed surveys to all the nurses on that unit and on my unit and requested that they anonymously rate their work environment. I found that the scores given by nurses on my unit were significantly higher than the scores given by nurses on the other unit.

Humans use inductive and deductive reasoning informally to answer day-to-day questions but seldom need to consider the steps involved. To develop the new skill of diagnostic reasoning, however, understanding the steps is essential. In diagnostic reasoning, both inductive and deductive processes are applied, and depend in part on the providers' experience level and expertise in gathering key clinical information. For instance, an experienced internist sees a patient with ear pain, and prior to entering the examination room, establishes a theory that the patient has otitis media. During the appointment, the internist asks questions and conducts an examination to gather evidence to support that theory—a deductive approach. If the information gathered does not support the theory that the patient has otitis media, then the internist must return to an inductive approach, gathering more information and making further observations to see if a different pattern consistent with a different disease process emerges (Table 1).

Sensitivity and Specificity

The concepts of specificity and sensitivity are essential in the diagnostic reasoning process. These concepts guide the diagnostician in weighing the impact of pertinent information and diagnostic test results on possible diagnoses. Sensitivity and specificity are expressed in percentages. Sensitivity is the ability of the measurement to detect those who have the condition (ie, a true positive). In contrast, specificity is

Table 1 **Examples of Inductive and Deductive reasoning**

1. "What is the cause of my headache?"

   INDUCTIVE: I had a headache like this last week when I did not have any coffee with breakfast. I did not have coffee today. I think the headache is from caffeine withdrawal.

   DEDUCTIVE: I think the headache is from not having caffeine. I will drink a cup of coffee and see if it goes away. Tomorrow, I will have coffee in the morning and see if this prevents a headache.

2. "Is this patient taking his medications correctly?"

   INDUCTIVE: The patient's blood pressure and blood glucose are consistently high, unchanged despite increases in medication doses. The patient does not recall the names of his pills or how often he takes them. The patient denies any side effects from the prescribed medications. I think the patient is not adhering to his medication regimen.

   DEDUCTIVE: I believe the patient is not taking his medication regimen as prescribed. To test this, I will check the refill dates on the pill bottles and the number of pills in the bottles. I will also call the pharmacy to verify if the patient is picking up refills appropriately.

3. "Does this patient have dementia?"

   INDUCTIVE: The patient is wearing a heavy sweater and boots when it is 80 degrees outside. When I ask the patient questions, she looks at her adult daughter to give the answers. The patient went to the restroom to leave a urine specimen and had trouble finding her way back to the examination room. I think the patient has developed dementia.

   DEDUCTIVE: I believe the patient has dementia. To test this I will administer a tool such as the Mini-Mental Status Examination or the Montreal Cognitive Assessment to score her cognitive function.

the ability of the measurement to detect those who do not have the condition (ie, true negatives). The accuracy of the test includes both of these concepts.

An interesting example of sensitivity and specificity is the troponin level for diagnosing a myocardial infarction (MI). The troponin test was developed because creatinine kinase levels, previously the gold standard test for an MI, were time consuming to measure, resulting in delays in treatment.[1] Troponin levels could be run more quickly and in addition were detectable for a longer period after infarction. Early versions of the troponin test had a sensitivity of 89% and specificity of 97%.[2] This meant that the troponin level was valuable in ruling in an MI 89% of the time but would not detect 11% of those who actually had an MI. The specificity of 97% indicated that only 3% who tested positive were false positives. So if the troponin level was elevated, the patient likely had an MI but due to the test's sensitivity, 11% of patients with an MI would not be detected by the test.

To address this, laboratories have developed more sensitive troponin assays. Newer, highly sensitive tests have a sensitivity as high as 95% on admission, and 99% for samples taken 3 to 6 hours after admission.[2] These newer tests are more effective in ruling out an MI. If the test is negative, the patient did not have an MI because the rate of true positives is almost 100%. However, with increased sensitivity, came less specificity, which is estimated to be 80% to 85%.[2] This means that when a patient tests positive with these newer tests, there is a greater chance that in fact they did not have an MI. This increased sensitivity increases the chances of detecting an MI, but the lower specificity decreases the ability of the test to detect true negatives. This can lead to invasive and costly procedures that do not benefit the patient.

Because of the sensitivity and specificity of the troponin test, the diagnosis of an MI requires serial testing and the measurement of the change in the troponin level between the admission value and a value drawn 3 to 6 hours later. This change in troponin, rather than the value at a single point in time, supports the diagnosis of MI and is essential to ruling in or out the diagnosis.[3] Results of a troponin test should always be analyzed in the context of the clinical picture. The patient may have other conditions, such as sepsis, heart failure, or chronic kidney disease that can contribute to elevations in the troponin level even in the absence of myocardial injury. Factors such as the patient's symptoms, ECG tracing, and risk factors for coronary artery disease are essential to guiding the decision to send the patient for cardiac imaging or catheterization versus monitoring the patient and repeating the troponin assay at a later time.

While certain diagnostic tests, including the troponin test, are accepted as gold standard tests for establishing a particular diagnosis, the clinician must always recognize the necessity of gathering all relevant information before arriving at a conclusion about the cause of the patient's presenting complaint. In some cases, by applying inductive reasoning, all the details taken together may lead to a clear conclusion as to that existing pathology. In other cases, it is more appropriate to formulate a theory and then gather information that supports or refutes it, a deductive reasoning process. With either approach, it is rarely possible to establish a diagnosis on the basis of a single piece of information. See *Figure 1* for more on sensitivity and specificity: http://www.straighthealthcare.com/sensitivity-specificity-figure.html.

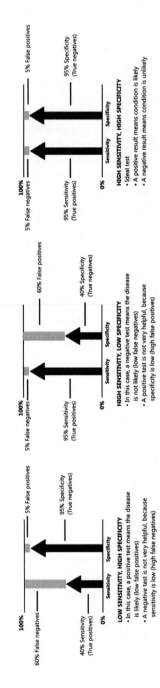

Figure 1 Sensitivity versus specificity. Reproduced with permission of StraightHealthcare.com.

A Stepwise Approach to Diagnosing Reasoning

1. IDENTIFY THE CHIEF COMPLAINT:

   The first step is recognizing the patient's chief complaint. What is the main problem, the reason the person is seeking care or asking for help? In medical notes, often the chief complaint is given in the patient's own words because framing the symptom with the meaning that the patient attaches to it assists in the diagnostic reasoning process.

   (Examples: "My back hurts so much that I called out from work." "My breathing has been getting worse and now I can't even get to the bathroom." "I couldn't wake my father up this morning.")

2. FORMULATE A DIFFERENTIAL DIAGNOSIS:

   There are several approaches to developing a differential diagnosis, a list of all the possible causes of particular complaint. One strategy is to consider in turn each body system—cardiac, pulmonary, gastrointestinal, genitourinary, integumentary, musculoskeletal, neurological, endocrine, vascular—then to identify pathologies in each system that might cause the patient's current symptoms. Another approach is to consider categories of pathology such as infection, malignancy, immunological, adverse medication event, and the conditions might produce this particular complaint. Always, in generating a differential diagnosis, consideration is given to what is MOST likely and to what is MOST life threatening. For obvious reasons, ruling in, or ruling out, life-threatening disease states is an early step in the process of diagnostic reasoning. There are web-based resources and applications for handheld devices that provide lists of differential diagnosis for different symptoms.

3. GATHER THE STORY OF THE ILLNESS:

   Use an algorithm such as OLDCARTS (Onset, Location, Duration, Characteristics, Aggravating factors, Relieving factors, Temporal factors, Severity) or COLDSPA (Character, Onset, Location, Duration, Severity, Pattern, Associated factors) to get more information about the patient's experience with this symptom. Ask about past experiences with the symptom, and determine if the patient has chronic health problems that make certain diagnoses more likely.

   Patients presenting in acute care settings may be unable to communicate their story, in which case it is gathered from family, friends, or other health care professionals who have observed the patient. While a novice nurse practitioner sometimes struggles to decide what questions to ask in order to obtain this key information, experienced nurses often already possess strong skills in listening. Hearing the story of the illness is a crucial step in diagnostic reasoning.

4. ANALYZE THE STORY:

   Consider the list of possibilities generated in the first step and the information gathered in the second step and sort the information into pertinent positives and significant negatives. What information is most applicable to ruling out or ruling in the variety of possible causes for this patient's illness? A patient presenting with shortness of breath might report no history of COPD or CHF (significant negatives) and also report that the problem is associated with a productive cough and a fever (pertinent positives).

Try to summarize key information into a single statement—a problem representation—that narrows the search and guides the next steps.[4] At this point, also consider which items can be crossed off the list of potential diagnoses. For example, when a patient with abdominal pain tells the story of their illness and describes undergoing appendectomy years ago, the diagnosis of appendicitis is safely ruled out.

5. PERFORM A HISTORY, REVIEW OF SYSTEMS, AND PHYSICAL EXAMINATION:

Additional information is gathered about the patient's past medical history, past surgical history, relevant family and social history. The review of systems involves questions that address the patient's overall health for the presence of additional information that might be related to the presenting symptom. This step is helpful in uncovering information the patient may not have connected to the presenting symptom but that is in fact pertinent to the diagnosis. For instance a patient with nausea and vomiting may not mention that urination is painful but this information is a pertinent positive for one of the items on the differential, urinary tract infection. Many electronic medical records or paper chart forms provide a template for the review of systems.

Physical examination of the patient follows the process established by the provider and should be accomplished in a systematic manner. In an acute situation, this step may be abbreviated so that only information pertinent to the patient's story is collected. While a focused physical examination saves time, a more thorough examination ensures that additional findings are not missed. For instance, if an examination of a patient with back pain focused only on the musculoskeletal system, then ruling out a spinal abscess or a myocardial infarction, both of which can cause back pain, is impossible.

6. SORT THE INFORMATION AND EVALUATE:

Again taking into consideration the list generated in step 2, sort the new information into pertinent positives and significant negatives. This analysis helps the practitioner identify the need for any additional information either from the patient or from diagnostic testing. In acute care settings, multiple health care professionals are involved in the care of a single patient and some laboratory or radiology testing take place according to protocols. Any additional diagnostic testing should be ordered and analyzed at this stage. Then, looking at all the details given and all the observations made, arrive at a theory regarding the cause of the illness in this patient.

7. IDENTIFY A DIAGNOSIS AND DEVELOP A TREATMENT PLAN:

Using the data gathered, determine the most likely condition or conditions as the cause of the patient's symptoms or complaints and initiate a treatment plan. While evidence-based guidelines are essential in selecting appropriate therapy, treatment must also take into consideration patient-specific factors such as any allergies, interactions with existing medications, or disease-specific contraindications. Consider using an online resource such as the National Institute of Health for evidence-based practice guidelines when seeking a treatment plan (http://www.nlm.nih.gov/hsrinfo/literaturesites.html.)

Then use the information gathered in step 5 to select the option most appropriate for this patient.

In some cases, a trial of treatment may be needed to confirm a diagnosis. For instance, a patient with dizziness where physical pathology is ruled out, and medication side effect is the suspected cause, discontinuation of the medication for a trial period followed by a reevaluation may be necessary to confirm or rule out this diagnosis. In such cases, deductive reasoning is applied—the theory formed and then tested.

Another potential situation is when the patient's clinical status warrants treatment prior to establishing a firm diagnosis. The best example is when a patient meets criteria for sepsis but blood cultures and other data are not yet available. To prevent complications, treatment with intravenous fluids and broad-spectrum antibiotics is warranted and the patient is reevaluated to determine the response to this treatment. However, the diagnostic reasoning process is not skipped. Even through treatment is initiated, the steps above are applied so appropriate adjustments to therapy, such as narrowing the antibiotic coverage, can be made.

Conclusion

In the subsequent chapters of this book, the reader will have the opportunity to listen as experienced nurse practitioners "think out loud" about a particular case. The authors will walk the reader through the diagnostic reasoning process step by step, though in the actual situation they may have followed these steps swiftly and without conscious intent.

References

1. Landenson JH. Troponin 1, the story. *Clin Chem*. 2010;56(3):482-483. doi: 10.1373/clinchem.2009.
2. Gamble JH, Carlton E, Orr W, Greaves K. High sensitivity troponin: six lessons and a reading. *Br J Cardiol*. 2013;20(3):109-112.
3. Thygesen K, Alpert JS, Jaffe AS, Simoons ML, Chaitman BR, White HD. ESC/ACCF/AHA/WHF Expert Consensus Document: Third universal definition of myocardial infarction. *Circulation*. 2012;126:2020-2035. doi: 10.1161/CIR.0b013e31826e1058.
4. Bowen JL. Educational Strategies to promote clinical diagnostic reasoning. New Engl Jo Med. 2006;355(21): 2217-2225. Accessed online at http://www.bumc.bu.edu/facdev-medicine/files/2010/06/Bowen-clinical-reasoning-NEJM.pdf.

CASE 1

Lynn A. Kelso

Lynn A. Kelso is an Assistant Professor of Nursing at the University of Kentucky College of Nursing in Lexington where she started the ACNP program and served as its coordinator for a number of years before focusing on undergraduate education. She holds a clinical appointment with the Department of Pulmonary, Critical Care, and Sleep Medicine, practicing in the Medical ICU at the University of Kentucky Chandler Medical Center.

CASE INFORMATION

Chief Complaint

A 39-year-old male is brought to the emergency department (ED) by emergency medical services (EMS) with confusion and decreased responsiveness.

❓ What is the potential cause?

Case Analysis: Confusion is a very nonspecific symptom and decreased responsiveness is not very telling about the patient's current neurological status. There are a number of causes that may initially be considered; however, given the patient's age, the most likely causes include drug toxicities and overdose, acute neurological events or infection, trauma, and acute organ dysfunction.

Initial, emergent considerations include:

- Oxygenation, ventilation, and airway protection: If the patient is too confused to control his secretions or maintain a patent airway, or is not breathing adequately, emergent intubation and ventilation may be necessary.

- C-spine protection: If there is any indication of trauma, the C-spine should be immobilized until we are able to establish if there is any spinal injury.

Differential Diagnoses for Patient With Confusion[1]

- Life threatening: hypoxia, hypoglycemia, hypertensive encephalopathy, sepsis, Wernicke encephalopathy, overdose, meningitis, intracranial hemorrhage, nonconvulsant seizures
- Common causes: infection (particularly urinary tract infection or pneumonia, especially in the elderly), electrolyte abnormalities, medications (adverse effects, withdrawal, polypharmacy), psychiatric conditions
- Other conditions: endocrine disorders, stroke, and brain lesion

CASE INFORMATION

General Survey and History of Present Illness

While the list of diagnoses in the differential is extensive, the most important next step is to complete a preliminary evaluation of the patient. Because EMS personnel are still in the ED, I ask them about the patient's surroundings when they arrived at the scene. They noted that he was found at home sitting in a chair and his brother was present. He had not been incontinent and there was no evidence that he had fallen or had a seizure. They also report that no prescription bottles were found in the home; however, there was a half-filled bottle of acetaminophen found in the bathroom, as well as a couple bottles of over-the-counter (OTC) cold medicines. There was no smell of alcohol but they did not look for any empty bottles. They asked the patient's brother to check the garbage for any empty alcohol containers.

These answers help me refine the evaluation of my patient; however, the most important data are obtained by examining the patient. Initially I am especially interested in anything that requires emergent interventions. I need to make sure that he is breathing adequately and able to protect his airway. I also need to do a rapid neurological evaluation to determine whether he may have had stroke.

Upon entering the examination room, I see that the patient is a well-developed adult male who appears to be sleeping. He is arouseable to light tactile stimulation, is oriented to person only, has slurred speech, a moderate cough, and adequate air movement with clear breath sounds. He moves all extremities slowly but his strength is equal bilaterally in both his upper and lower extremities and his face is symmetric. Although his skin is tan, it appears jaundiced and I note that his scleras are icteric. He has no evidence of injury to his head or upper body. Although he has been changed into a hospital gown, the ED staff reports he has not been incontinent. His bedside monitor shows a sinus tachycardia at 105 beats per minute and a pulse oximetry reading of 96% on room air. His brother and mother arrive in the ED and are able to provide additional information related to history.

His brother tells me, "When I talked to him this morning he was fine. I didn't notice anything strange. We were supposed to go to the gym together after work but he didn't show up there and didn't answer his phone. That concerned me because he had been having trouble at work recently and last month his divorce was finalized. When I got to his house, I found him just sitting in a chair in his bedroom. He couldn't look at me, and I'm not sure he even recognized me. He didn't remember anything about going to the gym. He was kind of slurring his words and when he finally looked at me his eyes looked really funny, almost yellow." Upon asking further questions I discover that he does not go hiking or camping. He has not traveled out of the country recently.

Because he has scleral icterus and is jaundiced I am especially interesting in hearing about any known history of liver disease and/or alcohol use. The jaundice does make me concerned that liver failure may be responsible for his confusion but I need to collect more data to confirm this hypothesis. Between his mother and his brother, I am able to put together additional pieces of the patient's history.

CASE INFORMATION

Past Medical History

He has hypertension, but is not currently on any medication; he had his appendix removed as a teenager and surgery on his left ankle after breaking it playing softball. His ankle causes him a lot of discomfort at times, especially with changes in the weather. Family denies history of liver disease.

Allergies

No known drug allergies; he does have seasonal allergies.

Social History

In college he drank heavily and smoked marijuana. Since that time he rarely drinks, he has no other illicit drug use, and he has never smoked. He currently manages a convenience store but has had financial problems related to the business for the last year. He was married for 18 years. Although they separated 4 years ago, it was only last year that his wife filed for divorce. The divorce was finalized a month prior to this admission.

Medications

The family is not aware of any regular medication use; however, he is not opposed to taking over-the-counter medications for colds, allergies, and pain.

Review of Systems

Because of the patient's current mental state, I am unable to do a complete review of systems. However, the family is able to tell me that he had complained that he thought he was getting a cold. Thinking back over the last few weeks, they confirm that it seemed he was more withdrawn and may have had some depression which they attributed to his reaction to his divorce.

❓ What are the pertinent positives from the information given so far?

- Confusion of acute onset, patient in usual mental state earlier in the day
- Icteric sclera

- Facial symmetry, (+) cough
- Trouble at work and recently divorced after an 18-year marriage
- Cold symptoms
- Ankle pain, especially with changes in the weather
- Moves all extremities
- Has been more withdrawn and depressed
- Takes over-the-counter medications for colds, allergies, and pain (bottles of over-the-counter medications found by EMS)
- Remote history of excess alcohol and marijuana use

? What are the significant negatives from the information given so far?

- No evidence of incontinence
- Has not traveled out of the country
- Does not go camping or hiking
- Has no history of liver disease
- Does not consume a large amount of alcohol or use illicit drugs

---

? How does this information affect the problem representation and the list of possible causes?

Case Analysis: This patient is a 39-year-old male with acute onset of confusion and jaundice most likely related to acute liver failure of unknown etiology.

The appearance of jaundice initially narrows my evaluation to the diagnosis of liver failure. Laboratory tests and diagnostics may show another contributing cause and I still need to do a comprehensive examination, but I am now going to try to determine whether he has acute liver failure (ALF), or an acute complication of chronic liver failure. He is too confused to give appropriate responses to questions related to his history; however, with information provided by the family I believe he is suffering from ALF, defined as:

- International normalized ratio (INR) ≥1.5
- Encephalopathy
- No preexisting liver disease or cirrhosis
- Illness <26 weeks in duration

The next stage of evaluation is threefold. First, I need to make every attempt to identify the cause of the ALF so that appropriate treatment decisions can be made. Second, I need to determine the severity of the liver failure and provide supportive care. And third, I need to alert the hepatologist and transplant team on call. For patients with ALF who present to facilities without a liver transplant program, transport to a transplant center is a crucial consideration. As I continue to evaluate my patient for other potential causes of confusion I keep in mind a comprehensive differential for ALF.

Differential Diagnoses of ALF[2]

- Drug induced: acetaminophen, carbon tetrachloride, *Amanita phalloides* (mushrooms), alcoholic hepatitis
- Infectious: hepatitis viruses A, B, E; herpes simplex virus, cytomegalovirus, Epstein- Barr virus, adenovirus, hemorrhagic fever viruses
- Ischemic/vascular: right heart failure, Budd-Chiari syndrome (acute hepatic vein thrombosis), veno-occlusive disease, shock liver
- Metabolic: Wilson disease (additional causes would include acute fatty liver of pregnancy and HELLP syndrome in women of childbearing age, and Reye syndrome in children)
- Miscellaneous: malignant infiltration, autoimmune hepatitis

---

CASE INFORMATION

Physical Examination

- Vital signs: pulse 102 beats per minute, blood pressure 126/72 mm Hg, respiratory rate 18 breaths per minute, oral temperature 99.4°F
- Bedside monitoring: pulse oximetry 96% on 2 L O_2 via nasal cannula (NC), telemetry—sinus tachycardia
- Constitutional: well-developed adult male, who appears his stated age, lethargic in bed
- Head/eyes/ears/nose/throat: head normocephalic and atraumatic, pupils equal, round, reactive to light and accommodation at 2 mm, sclera icteric, ears, nose, and oropharynx unremarkable with good dentition, mucous membranes pale and slightly jaundiced, but with no evidence of bleeding
- Neck: neck is supple with no nuchal rigidity, trachea appears to be midline, no appreciable thyromegaly, no jugular venous distention (JVD), no lymphadenopathy
- Cardiovascular: normal S_1S_2, no murmur, gallop or rub appreciated, peripheral pulses palpable, no peripheral edema
- Pulmonary: symmetric chest expansion, no retractions or accessory muscle use, bilateral breath sounds clear throughout all lung fields, cough intact with no sputum production
- Gastrointestinal: abdomen soft, nondistended with no organomegaly or masses palpated, patient grimaces to palpation of right upper quadrant (RUQ) but no other evidence of abdominal tenderness, normoactive bowel sounds

- Genitourinary: Foley catheter in place and draining dark yellow urine; normal male genitalia
- Integumentary: color jaundiced, warm and dry, no visible marks, lesions, or tattoos, no petechiae or spider angiomas
- Neurological: arouseable to touch, does not respond to voice, speech slurred, does not follow commands, oriented to person only, able to elicit asterixis in feet bilaterally, reflexes present bilaterally

---

? **Given the information to this point, what elements of the physical examination should be added to the list of pertinent positives? What elements should be added to the list of significant negatives?**

- **Pertinent positives:** asterixis, right upper quadrant tenderness to palpation, dark urine, jaundiced mucous membranes
- **Significant negatives:** no petechiae, spider angiomas, or evidence of bleeding in the mucous membranes, no abdominal distention, no marks or tattoos on the skin, no evidence of neurofocal deficits, no nuchal rigidity

---

? **How does this information affect the list of probable causes?**

Case Analysis: Because the patient is only arouseable to tactile stimulation and is only oriented to person, I am unable to get any additional review of systems other than what the family is able to tell me. I have to rely on my physical examination findings to help me narrow the list of possible causes.

The patient's facial symmetry, intact cough reflex, absence of focal neurological defects, and lack of nuchal rigidity make a neurological event, such as acute stroke or meningitis less likely. He has no signs of trauma. Because there was no evidence of incontinence, a seizure seems less likely as well. These findings move a neurological event or infection further down my list of differential diagnoses. The asterixis, dark urine, jaundiced mucous membranes, and right upper quadrant tenderness support the diagnosis of ALF. There is no evidence of ascites, which may be present if there is any underlying liver disease. The lack of markings on the skin—tattoos and marks of injection—moves hepatitis B and C lower on my list of possible causes but I cannot eliminate these from the list yet.

Acute liver failure seems most likely because of the sudden onset of confusion and jaundice. At this point I am beginning to think about acetaminophen toxicity as the cause of his ALF. Because he does not go camping or hiking and has not traveled out of the country, mushroom poisoning and hepatitis A are lower on my list. Also, although families do not always know of alcohol or drug use in a family member, alcohol toxicity is lower on my list of differentials because of their report and the information from EMS. He has no history of

Table 1-1   Clinical Manifestations of Encephalopathy by Level of Severity

Grade	Clinical Manifestations of Encephalopathy
1	Mild personality changes, decreased attention span
2	Asterixis with dorsiflexion, disorientation, lethargy, impaired ability to do simple math equations such as serial 7s (subtracting 7 from 100 and continuing as long as it is correct)
3	Stuporous but arouseable with noxious stimulation, incoherent speech, noticeable asterixis, marked confusion
4	Comatose, unresponsive to stimulation, may see either decerebrate or decorticate posturing

liver disease so I am not thinking about an acute complication of chronic liver disease at this point.

Acetaminophen is the most common cause of ALF in the United States.[3] Toxicity can occur secondary to intentional ingestion of acetaminophen, or can be inadvertent as many people do not recognize that multiple over-the-counter medications contain acetaminophen and if they take multiple drugs without this consideration, toxic levels of acetaminophen may result. Because the ALF associated with acetaminophen toxicity can be reversed if discovered and treated early enough, it is important to begin treatment as soon as ALF is recognized and even before acetaminophen toxicity has been confirmed.

The hallmarks of ALF include encephalopathy and coagulopathy with a prolonged INR. I found no evidence of bleeding so I have time to evaluate lab work and do not need to consider an emergent transfusion of fresh frozen plasma (FFP). From his physical examination, I am also able to determine his level of encephalopathy. He does not have evident asterixis, although I can elicit it. His speech is slurred and he is oriented to person only. However, he only arouses to tactile stimulation. This tells me that he is between Grade II and Grade III level encephalopathy so I have to consider that his encephalopathy is worsening. I will need to closely monitor his respiratory status and I will have a very low threshold for intubation (Table 1-1).

❓ What diagnostic testing should be done and in what order?

The initial blood work has been ordered and sent while I was completing the examination of the patient. The extensive blood work is essential to help establish a diagnosis, as well as the severity of the liver failure, and to begin the evaluation for possible transplantation. Although an arterial blood gas and an arterial ammonia level are preferred, until I know the level of coagulopathy, I do not want to perform an arterial stick.

The initial labs include a hemogram (complete blood count) with differential, comprehensive metabolic profile including magnesium and phosphorus levels, prothrombin time (PT), partial thromboplastin time (PTT) and INR, ammonia, lactate, toxicology screen, acetaminophen level, acute hepatitis profile, herpes virus serology, blood type and screen, autoimmune markers, HIV-1 and HIV-2, amylase, and lipase. Blood, sputum, and urine cultures are sent to evaluate for any infection which may also be contributing to his mental state.

A CT scan of the head will be important once initial therapy is initiated. Cerebral edema is a potentially fatal complication of ALF and should be monitored closely. At the same time, a CT scan of the abdomen, focusing on liver volume and any abnormal abdominal process should be done. This will be very important if the patient progresses to the need for liver transplantation. An ultrasound of the liver can also be helpful, for potential transplantation, to evaluate blood flow and to detect any biliary obstruction.

CASE INFORMATION

Diagnostic Testing Results

The comprehensive metabolic panel shows the following abnormal valves:
• Potassium 5.2 (normal 3.7–4.8 mmol/L)
• CO_2 13 (normal 22–29 mmol/L)
• Blood urea nitrogen or BUN 32 (normal 7–21 mg/dL)
• Creatinine 2.1 (normal 0.6–1.1 mg/dL)
• Total bilirubin 23 (normal 0.2–1.1 mg/dL)
• Alanine transaminase or ALT 3627 (normal 11–41 U/L)
• Aspartate aminotransferase or AST 5623 (normal 12–40 U/L)
• Alkaline phosphatase 326 (normal 40–115 U/L)

The rest of his electrolytes and his hemogram are within normal limits.

PT is increased to 29.8 (normal 9.6–12.5 s) and his INR is elevated at 3.4 (normal 1).

The urinalysis is unremarkable so there is no need to send a urine culture.

The ammonia level is 106 (normal 11–51 μmol/L) and the venous lactate 12.6 (venous normal 0.5–2.2 mmol/L).

The toxicology screen, acetaminophen level, viral serologies, HIV status and cultures are not immediately available. Although they are important, treatment decisions can begin with the results that are available.

ALF due to Acetaminophen Toxicity

Diagnosis and Treatment

The lab results support the diagnosis of ALF and the transaminase levels >3500 U/L are highly suggestive of acetaminophen toxicity.[4] Even if the acetaminophen level comes back low, I still need to consider, and treat, acetaminophen toxicity based on the ALT and AST levels, and his history including cold symptoms, ankle pain, and possible depression because of his recent divorce and difficulties at work. Activated charcoal is often used in patients who have recently ingested a large quantity of acetaminophen or other toxin. However, this is only effective with ingestion occurring within the last 1 to 3 hours, and in this case, I do not have the details regarding this patient's acetaminophen misuse. I choose not to give activated charcoal. In cases of acute acetaminophen overdose, an acetaminophen toxicity nomogram is helpful in directing treatment. However, for the nomogram to be helpful, knowing the time of ingestion is essential; in this case we do not know when he took the drugs.

N-acetylcysteine (NAC) is the antidote for acetaminophen toxicity and is started as soon as the condition is diagnosed. Although it can be given orally, it has to be given every 4 hours for a total of 17 doses. Because this may be difficult, especially if the patient is confused or not alert, the most accepted route for NAC administration is intravenous (IV). In the case of my patient, I order the standard IV dosing—150 mg/kg loading dose over 15 minutes followed by 50 mg/kg for 4 hours and then a maintenance dose of 6 mg/kg/h.[4] Although the maintenance dose may be stopped after 16 hours, many providers now continue NAC infusion until liver labs improve, the patient receives a transplant, or death occurs. At this time I do not have to consider a stop time and can base it on the patient's condition and recommendations made by the hepatology or transplant teams.

Addressing coagulopathy in patients with ALF is essential, particularly because many medical interventions introduce a risk of bleeding. Any invasive procedures will require transfusion with fresh frozen plasma (FFP) to prevent bleeding complications if the INR is elevated. In some cases, vitamin K is used to reverse coagulopathy and bring the INR back to normal range. However, for this patient, vitamin K is not a viable option since he cannot receive an intramuscular injection in the setting of an increased INR and oral vitamin K may not be properly absorbed. The most effective route for vitamin K, in this situation, is intravenous, which is not without risk. The benefit of intravenous vitamin K is limited given that the synthetic functioning of the liver is compromised. In the case of this patient, because FFP is readily available, I will monitor the PT/INR every 6 to 8 hours and consider transfusion if his anticoagulation worsens.

Another consideration in the management of ALF due to acetaminophen toxicity is the management of encephalopathy. Ammonia levels >200 μg/dL are associated with cerebral edema and herniation.[4] Oral, or rectal, lactulose is frequently used to increase bowel elimination of ammonia, and prevent progressive hyperammonemia. However, in the case of my patient, I do not want to order oral lactulose because increased gaseous distention of the bowel increases the technical difficulty of liver transplantation surgery. Lactulose enemas, in order to be effective, need to be retained, and in this patient, with severe coagulopathy, I will not order a rectal catheter, which can cause bleeding. So though his current level of 106 μmol/L, which converts to 148 μg/dL, warrants treatment, lactulose is not ideal for this patient. Therefore, I order rifaximin to be given through his nasogastric tube twice a day. This antibiotic alters the gastrointestinal flora, limiting ammonia production.

ALF from any cause can lead to acute renal failure. Maintaining renal perfusion through fluid replacement, or if necessary vasopressors, is essential. In some cases, continuous renal replacement therapy may be necessary. Patients with ALF also develop electrolyte disturbances and are prone to hypoglycemia because of the liver's role in maintaining normal glucose levels. Interventions to address this include monitoring blood sugar by fingerstick and providing enteral nutrition or intravenous infusion of supplemental glucose.

Along with standard care provided to any critically ill patient, families of patients with ALF due to acetaminophen toxicity need careful explanation of the patient's prognosis. There are three possible outcomes—full recovery, liver transplantation (which is a life changing surgery), or death. In the case of this patient, if he survives, we will need to determine if his acetaminophen toxicity is from an intentional overdose, or an accidental ingestion. He will require psychiatric evaluation for suicidal intentions, and may require treatment for depression.

CASE INFORMATION

Intensive Care Unit Stay

Patients with ALF can deteriorate very rapidly so in my approach to this patient, I need to think ahead. It is unclear how he will respond to IV NAC, but I have already determined that he is transitioning to Grade III encephalopathy, so I choose to intubate him and begin mechanical ventilation before he is severely compromised and the need to do so becomes emergent. I also order 4 units of FFP so that I can safely insert a central venous catheter and an arterial line. I do not recheck the PT/INR but place the arterial line while the FFP is infusing and place an internal jugular triple lumen catheter immediately after the FFP has been infused.

Once the patient's airway is secure, and I have adequate IV access, I order a CT scan of the head and abdomen. There is minimal cerebral swelling at this time and no acute intracranial process is seen although I make sure to notify the neurosurgery team in case there is a need for intracranial pressure monitoring which is a recommendation for patients with ALF who have Grade III or Grade IV encephalopathy.[5]

Over the next few days, I monitor the patient in the intensive care unit. His synthetic liver function, namely the PT/INR, is a key indicator of his response to treatment. This may show either improvement or the need for further FFP infusion. Transaminase and bilirubin levels are also checked on a daily basis to evaluate the patient's progress. I closely monitor the patient's ammonia level to determine if additional therapy is needed to maintain the level <200 µg/dL, which for my lab converts to <143 µmol/L. I assess his renal function with his daily labs, and his blood glucose is stable on enteral feedings through a nasogastric tube.

During this time I also monitor the patient carefully for infection. Because the liver is not functioning properly, he is at higher risk of developing an infection. Because of his ALF, he may not show typical signs of infection such as a high fever, or an elevated white blood cell count. Therefore, a careful daily examination is warranted, and I have a low threshold for starting antimicrobial therapy. If an infection develops, liver transplantation will no longer be a treatment option.

Case Follow-up

With appropriate and aggressive therapy, the patient's liver function improves within the first 24 hours. As his liver function continues to improve, his neurological status returns to normal. On day 4 he is extubated. A psychiatric evaluation determines that he is indeed depressed but not suicidal. On day 5 he is transferred to the medicine ward and he discharges home on day 7.

References

1. Huff JS. Evaluation of abnormal behavior in the emergency department. UpToDate. 2013. http://www.uptodate.com/contents/evaluation-of-abnormal-behavior-in-the-emergency-department.
2. Goldberg E, Chopra S. Acute liver failure in adults: etiology, clinical manifestations, and diagnosis. UpToDate. 2014. http://www.uptodate.com/contents/acute-liver-failure-in-adults-etiology-clinical-manifestations-and-diagnosis.
3. Bernal W, Wendon J. Acute live failure. *NEJM*. 2013;369(26):2525-2534.
4. Lee WM, Larson AM, Stravitz RT. AASLD position paper: the management of acute liver failure: update 2011. https://www.aasld.org/sites/default/files/guideline_documents/alfenhanced.pdf. Accessed 7/29/15.
5. Wang D-W, Yin Y-M, Yao Y-M. Advances in the management of acute liver failure. *World J Gastroenterol*. 2013;19(41):7069-7077.

CASE 2

Julie A. Grishaw

Julie Grishaw is an ACNP in the Medical ICU at the University of Virginia in Charlottesville. She is also a senior editor for McGraw-Hill Education's ClinicalAccess.

CASE INFORMATION

Chief Complaint

A Medical Intensive Care Unit (MICU) Acute Care Nurse Practitioner (ACNP) consult was called to request evaluation of a 60-year-old male with increasing oxygen requirements and altered mental status. He was admitted 3 days ago for treatment of community-acquired pneumonia (CAP). The consulting physician reports the patient has a history of chronic obstructive pulmonary disease (COPD) and currently smokes 3 packs of cigarettes per day.

❓ What is the potential cause?

Case Analysis: Acute changes in mental status and hypoxemia are concerning developments in a hospitalized patient. The cause must be determined quickly, with initiation of proper treatment, to ensure a positive outcome. Hypoxemia can lead to altered mental status. And some neurologic disorders, such as acute stroke, can lead to hypoventilation and result in hypoxemia. Thus, the differential for altered mental status with hypoxemia is broad. A systems-based approach is useful to ensure that all possible causes are considered.

Comprehensive Differential Diagnoses for Patients With Altered Mental Status and Hypoxemia[1]

- Neurologic: acute stroke, subarachnoid hemorrhage, administration of a CNS depressant, seizure with a postictal state, meningitis, encephalitis, central sleep apnea
- Cardiovascular: left ventricular (LV) dysfunction, cardiogenic pulmonary edema, dysrhythmia, hypertensive emergency, myocardial infarction, cardiogenic shock
- Pulmonary: pulmonary embolism, worsening pneumonia, acute respiratory distress syndrome (ARDS), COPD exacerbation, untreated obstructive sleep apnea, aspiration
- Gastrointestinal: ischemic colitis, intra-abdominal infection leading to sepsis

- Genitourinary: urinary tract infection
- Metabolic/Systemic: adrenal insufficiency, lactic acidosis, hypoglycemia, metabolic disturbance, hepatic encephalopathy, severe sepsis
- Psychiatric disorder: new onset psychosis

Case Analysis: After quickly considering the long list of differential diagnoses, I use the information gathered during the history and physical to order the differential. This allows me to quickly determine which diagnoses are more or less likely. This is paramount in cases in which the patient may be unstable and decisions need to be made in a timely fashion.

CASE INFORMATION

General Survey and History of Present Illness

I arrive at the patient's bedside after receiving the consult. The patient is a well-nourished, well-developed male, appearing slightly older than his documented age. The head of bed is at 45 degrees and he is sitting quietly with his eyes closed. A 100% nonrebreather mask is in place. He is taking rapid, shallow breaths. His wife and his nurse are at his bedside.

I attempt to wake him. I rub his arm and say his name, but he does not respond. I lightly squeeze his hand, and he murmurs something unintelligible. I ask if he can open his eyes, which he does for a few moments. He does not follow any additional commands. I ask his wife and the nurse if this is his usual mental status. His nurse reports that he was appearing anxious and slightly tachypneic at the beginning of her shift, 8 hours ago. At that time his pulse oximeter oxygen saturation (SaO_2) was 85% on 2 liters (L) nasal cannula (NC). He was able to follow all commands and his symptoms improved when his oxygen was increased from 2 L NC to 5 L NC, and his SaO_2 increased to 94%. Thereafter, he was able to eat his lunch, and asked to take a nap. When the nurse came back in to take afternoon vital signs, she noted that he was much more somnolent and not responding well to commands. His wife reports that he has never had an episode like this before, and that he is normally very interactive and able to care for himself without assistance.

During my conversation with the patient's wife, the nurse obtains another set of vital signs, which are as follows: heart rate (HR) 104 beats per minute, blood pressure (BP) 110/60 mm Hg, respiratory rate (RR) 40/min, SaO_2 89% on 100% nonrebreather. Based on this information alone, I realize that the hypoxemia is severe. In a healthy patient, the SaO_2 should be 100%. Even more significant, the PaO_2 should be over 500 mm Hg. While an ABG is not yet available, I know that the patient's PaO_2 is around 60 mm Hg, given the SaO_2 of 89% on 100% nonrebreather. Therefore, I need to gather additional data quickly and efficiently to expedite appropriate clinical decision making. I order a stat chest x-ray, arterial blood gas (ABG), complete blood count (CBC), basic metabolic panel (BMP), lactic acid, and coagulation studies to be drawn while I gather information about the patient from his wife. I ask about past medical history, medications, family history, and the current illness. I keep the differential in mind as I ask questions, as I need to quickly narrow down causes and create a plan of action.

Review of the electronic medical record (EMR) shows that all sputum cultures in the past have been negative and that his chest x-ray from 1 year ago showed evidence of COPD, but no infiltrates. The chest x-ray from this admission showed a right middle lobe infiltrate. Sputum cultures during this admission were unable to be obtained due to scant sputum production. He was not prescribed narcotics or sedatives during this admission and his nurse confirms that he had received no such medications.

Past Medical History

The patient's wife reports that he was diagnosed with moderate COPD about 5 years ago and sees a pulmonologist, but continues to smoke 3 packs of cigarettes per day. She says, "he really doesn't have any other health problems," and noted that the diagnosis with COPD was a shock for them. She states that he has never needed home oxygen, and takes a purple inhaler-type medication every day. She denies any history of stroke, seizure, cardiovascular disease, dysrhythmias, cirrhosis, renal failure, or recent exposure to toxic inhalants, and no recreational drug use. She reports that "he had his gallbladder removed about 10 years ago because of gallstone attacks" but has not had any other hospitalizations. I ask if he has an advanced directive, and his wife states they have discussed it many times and that he wants life support if needed.

Case Analysis: At this point, I have new data available. I review the x-ray on the portable viewer, and note diffuse, bilateral infiltrates. This change from his admission chest x-ray is consistent with acute respiratory distress syndrome (ARDS). The ABG reveals a respiratory acidosis with the following values: pH 7.30, Pa_{CO_2} 49, Pa_{O_2} 59, HCO_3 25. The patient's breathing pattern is rapid and shallow, which contributes to ineffective clearance of carbon dioxide, and the resulting respiratory acidosis. He is also profoundly hypoxemic. Due to the patient's quickly decompensating condition, I make the decision to intubate and ventilate him on a volume mode of ventilation with a set rate. I also transfer him immediately to the MICU. While some may consider a trial of noninvasive positive pressure ventilation (NIPPV), I recognize that it is not a reasonable option due to the patient's somnolent state and inability to protect his airway. In addition NIPPV is a poor choice for patients with ARDS due to the prolonged duration of the disease. It is unlikely, given his oxygen requirements, that noninvasive ventilation will be adequate.

Immediate stabilization is necessary before additional diagnostics can be obtained. After stabilizing the patient, I can further narrow the list of differential diagnoses and initiate appropriate treatment.

❓ What are the pertinent positives from the information given so far?

- The patient was admitted for CAP, has a diagnosis of COPD, and smokes.
- Oxygen requirements have gone from 1 L NC to 100% nonrebreather over 12 hours.
- Bilateral infiltrates noted on chest x-ray (a significant change from admission).
- Respiratory acidosis is present.
- The patient requires intubation for hypoxemia and altered mental status.
- Altered mental status seems to have occurred following the hypoxemia.

❓ What are the significant negatives from the information given so far?

- The patient does not have a history of cognitive impairment.
- History is negative for cardiovascular disease, neurologic disease, renal impairment, cirrhosis, metabolic disturbance, or malignancy.
- No recent exposure to toxic inhalants, other than cigarettes.
- The patient did not receive narcotics or sedatives.

❓ Can the information gathered so far be restated in a single sentence highlighting the pieces that narrow down the cause?

Putting the information obtained so far in a single statement—a problem representation—sets the stage for gathering more information and determining the cause.

The problem representation in this case might be: "a 60-year-old male with a history of COPD admitted with a right middle lobe pneumonia, now presenting with severe hypoxemia and altered mental status requiring intubation."

❓ How does this information affect the list of potential causes?

Case Analysis: I was initially concerned that the altered mental status may signify an acute stroke. However, given that the patient presented with pneumonia, has a history of COPD, now has bilateral infiltrates on chest x-ray, and that the somnolence occurred after severe hypoxemia all make this less likely and much lower on the differential. The patient is afebrile, which in conjunction with a lack of reported neurologic abnormalities makes neurologic infection less likely. Additionally, the lack of administration of narcotics or sedatives significantly lowers the possibility of medication overdose as a cause for the somnolence.

Given that the altered mental status followed the hypoxemia, and that his x-ray now shows bilateral diffuse infiltrates, I am thinking that this is primarily a pulmonary problem. However, I cannot rule out a metabolic or cardiac etiology at this time. I believe a metabolic cause to be much less likely, as the patient does not have a history of diabetes, malignancy, or metabolic disturbances. While the differential is still quite long and pulmonary is highest on my list, I must also consider cardiac conditions until I definitively rule them out.

My concern is that the patient may have developed a dysrhythmia, or may have an undiagnosed cardiac disease. Unfortunately my early review of the EMR did not have an electrocardiogram (ECG) listed and his wife did not recall him having a recent ECG. Following his transfer to the MICU, he is monitored continuously. The rhythm appears regular, with a rate of 98 beats per minute. I order a stat ECG as this is the first step to ruling out cardiac etiology.

CASE INFORMATION

Review of Systems

The patient is intubated and sedated, and the information was obtained from his wife.
- Constitutional: Denies fever, his appetite is good, but took very little of his lunch, as he seemed tired. Denies recent falls or trauma.
- Cardiovascular: Denies chest pain, swelling of extremities, palpitations, lesions on extremities, cold or numbness of extremities.
- Pulmonary: Shortness of breath started approximately 2 days before hospitalization. Frequent, nonproductive cough. Denies bloody sputum. New difficulty walking to the end of the driveway to get the mail. He needed to stop half way to catch his breath. The day before being admitted to the hospital, he had shortness of breath at rest.
- Gastrointestinal: Denies nausea/vomiting, reports he had a bowel movement day before yesterday, which is his normal schedule.
- Genitourinary: Denies blood in his urine, change in urine smell, frequency, or amount. Denies urinary discomfort.
- Musculoskeletal: Reports a sore elbow, thought to be strained from playing golf 2 weeks ago.
- Neurological: Denies headache, falls, history of seizure disorder or stroke, numbness, tingling, or extremity weakness, changes in speech, difficulty swallowing.
- Endocrine: Not pertinent.
- Psychiatric: Mood is unchanged from normal. Reports being very social and denies depressive symptoms.

Physical Examination

- Vital signs: heart rate 97, blood pressure 130/60 mm Hg, respiratory rate 25, and temperature 37°C oral, SpO_2 93% on volume control (VC) mechanical ventilation with settings of 60% fraction of inspired oxygen (FIO_2), RR 25, PEEP 7, tidal volume (TV) 300, and a fingerstick blood glucose 118.
- Intubated male, appearing slightly older than stated age. Sedated, and unable to participate in examination.
- Head/eyes/ears/nose/throat: Pupils are equal, round, reactive to light, buccal mucosa moist, oropharynx is moist, native teeth appear in good condition, with no looseness or decay noted
- Cardiovascular: Heart rate and rhythm regular, no murmurs, rub, or gallops. No edema noted. Nail beds are pink, cool to touch; brisk capillary refill.
- Pulmonary: Intubated on VC mechanical ventilation, appears comfortable on mechanical ventilation, not breathing over set rate, no auto-PEEP. Diffuse crackles and rhonchi throughout all lung fields.
- Gastrointestinal: Normoactive bowel sounds, tympanic on percussion, abdomen soft and nontender.
- Genitourinary: Urinary catheter in place draining urine to gravity.
- Skin: Intact, no rashes, lesions, or ulcerations; normal skin turgor.
- Neurological: Unable to participate in physical examination due to being intubated and sedated. No focal neurologic deficits noted, face symmetric, reflexes intact and symmetric, appropriate blink reflex and response to painful stimuli
- ECG: Normal sinus rhythm, with possible left ventricular hypertrophy. No findings suggested a bundle branch block or ischemia.

? **What elements of the review of systems and the physical examination should be added to the list of pertinent positives?**

- Diffuse crackles and rhonchi throughout all lung fields noted on examination, dyspnea worsening over the past week in conjunction with a diagnosis of pneumonia.

? **Which items should be added to the list of significant negatives?**

- Review of systems and the physical examination are both negative for focal neurological deficits, or signs of neurologic infection. The ECG is negative for dysrhythmia or ischemic changes. The review of systems, though obtained from the patient's wife, reveals no complaints pointing to a vascular cause, such as abdominal pain.

Case Analysis: The physical examination and review of systems are furthe. reassurance that this is not a stroke or neurologic condition. Though computed tomography (CT) scan of the head is always a consideration in the patient with altered mental status, the current history indicates that the altered mental status occurred after the hypoxemia, making this much less likely. The absence of abdominal pain, an unremarkable abdominal examination, and lack of fever make intra-abdominal infection a less likely cause. It is also reassuring that the patient had a cholecystectomy, though there are many other potential sources of intra-abdominal infection. The absence of palpitations, edema, nonhealing ulcers, and signs of venous stasis make a cardiac origin or vascular insufficiency much less likely. The unremarkable ECG and continued normal sinus rhythm on telemetry further exclude a cardiac origin. The patient does not have a history of alcoholism or cirrhosis, making hepatic encephalopathy unlikely.

The most likely origin is a pulmonary cause. In my differential, I listed worsening pneumonia, COPD exacerbation, pulmonary embolism, and ARDS. ARDS and pulmonary embolism cause acute hypoxemia. I cannot completely rule out a pulmonary embolism without a computed tomography pulmonary angiogram (CTPA). However, the patient's presentation and chest x-ray findings make this very unlikely. Given the pneumonia, acute hypoxemia, and bilateral infiltrates, my working diagnosis is ARDS. The diagnosis of ARDS requires that specific guidelines are met. I must examine all aspects of the situation to make sure the patient fits within these criteria.

Diagnosis: ARDS

A diagnosis is established when patients meet the ARDS Berlin definition. This was published in 2012, replacing the American-European Consensus Conference on ARDS definition, published in 1994.[2,3] According to the ARDS Berlin definition, patients must meet the following criteria to be diagnosed with ARDS: Acute hypoxemia with an onset of less than 1 week, bilateral infiltrates on chest imaging that are not otherwise fully explained by other pulmonary pathologies such as effusions, atelectasis, or nodules, and respiratory failure that is not explained by a cardiac etiology or volume status.[2,4] Additionally, the ARDS Berlin definition gives specific criteria for determining the severity of ARDS:

- Mild: $200\,mm\,Hg < PaO_2/FIO_2 \leq 300\,mm\,Hg$ with PEEP or CPAP $\geq 5\,cm\,H_2O$
- Moderate: $100\,mm\,Hg < PaO_2/FIO_2 \leq 200\,mm\,Hg$ with PEEP $\geq 5\,cm\,H_2O$
- Severe: $PaO_2/FIO_2 \leq 100\,mm\,Hg$ with PEEP $\geq 5\,cm\,H_2O$[4]

It is noteworthy to mention that acute lung injury (ALI) is no longer an appropriate diagnostic term. This has been replaced by mild ARDS, using the Berlin definition as noted above.[2,4]

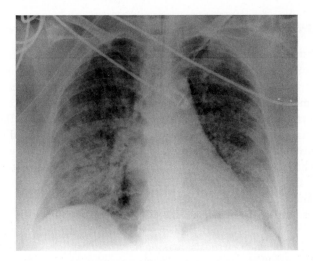

Figure 2-1 Diffuse bilateral infitrates in ARDS patient. Reproduced, with permission, from Longo DL, Fauci AS, Kasper DL, et al. *Harrison's Principles of Internal Medicine.* 18th ed. New York: McGraw-Hill Education; 2012. Figure 268-2.

I obtained a chest x-ray prior to intubating the patient, and obtain another shortly after intubation. At the time of the postintubation chest x-ray, the ventilator settings were as follows:

Volume Control Mode: FiO_2 -60%, Rate- 20 (total rate 25), PEEP-7cm H_2O, TV-300 mL. I view the chest x-ray to confirm that the endotracheal (ETT) is placed appropriately and I also note the presence of bilateral alveolar infiltrates (see Figure 2-1)[5].

I know that the duration of my patient's acute hypoxemia has been less than 1 week and the infiltrates are not explained by any other pulmonary pathology. The patient does not have a history of interstitial lung disease, which could cause a persistent appearance of infiltrates. The infiltrates are new from this admission, and were not visible on the initial admitting chest x-ray. The patient has no history of cardiovascular disease, and the physical examination and diagnostics do not support a potential cardiac etiology of the infiltrates. A review of volume status shows that the patient is net negative 1 L since admission, and hypervolemia is not suspected based on this and the lack of associated physical examination findings. So, I have now determined that the patient meets at least two of the three criteria for diagnosis of ARDS. I must now determine the PaO_2/FIO_2 (P/F) ratio. I obtain another ABG following intubation on the previously mentioned ventilator settings. The results are: pH 7.32, Pa_{CO_2} 40, Pa_{O_2} 67, HCO_3 25. We calculate the P/F ratio by dividing the Pa_{O_2} by the FIO_2.

$$\frac{Pa_{O_2} (67)}{FIO_2 (0.6)} = \frac{P}{F} \text{ ratio of } 112$$

I can now confirm the diagnosis of moderate ARDS.

ARDS Management

The treatment of ARDS consists largely of supportive care. The first task is to stabilize the patient, ensuring adequate oxygenation and perfusion. This is achieved successfully in this case with intubation, initiation of mechanical ventilation, and transfer to the MICU. Patients with ARDS are often in septic shock; though this patient is not and he is also hemodynamically stable.

Achieving and maintaining adequate oxygenation in patients with ARDS, while also avoiding barotrauma, is paramount. In order to achieve this fine balance, numerous studies have examined the most appropriate ventilator settings for ARDS. This has led to the development of lung protective mechanical ventilation. This strategy consists of using small tidal volumes of 6 mL/kg to prevent volutrauma (large volumes translate into high distending pressures), and higher PEEP levels to recruit alveoli. The FIO_2 should be set to achieve a goal Pa_{O_2} of 60 mm Hg or greater. To avoid oxygen toxicity, the lowest level of FIO_2 necessary to achieve adequate oxygenation is used.[6] The ventilator settings I chose were in accordance with these strategies. While these initial settings were appropriate for the patient, I kept in mind other more aggressive options should his oxygenation not improve or further decline. In these cases I would increase PEEP to further "recruit" the lung. I would also consider other "recruitment" strategies such as to change the mode of ventilation to airway pressure release ventilation (APRV), which allows for patient spontaneous breathing while maintaining a high level of CPAP.

 CASE INFORMATION

The patient is maintained on mechanical ventilation after being transferred to the ICU. Initially "as-needed" IV injections of midazolam are used to achieve patient/ventilator synchrony but this proves unsuccessful. To improve synchrony, ensure patient comfort, and maintain a consistent oxygen supply, the patient is sedated with continuous fentanyl and midazolam infusions. Two 18-gauge IVs were placed, along with an orogastric tube (OGT) and sequential compression devices. The nursing staff inserts a urinary catheter.

As these MICU admission procedures are performed, I examine the medication administration record more closely. I am interested in reviewing details related to the source of his infection (which may have been the etiology of his evolving ARDS). I find that the patient received 3 days of azithromycin and 4 days of ceftriaxone for treatment of CAP. No sputum cultures were obtained due to the lack of sputum production. Blood cultures taken at the time of admission were negative. I ordered new blood cultures upon MICU transfer. While I recognize that blood cultures have a relatively low yield rate of 5% to 15% in febrile patients and the accuracy varies with specific organisms, a positive yield will help focus his antibiotic therapy. A urine culture is also ordered at the time of transfer to ensure that a urinary tract infection, if present, is identified.

Due to the patient's respiratory decompensation, it is essential that I assure adequate antibiotic coverage, and to that end, I order another sputum sample, discontinue the ceftriaxone, and broaden coverage with the addition of cefepime. The patient had received 3 days of azithromycin, which was appropriate coverage for atypical organisms. His MRSA swab was negative, and at this point empiric coverage for MRSA-associated respiratory infection is unnecessary. Additionally, he does not have any central lines, which makes a systemic MRSA infection less likely. I also decide against administering vancomycin at this time. Instead, I selected cefepime, a fourth-generation cephalosporin, because it offers more broad antibiotic coverage as opposed to ceftriaxone, a third-generation cephalosporin. If my patient does not demonstrate improvement, or worsens in the next 24 hours, I will consider adding vancomycin.

In addition to the critical elements of care noted above, I order appropriate prophylactic measures, such as oral care with chlorhexidine, elevation of the head of bed at 30 degrees, histamine-2 blockers via OGT, and frequent turning. I also initiate the standard ICU order set, which includes continuous telemetry, every 1 hour vital signs, and suctioning as needed.

Over the next 4 hours, the patient remains hemodynamically stable. Auscultation reveals coarse rhonchi throughout all lung fields. Labs reveal normal renal function and no electrolyte disturbances. Studies have suggested that administration of diuretics with resultant net negative fluid status may reduce the duration of mechanical ventilation needed for management of ARDS.[7] I administer 40 mg IV furosemide (Lasix) and instruct the bedside nurse to closely evaluate the heart rate and blood pressure every 30 minutes, and urine output every hour.

Over the course of the next 24 hours, I closely monitor the patient's hemodynamic status. I continue IV furosemide every 6 hours, providing the patient is hemodynamically stable and does not have electrolyte disturbances. Labs are drawn every 8 hours and the patient requires several doses of potassium and phosphorus via OGT. He continues to respond well to 40 mg IV furosemide (Lasix).

On his second day in the MICU, the patient remains hemodynamically stable. His volume status is 1.5 L net negative over the last 24 hours. ABG is as follows: pH 7.34, Pa_{CO_2} 38, Pa_{O_2} 63, HCO_3 22 on VC mechanical ventilation with settings of VC 40% FIO_2, RR 25, PEEP 5, TV 300. Blood, urine, and sputum cultures continued to be negative at this time. His basic metabolic panel shows sodium of 148 mEq/L. The next dose of furosemide (Lasix) is held, and free water 40 mL every 4 hours is given was via OGT and a repeat level drawn later that shows a normal sodium level of 140 mEq/L. I resume periodic diuresis.

During the latter part of MICU day 2, the patient is transitioned to pressure support (PS) mechanical ventilation with settings of 40% FIO_2, PEEP 5, PS 10. An ABG collected after 4 hours on the new settings shows pH 7.36, Pa_{CO_2} 37, Pa_{O_2} 68, HCO_3 24. The patient continues to be hemodynamically stable, afebrile, and exhibits an unlabored respiratory rate of 14 breaths/minute with good tidal volumes of 250 to 500 mL. The patient is started on high protein tube feedings at 30 kcal/h to provide nutritional support.

On MICU day 3, sedation is weaned given the improvement in ventilator requirements. The patient is taken off the midazolam infusion and given midazolam pushes as needed instead. He continues on the fentanyl infusion but the dose is weaned to 25 μg/h. He begins to wake up and follow a few simple commands. He is able to shake his head yes and no to questions, much to the delight of his wife, who remains at the bedside to comfort him. He denies pain or dyspnea.

His intake and output record shows an additional 2 L net negative with continued administration of furosemide (Lasix). His cultures remained negative.

On MICU day 4, the patient is placed on a continuous positive airway pressure (CPAP) trial with settings of FIO_2 40%, PEEP 0, and PS 0 for a period of 2 hours. His ABG reveals pH 7.38, Pa_{CO_2} 39, Pa_{O_2} 78, HCO_3 25. The patient continues to be hemodynamically stable. His respiratory pattern is unlabored, with a normal rate of 15 breaths/minute. He is alert and able to follow simple commands, including coughing. When the endotracheal tube cuff is deflated, an air leak is present on exhalation. Rhonchi are still present throughout lung fields but are much less and more scattered than upon admission. He denies pain, anxiety, or dyspnea. These all suggest that the patient is ready for extubation.

The patient is successfully extubated and placed on 4 L NC. He is able to softly state his name, date of birth, and month of the year. He is unsure of the date. He recognizes his wife at the bedside. He denies pain or dyspnea. He is closely monitored, and continues to be hemodynamically stable, alert, and appropriate, with a eupneic respiratory pattern.

The patient remains in the MICU following extubation. I prescribe physical therapy and the therapists get him out of bed to the chair. He is able to take food by mouth with no difficulty swallowing or coughing. He continues to have an occasional, nonproductive cough. Cultures are still negative. I therefore scale back his antibiotic regimen to ceftriaxone and closely monitor him for decompensation.

Because he continues to exhibit hemodynamic stability, improved oxygenation (oxygen now at 3L NC), and decreased dyspnea on oxygen, I transfer him to the General Medicine service. I continue to follow him as a pulmonary consult.

He continues to show improvement on the General Medicine floor. He spends an additional 3 days in the hospital, at which point antibiotics are discontinued. He completed a 14-day course of antibiotics for treatment of his CAP, and no additional antibiotics are needed as an outpatient. He continues physical therapy, and is able to ambulate and able to go up three to four stairs, which is necessary to enter his home. He remains afebrile, hemodynamically stable, and denies dyspnea. He states that he felt much improved and his wife agreed completely.

Case Follow-up

After 2 weeks in the hospital, the patient is discharged to home. He is instructed to use his fluticasone/salmeterol (Advair) as previously prescribed. He has a follow-up appointment with his primary care provider in 3 days. I also arrange a follow-up appointment with him in the pulmonary clinic in 3 months.

References

1. Zeiger RF. McGraw-Hill's Diagnosaurus 4.0. http://accessmedicine.mhmedical.com/diagnosaurus.aspx.
2. ARDS Definition Task Force, Ranieri VM, Rubenfeld GD, et al. Acute respiratory distress syndrome: the Berlin definition. *JAMA*. 2012;307(23):2526-2533.
3. Bernard GR, Artigas A, Brigham KL, et al. The American-European Consensus Conference on ARDS: definitions, mechanisms, relevant outcomes, and clinical trial coordination. *Am J Respir Crit Care Med*. 1994;149(3, pt 1):818-824.
4. Fanelli V, Vlachou A, Ghannadian S, Simonetti U, Slutsky A, Zhang H. Acute respiratory distress syndrome: new definition, current and future therapeutic options. *J Thorac Dis*. June 2013;5(3):326-334.
5. Longo DL, Fauci AS, Kasper DL, Hauser SL, Jameson JL, Loscalzo J. *Harrison's Principles of Internal Medicine*. 18th ed. www.accessmedicine.com.
6. What are treatments for ARDS? ClinicalAccess. http://clinicalaccess.mhmedical.com/content.aspx?gbosId=113616&searchterms=treatment%2520ARDS&SRO=0&ResultClick=1. Published September 2014. Accessed September 20, 2014.
7. Wiedemann HP, Wheeler AP, Bernard GR, et al. Comparison of two fluid-management strategies in acute lung injury. *N Engl J Med*. 2006;354:2564-2575.

CASE 3

Suzanne M. Burns

Suzanne M. Burns is a Professor Emerita at the University of Virginia in Charlottesville. Prior to her retirement from the University of Virginia she was the clinical coordinator and a clinical instructor for the ACNP and CNS programs. Currently she consults on acute and critical care practice and clinical research.

CASE INFORMATION

Chief Complaint

JR is a 24-year-old female college graduate student with a history of asthma, who is admitted to the emergency department (ED) with "wheezing, shortness of breath, and chest tightness." Her fiancé accompanies her.

? What is the potential cause?

Case Analysis: Wheezing, shortness of breath, and chest tightness are concerning symptoms in a young adult and I am already considering potential life-threatening diagnoses that may be the cause of these symptoms. Given the patient's known history of asthma and the constellation of symptoms she is experiencing, an acute severe asthma episode is the likely diagnosis. Regardless, it is essential that I also consider other potential life-threatening causes such as anaphylaxis, pulmonary emboli, pneumothorax, and even an MI or aortic dissection, and I must do so quickly. I begin with a survey of the patient as I walk into the ED room. The ED nurse introduces me to the patient and her fiancé Bob, and clarifies that the patient has requested that Bob stay with her at all times and act as her spokesperson as she is very short of breath. He is currently at the bedside holding her hand.

CASE INFORMATION

General Survey and History of Present Illness

I see an alert, fit appearing young woman who is sitting upright in the bed. I hear wheezing from across the room. Her respiratory pattern appears rapid (25/min) and labored, she is using accessory muscles, and she looks frightened. Her bedside monitor shows a sinus tachycardia of 140 beats per minute with a pulse oximetry reading of 92% on a 100% nonrebreathing oxygen mask. A noninvasive blood pressure cuff is on her right arm and the last reading taken 3 minutes before I arrived was 150/90 mm Hg. The nurse also noted a 15 mm Hg pulsus paradox on her admission BP of 148/89.

After I introduce myself as the ACNP who will be caring for her, the patient tries to talk to me but cannot speak in a whole sentence. She tells me, in very short phrases, that she has asthma and has already used her inhaler twice but that it did not work this time. Bob states: "She has been this way for the last half hour or so. She said her chest was tight and that she just couldn't get her breath. I told her I needed to take her to the ED because I was scared when she got so short of breath and her inhaler just didn't seem to help even though she used it twice." He states further: "Whenever her asthma acts-up she takes a puff or two of her inhaler and it usually helps but this is the worst I've ever seen her. She was using the inhaler yesterday too but her breathing wasn't as bad as now."

Given her extreme respiratory status I do a rapid cardiac and pulmonary examination. With the exception of a rapid heart rate, her heart sounds are normal. Upon auscultation of her upper airway and lungs I hear profound expiratory wheezing throughout both lung fields but no upper airway stridor. While I have other potential life-threatening causes to consider, I must first attend to her breathing. Given her history of asthma, and the information from Bob that her handheld inhaler has been less effective than usual, I order a stat continuous albuterol treatment and every 20 minute ipratropium treatments. I also order a peripheral IV of normal saline to be started at 75 mL per hour, 125 mg of methylprednisolone IV, a stat portable chest x-ray, peak expiratory flow rate (if she can tolerate performing the test), ECG, and the following laboratory tests: arterial blood gas, complete blood count (CBC) with differential, metabolic panel, and sputum for gram stain and culture (if she can produce sputum).

At this point I believe that the patient is experiencing an acute severe asthma exacerbation (formerly referred to as status asthmaticus) and my priority is to treat her severe bronchoconstriction immediately and aggressively while I consider the need for intubation should she not respond. As I complete a history and physical examination and evaluate my findings, I will keep in mind the following differential for wheezing, shortness of breath, and chest tightness.

Comprehensive Differential Diagnoses for Patient With Wheezing, Shortness of Breath, and Chest Tightness

- Head/eyes/ears/nose/throat: aspiration with obstruction (ie, foreign body), chronic sinusitis with postnasal drip, tracheomalacia, upper respiratory infection, vocal cord dysfunction
- Cardiovascular: acute coronary syndrome, aortic dissection, Churg-Strauss syndrome, heart failure, pericarditis
- Pulmonary: asthma, bronchiolitis, cystic fibrosis, pleurisy, pneumonia, pulmonary embolus, pulmonary eosinophilia, pulmonary fibrosis, sarcoidosis
- Exogenous: drug-induced or ingestion-induced bronchoconstriction/anaphylaxis, inhalation injury of toxic substances

CASE INFORMATION

With the list of all possible causes in mind, I continue to gather additional data. While the patient is receiving her respiratory treatments and diagnostics are performed at the bedside, I ask JR's fiancé to tell me a bit more about the patient's condition. He states that he and JR arrived in Charlottesville 2 weeks ago to attend graduate school together. "JR has always had asthma but generally only needs her inhaler when she exercises and when she gets a cold." He states: "she is very fit, works out regularly, and is rarely sick with anything! I've never seen her this bad before! I really got scared because this is so unusual for her and she was really wheezing a lot and having trouble breathing." Bob also notes that since they moved here the pollen counts have been very high and she has had to use her albuterol inhaler every day and sometimes multiple times per day. He states that she has not been sick with a cold or any other condition for months and months. Today they were out for a walk because it was a pretty day, if a bit windy, and she started wheezing again. I ask JR if there is anything else to add to the report from Bob and she shakes her head "no." I ask if she has ever been to the ED or hospitalized for her asthma in the past, if she has had any recent infections, has any known chronic diseases or conditions in addition to her asthma, taken any recent drugs (over the counter or illicit), whether she smokes or is regularly exposed to cigarette smoke, and if she takes anything else for her asthma. She shakes her head "no" to these questions but haltingly states: "I sometimes have some allergies in the summer. I take Claritin for them." As she is new to the area, no medical records are available to review.

❓ What are the pertinent positives from the information given so far?

- The patient is fit appearing and fully conscious.
- The patient has severe wheezing and shortness of breath—speaks in short phrases.
- Able to answer questions with short phrases or "yes," "no" head gestures.
- The patient has a history of asthma.
- She takes albuterol by handheld inhaler when she wheezes, which is usually only when she exercises or with an upper respiratory infection.
- She takes no other medications or products for her asthma but takes an antihistamine for her "summer allergies."
- Since moving to the area 2 weeks ago she has escalated her inhaler use.

- Vital signs demonstrate no signs of anaphylaxis but do support severe distress.
- Pulse oximeter reading is 92% on 100% FiO_2.
- She has a 15 mm Hg pulsus paradox on inspiration.

? What are the significant negatives from the information given so far?

- No recent infections or illnesses
- Denies chronic health issues or conditions in addition to asthma
- Denies any recent use of drugs, illicit substances, is a nonsmoker, and no regular exposure to second-hand smoke
- Has never been to the ED or hospitalized for her asthma

? Can the information gathered so far be restated in a single sentence highlighting the pieces that narrow down the cause?

Putting the information obtained so far in a single statement—a problem representation—sets the stage for gathering more information and determining the cause.

The problem representation in this case might be: "a 24-year-old female with a history of asthma presents to the ED with an acute severe asthma exacerbation."

? How does this information affect the list of possible causes?

Case Analysis: The patient's age, overall fitness, good health, and absence of chronic conditions or diseases other than her asthma make many of the diagnoses on my differential unlikely. But she does endorse summer allergies for which she takes an antihistamine and has recently moved to this community to attend graduate school. I am highly suspicious that her asthma exacerbation has an allergic component and has been triggered by the high pollen count this summer. Her vital signs and presentation do not suggest other immediate life-threatening conditions such as anaphylaxis, pulmonary emboli, pneumothorax, acute coronary syndrome, or aortic dissection but I move quickly to definitively rule these out along with other potential causes as I monitor and manage the patient's respiratory status.

The albuterol aerosol treatment has been continuous now for approximately 15 minutes and JR appears to be in less distress. Her breathing appears less labored and she states that the aerosol treatment is working. She says her chest tightness is gone and she is much less short of breath. She looks better and is speaking quietly to Bob. I begin a comprehensive history and physical while I await the results of her diagnostics.

CASE INFORMATION

Family and Social History

The patient denies any relevant family history. Denies ever using cigarettes or other substances, drinks occasionally.

Medications

- Prescribed: albuterol(ProAir) inhaler: two inhalations every 4 to 6 hours if needed, two inhalations 15 to 30 minutes before exercise
- Over the counter: loratadine/pseudoephedrine (Claritin D): as needed every 12 hours for allergies, daily multivitamin, occasional ibuprofen (Advil) for headache and "aches and pains" due to exercise

Review of Systems

The patient is much improved and is able to answer all questions. She first affirms her wish that her fiancé be present throughout the history and physical.

- Constitutional: denies fever or recent infections, eats well, exercises regularly
- Head/eyes/ears/nose/throat: wears reading glasses (farsighted), denies sinusitis, endorses rhinitis and sneezing since moving here, denies sore throat but unsure if she has postnasal drip
- Cardiovascular: denies chest pain and relates "chest tightness" to wheezing, denies leg swelling, or difficulty breathing when lying down except with this episode of wheezing
- Pulmonary: affirms shortness of breath, and nonproductive cough with wheezing. Does not use peak expiratory flow rate (PEFR) meter, and does not know her "personal best" value
- Gastrointestinal: denies gastroesophageal reflux disease (GERD) or burning in her chest. Normal digestion, eating and bowel patterns
- Genitourinary: normal
- Musculoskeletal: normal
- Integumentary: normal
- Neurological: alert, oriented, anxious. Otherwise normal
- Endocrine: normal.
- Psychiatric: denies any psychiatric problems

Physical Examination

- Vital signs: pulse is 108 beats per minute, blood pressure: right arm: 130/74 and left arm: 132/75 mm Hg with a pulsus paradox of 10 mm Hg on inspiration (both arms), respiratory rate: 20 breaths per minute, temperature: 37°C—tympanic, pulse oximetry: 100% on 3 L nasal prongs (was changed from 100% nonrebreather mask by respiratory therapist because saturation improved while giving albuterol treatment). Height 5'4", weight 118 lb, BMI 20.3

- Constitutional: improving status, appears less anxious, talking in whole sentences. Still receiving continuous albuterol treatment
- Head/eyes/ears/nose/throat: no nasal discharge, nasal polyp in right nare, no throat redness or exudate. Normal head, eyes, and ears examination
- Cardiovascular: heart rate and rhythm regular, no murmurs, rubs, or gallops, brisk capillary refill in all extremities and without any edema. Bedside telemetry shows sinus tachycardia at 108 beats per minute
- Pulmonary: respiratory rate and rhythm are synchronous, slight accessory muscle use but greatly improved from initial encounter. Hyperresonant percussion notes throughout lung fields. Voice sounds: negative E to A sounds. Auscultation: moderate expiratory wheezing throughout lung fields
- Gastrointestinal: normal
- Musculoskeletal: normal except for tremor of hands (secondary to β-agonist)
- Neurological: normal neurologic examination. Oriented and appropriate though still anxious. Able to speak in whole sentences
- Integumentary: no central or peripheral cyanosis, normal skin turgor and integrity
- Endocrine: normal

Diagnostics Obtained 15 to 20 Minutes Ago

- Portable chest x-ray: hyperinflation, normal heart size and no mediastinal widening, no infiltrates
- Peak expiratory flow rate (PEFR): initial 150 L/min, repeat PEFR now is 360 L/min (average PEFR for adult woman 5'4" is ~450 L/min)
- ECG: sinus tachycardia, no ischemic changes noted
- Arterial blood gas (ABG): pH 7.33, $PaCO_2$ 50 mm Hg, PaO_2 68 mm Hg (taken while on 100% nonrebreathing mask, prior to albuterol treatment)
- Complete blood count (CBC) with differential: normal red cell count, normal white blood cell count, differential normal except for slightly elevated eosinophil count: 5% (normal = 1%–3%)
- Metabolic panel: normal
- Sputum: unable to obtain because cough is minimal and nonproductive

❓ What elements of the review of systems and the physical examination should be added to the list of pertinent positives?

- Initial ABG: uncompensated respiratory acidosis with moderate hypoxemia on 100% O_2.
- Current findings suggest rapid improvement of bronchoconstriction and include improving oxygenation, ability to speak in whole sentences, decreased accessory muscle use, and improving PEFR.
- Nasal polyp noted (polyps often result from chronic inflammation due to asthma and allergies).
- Chest x-ray shows hyperinflation consistent with asthma.
- ECG normal except for tachycardia, pulsus paradox decreased to 10 mm Hg both arms.

❓ Which items should be added to the list of significant negatives?

- Gastrointestinal, neurological, and endocrine examinations are all normal.
- No signs of sinusitis or sore throat.
- Negative for history of gastroesophageal reflux disease (GERD).
- Chest x-ray negative for infiltrates, foreign body obstruction, mediastinal widening.
- CBC normal except for eosinophils as noted.

❓ How does this information affect the list of possible causes?

Case Analysis: The findings to this point rule out the vast majority of potential causes on my differential. Aspiration with obstruction (ie, foreign body) and chronic sinusitis with postnasal drip can be eliminated from my differential, as her history and physical and diagnostics do not support these diagnoses. Tracheomalacia is unlikely and not supported by her history or her presentation. She had no stridor on examination, which is more common with tracheomalacia than is wheezing. It is most common in infants but can be a sequel of prolonged intubation, tracheostomy, chest trauma, or recurrent tracheobronchitis, none of which are consistent with JR's history. Vocal cord dysfunction often appears much like asthma and is often triggered by such things as allergies but generally the difficulty breathing, and subsequently the associated wheezing, is during inspiration versus expiration.

Pulmonary embolism (PE) is highly unlikely as she is an active and healthy young woman and her history and examination reveal no potential site of deep vein thrombosis. There are also no signs of PE on her ECG such as low amplitude or ST changes. Her cardiac examination and ECG are normal except for a sinus tachycardia, which is consistent with her stress state and is an expected side effect of the bronchodilator. Though albuterol is β_2-specific bronchodilator, the drug does have some β_1 activity as well, which both increases heart rate and results in tremors and shakiness.

I can rule out pericarditis as her ECG shows no signs suggestive of pericarditis (ST and T wave changes), she does not have a pericardial fiction rub, and her x-ray shows a normal cardiac silhouette. In addition, she is no longer complaining of chest tightness as her bronchoconstriction has improved. Her examination and chest x-ray also rule out heart failure and aortic dissection, as both her heart size and mediastinum are normal and her lungs, though hyperinflated, are clear.

I am also comfortable ruling out bronchiolitis and pneumonia, since she has not reported any past febrile illnesses, has a nonproductive dry cough, examination findings are not consistent with areas of consolidation, and her chest-x ray is clear. Pleurisy generally follows a pneumonia and is often associated with chest pain during inspiration on the affected side; I also rule this out as a cause of her symptoms. She does not have a history of cystic fibrosis (CF) and it is extremely rare for such a diagnosis to appear at the age of 24. I eliminate CF from my differential. I also eliminate pulmonary fibrosis, sarcoidosis, and pulmonary eosinophilia as these would have interstitial findings on the x-ray and symptoms would likely develop more slowly than the patient's history describes. And, given her history, I also eliminate drug-induced ingestions and inhalations as causes.

Churg-Strauss syndrome is also known as eosinophilic granulomatosis with polyangiitis. It is a condition that results in inflammatory vascular changes and acute asthma is a common finding. Eosinophilia is present with the condition, and JR does have a mild serum eosinophilia; however, she also has a history of seasonal allergies, which is a more common cause of elevated serum eosinophils. Other diagnostic criteria for the condition include sinusitis, pulmonary infiltrates, and polyneuropathy, none of which are present. I eliminate this diagnosis from my differential.

Given JR's rapid improvement, H & P findings, and diagnostics, I am confident that the diagnosis of acute severe asthma exacerbation, likely triggered by seasonal allergies, is accurate. She reports a history of asthma and has chronic allergies supported by her history and the presence of a nasal polyp, which is suggestive of chronic inflammation. Despite her improvement I am concerned that her asthma is not well controlled; she does not use an inhaled corticosteroid or leukotriene receptor antagonist such as montelukast (Singulair). In consultation with the ED team, we decide to keep her in the ED for up to 6 hours to ensure she does not experience a late airway response, which is generally of slower onset (ie, 4–6 hours) and is mediated by eosinophils.[1] I also must consider potential admission to the hospital versus discharge and will discuss this and a follow-up plan of care with her as well.

Diagnosis: Acute Severe Asthma

Description

The Global Initiative for Asthma (GINA) report defines asthma as: "A characteristic pattern of respiratory symptoms such as wheezing, shortness of breath, chest tightness or cough, and variable airflow limitation."[2] The pathophysiology and pathogenesis of asthma is airflow obstruction due to inflammation, bronchoconstriction, and mucus plugging. Thus, it is recognized as primarily an inflammatory condition rather than a disease involving primary bronchoconstriction. Mediators of inflammation include eosinophils, macrophages, T lymphocytes, and mast cells that release histamine, prostaglandins, thromboxanes, and leukotrienes to name a few.[2,3] The profound bronchoconstriction results in difficulty exhaling, dynamic hyperinflation, and a very high work of breathing. If not reversed, the patient fatigues and respiratory arrest ensues.

Proposed causes of asthma include changes in innate immunity (the hygiene hypothesis), genetic predisposition, and environmental factors such as allergies and other exposures.[2,3] Asthma "triggers," while not causal, stimulate or trigger bronchoconstriction in airways that are chronically "inflamed." Common triggers include infections, allergens, smoke and other toxic inhalants, animals, foods, medications, exercise, sinusitis, and gastroesophageal reflux disease.[2,3]

GINA notes that asthma is a common chronic disease affecting between "1% and 18% of populations in different countries."[2] Asthma exacerbations account for 497,000 hospitalizations annually and significant morbidity and mortality.[4] The condition is most common in females, children, and minorities and deaths in these groups are also higher.[4] Guidelines from the National Asthma Education and Prevention Program (NAEPP) of the Heart, Lung and Blood Institute, National Institutes of Health, suggest that asthma deaths may be attributed to inadequate control of the disease, late ED arrival, underuse of corticosteroids, and lack of aggressive pharmacotherapy.[3]

While the diagnosis of asthma is best done in a pulmonary function laboratory, many are seen first in a health care facility such as an ED or clinic during an acute exacerbation. In these settings, they are urgently or emergently treated with bronchodilators and corticosteroids and their response to these therapies suggests the diagnosis of asthma. Regardless, follow-up outpatient care is recommended to determine the severity of the disease, and develop a long-term treatment plan to prevent recurrent exacerbations.

Management of Acute Severe Asthma Exacerbations: ED, Acute and Critical Care Units

As in JR's case, patients experiencing acute severe exacerbations of asthma often seek help in EDs. For these patients the priority is to accomplish a rapid assessment of their respiratory status while their bronchoconstriction is treated. Management needs to be aggressive as deterioration and cardiopulmonary arrest may rapidly ensue. Physical signs and symptoms suggesting moderate to severe asthma include disturbances in consciousness, inability to say whole sentences, anxiety, tachypnea, tachycardia, respiratory muscle recruitment, prolonged expiratory phase, pulsus paradox (>15 mm Hg), paradoxical respirations, central cyanosis, profuse diaphoresis, agitation, O_2 saturation of 90% to 95% (or less) on room air, PEFR <50% estimated or personal best. While JR experienced many of these signs and symptoms she was fully alert and able to cooperate with therapies. Had she not been alert and had quiet breath sounds (ie, silent chest) intubation would be a necessary first step.

Pharmacotherapy is the mainstay of acute severe asthma exacerbation management and should be provided rapidly and aggressively. The two most important initial drugs (first line) are short-acting β-agonists (SABAs) such as albuterol (commonly referred to as "rescue" drugs) and corticosteroids (referred to as controllers).[2,3] Epinephrine in adults is not given except in cases of anaphylaxis or angioedema and when bronchospasm is so severe that inhaled drugs cannot be effectively provided.[2] The use of continuous nebulization of β_2 agonists is both efficient and effective in the short term and can be decreased to intermittent or on-demand dosing with handheld nebulizers or metered dose inhalers with improvement, and during subsequent hospitalization.[2,3] Doses of albuterol (or other agents in this β_2-specific class of drugs) mixed with a diluent are calculated to provide 2.5 mg of albuterol over 4 to 6 hours.[5] During an acute exacerbation, the addition of ipratropium (an anticholinergic) 500 µg every 20 minutes for three doses, then as needed, may enhance bronchodilation while in the ED.[5] Efficacy has not been proven for the use of ipratropium after the acute severe exacerbation is resolved.[2,5]

Steroids should be given as soon as possible within the first hour of admission as they speed resolution of the episode and prevent relapse, particularly if the patient was not taking oral steroids prior to arriving in the ED.[2,3,6] Steroids may be provided orally as they are equally as effective as steroids given IV.[2,3,6] However, the IV route is preferred if the patient is extremely dyspneic, nauseated, or drowsy. The patient may be transitioned to the oral route once the acute severe stage is resolved. The exact dose of glucocorticoids to use for acute severe asthma exacerbations is undetermined and largely based on experience and preferences.[2] It is common for a large dose of methylprednisone (125 mg IV) to be given initially, and every 6 hours for 4 doses. However, the data suggest that lower doses (ie, 60–80 mg every 6–12 hours) are appropriate in both acute and critical care settings and even lower doses (40–60 mg every 12–24 hours) may be adequate for those not in intensive care.[6]

Management and Placement Decisions: ED, Acute Care, or ICU

Decisions related to placement following ED admission are largely dependent on the severity of the patient's condition and the intensity of the therapies required. Most patients who have experienced an acute severe asthma exacerbation may be quickly reversed with bronchodilators and steroids provided immediately in the ED setting. However, decisions about discharge from the ED and when to admit to the hospital are made by considering the patient's risk of experiencing another exacerbation or fatal episode, availability of care if needed, the baseline status of the patient and response to therapy, and the patient's past history, especially the past need for intubation and ICU care. The patient's ability to lay flat plus a comparison of lung function measurements from admission to an hour after the start of bronchodilator and steroid therapy are reliable indicators associated with prognosis and the need for further hospitalization and ICU care.[2] If the posttreatment FEV_1 or

PEFR are <40% predicted (or personal best), hospitalization is recommended. And, if posttreatment FEV_1 and PEFR are 40% to 60% of predicted (or personal best) discharge may be considered if there are no risk factors and follow-up health care is available.[2] However, if after the first hour, improvement is not noted and/or the patient's oxygen saturation and clinical status have declined, the patient should be transferred to an ICU. Intubation may be necessary before doing so.

The initial care of an acute severe asthma exacerbation focuses on airway, breathing, and circulation. Stabilizing the patient by improving lung function with the aggressive use of corticosteroids, bronchodilators, and oxygen are the mainstays of therapy. Management in the acute care setting generally includes the same therapies but in gradually decreasing doses (such as a 5–7 day steroid taper), and transitioning to handheld metered dose inhalers for both bronchodilators and steroids.

Critical care management generally includes steroids (as described), increasing doses of bronchodilators, and often intubation and mechanical ventilation to break the cycle of airway inflammation and bronchoconstriction and to support oxygenation and ventilation. If intubation ensues, the general approach is to decrease the potential for barotrauma secondary to auto-PEEP (and dynamic hyperinflation) caused by profound bronchoconstriction. The use of small tidal volumes, low rates, and long expiratory times allow for better exhalation and decompression of the lungs. Narcotics, sedatives, and paralytic agents are necessary to ensure patient/ventilator synchrony with this technique and to address patient comfort. Because the goal is to prevent barotrauma while supporting oxygenation and ventilation until the airways respond to pharmacotherapy, a higher than normal $PaCO_2$ is expected with this ventilator technique and is referred to as "permissive hypercarbia." A pH of ~7.20 is generally considered acceptable provided the patient does not have a neurological condition or myocardial instability. Other ventilator adjuncts have been used such as Heliox (helium/oxygen mix) and noninvasive ventilation but there is little evidence to recommend their use in the emergent treatment of asthma.

Patient Follow-Up

JR was transferred from the ED to a medical floor for further follow-up. She had many risk factors for an exacerbation (female, not on corticosteroids or other "controllers" prior to admission, frequent bronchodilator use prior to the exacerbation, no primary care or pulmonary physician), and after the initial improvement in her PEFR (320 L/min) she plateaued at that level and continued to wheeze. We continued her steroids and intermittent bronchodilators throughout the night and by morning her PEFR was 420 L/min (close to estimated value); she was greatly improved and comfortable. The medical team and I prepared her for discharge. Her discharge medications, which included albuterol and prednisolone (1 mg/kg/day with a 5–7 day taper to start the following day) were discussed. Because JR did not know her "personal best" peak flow rate, I taught her how to use the PEFR meter and instructed her to measure her peak flow every 4 hours, and as needed if she felt her pulmonary status was changing. If her peak flow decreased by 20% from her peak flow of 420 despite bronchodilator use, or if her symptoms got worse, she was directed to call the "on-call" medical team at the hospital immediately. She was discharged that afternoon with a follow-up appointment in 2 days with the pulmonary service. JR did well and was eventually transitioned to an oral "controller" and a prn "rescue" inhaler with the guidance of her pulmonary physician. She has fully resumed activities, enjoys her graduate studies, and is planning her wedding to Bob.

References

1. Late airway response. The Asthma Center. http://www.theasthmacenter.org/index.php/disease_information/asthma/what_is_asthma/definition_of_asthma/hyper-responsiveness_of_the_airways_/. Accessed April 30, 2015.
2. The Global Initiative for Asthma (GINA) report: Global Strategy for Asthma Management and Prevention. 2015. http://www.ginasthma.org/documents/4. Accessed April 28, 2015.
3. NAEPP Expert Panel Report: Guidelines for the Diagnosis and Management of Asthma-update on selected topics. 2007. http://www.nhlbi.nih.gov/health-pro/guidelines/current/asthma-guidelines. Accessed April 28, 2015.
4. National Center for Health statistics. http://www.cdc.gov/nchs/. Accessed April 28, 2015.
5. Fanta CH. Treatment of acute exacerbations of asthma in adults. UpToDate. http://www.uptodate.com/contents/treatment-of-acute-exacerbations-of-asthma-in-adults. Accessed April 29, 2015.
6. Manser R, Reid D, Abramson M. Corticosteroids for acute severe asthma in hospitalised patients. *Cochrane Database Syst Rev.* 2001;(1):CD001740.

CASE 4

Tonja M. Hartjes

Tonja Hartjes is an Clinical Associate Professor at the University of Florida, College of Nursing in the AG-ACNP Program and has extensive work experience in surgical critical care.

CASE INFORMATION

Chief Complaint

Mrs P is a 77-year-old Caucasian female who underwent a left upper lobe wedge resection of a non-small-cell cancer 36 hours ago and is currently experiencing mild confusion, fatigue, abdominal pain, and weakness. The nurse calls me to her bedside in the intensive care unit (ICU).

❓ What is the potential cause?

Case Analysis: When I receive the call from the bedside nurse, I know I need more information, as the symptoms Mrs P is experiencing may have many causes. While I will consider all the patient's symptoms in my evaluation, I begin with a focus on confusion. I start by asking the nurse additional questions such as: "When did the symptoms appear" and "what was she like prior to the onset of the symptoms?"

After talking to the nurse, my priority is to rule out potentially life-threatening etiologies. These include cerebrovascular accident (CVA), acute myocardial infarction (AMI), severe hypoxemia and hypercarbia, hypovolemia, hypotension, pulmonary embolus (PE), cardiac dysrhythmias, hypoglycemia, sepsis, electrolyte imbalance, and drug effect, overdose, or withdrawal.[1] Should my early survey suggest cardiopulmonary instability, I will initiate advanced cardiac life support (ACLS) guidelines for intubation.

CASE INFORMATION

General Survey

I must evaluate these possible conditions simultaneously and efficiently. In order to do this, I consider the adage, "A picture is worth a thousand words," and visit the patient to obtain a general survey. The patient appears mildly anxious; however, her breathing is quiet and unlabored and she does not appear to be in any acute distress. She greets me and states: "I want to go home, and they won't let me go home." I note she is on oxygen by nasal cannula at 2 L/min and her oxygen saturation is 98%. On the monitor I note she is in sinus tachycardia at 105 beats per minute.

❓ What are the pertinent positives from the information given so far?

• Recent left upper lobe wedge resection for non-small-cell cancer
• Currently experiencing mild confusion, fatigue, abdominal pain, weakness and is in sinus tachycardia

❓ What are the significant negatives from the information given so far?

• The patient is awake, alert, and is aware of her surroundings.
• Her speech is clear.
• Her respirations are unlabored, and oxygen saturation level is 98% on 2 L/min nasal cannula.

Case Analysis: Based on the information obtained in my general survey, I determine her level of consciousness (LOC) and overall condition. Because the patient is calm, alert, and following commands, the diagnoses of CVA, severe hypoxemia and hypercarbia, significant hypoglycemia or hypotension, sepsis, or drug effect move lower on my differential. I recognize that patients do not always present with expected textbook symptoms for these conditions so I do not rule these out yet. Additional clinical data will help me eliminate these and other potential etiologies.[1]

Now that I have seen the patient I develop a comprehensive mental checklist of potential differential diagnoses for her primary symptom, confusion, as it is nonspecific and may have multiple etiologies. Because I determine that Mrs P's condition is urgent, but not critical, I can proceed with creating a complete differential diagnosis and obtaining more data. I suspect the patient's other presenting symptoms (fatigue, abdominal pain, and weakness) are related to the cause of her confusion. A comprehensive, systems approach and attention to detail will provide vital information necessary to ensure this is the case.

Differential Diagnoses for Confusion[1]

• Neurologic: CVA (embolic or hemorrhagic), vasospasm, traumatic head injury, seizure with postictal state, seizure, brain tumor, meningitis, delirium
• Cardiovascular: myocardial infarction, cardiac dysrhythmias, congestive heart failure (CHF) exacerbation, hypertensive encephalopathy, hypotension, pericardial effusion, cardiac tamponade
• Pulmonary: hypoxia, hypoventilation resulting in hypercapnia, carbon monoxide poisoning, pulmonary embolism, pneumonia, chronic obstructive pulmonary disease (COPD) exacerbation
• Gastrointestinal: ischemic bowel, cholecystitis, appendicitis, diverticulitis, constipation, gastritis, colitis

- Genitourinary: renal failure, urinary tract infection, urinary retention or obstruction
- Hematologic: anemia, infection/sepsis
- Musculoskeletal: fracture, rhabdomyolysis
- Endocrine: adrenal insufficiency, myxedema, thyrotoxicosis, hypoglycemia
- Psychiatric disorder: depression, new onset or exacerbation of bipolar disorder, psychosis
- Metabolic: dehydration, electrolyte imbalance, hyperglycemia, hypoglycemia, hypernatremia, hyponatremia, hepatic encephalopathy, metabolic acidosis or alkalosis
- Exogenous: medication side effect or interaction or withdrawal, drug overdose, alcohol withdrawal, pain

Case Analysis: I will continue to evaluate my patient for the emergence of life-threatening conditions in conjunction with a thoughtful evaluation of all potential differential diagnoses for confusion. To that end, my next steps include a review of current vital signs, her home and hospital medication lists, and recent diagnostics. I will also perform a focused health history and physical examination.

CASE INFORMATION

Obtained from medical record review, nurse's report, and patient interview.

Past Medical History

Significant for left upper lobe mass for non-small-cell cancer, chronic obstructive pulmonary disease (COPD), hypertension, and hyperlipidemia

Past Surgical History

Left upper lobe wedge resection this hospitalization, 1999 blepharoplasty, 2009 lumbar surgery, and 2013 C5-C7 anterior cervical discectomy and fusion

Allergies/Reaction

Sulfa/rash, tetracycline/nausea, ampicillin/rash, and citrus/"sores in mouth"

Home Medications

- Furosemide 20 mg by mouth daily
- Salmeterol two inhalations twice a day
- Ipratropium bromide two inhalations twice a day
- Albuterol two puffs as needed every 4 hours

- Prednisone 10 mg by mouth daily
- Atorvastatin 40 mg by mouth daily

In-Hospital Medications

- Furosemide 20 mg by mouth daily
- Salmeterol two inhalations twice a day
- Ipratropium bromide two inhalations twice a day
- Albuterol two puffs as needed every 4 hours
- Atorvastatin 40 mg by mouth daily
- Heparin 5000 units subcutaneously twice a day
- Morphine via patient-controlled analgesic pump 1 mg every 6 minutes, lockout 10 mg/h (patient has used 4 mg in the past 8 hours)
- Famotidine 20 mg by mouth twice a day

Social History

Current smoker with 40 pack-year history. Drinks wine occasionally. Denies any illicit drug use.

Review of Systems

- Constitutional: reports mild weakness, denies recent weight change, fever, chills, or malaise, no sweating
- Cardiovascular: denies chest pain, denies left arm pain, discomfort or palpitations
- Pulmonary: denies breathing difficulties, complains of pain at incisional line and chest tube insertions sites
- Gastrointestinal: complains of mild generalized abdominal pain and nausea, which started last night, denies emesis, diarrhea, or constipation
- Genitourinary: denies pain with urination, denies hematuria, notes urinary frequency with taking furosemide
- Musculoskeletal: denies tremors or involuntary movements, denies muscle cramps in arms or legs
- Neurological: denies syncope, loss of consciousness, or seizures. Nurse reports the patient has been confused since last evening

Physical Examination

- Vital signs: Blood pressure 105/59 mm Hg, heart rate 105 beats per minute, temperature 37.9°C, respirations 22 breaths per minute, oxygen saturation 98% on 2 liters per minute via nasal cannula. Height 63 inches, weight 81 kg, body mass index 32.
- Constitutional: Alert, mildly anxious (looking around, wringing hands), some difficulty maintaining conversation and train of thought.
- Head/eyes/ears/nose/throat: No obvious deformity or signs of trauma. Pupils equal, round, reactive to light, no nystagmus, extraocular movements intact.

- Neck: Trachea palpable at midline, no jugular venous distension noted with head of bed at 20 degrees, carotid pulses +2 bilaterally, no carotid bruit.
- Cardiovascular: Point of maximal inspiration at left fifth intercostal space, S1, S2, regular, no murmur, rubs, or gallops. Extremities are warm, dry, no clubbing, normal tone, no peripheral edema, peripheral pulses are +2 in all extremities.
- Pulmonary: Respirations even, and unlabored with mild tachypnea, breath sounds are absent in left upper lobe, crackles noted bilateral lower lobes. Lungs are resonant to percussion bilaterally.
- Gastrointestinal: No visible masses, pulsations, or wounds, hypoactive bowel sounds in all four quadrants, soft, nontender to light and deep palpation, no hepatosplenomegaly.
- Integumentary: Skin is pale, warm and dry, mild tenting. No masses, rashes, or bruising. Left thoracotomy incision approximated, without redness or drainage, no masses noted, no crepitus.
- Neurological: Awake, oriented only to self, normal language and comprehension, no neglect, follows simple commands, GCS 15, mild confusion is noted.
- Cranial nerves: 3–12 Intact, extraocular eye movements intact, visual fields full to confrontation, smile symmetric, speech clear, shoulder shrug symmetric, tongue midline.
- Motor: 4/5 strength bilateral upper and lower extremities, bilateral radial, brachioradialis, and Achilles reflexes are brisk 2+.
- Lymphatic: Absence of lymphadenopathy.
- Lines and drains: Indwelling urinary catheter removed postoperative day 1, no central venous access during hospitalization, left chest tube in place on water seal with serosanguineous drainage 150 mL/24 hours, small intermittent air leak is present in the first air chamber, which is stable from yesterday. 24-hour intake 1250 mL/output 1440 = negative 190 mL.

Recent Diagnostics

Portable chest x-ray (CXR), taken 6 hours ago: absence of hilar engorgement, normal heart size, bilateral lower lobe alveolar edema present with partial resolution from yesterday, left chest tube in place, small apical pneumothorax noted and stable from yesterday
- 12-Lead ECG, 5 hours ago: sinus tachycardia rate 105 without any ST/T wave abnormalities. Review of bedside telemetry shows no arrhythmia.
- Labs drawn this morning: sodium 131 mEq/L (normal 135–145 mEq/L), potassium 3.3 mEq/L (normal 3.5–5.0 mEq/L), glucose 73 mg/dL (normal 70–100 mg/dL), hemoglobin 10.9 g/dL (baseline 11.5 g/dL) (normal 12.1–15.1 g/dL), blood urea nitrogen 9 mg/dL (normal 5–20 mg/dL), creatinine 0.9 mg/dL (normal 0.5–1.1 mg/dL).

What elements of the review of systems, physical examination, and diagnostic information should be added to the pertinent positives and significant negatives?

Pertinent Positives

- Mild confusion
- History of lung cancer, COPD, and hypertension
- Postoperative day 2 from left upper lobe wedge resection
- Afebrile, mild sinus tachycardia, hypotension
- Mild tachypnea, absent breath sounds left upper lobe, crackles noted bilateral lower lobes, oxygen saturation on 2 L/min is 98%
- Chest tube present with air leak
- Mild tenting of skin
- Mild nausea, mild generalized abdominal pain, and weakness
- Labs: hyponatremia (sodium 131 mEq/L), hypokalemia (potassium 3.3 mEq/L), normal glucose (73 mg/dL), anemia (hemoglobin 10.9 g/dL)
- Chest x-ray shows resolving bilateral lower lobe edema and small stable apical pneumothorax
- The patient was on daily prednisone at home but is not receiving this in the hospital

Significant Negatives

- No neurologic deficits except mild confusion
- Denies chest pain, shortness of breath, left arm pain, and diaphoresis
- Gastrointestinal assessment normal
- Normal cardiovascular examination, no swelling or change in peripheral pulses
- No abnormalities on ECG except tachycardia
- Fluid balance shows negative 190 mL 24/hour
- Normal kidney function on labs drawn this morning
- BP stable for past 24 hours
- No obvious signs of infection sources: warm and dry left thoracotomy incision and CT insertion sites are approximated, without redness, swelling, or drainage; no urinary catheter present; no central venous access
- The patient denies a history of illegal drug use

How does this information affect the list of possible etiologies?

Case Analysis: During my primary survey at the bedside, I was able to determine that the patient was relatively stable. Her condition has not changed much over the past 24 hours, and her confusion gradually emerged overnight. In the course of completing a comprehensive history and physical, I am able to rule out the life-threatening etiologies as I also sort other potential causes for confusion listed on my confusion differential.

Neurologic

I am able to rule out CVA[1] as a life-threatening cause because Mrs P is alert, awake, and oriented to self and has no focal neurological deficits. Her neurologic examination is normal with the exception of her confusion. Currently she does have difficulty maintaining conversation and train of thought. Potential causes such as meningitis and brain tumor are unlikely as she is afebrile and has no focal neurological changes or rash. Delirium is a potential cause of her confusion and will need to be considered.

Cardiac

Acute myocardial infarction (AMI) and cardiac dysrhythmias, both potentially life threatening, are now lower on my differential as the patient denies chest pain, left arm pain, shortness of breath, nausea, and diaphoresis. There is no evidence of rhythm disturbances on the bedside monitor or on her ECG. Her ECG is normal with the exception of a sinus tachycardia. AMI is unlikely, but until I can repeat the ECG and compare to prior ECGs, as well as obtain a set of cardiac enzymes, it cannot be completely ruled out. Other cardiac conditions such as an exacerbation of heart failure (HF), pericardial effusion, or tamponade are unlikely based on her normal cardiac examination. Her chest x-ray shows a normal heart size, improved bilateral pulmonary edema, and no hilar engorgement. These findings do not support heart failure exacerbation, pericardial effusion, or tamponade. Hypotension is low on my differential as a cause of her confusion but can be life threatening. She has a history of hypertension so her blood pressure (105/59) while not severely low may be lower than her baseline blood pressure. I will need to follow her blood pressure closely.

Pulmonary

I am able to rule out hypoxemia based on her normal oxygen saturation. Her chest x-ray does not indicate a new pulmonary process, such as a consolidation or worsening infiltrates. Trending or comparing the patient's condition and the chest x-ray helps me evaluate progression of abnormalities. Interstitial edema, pneumothorax, and presence of an air leak are not normal but by comparing the x-ray to one taken yesterday, I know these do not represent a change that would contribute to her recent confusion. Additionally, the patient denies shortness of breath, though her respiratory rate is 22, due to pain or possibly due to atelectasis. The patient is receiving bronchodilators for her COPD. I do not know the patient's $PaCO_2$ level so I cannot rule out hypercapnia as a cause of her confusion. I will consider drawing an arterial blood gas to further evaluate her ventilation, and obtaining another CXR to review for a new atelectasis, increased edema, or extension of her apical pneumothorax.

Using the Wells Criteria, which is a predictive model for suspected pulmonary embolism (PE), I consider this patient to be at low-moderate risk for PE.[2] The negative criteria for this patient include that she has no history of deep vein thrombosis (DVT) or PE, and she has no signs or symptoms consistent with a DVT or PE at present—no leg swelling, no shortness of breath, no hemoptysis. Positive Wells criteria for this patient include heart rate greater than 100, and risk factors including her age over 65, history of malignancy, and recent surgery. In addition, while not an absolute preventive strategy, she is covered for DVT prophylaxis with subcutaneous heparin. Based on this information, I lower DVT and PE on my differential.

Gastrointestinal

Given the patient's normal gastrointestinal examination, I doubt that her symptoms are caused by cholecystitis, appendicitis, diverticulitis, gastritis, or colitis. She denies constipation and the nursing notes indicate a normal bowel movement 1 day ago. Ischemic bowel seems very unlikely given that her discomfort is relatively mild and she does not appear in any distress.

Genitourinary

Her lab work shows that she is not in renal failure. I will need to do a urinalysis to rule out urinary tract infection, which is a common nosocomial infection and a common cause of acute confusion in older adults. Given the absence of urinary symptoms, and her normal urine output, urinary retention and obstruction are unlikely to be causing her confusion.

Hematological

Bleeding is always a concern after surgery but there is no sign of this on my examination and while she is anemic, she does not require transfusion, and her hemoglobin is actually stable when compared to labs drawn yesterday. At this point she does not meet criteria for sepsis but may be transitioning from systemic inflammatory response syndrome (SIRS) to sepsis, which could cause acute confusion. Her white blood cell (WBC) count is not available for review but there are no obvious sources of infection in my history and physical. I need more information, including a WBC count, a urinalysis, and blood cultures to definitively rule out infection leading to SIRS and sepsis as the cause of her symptoms.

Metabolic

While many electrolyte abnormalities can affect mental status, I must rule out hypoglycemia first as this is a potentially lethal abnormality. Mrs P's morning glucose is normal at 73 mg/dL and she is not receiving insulin. Hypoglycemia is ruled out. An arterial blood gas is needed to determine if acidosis is contributing to her confusion. Dehydration is also a consideration particularly given the physical examination finding of skin tenting. However, there is no source of volume loss as her chest tube drainage is in the expected range at this point in her postoperative recovery, her fluid balance for the last 24 hours is only 190 mL negative, and there are no other fluid losses reported, such as diarrhea or vomiting. While I do not have a complete set of electrolytes to review I know that her sodium and potassium are slightly low. This degree of alteration is unlikely to cause her symptoms, but these abnormalities do suggest possible adrenal insufficiency.

Exogenous

I review the patient's medication list to determine the frequency and doses of her morphine PCA and benzodiazepine's as these medications are sometimes implicated in postoperative confusion. I also review the patient's medication list to determine if she is receiving all of her medications from home. Patients with chronic health conditions such as COPD or depression may be on steroids, selective serotonin reuptake inhibitor medications, antianxiety medication, or narcotics for chronic pain. Abruptly discontinuing any of these medications can precipitate severe and sometimes life-threatening withdrawal reactions. I note that this patient was taking daily prednisone for her COPD at home but is not receiving it since admission. I now put adrenal insufficiency at the top of my differential.

I will need to gather additional diagnostic information to complete my assessment and rule out or in, my top diagnosis, which at this point is adrenal insufficiency from the withdrawal of her daily steroids.

❓ What other diagnostic testing should be done and in what order?

Case Analysis: A current CXR will ensure there are no changes from the morning in regard to progression of her pulmonary edema, pneumothorax, and atelectasis. A current 12-lead ECG will affirm there is not recent myocardial injury or ischemia. Additionally, the ECG may provide evidence of right heart strain, which may be consistent with PE. Laboratory studies, as discussed above, include (1) arterial blood gas (ABG) to assess acid-base balance and determine if she has hypercapnia, (2) serial troponin levels to definitively rule out cardiac injury, (3) complete blood count (CBC) with differential to check for the presence of a new anemia and potential infection, (4) repeat metabolic profile to assess electrolytes, glucose, calcium, and magnesium levels, (5) current point of care glucose level, (6) urinalysis to determine if leukoesterase and white blood cells are present, which are indicative of a urinary tract infection, (7) adrenocorticotropic hormone (ACTH) and plasma cortisol levels. It is preferable to measure ACTH and cortisol in the morning; however, if a random ACTH and cortisol level is low, this is often enough to make a preliminary diagnosis of adrenal insufficiency.

To help rule out PE, I may order a Doppler ultrasound of the bilateral lower extremities depending on the results of other diagnostics (above).[2] The majority of pulmonary emboli arise due to DVT in the lower extremity and the ultrasound to rule out lower extremity DVT is noninvasive and easily completed at the bedside. If the patient has further signs or symptoms of PE, I will obtain a spiral computed tomography (CT) scan of her chest. In addition, if her neurologic status worsens, a CT scan of the head with and without contrast may be warranted.[1]

Although I have pending diagnostic tests, adrenal insufficiency from corticosteroid drug withdrawal at this point seems to be the most likely etiology for Mrs P's confusion.

CASE INFORMATION

Results of Diagnostics

The patient's cortisol level is 5 μg/dL (normal 7–28 μg/dL), confirming my diagnosis of adrenal insufficiency.[3-7] Her arterial blood gas and other lab tests are all normal so I am able to rule out the remaining differential diagnoses of AMI, electrolyte disturbances, and hypoventilation.

Diagnosis: Acute Adrenal Insufficiency

Assessment and Treatment

A functional or relative adrenal insufficiency (AI) can occur if patients undergo serious illness or injuries. Surgery can increase this occurrence by five- to sixfold.[6] This causes a defect in the function of the hypothalamic pituitary (HPA) axis and decreases levels of glucocorticoid production or causes resistance to glucocorticoid in the target cells in the adrenal gland. Because Mrs P was on chronic steroid therapy, the abrupt withdrawal results in adrenal crisis, which is a medical emergency.

Ideally, this patient, whose steroid use exceeded 3 weeks and therefore is considered chronic use, should have received "stress dose of steroids," such as 125 mg of hydrocortisone intravenously, prior to surgery. Then her home prednisone dose of 10 mg could be restarted. If she is unable to take oral medications, an intravenous steroid may be given for 1 to 3 days postoperatively prior to reinstituting the daily 10 mg dose of oral prednisone.[3-7]

Diagnosis of AI can be difficult especially in critically ill patients. Typically, random serum cortisol levels of less than 3 μg/dL (80 nmol/L) suggest absolute adrenal insufficiency. However, values of less than 10 μg/dL (275 nmol/L) are diagnostically probable for AI. To determine if the AI is primary, secondary, or tertiary, an ACTH stimulation test is recommended. Various protocols are available for the ACTH stimulation test, and it is important to check your facility's protocol. One example includes: draw a baseline cortisol level, and then administer 250 μg of intravenous ACTH. Following the baseline blood draw, cortisol levels are obtained at 30 and 60 minutes following the ACTH administration. A rise in serum cortisol levels to 18 to 20 μg/dL (500–550 nmol/L) is considered a normal result.[3-7]

Treatment includes determining the etiology of the AI (eg, tumor, infection, medications, etc). In this patient, it is important to investigate the use of her steroid medication, especially the dose, frequency, and timeframe of use. If the patient is hemodynamically unstable, immediate treatment with dexamethasone (1 mg every 6 hours IV) may be given prior to the ACTH stimulation testing as it will not interfere with test results.[3-7]

The patient in this case is treated with hydrocortisone. Continuous infusions of 10 mg/h, or intermittent doses of 50 mg IV every 4 hours or 75 to 100 mg IV every 6 hours may be given for a total dose of 240 to 300 mg per day. Patients with AI may also require isotonic IV fluids for dehydration and low sodium levels. Dextrose may also be added to prevent hypoglycemia.[3-7]

Mrs P responded well to treatment with intermittent intravenous hydrocortisone for 3 days. She was then transitioned to oral prednisone and discharged on her maintenance dose of 10 mg within the week.

References

1. Darby J, Anupam A. Sudden deterioration in neurologic status. In: Vincent J-L, Abraham E, Kochanek P, Moore F, Mitchell P, eds. *Textbook of Critical Care.* 6th ed. Philadelphia, PA: Elsevier Saunders; 2011:3-7.
2. Konstantinides S, Torbicki A, Agnelli G, et al. Guidelines on the diagnosis and management of acute pulmonary embolism. The Task Force for the Diagnosis and Management of Acute Pulmonary Embolism of the European Society of Cardiology (ESC). *Eur Heart J.* 2014;35:3033-3080. doi:10.1093/eurheartj/ehu283.
3. Li-Ng M, Kennedy L. Adrenal insufficiency. *J Surg Oncol.* 2012;106(5):595-599.
4. Boysen T, Drayton-Brooks S, Smith M. Endocrine disorders. In: Smith P, Boysen T, Davey J, Moser H, Smith M, eds. *Acute Care Nurse Practitioner.* Silver Spring, MD: American Nurses Credentialing Center; 2011:180-183.
5. Gerlach H. Part 10: Chapter 165: Adrenal insufficiency. In: Vincent J-L, Abraham E, Kochanek P, Moore F, Mitchell P. eds. *Textbook of Critical Care.* 6th ed. Philadelphia, PA: Elsevier Saunders; 2011:1215-1234.
6. Dello Stritto R, Barkely TW. Primary AI and adrenal crisis. In: Barkley TW, Myers C, eds. *Practice Consideration for Adult-Gerontology Acute Care Nurse Practitioners.* West Hollywood, CA: Barkley & Associates; 2014:616-619.
7. Falorni A, Minarelli A, Morelli A. Therapy for adrenal insufficiency: an update. *Endocrine.* 2013;43:514-528.

CASE 5

Caroline Austin-Mattison

Caroline Austin-Mattison is a certified Family NP who has worked in cardiac telemetry and cardiac catheterization units. She is currently working toward a DNP at Yale University.

CASE INFORMATION

Chief Complaint

Ms A is 45-year-old African American female with history of hypertension, hyperlipidemia, and end-stage renal disease (ESRD) managed with hemodialysis three times per week who now presents to the emergency department with the complaint of "feeling very tired" and having a low blood pressure after dialysis.

Differential Diagnoses for Fatigue[1]

Fatigue is a common complaint and there are both acute and chronic causes. But in this patient, the fatigue is new and associated with hypotension during and following dialysis. I immediately consider a differential for fatigue especially those that could potentially cause hypotension as they may be life threatening.

- Hypovolemia
- Anemia
- Acute coronary syndrome, including myocardial infarction
- Acute bleed, such as gastrointestinal or aneurysm rupture
- Cardiac arrhythmias
- New onset infection including sepsis or pneumonia
- Endocrine disorders: diabetes, hypothyroidism
- Autoimmune disorder
- Viral infection
- Sleep disturbances: sleep apnea
- Medication side effects
- Adrenal insufficiency
- Malignancies (rare presentation acutely)

CASE INFORMATION

General Survey and History of Present Illness

Ms A has been an outpatient hemodialysis patient for 2 years due to a history of uncontrolled hypertension and today received her usual hemodialysis without complications during the treatment, but toward the end of the dialysis, and following completion, she complained of feeling exceptionally tired and weak. She had a total of 1000 mL of fluid removed, which was a usual amount removed during previous dialysis treatments. Her blood pressure at the end of dialysis was 70/50 mm Hg and she was given a fluid bolus of normal saline (500 mL) that increased her BP to 92/48 mm Hg. She continued to complain of severe fatigue following the fluid bolus and so she was sent from the outpatient unit to the emergency department (ED).

I was called to the ED to evaluate the patient. When I arrive, my bedside survey reveals an obese, well-developed, well-groomed, and very pleasant woman in no acute distress. She is semirecumbent in bed and is awake, alert, and oriented to person, place, and time. Her speech is clear and she is appropriate in her responses. She is moving all extremities. The patient is asked about whether she monitored her blood pressure at home and she states that she measures and records her blood pressure sometimes. She was asked about her baseline blood pressure and stated it ranges from the 130 to 140/80s. She states: "I forgot to take my medication yesterday so my blood pressure was very high when I woke up this morning. It was 160/95 and that is high for me. I took two of my lisinopril tablets because my dialysis wasn't scheduled until 6 PM. I planned to take my other pressure pill, amlodipine after dialysis if my pressure was still high." She went on to say, "I hate when my pressure gets high, because I don't want to have a stroke like my mother did."

The patient verbalizes feeling very faint, nauseous, and diaphoretic toward the end, and following, her dialysis treatment but completed the whole cycle. She received intravenous fluids as noted, and felt somewhat better following the infusion but was still not her "usual self." The nephrologist at dialysis recommended that she go to the emergency department for further evaluation. She stated she is usually a bit tired after dialysis but has never felt so weak in the past.

The nurse at the dialysis unit calls the ED to report a postdialysis hemoglobin and hematocrit of 7 g/dL and 23%, respectively. On review of the electronic medical record, I learn that 1 week ago her hemoglobin and hematocrit were 9 g/dL and 27%, respectively, and that these values are at baseline for this patient.

Medical History (From Patient and Confirmed by Electronic Medical Record)

• Hypertension
• End-stage renal disease

- Obesity
- Chronic anemia
- Denies any history of heart disease

Family and Social History

- Nonsmoker, lifetime
- No alcohol or illicit substance use
- Father and siblings alive and well, mother with a cerebrovascular accident at age 65

Medication List (Patient Denies Any Medication Allergies)

- Amlodipine 10 mg daily
- Lisinopril 40 mg daily
- Rosuvastatin 10 mg daily
- Alprazolam 0.5 mg three times a day as needed

❓ What are the pertinent positives in the information given so far?

- History of ESRD requiring outpatient hemodialysis three times per week
- Alert, oriented, and in no acute distress in semirecumbent position in bed
- Was hypotensive and required intravenous fluid boluses following dialysis
- BP improved somewhat with fluid boluses but is still low
- Record shows she is chronically anemic but posthemodialysis her hemoglobin and hematocrit are lower than baseline values
- Took a double dose of her lisinopril today
- African American descent

❓ What are significant negatives in the information given so far?

- No acute signs of distress, pain, or discomfort
- No neurological deficits
- No history of heart disease

❓ What is the potential cause of the patient's fatigue?

Case Analysis: From the information obtained so far, I believe that Ms A suffers from a chronic anemia that is secondary to her renal failure. But it is concerning that she is more anemic than previously and is hypotensive, weak, and fatigued. Her hypotension has responded to fluid repletion and now she is alert, comfortable, and sitting in a semirecumbent position, which makes me less concerned about an emergent crisis. Her response to fluid resuscitation is suggestive of hypovolemia post hemodialysis. At this point the low hematocrit makes me think that the symptoms of hypotension and fatigue may be related to her anemia. However, other potential life-threatening causes of her hypotension and fatigue such as a cardiac event, adrenal insufficiency, a gastrointestinal or other occult bleed or sepsis must also be ruled out. In addition she has taken a double dose of her blood pressure medication and unless the drug was eliminated during dialysis, her hypotension and fatigue may be due to drug effect. I check the clearance of lisinopril and learn that it is significantly reduced in the plasma (30% or more) during dialysis.[2] So while the lisinopril may not be the entire reason for her fatigue and hypotension, it may have contributed.

While I gather more information to help me determine the cause of Ms A's symptoms, I will keep a complete differential of potential diagnoses for acute fatigue in mind; one of which is anemia. Severe anemia is a medical emergency as potential negative outcomes precipitated by an acute severe anemia include life-threatening conditions such as a myocardial infarction. I need to quickly gather more information and as I do so I will keep in mind my differential diagnoses.

? What is the problem representation in this case given the information so far?

A 45-year-old female with history of hypertension, ESRD, and chronic anemia is referred to the ED by her nephrologist following routine outpatient hemodialysis with new onset fatigue and hypotension, requiring fluid repletion. Her current postdialysis hematocrit is lower than her baseline hematocrit.

Given her obesity, history of hypertension, hyperlipidemia, family history of CVA, and her low hematocrit with hypotension, I order a stat ECG and serial cardiac enzymes to rule out acute coronary syndrome (ACS). This requires early intervention for successful outcome so must be addressed immediately. I also order a stat portable chest x-ray to evaluate for thoracic aneurysm and pneumonia, which are possible sources of sepsis. Keeping my differential diagnosis in mind, I proceed to the review of systems and physical examination.

CASE INFORMATION

Review of Systems

The patient is a reliable source for health history.
- Constitutional: Denies recent fever, infection, sleep disorder, and any evidence of active bleeding. Her appetite has been good and she states she eats a well-balanced diet.

- Head/eyes/ears/neck/throat: Denies headache, earache, drainage from ears or nose, nosebleeds, or bleeding gums.
- Cardiovascular: Denies chest pain, rapid or irregular heart rate, lower extremity edema, paroxysmal nocturnal dyspnea, or shortness of breath while lying flat.
- Pulmonary: Shortness of breath when climbing stairs or walking fast and denies cough.
- Gastrointestinal: Denies nausea, vomiting, constipation, or diarrhea and denies bloody or dark stools. Endorses that she has previously been prescribed iron supplements but stopped taking the iron recently due to constipation. She states she now has regular bowel movements.
- Genitourinary: Denies urinary frequency, dysuria, hematuria, or abnormal odor.
- Integumentary: Denies skin rashes, bruising, recent bug bites.
- Musculoskeletal: Denies joint pain, no history of fractures, recent trauma or falls.
- Neurological: Denies headache, dizziness, falls; history of stroke, seizure disorder, numbness, tingling, or weakness (except for the fatigue and weakness experienced today). Endocrine: denies increased hunger, thirst, urinary frequency and endorses she has eliminated simple sugars from diet.
- Lymph: Denies any swollen or sore glands.

Physical Examination

- Vital signs: Temperature 36.4 (tympanic), pulse 74, blood pressure 92/48 supine, sitting 100/50, standing 95/50, and oxygen saturation 100% on room air. Weight 165 lb, body mass index (BMI) 30 kg/m^2.
- The patient appears well and her stated age. She is calm and maintains eye contact during provider-patient interaction.
- Neurological: No focal neurological deficits, awake, alert oriented to place, person, and time.
- Head/eyes/ears/nose/throat: Pupils are equal, round, reactive to light, buccal mucosa pale pink, moist, neck is supple, no jugular venous distension, oropharynx is moist and rises symmetrically.
- Cardiovascular: Heart rate and rhythm is regular, normal S1, S2, no murmurs, gallops, rubs, or clicks. Skin warm, nail beds are pale, capillary refill brisk, positive pulses. Left AV fistula site clean, scant old blood on dressing, a palpable bruit and thrill.
- Pulmonary: Chest rises symmetrically; lungs clear to auscultation bilaterally and no use of accessory muscles.
- Gastrointestinal: Bowel sounds present in all four quadrants, tympanic on percussion, abdomen soft, nondistended, and no tenderness. Rectal

examination negative for blood, fissures, or hemorrhoids. Smear for occult blood at bedside was guaiac negative.

• Integumentary: Intact, no rashes, lesions or sores, skin turgor normal, no bruises noted.

• Lymph: No lymphadenopathy noted in neck or under arms, body mass precludes detection of nodes in groin.

Diagnostic Testing Results

The electrocardiogram shows normal sinus rhythm and the first troponin is normal.

The portable chest x-ray shows no acute cardiopulmonary disease.

❓ What elements of the review of systems and physical examination should be added to the pertinent positives?

• Obese with BMI of $30 \, \text{kg/m}^2$.

• Blood pressure remains low compared to patient's reported baseline.

• Pale pink mucosal membrane and nail beds.

• Noncompliant with iron supplement due to constipation.

❓ What elements of the review of systems and physical examination should be added to the significant negatives?

• Orthostatic blood pressure normal.

• The ECG is normal and there is no evidence of ischemia or arrhythmias.

• Chest x-ray is normal.

• No elevation of first troponin.

• Denies bleeding and no evidence of bleeding on examination.

• Afebrile, with no signs or symptoms or infection.

❓ How does this information affect the list of possible causes?

Case Analysis: Her review of systems and physical examination are essentially normal with the exception of her chronic renal failure and dialysis requirements. They do not elucidate a cause of her current fatigue nor the hypotension. Fluid boluses did improve her hypotension and she is not orthostatic despite a fairly low blood pressure.

I am concerned about identifying life-threatening issues first. At this point I am comfortable ruling out acute coronary syndrome as she denies chest pain, and the ECG, first troponin, and cardiovascular examination are all normal. There is no indication in the data thus far that her symptoms are related to a neurological event and her neurologic examination is normal. I eliminate this from my differential. All other systems are also normal; there are no signs of infection or endocrine disorders. Adrenal insufficiency is not ruled out yet but this is less likely as her blood pressure did respond to very modest fluid resuscitation. These potential causes are unlikely and will move lower on my differential for now.

While the patient denies a sleep disorder, she is obese. I will keep this on my differential, as patients with obstructive sleep apnea are often fatigued. Usually though, this would present as chronic fatigue, not an acute onset. In addition, obstructive sleep apnea usually results in poorly controlled hypertension and this patient presents with low blood pressure. Malignancy is also a possibility but low on the list in the absence of unexplained weight loss, pain, or bleeding. In addition, a person with malignancy usually has ongoing symptoms not the abrupt onset described by this patient.

Because the history and physical and some key diagnostics have eliminated several of my urgent concerns and because she is also chronically anemic, I need to carefully evaluate her current drop in hemoglobin and hematocrit as these are the most obvious source of her fatigue as well as her hypotension. Patients with chronic anemia generally tolerate low blood counts relatively well but an additional drop in hemoglobin from the low baseline, especially if acute, may result in a very generalized fatigue, hypotension, and weakness. At hemoglobin levels of 6-7 g/dL, transfusion is often indicated.[3]

I consider a differential for her recent lower hemoglobin level and also how I will approach the workup. In general, anemia occurs due to one, or a combination of the following causes: blood loss (acute or chronic, or both), deficient erythropoiesis, causing low or abnormal production of red blood cells, or excessive red blood cell destruction, hemolysis, that is intrinsic and extrinsic to the red blood cell. An anemia workup generally focuses on determining the etiology by evaluating the reticulocyte response to the anemia, the complete blood count components, and the morphology of red blood cells. An algorithmic approach to the anemia workup is helpful. An example may be found at: http://www.arupconsult.com/Algorithms/Anemia.pdf.

❓ What diagnostic tests or other information are necessary at this point?

Further diagnostic testing is needed to determine if my patient's recent drop in hemoglobin is acute or part of her chronic disease. To that end I order the following labs:

1. Complete blood count (CBC) with differential so I can evaluate her mean corpuscular volume (MCV) and mean corpuscular hemoglobin (MCH) and identify the type of anemia.
2. Reticulocyte count: These are newly released cells from the bone marrow and if elevated, generally represent a response to active bleeding, though in situations of deficient erythropoiesis, the reticulocyte count might not elevate.

3. A peripheral blood smear to look for abnormal cell fragments, which can occur with hemolysis and for abnormal cell sizes and shapes, found in some blood dyscrasias.
4. Iron, ferritin, total iron binding capacity, folate, and B_{12} levels will help me identify if this is iron-deficient anemia, which is likely given that she is not taking iron as prescribed.

Other important labs to draw include a metabolic profile, coagulation times, and liver function tests. I need these results to determine her risk of bleeding, and if any electrolyte abnormality is contributing to her symptoms. Lastly, a thyroid-stimulating hormone (TSH) level is indicated, as hypothyroidism is associated with fatigue.

CASE INFORMATION

Results of Diagnostics

CBC with Differential, Coagulation Studies and Liver Function Tests
The patient's CBC confirms her anemia with a hemoglobin and hematocrit of 8 g/dL and 24%, respectively. She does not have reticulocytes. Her mean red cell volume (MCV) was 83 (normal: 82–98) and her MCHC% was 34 (normal: 30–34), which classifies her anemia as a normocytic normochromic anemia. This finding is consistent with bone marrow hypoproliferation of red cells and thus an anemia of chronic illness. Her peripheral smear does not show abnormal (or lysed) cells that would suggest hereditary spherocytosis or other hematologic abnormalities as causes of her anemia. Her WBC, platelets, coagulation studies, liver function tests are normal. These findings combined with findings from her history and physical examination put infection and acute bleeding very low on my differential.

Iron Studies
Next I look at the iron studies. If this patient has iron deficiency, then I would expect that the total iron binding capacity (TIBC) would be high (an attempt to hold on to the available iron) and her iron and ferritin values would be low. Her TIBC is normal, at 322 μg/dL (normal: 250–420 μg/dL), her iron level is normal at 142 (65–150 μg/dL) but her ferritin is high at 434 (normal range 13–300 ng/mL). While initially this finding puzzled me, I then find that elevated ferritin levels may be present in patients with ESRD receiving hemodialysis because ferritin may be acting as an acute phase reactant.[4] Ferritin levels reflect iron storage and lower levels, even within the normal range, are indicative of a lack of iron storage. A level of 30 ng per milliliter signifies iron deficiency in 92% to 98% of people studied.[5] Patients with anemia of chronic disease can have normal or increased ferritin levels. Elevated ferritin levels reflect storage and retention of ferritin in the reticuloendothelial system. The increased level is a result of immune activation.[6]

Metabolic Profile, TSH, B$_{12}$, and Folate Studies
Her metabolic profile is notable for a normal potassium of 4.2 (normal: 3.5–5.0 mEq/L) and a BUN of 70 (normal: 7–30 mg/dL) and a creatinine of 4.8 (normal: 0.7–1.4 mg/dL), respectively, post dialysis. The BUN and creatinine are a bit higher postdialysis values than I would expect but consistent with her chronic renal failure. Other metabolic values are normal.

Her TSH is 2.1 (normal: 0.5–4.5), which rules out hypothyroidism as a cause of her symptoms. Her B$_{12}$ is 283 (normal: 150–300 ng/L) and folate is 15 (normal: 2–20 ng/mL), ruling out B$_{12}$ and folate deficiencies as reasons for her anemia.

Case Analysis: Given the combined results of the patient's history and physical and diagnostic studies I can reasonably assume her acute symptoms of fatigue and hypotension are related to a worsening of her anemia of chronic disease prior to this most recent dialysis. Her additional dose of lisinopril, even though some was dialyzed out, may have magnified the symptoms. The last few conditions on my differential while not completely ruled out are much lower because of negative findings in the diagnostics and history and physical. These include aplastic anemia, autoimmune disorders, or a viral infection. At this point the patient's blood pressure is improved though she is still very tired. Because I continue to be unsure of her status, I inform her of all diagnostic test results and admit her to the medicine unit for overnight observation and further evaluation.

Diagnosis: Anemia of Chronic Disease

Treatment

Anemia of chronic disease (ACD) or anemia of inflammation is frequently seen in patients with systemic illness or those causing inflammation. ACD is the second most common type of anemia and is usually the cause of anemia in people with chronic illnesses such as chronic kidney disease.[6] ACD is also seen in patients with active infections, cancer, and autoimmune conditions. Management guidelines suggest there are several reasons that ACD should be corrected. They include

1. Anemia may have a harmful effect on the cardiovascular system that is needed to maintain tissue oxygenation.

2. Anemia may result in poorer prognosis in patients with chronic diseases.[7,8]

3. Treating the anemia may improve the patient's quality of life while living with chronic conditions.[9]

Managing the chronic health conditions that cause ACD can improve the degree of anemia. For example, inflammatory diseases such as rheumatoid arthritis and inflammatory bowel disorders may be improved with medications such as corticosteroids and human immunodeficiency (HIV) anemia may improve with antiretroviral medications. Treatment of chronic diseases affecting the heart, such as congestive heart failure or chronic renal failure affecting the kidneys, requires a different approach but must be addressed to ensure a good quality of life. Patients undergoing hemodialysis with levels of hemoglobin 8 g/dL or less have been shown to have an increased mortality up to two times more than those above 8 g/dL.[7]

Current guidelines recommend that providers should first treat the underlying disease in patients with ACD. When it is not feasible, other options include:

1. Blood transfusion is an option widely used as a rapid and effective therapeutic intervention. This treatment is recommended for those with severe anemia defined as a hemoglobin less than 8 g/dL or a life-threatening anemia less than 6.5 g/dL. The guideline for management of ACD in patients with chronic kidney disease does not recommend long-term transfusion therapy due to increased risk of iron overload.[6]

2. Iron therapy should be used in patients with ACD when there is an absolute iron deficiency. Supplemental iron may also be used in patients who do not respond to erythropoietic agents because of functional iron deficiency. A high transferrin level and low transferrin saturation level (TSAT <16%) suggests iron deficient erythropoiesis and a treatment target would be a TSAT >20%. However, iron therapy is not recommended for patients with ACD that have a normal or high ferritin level.

3. Erythropoietic agents are approved for patients with ACD who have cancer and are undergoing chemotherapy, those with chronic kidney disease, and in patients with HIV infection undergoing myelosuppressive therapy. Ninety-five percent of patients diagnosed with a rheumatoid disorder and chronic kidney disease respond to erythropoietic agents.[9]

Patient Course

Ms A's inpatient treatment for her symptomatic anemia was the infusion of two units of packed red blood cells to a goal hemoglobin of 8 g/dL. A recommendation was made to the PCP to start epoetin alfa as an outpatient three times weekly with hemodialysis and to obtain follow-up iron studies every 1 to 3 months. The patient was discharged with follow-up appointments arranged with her nephrologist and primary care physician in the next 2 weeks.

References

1. Ponka D, Kirlew M. Top 10 differential diagnosis in family medicine: fatigue. 2007;53(5):892. http://www.ncbi.nlm.nih.gov/pmc/articles/PMC1949177. Accessed February 5, 2015.
2. Dialysis and drug clearance. http://renalpharmacyconsultants.com/assets/2013dodbooklet.pdf. Accessed November 18, 2014.
3. Carson J, Silvergleid A, Tirnauer J. Indications and hemoglobin thresholds for red blood cell transfusion in the adult. UpToDate. http://www.uptodate.com/contents/indications-and-hemoglobin-thresholds-for-red-blood-cell-transfusion-in-the-adult. Accessed December 2014.

4. Weiss G, Goodnough LT. Anemia of chronic disease. *N Engl J Med*. 2005;352:1011-1023. DOI: 10.1056/NEJMra041809.
5. Camaschella C, Poggiali E. Towards explaining "unexplained hyperferritinaemia." *Haematologica*. 2009;94:307-309.
6. Lee M, Means R. Extremely elevated serum ferritin levels in a university hospital: associated diseases and clinical significance. *Am J Med*. 1995;98:566-571.
7. Ma JZ, Ebben J, Xia H, Collins AJ. Hematocrit level and associated mortality in hemodialysis patients. *J Am Soc Nephrol*. 1999;10:610-619.
8. Caro JJ, Salas Mm, Ward A, et al. Anemia as an independent prognostic survival in patients with cancer. *Cancer*. 2001;91:2214-2221.
9. Moreno F, Sanz-Guajardo D, Lopez-Gomez JM, Jofre R, Valderrabano F. Increasing the hematocrit has a beneficial effect on quality of life and is safe in selected hemodialysis patients: Spanish Cooperative Renal Patients Quality of Life Study Group of the Spanish Society of Nephrology. *J Am Soc Nephrol*. 2000;11:335-342.

CASE 6

Joan E. King

Joan King is the Program Director for the AG-ACNP program at Vanderbilt University and also practices as an ACNP in the Pre-anesthesia Evaluation Clinic at Vanderbilt.

CASE INFORMATION

Chief Complaint

A 50-year-old woman presents with the chief complaint of: "I am worried. I am so tired and fatigued."

General Survey and History of Present Illness

This 50-year-old female presents to the emergency department with a chief complaint of fatigue. She states that over the past 2 months she has become increasingly tired. And while she does not relate the fatigue to any specific activity over the past month, she does state that if she walks upstairs she becomes short of breath. She denies fevers, chills, chest pain, nausea, vomiting, or changes in her stool. She also denies any changes in her diet, but notes that she has lost 8 lb unintentionally over the past 2 months. She indicates that her family has commented that she appears pale. Vital signs are HR 98 beats/min, RR 12/min, BP 130/78 mm Hg, and oral temperature = 98.6°F.

❓ What is the potential cause of this patient's symptoms?

Case Analysis: There are many reasons for the chief complaint of fatigue and the patient's symptoms seem to have progressed over months. She has lost weight and also complains of shortness of breath with activity. I suspect all these symptoms are related but will start with a differential list for fatigue.

Differential Diagnoses for Fatigue and Tiredness

- Hematological: anemias such as anemia of chronic disease, iron deficiency anemia, thalassemia, vitamin B_{12} deficiency, or folic acid deficiency
- Malignancy: leukemias or multiple myeloma, lymphomas, colorectal cancers, lung cancer, breast cancer, uterine or ovarian cancer
- Infection: sepsis, urinary tract infection, pneumonia, or other viral, bacterial or fungal infections
- Gastrointestinal: peptic or gastric ulcer, Crohn disease, ulcerative colitis, diverticulosis

- Pulmonary: chronic obstructive lung disease, obstructive sleep apnea, asthma
- Cardiac: systolic or diastolic heart failure, coronary artery disease, arrhythmias
- Gynecological: pregnancy, menorrhagia, uterine fibroids, postmenopausal bleeding

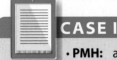

CASE INFORMATION

- **PMH:** anemic (1970), no recurrence to her knowledge. Pneumonia: 1990
- **Medications:** Aspirin 325 mg once daily
- **Last menstrual period:** perimenopausal with last period 2 months ago
- **Allergies:** none
- **Social history:** sales manager, married for 25 years, former smoker with a 15 pack-year history. Diet: vegetarian
- **Family history:** coronary artery disease: father (fatal MI age 50), mother (CABG age 70), no family history of chronic anemias, no family history of thalassemia

❓ What are the pertinent positives from the information given so far?

Fatigue over a 2-month period, short of breath walking up stairs, 8 lb weight loss, pallor, vegetarian diet, history of anemia, history of pneumonia, perimenopausal, former smoker, family history of coronary artery disease

❓ What are the significant negatives from the information given so far?

No chest pain, no nausea, no vomiting, no change in diet or stools, stable vital signs, no family history of anemia

❓ How does the information affect your list of potential causes?

Case Analysis: At this point in the history, I believe her fatigue could be caused by pregnancy (despite being perimenopausal), the family of anemias (iron deficiency anemia, anemia of chronic disease thalassemia, vitamin B$_{12}$ or folic acid deficiencies), peptic or gastric ulcer, ulcerative colitis, diverticulitis, Crohn disease, or a malignant process. While including cancer on the list of differentials may seem like a "zebra," fatigue is a symptom that 80% of patients with cancer report.[1] She has also lost 8 pounds. In addition, cancer is a life-threatening disease in which early identification and treatment affects prognosis. Hence cancer is an important differential to consider. The possible types of cancer may be narrowed through a thorough review of systems and physical examination. Pregnancy is also high on my list and is important to diagnosis early as it impacts her treatment so I will order a blood test for human chorionic gonadotropin (hCG). Given the duration of her symptoms, and the absence of fever, I am less inclined to think there is an infectious cause and this would certainly be an atypical presentation of coronary artery disease. I will not order an ECG or a sepsis workup until I get more information.

She reports being a vegetarian and has a previous history of anemia as a teenager; iron deficiency anemia is high on my list of differentials for this patient's fatigue.[2] Iron deficiency anemia is fairly common, making it a likely diagnosis, and it is generally a benign disease. I am careful, however, not to let this diagnoses overshadow the possibilities of other more significant and life-threatening diagnoses, especially colorectal cancer. A bleeding peptic ulcer also needs to be considered, as well as ulcerative colitis or bleeding from diverticulitis. A more detailed discussion with the patient of gastrointestinal signs and symptoms may help focus on one of these potential diagnoses. The associated symptom of shortness of breath could be an additional indication that she is anemic or an early sign of a chronic cardiopulmonary disease, such as chronic obstructive pulmonary disease (COPD) or congestive heart failure (CHF). These are less likely diagnoses in a patient of this age but they will be considered as I complete a full history and physical. I start with a review of systems and focus on specific questions to narrow the list of differential diagnoses. My physical examination will be looking for specific physical findings that support a final diagnosis.

CASE INFORMATION

Review of Systems

- Constitutional: As per history of present illness.
- Cardiac: The patient notes that over the past month she has felt like her heart was racing, particularly when walking at work, but she denies any chest discomfort, symptoms of angina, or any presyncope. The patient has never had a 12 lead ECG obtained when she felt her heart racing. The patient denies any history of hypertension, murmurs, myocardial infarction, or heart failure. The patient does state that she takes an adult aspirin (325 mg) daily since both of her parents died of coronary artery disease. The patient states that she has never been advised to take aspirin by any health care provider.
- Pulmonary: New onset shortness of breath over the past month when climbing stairs (see HPI). The patient indicates she has no shortness of

breath when walking on level ground, and she is able to do her housework without having to rest between activities. The patient was diagnosed with pneumonia in 1990, and was treated as an outpatient with no recurrence. Patient does have a 15 pack-year history of smoking, but she quit 10 years ago and she denies a history of asthma, COPD, emphysema. The patient indicates she has never been told that she snores, and states that her husband has never indicated she has any symptoms of sleep apnea.

- Gastrointestinal: the patient denies any change in bowel habits (no melena), any abdominal pain or cramping, or changes in her stool or any melena. The patient denies any symptoms of heartburn or GERD, or any prior history of peptic ulcers, ulcerative colitis, Crohn disease, or diverticulosis. The patient denies a history of constipation or diarrhea or any food intolerances, and the patient denies any previous GI surgeries such as gastric bypass or bowel resections.

- Genitourinary: Denies any voiding problems, blood in urine, denies use of birth control since her husband's vasectomy 2000. The patient states that she has a period about every 3 or 4 months over the past year. The patient describes her periods as light, and denies any spotting in between periods.

- Hematological: The patient was anemic at the age of 17, but anemia resolved after increasing intake of vegetables and dried fruits and she has remained on her vegetarian diet. The patient denies having had any transfusions, and she has never been diagnosed with leukemia or multiple myeloma. Denies abnormal bruising or bleeding. Denies nodes.

- Musculoskeletal: The patient states she has full range of motion of all extremities and she denies any bone pain or soreness. She denies any symptoms of osteoarthritis.

- Neurological: Patient denies a history of stroke, TIA, or seizures.

Physical Examination

Weight 130 pounds, height 5′4″, BMI 22.3. Vital signs: heart rate 98 beats/min, blood pressure 130/78 mm Hg, respiratory rate 12/min, SaO$_2$ 98% on room air.

- Constitutional: Well-developed well-nourished female in no acute distress.

- Head/eyes/ears/nose/throat: Mucous membranes are pale, no palpable lymphadenopathy.

- Cardiac: Rate and rhythm regular, PMI fifth intercostal space midclavicular line. No murmurs, gallops, or rubs noted. No jugular venous distension noted. Carotid pulses strong bilaterally, no carotid bruits noted. No peripheral edema.

- Pulmonary: Breath sounds clear in all lobes both anteriorly and posteriorly. No wheezes or stridor noted. Anteroposterior diameter is less than transverse diameter.

- Gastrointestinal: Bowel sounds active in all four quadrants, tympany noted in all four quadrants. No abdominal tenderness noted on light or deep palpation. No hepatosplenomegaly. No tenderness noted at the xiphoid process. Stool guaiac positive using current guaiac-based fecal occult blood test. Fecal immunochemical test (FIT) pending. No hemorrhoids noted.

- Hematological: No bruising or petechia noted.
- Neurological: Awake, alert, and oriented × 4. Pupils react briskly to light. No focal neurological deficits.

❓ What diagnostic tests are necessary at this time?

Case Analysis: I first need to assess her CBC with differential, iron studies, electrolytes, and a pregnancy test. Other diagnostics will be ordered based on the results of these tests.

CASE INFORMATION

Results of Laboratory Values

Initial hematocrit 32 (N = 36%–47%), hemoglobin 11 (normal = 12–16 g/dL), platelets 140,000. MCV 75 (N = 82–98), MCHC 29 (31%–37%).

Ferritin level 9 µg/L (N = 15–200 µg/L), TIBC 350 µg/dL (250–460 µg/dL), serum iron 25 µg/dL (65–150), folic acid and vitamin B_{12} pending.

WBC 4.5 × 103 (N = 3.9–10.7 cells/mm³) bands 3%.

hCG: negative.

Na 140 (136–145 mEq/L)	Cr+ 1.1 (0.7–1.3)	Albumin 4.0 (3.5–5.5 g/dL)
K 4.2 (3.5–5.0 mEq/L)	Glucose 104 (fasting < 110 mg/dL)	Calcium 8.8 (8.8–10.3 mg/dL)
Cl 102 (98–106 mEq/L)	ALT 20 (0–35 U/L)	
CO_2 24 (23–28)	AST 30 (N = 0–35 U/L)	
BUN 20 (8–20 mg/dL)	SED Rate 20 (N = 0–22 mm/h)	

❓ Given the new information above, what additional pertinent positives and significant negatives can be added to your list?

- **Pertinent positives:** Low hematocrit, low hemoglobin, low mean corpuscular volume (MCV), low ferritin, pale mucous membranes.
- **Significant negatives:** Review of systems and physical examination are negative for respiratory or cardiac or gastrointestinal disorders. Her WBC and vital signs are normal and her hCG is negative.

Case Analysis: Combining the review of systems and the physical examination, I can now reprioritize and narrow the list of differentials. With her hCG negative, I can conclude that she is not pregnant, and she does not present with any history of abnormally heavy menses or spotting, ruling out the other gynecologic conditions on my list. In performing the respiratory physical examination, I find no wheezing, a normal anteroposterior diameter, and her SaO$_2$ remains within the normal range on room air. Given her negative pulmonary history along with a normal physical examination, COPD, emphysema, and asthma can be ruled out. Her cardiac examination was also normal. She had no jugular venous distension and no bruits, her PMI is within normal limits and her rhythm is regular although a heart rate of 98 is close to being defined as tachycardia. Because these findings are all within normal limits, I decide not to obtain a 12-lead ECG or a chest x-ray as my history and examination are sufficient to rule out cardiopulmonary disease in this patient.

The fact that her hemoglobin and hematocrit are low supports the initial conclusion that she is anemic. Two broad classifications of anemia are microcytic and macrocytic anemias. Subclassifications of microcytic anemias include iron deficiency anemia, anemia of chronic diseases, anemia of acute blood loss, and blood dyscrasias such as thalassemia. Subclassifications of macrocytic anemia include vitamin B$_{12}$ deficiency and folic acid deficiency. In obtaining the gastrointestinal (GI) history, specific questions were asked about previous colon surgeries or gastric bypass since these procedures can lead to either vitamin B$_{12}$ deficiency or an inability to absorb iron. In this case the patient denied any colon or bypass procedures, and she had no family history of chronic anemias including no history of thalassemia. The mean corpuscular volume (MCV) provides data about the size of the red blood cells. The normal MCV is 82 to 98 mm.[3] This patient's MCV is 75, indicating a microcytic form of anemia. While the MCV helps differentiate between macrocytic and microcytic anemia, it is still key to identify the cause of her anemia.[3]

Analyzing her MCV, MCHC, ferritin, and TIBC levels together can also help narrow the type of anemia that is present. While the MCV looks at the size of the red blood cells, the MCHC represents the average hemoglobin concentration in the red blood cells. In iron deficiency anemia, the red blood cells are small and pale, hence the MCV is typically below 80 and the MCHC is typically below 30. Serum ferritin levels and serum iron levels are also decreased in iron deficiency anemia, typically below 12 µg/L, and below 30 µg/L, respectively. While the transferrin saturation is often less than 15% in iron deficiency anemia, the *total iron binding capacity* (TIBC) is usually elevated.[4] In anemia of chronic diseases, the MCV may be normal or slightly decreased, the transferrin saturation levels are low and the serum iron levels are very low (Table 6-1). To distinguish between anemia of chronic disease and iron deficiency anemia, the iron level needs to be evaluated as well as the total iron binding capacity. This patient's iron stores are low as indicated by her ferritin level below 12 µg/L, but her TIBC is high, indicating that there are still binding sites available. With anemia of chronic disease, the TIBC is low because fewer binding sites are available for transferrin to bind with iron. In other words, if the TIBC

Table 6-1 Laboratory Values found in Iron Deficiency Anemia versus Anemia of Chronic Diseases

Lab	Iron Deficiency Anemia	Anemia of Chronic Diseases
Ferritin	Decreased (less than 10 µg/dL)	Normal or increased
TIBC	Increased (greater than 300 µg/dL)	Decreased
Serum Fe	Decreased (less than 30 µg/L)	Decreased
Transferrin saturation ratio	Decreased (less than 15%)	Decreased (very low)
MCV	Decreased	Normal or slightly low

is low, transferrin is becoming saturated with iron; if the TIBC is high, transferrin is not fully saturated with iron. In this case scenario, the patient's TIBC is elevated, and her serum iron levels were low. This indicates that she has an iron deficiency.

The challenge now is to focus on possible causes of her iron deficiency anemia. This patient's anemia may be stemming from her vegetarian diet. Another differential to consider is anemia of acute blood loss from gastrointestinal bleeding; however, her vital signs are stable and she does not provide a history of melena. If she is losing blood from her GI tract, it has not caused her to become hemodynamically unstable. More insidious causes of a lower GI bleed such as ulcerative colitis, Crohn disease, diverticulitis, or colorectal cancer also need to be considered, as well as other cancers such as leukemia and multiple myeloma. Neither her history nor her physical examination support the diagnosis of ulcerative colitis, Crohn disease, or diverticulitis. She provides no history of abdominal pain, abdominal distension, constipation, or diarrhea. Given her normal white blood cell count and bands, infection and leukemia can be ruled out. Her erythrocyte sedimentation rate is normal as well as her calcium levels and she denies any bone pain or areas of tenderness. Given these negative findings, along with her age, of 50 versus 65, multiple myeloma is very unlikely.[3]

Because her stool test for guaiac is positive, both colorectal cancer and a bleeding ulcer rise to the top of the list. And while certain vegetables such as cucumbers or cauliflower can produce false-positive results, her actual CBC indicates that she is anemic. The fecal immunochemical test (FIT), which also measures occult blood but is not affected by medications or food, is pending, and this is more specific for colon bleeding, so may provide additional data as to the source of the bleeding.[5]

However, I still need to explore her positive stool guaiac. Given her history of taking a daily adult aspirin, she is at risk for a bleeding peptic or gastric ulcer. While colorectal cancer is less likely, it is still a possibility that I cannot rule out at this time. While it would be easy to assume that she is experiencing an upper GI bleed, and treat her for both anemia and peptic or gastric ulcer disease, to do so would be falling into the trap of "satisfaction of search," or prematurely accepting a diagnosis without looking for other possible diagnoses. With this patient, cancer has been on the list of differentials from the onset, and both her weight loss as well as her positive stool guaiac keep cancer on the active list of diagnoses. In order to explore this diagnosis more thoroughly, a colonoscopy is necessary. As the nurse practitioner providing her care, it is my responsibility to refer her to a gastroenterologist and specifically arrange for a colonoscopy. It is my hope that the colonoscopy will be negative, but in order to ensure that she undergoes this examination, I need to take responsibility for making the necessary arrangements, rather than simply recommending to the patient that she have this done. Given her age and her symptoms of fatigue and the positive stool guaiac, a colonoscopy is essential.

Diagnosis and Treatment of Anemia

In the meantime, I will manage her anemia by asking the patient to stop her aspirin and order iron sulfate 325 mg three times daily once her colonoscopy has been completed. Also her diet should be reviewed in more detail. Given the fact that she is a vegetarian and does not eat beef, foods such as spinach, dried fruits such as raisins and apricots are good sources of iron. If the colonoscopy can be arranged within the next week, I will recommend that she not start the iron supplement until after the colonoscopy since iron is very constipating and may interfere with the bowel preparation. But now is an excellent time to begin patient teaching about dietary changes, as well as how to take the iron supplements. While it is recommended that iron be taken on an empty stomach to improve absorption, few patients can tolerate it this way. As a result, I advise the patient to take the iron with 250 mg of vitamin C to enhance the absorption of iron. It is also recommended to gradually increase the dosage in order to improve compliance.[3] Following her colonoscopy I recommend she start with one tablet per day for several days and gradually increase the dosage to help with compliance. Also I assure that she is informed that the iron tablets will change the color of her stools, and that the goal is for her to remain on the iron supplement for 3 to 6 months. As the nurse practitioner, I recommend reevaluating her hemoglobin in 4 weeks, anticipating that within 3 weeks, her levels should be responding.

As I work with this patient, I need to be aware of her psychosocial needs. She presented to the ED with a chief complaint of fatigue. And I have asked many probing questions including whether she might be pregnant in spite of her husband having had a vasectomy and whether she has any other symptoms of any chronic bowel problems. I continue to explore the possibility that she has colorectal cancer. I am also recommending that she stops her daily adult aspirin. She initiated this to "stay healthy" but at this point is not necessary and may be harmful. I know that I am also potentially raising her stress level by ordering a gastroenterologist consult and colonoscopy and order it myself to ensure it is done within the next week or 10 days. It is important that I realize that as she leaves my care, she is facing the possibility of a serious diagnosis such as cancer. As her nurse practitioner, I need to be able to allow her the opportunity to ask questions, and to explain the laboratory values to her, and incorporate her into the management of her care as an active team member. The hope is to increase her adherence to my recommendations for medication changes and dietary adjustments as well as additional diagnostic tests.

In addition I recognize that this is a great deal of new information for this patient to process and remember. To that end I put all instructions in writing so she can refer to the printed information as well. Given her history and use of aspirin, it is very conceivable that she has an upper GI bleed. Taking her off aspirin and prescribing both iron and dietary adjustments may resolve her symptoms and correct her anemia, but as noted earlier I know that anemia is not the final diagnoses but the result of the diagnoses.

Case Follow-up

In summary, this patient presented to the ED with symptoms of fatigue and shortness of breath when climbing stairs. These symptoms are definitely not life threatening, but still as the nurse practitioner, I needed to identify the cause. Fatigue, tachycardia, and shortness of breath with exertion frequently occur with anemia. But identifying the type of anemia is only part of the solution. Asking about family history of chronic anemias helped rule in or rule out the thalassemias and/or other blood dyscrasias. And by asking detailed questions about her medications I found she regularly took aspirin, which can result in bleeding. Many patients do not consider taking an aspirin as "taking medications," especially because it is available over the counter. Given her history of being a vegetarian, and also taking aspirin, one may quickly conclude that she has had an upper GI bleed. But her weight loss needs to be considered as well.

As this case study unfolded, the colonoscopy revealed a Stage I colon cancer with no lymph node involvement and a partial colectomy was performed. Had I assumed that her symptoms were related to her diet and her use of aspirin, and had a colonoscopy not been ordered, or delayed, this patient's long-term outcome would have been dramatically different.

References

1. Govindan R, Waqar S, Subramanian J. Medical management of malignant disease. Godara H, Hirbe A, Nassif M, Otepka H, Rosenstock A, eds. *The Washington Manual of Medical Therapeutics.* Philadelphia, PA: Lippincott Williams & Wilkins; 2014:796-848.
2. Zhang HY, Yu L, Liu BW, Yang GL, Qian W. How much is fatigue associated with anemia. *Value Health.* 2013;16(3):A44-A44.
3. Damon LE, Charalambos AC. Blood Disorders (chapter 13) In: Papadakis MA, McPhee SJ, Rabow MW, eds. *Current Medical Diagnosis and Treatment.* New York, NY: McGraw Hill Education, 2014.
4. Fischbach F, Dunning MB. Overview of basic blood hematology and coagulation tests. *A Manual of Laboratory and Diagnostic Test.* Lippincott Williams & Wilkins; 2009:56-183.
5. McQuaid KR. Gastrointestinal disorders (chapter 15). In: Papadakis MA, McPhee SJ, Rabow MW, eds. *Current Medical Diagnosis and Treatment.* New York, NY: McGraw Hill Education, 2014.

CASE 7

Megan M. Shifrin

Megan Shifrin is ACNP faculty at the Vanderbilt University School of Nursing in the AG-ACNP program. Dr Shifrin's clinical background is in critical care with an emphasis on trauma and cardiac surgery.

CASE INFORMATION

Chief Complaint

CD is a 62-year-old white male who presents to the emergency department with a recent onset of "pain in the front part of my chest."

? What is the potential cause?

Case Analysis: In patients who present with anterior chest pain, immediate causes that need to be ruled out include those of an acute cardiovascular and pulmonary etiology. However, musculoskeletal or gastrointestinal etiologies are also possible causes of this kind of pain. A detailed history and physical examination coupled with appropriate imaging can assist in making a rapid and accurate diagnosis.

Comprehensive Differential Diagnoses in a Patient with Chest Pain[1]

- Cardiovascular: myocardial ischemia (myocardial infarction or coronary artery vasospasm); aortic valve stenosis; mitral valve stenosis; pericarditis; myocarditis; acute aortic dissection; aortic aneurysm rupture; cardiac tamponade; penetrating aortic ulcer; mediastinitis
- Pulmonary: pneumonia (bacterial, fungal, or viral); noninfective pneumonitis; pulmonary embolism; pneumothorax; pleural effusion; pulmonary tumor; pulmonary hypertension; pleuritis
- Gastrointestinal: gastroesophageal reflux disease; esophageal rupture or perforation; perforating peptic ulcer
- Musculoskeletal: costochondritis; rib or sternal fracture
- Psychiatric: panic disorder; anxiety, depression; hypochondriasis
- Exogenous: medication reaction/interaction/side effect

CASE INFORMATION

General Survey and History of Present Illness

When trying to narrow down the differential diagnoses in a patient presenting with chest pain, questions regarding the patient's past medical history and the details surrounding the onset of chest pain are extremely helpful. However, it is also important not to delay diagnostic testing in these individuals by spending an extraordinary amount of time completing the history and physical examination since many of the diagnoses associated with chest pain carry heavy morbidity and mortality rates if treatment is delayed.

The patient reports a past medical history of Marfan syndrome and hypertension. He states that he was outside working in his garage when he experienced a sudden, tearing sensation in his anterior chest lasting approximately 10 to 15 seconds. Since onset, his chest pain has been a constant ache that he rates as a 7 out of 10 on a 1 to 10 scale. His pain radiates from the anterior to the posterior aspect of his chest. Associated symptoms include new onset of shortness of breath and diaphoresis. He denies loss of consciousness, nausea, vomiting, and pain or numbness in his extremities.

He denies a history of coronary artery disease and use of illicit substances. He states that he has been consistently taking his prescribed lisinopril for hypertension. Concerned that he might be having a myocardial infarction, the patient took aspirin 81 mg PO ×1 while his wife drove him to the emergency room. However, he has not experienced any alleviation in symptoms following the aspirin ingestion.

? What are the pertinent positives from the information given so far?

- He has a past medical history of Marfan syndrome and hypertension.
- His chest pain had a sudden onset during physical activity.
- He described his chest pain as "tearing" followed by "aching" pain.
- He has associated shortness of breath and diaphoresis.
- His pain was not alleviated when he took aspirin.

? What are the significant negatives from the information given so far?

- He denies loss of consciousness, nausea, vomiting, and pain or numbness in his extremities.
- He denies use of illicit substances.

- The pain is not described as a "pressure."
- The patient does not have a history of coronary artery disease or illicit substance use.

? Can the information gathered so far be restated in a single sentence highlighting the pieces that narrow down the cause?

CD is a 62-year-old white male who has a history of Marfan syndrome and hypertension who now presents with an acute onset of "tearing" chest pain that occurred during activity.

? How does this information affect the list of possible causes?

Case Analysis: Due to the patient's past medical history and description of his chest pain, there are several diagnoses that should be prioritized in regard to diagnostic testing. First, his history of hypertension places him at risk for both a myocardial infarction and a Stanford type A aortic dissection.[1] Second, Marfan syndrome has been associated with a bicuspid aortic valve, aortic valve stenosis, and type A aortic dissections. Given these risk factors, quickly ruling out, or ruling in, a myocardial infarction and a type A aortic dissection is essential. Both of these conditions require immediate treatment for successful outcomes.

CASE INFORMATION

Past Medical History

- Current state of health: "good until this afternoon"
- Previous medical diagnoses: Marfan syndrome; hypertension
- Past surgical history: tonsillectomy at age 8 years
- Family history:
  - Marfan syndrome: father
  - Hyperlipidemia: mother
  - Denies family history of cardiovascular disease, hypertension, kidney disease, liver disease, and obesity
- Current medications: lisinopril 10 mg once daily
- Allergies: none

Social History

- Habits:
  - Alcohol intake: three to four beers weekly
  - Illicit substance use: denies
  - Tobacco use: denies

- Current occupation: retired. Previously worked as a mechanical engineer.
- Living situation: Lives with wife in a rural area.

Review of Systems (ROS)

- Constitutional: Denies weakness, fatigue, night sweats, and unintentional weight loss.
- Cardiovascular: See HPI regarding history of chest pain and shortness of breath. States that his shortness of breath and chest pain is exacerbated by activity. Symptoms are mildly alleviated by rest. Denies history of palpitations, orthopnea, heart murmurs, and lower extremity edema. No history of claudication or thrombophlebitis.
- Pulmonary: See HPI regarding history of shortness of breath. States that his shortness of breath is exacerbated by activity and partially alleviated by rest. Denies wheezing, hemoptysis, and cough.
- Gastrointestinal: Denies constipation, diarrhea, melena, hematochezia, and vomiting. No history of dysphagia, gastric reflux symptoms, or jaundice. The patient states he has a bowel movement one time per day and that they are normal for him.
- Genitourinary: Denies history of frequency, dysuria, hesitancy, urgency, polyuria, nocturia, hematuria, or incontinence. No history of renal calculi, recurrent urinary tract infections, or flank pain.
- Musculoskeletal: Denies history of muscle myalgia, recent trauma or injury, joint pain, swelling, stiffness, or erythema. Denies decreased range of motion in any of his joints.
- Neurological: Denies history of seizures, syncope, numbness, tingling, extremity weakness, or changes in speech. No headaches, memory changes, or forgetfulness.
- Psychiatric: Denies history of depression, anxiety, and other previous psychiatric diagnoses.
- Hematologic/lymphatic/immunologic: Denies history of fever, chills, easy bruising, bleeding, or enlarged/tender lymph nodes. No history of blood product administration. Denies previous history of frequent illness.

Physical Examination

- Vital signs: temperature 98.2° F oral; heart rate 113 beats per minute; respirations 24/min; blood pressure 158/94 mm Hg; O_2 saturation on room air 98%, weight 220 lb, height 80 inches, BMI 24.2 kg/m².
- Constitutional: CD is calm, demeanor appropriate for situation. He is well groomed and is alert, cooperative, answers questions appropriately.
- Cardiovascular: Heart rhythm is regular. S1 and S2 present; no S3 or S4 noted. Diastolic murmur (IV/VI) auscultated at the right sternal border, second intercostal space. No rubs, clicks, or gallops. No heaves, thrills, or

lifts noted upon palpation. Bilateral lower extremity edema (1+). Bilateral carotid pulses strong with smooth, regular pulsations; no carotid bruits noted. Capillary refill <3 seconds in upper and lower extremities bilaterally. No varicosities present. Radial, brachial, dorsalis pedis and posterior tibialis pulses 2+ and symmetrical bilaterally. No aortic, renal, iliac, or femoral bruits noted.

- Pulmonary: Regular respiratory rate and rhythm. No use of accessory muscles. Trachea midline. Chest wall expansion symmetrical bilaterally. Breath sounds clear bilaterally in all lung fields. No wheezes, rhonchi, or crackles noted.
- Gastrointestinal: Abdominal contour flat. No abdominal distention, pulsations, heaves, or masses noted. Bowel sounds normoactive in all four quadrants. Tympany heard with percussion in all quadrants. No rebound tenderness or guarding noted. Liver not palpable.
- Renal/Genitourinary: No costovertebral angle tenderness.
- Musculoskeletal: Skeletal frame consistent with previous diagnosis of Marfan syndrome. Spine midline without deviation or masses. No tenderness or crepitation upon palpation of upper and lower extremities. Muscle tone equal bilaterally with no masses or tenderness noted upon palpation.
- Neurological: Patient is calm, alert, and oriented to person, place, and time. Able to answer questions appropriately and respond without difficulty. Short-term memory intact as evidenced by ability to recall three words with no difficulty. Speech tone, volume, and clarity without abnormality.
- Psychiatric: Affect and behavior appropriate for situation. Thought process logical; speech is clear and easily understood. Demonstrates appropriate emotions and cognition.
- Hematologic/Lymphatic/Immune: No signs of active bleeding. No petechiae, purpura, or ecchymosis noted. No enlarged or tender lymph nodes. Spleen not palpable.

❓ What are the pertinent positives from the review of systems and physical examination?

- He is presently hypertensive and tachycardic.
- Activity increases his chest pain and shortness of breath; rest only partially alleviates symptoms.
- He has a new diastolic aortic valve murmur indicative of aortic valve insufficiency.
- He has mild lower extremity edema.
- Physical features of his musculoskeletal system are consistent with his previous diagnosis of Marfan syndrome.

❓ What are the significant negatives from the review of systems and physical examination?

- He exhibits normal findings in the review of systems and physical examination for the gastrointestinal, renal/genitourinary, neurological, psychiatric, and hematologic/lymphatic/immune systems.

- He has no past medical history of coronary heart disease, diabetes, or tobacco use.

Case Analysis: Based on the information gathered so far, I can now rule out a few differential diagnoses. First, it seems unlikely that an infectious disease process such as pneumonia or mediastinitis are causing the patient's symptoms. He denies a history of fever, chills, cough, nausea, and myalgia that are common in many infectious disease etiologies. Second, he denies having any recent trauma, thus eliminating a rib fracture or other traumatic injury from the list of differential diagnoses. He also has clear breath sounds bilaterally in all lobes and states that his recent dyspnea is related to increased activity. These findings make a large pleural effusion or tension pneumothorax unlikely diagnoses.

There are no significant symptoms or examination findings related to the gastrointestinal system. He denies having symptoms that would be consistent with gastric reflux, esophageal rupture, or a penetrating gastric ulcer. There is no relationship between his symptoms and food intake. His gastrointestinal examination is unremarkable, allowing me to eliminate several gastrointestinal differential diagnoses as sources for his symptoms.

The patient does not have a psychiatric past medical history, and his review of systems and physical examination do not reveal signs or symptoms consistent with the diagnosis of panic disorder, anxiety, depression, or hypochondriasis. Thus, these specific diagnoses are ruled out as primary source of the patient's symptoms.

Based on the information gathered so far, particularly the new aortic valve murmur in the setting of an acute onset of chest pain, make me concerned that the patient may have an acute type A aortic dissection. In addition, his past medical history of Marfan syndrome and hypertension predispose him to this particular diagnosis.[1]

CASE INFORMATION

An aortic dissection occurs when blood enters in between the intima and media layers of the vessel. If a dissection occurs in the ascending aspect aorta or the aortic arch, it is referred to as a Stanford type A aortic dissection (*Figure 7-1*). If it occurs distal to the left subclavian in the descending aorta, it is referred to as a Stanford type B aortic dissection. Rapid dissection identification is crucial, particularly since management of a type A aortic dissection differs from that of a type B aortic dissection.[2]

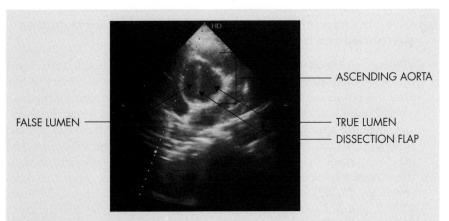

ASCENDING AORTA

FALSE LUMEN

TRUE LUMEN

DISSECTION FLAP

Figure 7-1 Type A dissection visualized within the ascending aorta on TEE. Used with permission from M. Shifrin.

When a type A aortic dissection occurs, the dissection flap may dilate the aortic valve annulus, thus causing misalignment or prolapse of the aortic valve leaflets, resulting in a new diastolic aortic valve murmur. This sign guides my prioritization of diagnostic testing.

Patients with type A aortic dissections may also present with neurological changes or deficits if the dissection flap has disrupted blood flow into the carotid arteries, causing syncope, stroke, or ischemic neurological changes. They may also show signs and symptoms of an acute coronary syndrome if the dissection flap extends into the coronary arteries and obstructs coronary blood flow. Other vascular complications that may result from a dissection include limb, renal, and mesenteric ischemia. Evaluating for pulse deficits, mottled extremities, decreased urinary output, abdominal pain, and nausea can be helpful in initially assessing for this possibility. If aortic rupture has occurred, patients may also present with signs and symptoms of profound hypotension or tamponade physiology.

Case Analysis: This patient's history and physical do not reveal the obvious sequelae of an aortic rupture or of overt ischemia as a result of a type A aortic dissection. However, the absence of these signs and symptoms does not rule out an acute aortic dissection. Since the dissection may have occurred recently, several of these complications may have not yet fully evolved.

Aside from the new murmur, there are few other physical examination findings that presently assist in ruling in or ruling out the other differential diagnoses. Therefore, prompt initiation of diagnostic testing must be used in order to rule out other rapidly lethal causes of acute chest pain and shortness of breath. Other priority differential diagnoses to rule out still include myocardial ischemia, contained aortic rupture, cardiac tamponade, and pulmonary embolism.

❓ Given the new information what diagnostic testing should be performed and in what order?

When addressing an urgent patient situation, the safest approach is to rule out the most life-threatening issues or diagnoses first. It is also important to consider which tests can be obtained quickly to assist in this process. In this case, a stat 12-lead ECG can be completed and read immediately. A stat chest x-ray and computed tomography (CT) scan of the chest with intravenous contrast while also essential for diagnostic purposes will take longer but will be useful for diagnosing aortic rupture, cardiac tamponade, pulmonary embolism, pneumothorax, and esophageal rupture or perforation. Furthermore, cardiac enzymes (troponin, CK-MB, and CPK), a CBC, complete metabolic panel, D-Dimer, PT/INR, and PTT are obtained in order to rule out myocardial infarction, pulmonary embolism, acute blood loss anemia, leukocytosis, and hypercoagulable or hypocoagulable states as well as establish baseline laboratory values for this patient.

However, if an aortic dissection is strongly suspected, echocardiography can be used to confirm the diagnosis. With transesophageal echocardiography (TEE), sensitivity for type A aortic dissections is 88% to 98% with a specificity of 90% to 95%.[2] Not only does TEE allow for visualization of the aortic dissection flap, but it can also be useful in identifying and quantifying aortic valve regurgitation, wall motion abnormalities caused by dissection into the coronary arteries, and cardiac tamponade physiology (Figure 7-1).

Rapid determination and classification of aortic dissections have direct implications for immediate management. Type A aortic dissections are considered to be surgical emergencies due to the high risk of lethal neurological and cardiovascular sequelae.[3] Type B dissections may be managed medically rather than surgically if vital organs have not been directly compromised as a result of the dissection.

CASE INFORMATION

Diagnostic Results

A 12-lead ECG was performed within a few minutes of arrival to the emergency department. It demonstrated sinus tachycardia but no acute ST-segment or T-wave abnormalities suggestive of a ST-elevation myocardial infarction. Lab work was drawn while the ECG leads are placed to rule out STEMI. The patient also underwent stat CT scan of the chest, which showed an intimal flap in the ascending aorta originating at the level of the aortic root and terminating prior to the takeoff of the brachiocephalic artery, thus confirming the diagnosis of a Stanford type A aortic dissection. Laboratory data was notable for a troponin I 0.8 ng/mL (N = <0.01 ng/mL), indicative of an NSTEMI and possibly due to extension of the dissection into the coronary arteries.

Diagnosis: Aortic Dissection Type A: Marfan Syndrome

Management

Immediate surgical repair of a Stanford type A aortic dissection is essential for both short- and long-term outcomes; however, medical management should be optimized until the patient can proceed to surgical intervention.[3] Placement of an arterial line and use of other forms of hemodynamic monitoring may be initiated preoperatively, though placement of these monitoring devices in the emergency department or in an intensive care unit setting should not delay surgical intervention.[4] Careful consideration should be paid to the placement sites of arterial lines as extension of the dissection flap into the brachiocephalic, subclavian, and femoral arteries may cause erroneously low blood pressure readings.

The current medical management of a patient with a Stanford type A dissection centers on rapid reduction of cardiac contractility and systemic arterial pressure in patients who present with tachycardia and hypertension. Intravenous β-blockade should be initiated and titrated to a heart rate of less than 60 beats per minute and a systolic blood pressure of 100 to 120 mm Hg.[5] Labetalol and esmolol are commonly used due to their ability to be easily and quickly titrated. However, in patients with acute aortic valve insufficiency, β-blockers are used cautiously because they can inhibit reflex tachycardia. For those patients who have contraindications to β-blockade, calcium channel blockers such as diltiazem can be used to achieve heart rate control. If the systolic blood pressure remains greater than 120 mm Hg after heart rate management is achieved using β-blockade or calcium channel blockers, then other intravenous vasodilators such as nitroprusside may be used to achieve hemodynamic optimization.[4]

In addition to achieving hemodynamic stability preoperatively, other steps are taken to prepare the patient for surgery. This includes obtaining a type and crossmatch and reserving blood products for potential administration in the operating room.[4]

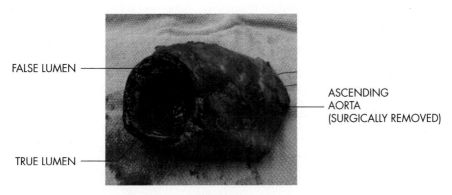

Figure 7-2 Photo of the type A dissection following surgical removal of the ascending aorta. Used with permission from James Greelish, MD, 2014.

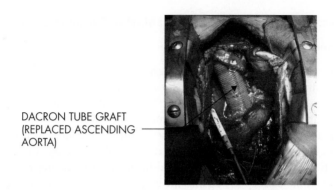

DACRON TUBE GRAFT
(REPLACED ASCENDING
AORTA)

Figure 7-3 Completed Bentall procedure. Used with permission from James Greelish, MD, 2014.

Case Follow-Up

In this case, the patient is optimized preoperatively in the cardiovascular intensive care unit. A left radial arterial line is placed, and the patient is started on an esmolol infusion to achieve hemodynamic stability. The patient is taken emergently to the operating room where TEE confirms the presence of a Stanford type A aortic dissection with severe aortic valve regurgitation. A successful Bentall procedure is performed. This involves replacement of the aortic valve, aortic root, and ascending aorta as well as reimplantation of the coronary arteries (Figures 7-2 and 7-3). The patient is transferred back to the cardiovascular intensive care unit postoperatively.

The patient's immediate postoperative course was complicated by coagulopathic blood loss and acute respiratory failure; however, after transfusion and hemostasis was achieved, he was successfully weaned from the ventilator on postoperative day 2. The remainder of his hospital course was relatively unremarkable, and he was discharged to home on postoperative day 6.

References

1. Patel PD, Arora, RR. Pathophysiology, diagnosis, and management of aortic dissection. *Ther Adv Cardiovasc Dis*. 2008;2(6):439-468. doi: 10.1177/1753944708090830.
2. Shiga T, Wajima Z, Apfel CC, Inoue T, Ohe Y. Diagnostic accuracy of transesophageal echocardiography, helical computed tomography, and magnetic resonance imaging for suspected thoracic aortic dissection: systematic review and meta-analysis. *Arch Intern Med*. 2006;10(166):1350-1356. doi: 10.1177/1753944708090830
3. Stevens LM, Madsen JC, Isselbacher EM, et al. Surgical management and long term outcomes of acute ascending aortic dissection. *J Thorac Cardiovasc Surg*. 2009;138(6):1349-1357.
4. Hiratzka LF, Bakris GL, Beckman JA, et al. ACCF/AHA/AATS/ACR/ASA/SCA/SCAI/SIR/STS/SVM guidelines for the diagnosis and management of patients with thoracic aortic disease. *J Am Coll Cardiol*. 2010;55(14):e27-e129.
5. Tsai TT, Nienaber CA, Eagle KA. Acute aortic syndromes. *Circulation*. 2005;112:3802-3813.

CASE 8

Kelly Godsey

Kelly Godsey has worked in the Advanced Heart Failure and Cardiac Transplant outpatient clinic at University of Virginia for 13 years. Prior to that she worked for many years as a medical intensive care unit nurse.

CASE INFORMATION

Chief Complaint

A 44-year-old white male with a history of heart transplant 22 years ago calls the office complaining of 4 days of upper abdominal and lower chest pain, nausea, and vomiting.

? What is the potential cause?

Case Analysis: Abdominal and lower chest pain and nausea have a broad list of potential causes. A systems approach to investigating the causes of these symptoms allows a quick review of the diagnoses beginning with the most critical. In this patient's case, his history of heart transplant makes the diagnosis of myocardial ischemia and rejection a high possibility. And given his immunocompromised state, infectious etiologies and malignancies are high on the list as well.

? Differential Diagnoses of Chest/Upper Abdominal Pain in an Adult

- Ischemic syndromes: coronary artery disease, angina, coronary artery dissection, valvular heart disease
- Nonischemic: aortic dissection, pericarditis, myocarditis
- Hyperadrenergic states: cocaine or amphetamine intoxication
- Chest wall: costochondritis, rheumatic disease, malignancy, herpes zoster (shingles), mediastinitis
- Pulmonary: acute pulmonary embolism, pleuritis, pneumonia, cancer, pneumothorax
- Gastrointestinal: esophageal reflux, spasm, rupture, or esophagitis, cholecystitis, pancreatitis, cholangitis, biliary colic, peptic ulcer disease
- Psychiatric: panic attack, anxiety

? Differentials of Abdominal Pain, Nausea, and Vomiting in an Adult[1,2]

Classification of pain by location[3]:

Right Upper Quadrant	Left Upper Quadrant
Hepatitis	Splenic abscess
Cholecystitis	Splenic infarct
Cholangitis	Gastritis
Biliary colic	Gastric ulcer
Pancreatitis	Pancreatitis
Budd-Chiari syndrome	**Left lower quadrant**
Pneumonia/empyema pleurisy	Diverticulitis
Subdiaphragmatic abscess	Salpingitis
Right lower quadrant	Inguinal hernia
Appendicitis	Nephrolithiasis
Salpingitis	Irritable bowel syndrome
Inguinal hernia	Inflammatory bowel disease
Nephrolithiasis	**Periumbilical**
Inflammatory bowel disease	Early appendicitis
Epigastric	Gastroenteritis
Peptic ulcer disease	Bowel obstruction
Gastroesophageal reflux disease	Ruptured aortic aneurysm
Gastritis	**Diffuse**
Pancreatitis	Gastroenteritis
Myocardial infarction	Mesenteric ischemia
Pericarditis	Constipation
Ruptured aortic aneurysm	Bowel obstruction
	Peritonitis
	Irritable bowel syndrome

CASE INFORMATION
General Survey and History of Present Illness

The patient reports to me by phone that he went to the emergency room (ER) when his symptoms started 4 days ago. A review of ER record shows that he presented with chest pain, flank pain, hematuria, nausea, and vomiting.

Evaluation in the ER included a chest x-ray which was unremarkable, an abdominal computed tomography (CT) scan which ruled out renal stones, and a normal ECG and serial troponins ruling out myocardial ischemia. His urine was negative except for moderate blood and small ketones. His blood work was normal except for a mildly elevated WBC at 12.2. The patient was discharged home but his symptoms have continued without any improvement. The pain is in his upper abdomen and lower chest but also moves around to his back. It is not associated with food intake or activity. He denies any fever or chills. The hematuria is intermittent and not associated with pain or urgency or changes in his stream. The nausea and vomiting also occur intermittently but have happened at least once a day since the symptoms started.

Past Medical and Surgical History

- Heart transplant 22 years ago
- Normal coronary arteries on routine posttransplant cardiac catheterization 6 months prior to ER visit
- Hypertension
- Hyperlipidemia
- Allergies: penicillin

Current Medications

Working with cardiac transplant patients, I am accustomed to an extensive medication list. In this patient's case, his list is fairly compact. It includes:
- Cyclosporine (Gengraf) 100 mg tabs, adjusted according to levels, to prevent rejection
- Azathioprine (Imuran) 75 mg daily to prevent rejection
- Lisinopril 5 mg daily for hypertension
- Diltiazem 120 mg once a day (extended release) for hypertension
- Potassium chloride 10 mEq daily
- Atorvastatin 40 mg daily in the evening for hyperlipidemia

The patient reports he takes his medications as prescribed with the exception of the lisinopril which he sometimes intentionally misses because it makes him dizzy, and he worries about this side effect when his work day includes climbing ladders. The patient denies taking any over-the-counter medications.

❓ What are the pertinent positives from the information given so far?

- The patient has had 4 days of chest and abdominal pain.
- The patient has hypertension which may be under erratic control.

- He has nausea and vomiting associated with his pain.
- He has hematuria without a clear diagnosis of renal involvement.

❓ What are the significant negatives from the information given so far?

- Normal troponins and normal ECG.
- Abdominal CT does not reveal an acute process.
- Urinalysis abnormal, but negative for infection.
- He is generally in excellent health.

Case Analysis: Situations such as this illustrate the way experience enhances the ability to quickly process data in order to safely develop a plan of treatment. I know that while heart transplantation was once thought to make anginal pain impossible because the cardiac muscle is denervated, it is now known that some nerve regrowth occurs, allowing transplant patients to experience ischemic pain. In addition, heart transplant patients far removed from their transplant, as this patient is, often develop graft vasculopathy, a chronic inflammatory process in which the intimal linings of the coronary arteries narrow. This narrowing is often diffuse and can cause ischemia and myocardial infarction. For this reason, ruling out myocardial infarction is a top priority. Based on the data I have so far, myocardial infarction is very unlikely. His catheterization several months ago showed clean coronaries and his troponins were normal in the emergency room.

An additional consideration in a transplant patient is infection with cytomegalovirus (CMV). This is a common childhood illness to which nearly 2/3 of the general population have been exposed. For those with normal immune systems, CMV is not an issue, but when an immunosuppressed patient presents with gastrointestinal symptoms such as vomiting and abdominal pain, early diagnosis and initiation of antiviral therapy is essential as CMV can causes severe illness. However, with a CMV infection you typically see severe leukopenia, which he did not have. CMV infection is also much less likely in someone this many years removed from transplantation, but it is still possible.

The fact that he is not consistently adherent to his antihypertensive medications and his blood pressure was high in the emergency room leads me to consider whether the uncontrolled hypertension is the cause of his symptoms. Patients with uncontrolled hypertension report symptoms of headache and vomiting, although abdominal pain and chest pain are not typically seen. One area of concern with abdominal pain and high blood pressure is a ruptured abdominal aneurysm, but there was no mention of abdominal bruit in the history and physical, he had a normal hemoglobin and hematocrit and his CT, done in the emergency department, was negative for any acute process.

The patient's overall good health and ability to continue working a physically demanding construction job plus the normal results from the ER make an acute process such as myocardial infarction, pulmonary embolus, dissecting aortic aneurysm, intestinal obstruction, cholecystitis, diverticulitis, and renal stones less likely. Given the diffuse, wandering element of his pain as well as the hematuria, an infectious component remains high on my list. This could also be a lingering virus or even a food-borne illness but he denies any similar symptoms in his close contacts. I will, however, keep this in the back of my mind as I decide what diagnostics to order. When someone has a significant history such as solid organ transplant, it is easy to be derailed by concerns of a critical medical event and overlook everyday causes such as community-acquired viruses or food-borne illnesses.

Given his normal ECG, and the associated symptoms of hematuria, other heart conditions such as angina and pericarditis or heart rejection are lower on my list at this point.

Quite a bit of my practice involves telephone triage due to factors such as the financial constraints of my patients and the distance they have to travel to our facility. With this case, I start out with the knowledge that he was seen and examined in the ED, and I have the ED provider's notes to go on (see case information below). Our practice has been caring for this patient for over two decades, so we know he rarely calls the office unless he needs a prescription refill. Understanding his reluctance to call with complaints and his normal state of excellent health heightens my concern that there is a more serious issue occurring. So I advise the patient by phone that he needs to come in for some additional diagnostic testing, including a right upper quadrant (RUQ) ultrasound, repeat urinalysis, blood draw for CMV viral load (though this is unlikely, it warrants ruling out because, as noted, it can become a devastating problem in an immunocompromised adult), a comprehensive chemistry panel (CMP), and a complete blood count (CBC) with differential.

CASE INFORMATION

Review of Systems (From ER and From Phone Triage)

- Constitutional: Denies fever, chills; appetite and oral intake is poor. Denies sick contacts, denies any recent trauma.
- Cardiovascular: Endorses lower diffuse chest pain but denies dyspnea on exertion, paroxysmal nocturnal dyspnea orthopnea, edema, and syncope.
- Pulmonary: Denies dyspnea, cough, and sputum production.
- Gastrointestinal: Complains of intermittent nausea and vomiting and epigastric pain, denies diarrhea or constipation, denies blood in stools, denies hematemesis.
- Genitourinary: Complains of flank pain and hematuria but denies dysuria or frequency
- Musculoskeletal: Complains of back pain.
- Neurological: Denies headache, falls, or seizure activity.
- Endocrine: Denies changes in thirst or urination.

Physical Examination (in the Emergency Room)

- Vital signs: pulse 88 beats per minute, blood pressure elevated at 155/100 mm Hg, respiratory rate 20/min, temperature 98.5°F orally, oxygen saturation 98% on room air
- Constitutional: well-nourished male who appears stated age, in moderate discomfort
- Head/eyes/ears/nose/throat: pupils equal and reactive, face symmetrical, trachea midline
- Cardiovascular: normal rate and rhythm, S1 and S2 without murmurs, gallops or rubs, no carotid bruit, no ankle edema, brisk capillary refill, skin warm and dry to touch
- Pulmonary: respiratory rate and pattern normal, clear to auscultation
- Gastrointestinal: normal bowel sounds, some mid upper abdominal tenderness
- Integumentary: no rashes, lesions, or sores
- Neuro: awake, alert, and oriented without focal deficits

Laboratory Results (Ordered by My Clinic After 4 Days of Symptoms)

Complete blood count shows a mildly elevated white blood cell count at 12,700 cells/µL, 81.9% neutrophils (within normal range).

Urinalysis reveals amber, cloudy urine with 3+ protein, negative glucose, large ketones, moderate bilirubin, large blood, positive nitrite, small leukocyte esterase, and high WBC (3) with few bacteria (culture pending)

Chemistry panel is within normal limits except for a total bilirubin of 2.0 (up from 0.4 three days prior) with normal liver enzymes.

His right upper quadrant ultrasound is normal.

❓ What elements of the review of systems and physical examination should be added to the list of pertinent positives?

- Loss of appetite, diffuse chest pain, intermittent abdominal pain, nausea, and vomiting, hypertension, flank and back pain, hematuria with a urinalysis showing leukocyte esterase, high white blood cell count, moderate blood and a few bacteria, blood serum with elevated WBC and elevated bilirubin.

❓ What elements of the review of systems and physical examination should be added to the significant negatives list?

- Negative for neurologic deficits, negative for dyspnea. No melena, no hematemesis, no diarrhea, no trauma, no sick contacts. Normal right upper quadrant ultrasound.

❓ How can this information be reconciled with the list of possible diagnoses?

Case Analysis: A cardiac cause for these symptoms appears to be unlikely given the negative troponins and normal ECG in the ER. Pulmonary issues appear to be ruled out as well given a normal chest x-ray, normal pulmonary examination, and normal oxygen saturation on room air. There is no report of chest or abdominal trauma, no ill contacts or anyone else in his family complaining of a food-borne illness. He denies any melena or hematemesis, making concerns for peptic ulcer disease less likely. He did endorse some upper gastric tenderness as well as flank and back pain but his renal stone CT did not reveal any sign of renal calculi.

This patient's urinalysis findings, positive nitrates and leukoesterase, as well as the presence of WBCs in the urine, suggest a urinary tract infection. Urinary tract infection (UTI) is uncommon in males under the age of 50 due to the anatomical protections such as a long urethra, a bladder capable of holding large amounts of urine, and several centimeters of tissue between the urethral opening and the rectum. It can be seen in males with a suppressed immune system or anatomical abnormalities. The causes can vary from prostatic hypertrophy, causing urinary reflux and cystitis, to prostatitis to pyelonephritis, which can occur if the ureter becomes inflamed, causing urine to reflux back into the kidney. As with females, the most common organism is *E coli*. I am not suspicious of epididymitis as he does not complain of scrotal edema or pain. Given the current information, I start a 10-day course of ciprofloxacin. Fluoroquinolones provide broad coverage, so they are the first-line therapy in complicated UTI (male UTI is typically considered to be complicated.). I also refer him to urology, as UTI in males can be indicative of a more serious anatomical issue requiring surgical intervention or a chronic problem such as sexually transmitted disease.[4]

CASE INFORMATION

Four days later, the patient calls back and requests to be seen in clinic because he is still unwell. He is not tolerating the ciprofloxacin due to side effects of restlessness and agitation, so he stopped it. The restlessness abated somewhat but he is having difficulty sleeping with some residual flank and shoulder discomfort, as well as mild tenderness to the right upper quadrant and left flank.

On examination, he is still hypertensive at 160/100, with regular pulse rate of 78. He has a nonradiating 2/6 systolic murmur (a fairly common finding in heart transplant patients due to repeated heart biopsies causing tricuspid valve damage and regurgitation). His breath sounds are clear, and he has normal bowel sounds in a soft abdomen and no frank hematuria. I consult with my attending and we still believe the most likely cause of these symptoms is a renal stone not seen on the CT, so we advise pushing oral fluids and keeping his appointment with urology in 2 weeks. In light of the two previous abnormal urinalysis tests and an incomplete course of ciprofloxacin, I prescribe Bactrim. There is a rare chance of a penicillin-allergic patient reacting to Bactrim, which is a combination of sulfamethoxazole and trimethoprim but this patient has taken Bactrim before without a problem, so I prescribe a 14-day course. Due to ongoing hypertension, I also increase his lisinopril from 5 mg daily to 10 mg daily, and encourage him to adhere to this regimen.

Just before his urology appointment, he returns to clinic again still complaining of feeling unwell. He has lost weight and notes worsening gastrointestinal symptoms of belching, a bad taste in his mouth, and abdominal fullness with an intermittent "boring" pain in the mid upper quadrant. His flank pain has resolved.

On examination, his weight is down another 5 lb and he appears pale and chronically ill. His vital signs are improved with blood pressure 124/70 mm Hg and regular heart rate of 80 beats per minute. Heart sounds reveal normal S1 and S2, with no murmurs auscultated today. Lungs remain clear and the abdominal and flank tenderness have resolved. With this examination, he appears to have more gastric complaints, which leads to concerns for gastroesophageal reflux disease or peptic ulcer disease. An 8-week course of a proton-pump inhibitor is prescribed with plans to reassess symptoms or need for gastroenterology referral after that course.

The following week he calls to report that the urologist scheduled him for a computed tomography scan with intravenous pyelogram (CT-IVP) to better visualize his genitourinary tract but he wants to cancel the study because his flank pain is gone and he has missed too many days of work and is fearful of losing his job. He reports continued abdominal complaints as well as further weight loss, so I strongly encourage him to keep this appointment for a CT-IVP as he still feels unwell and we are nearly 8 weeks into his illness without a definitive diagnosis. At the end of the call, the patient agrees to come into the radiology department for the study as scheduled the following day.

The following morning, the radiologist pages me to report findings of dissection of the abdominal aorta extending into the left common iliac artery, but the extent of the dissection was incompletely characterized in the study. The radiologist requests orders to extend the testing to a CT with reduced dose contrast to the chest, abdomen and pelvis, which I immediately approve. The reduced dose of contrast is given due the patient already having received IVP dye.

This further CT scan reveals a Stanford type A aortic dissection originating in the ascending aorta, not involving the coronary arteries, extending throughout the aorta into the left iliac artery. The dissection extends into the innominate, right subclavian, and right common carotid arteries. The left gastric artery and right renal artery arise from the false lumen but fortunately none of the affected arteries have significant compromise.

The radiology staff arranges for the patient to be transported directly to the ICU, where he is stabilized with tight blood pressure control, his nutritional status is optimized, and he undergoes surgical evaluation. He is taken to the OR 6 days later for complete arch reconstruction with anastomoses performed off of the graft to the brachiocephalic artery, left common carotid, and left subclavian arteries. He is discharged home on postoperative day 4.

Diagnosis: Aortic Dissection (Type A): Post-Heart Transplant

Management

A Stanford Type A dissection involves the thoracic aorta and can carry an 80% mortality rate if treated medically instead of surgically; the surgical mortality rate can be as high as 25%. "Tearing" chest pain is a common presenting symptom, with 20% of cases showing neurologic deficits from carotid artery obstruction, such as paresthesia or hemiparesis. Other potential complications include myocardial ischemia from coronary ostium involvement, congestive heart failure from severe aortic regurgitation, hypotension and shock from aortic rupture, flank pain, bowel or renal ischemia with acute renal failure from renal artery involvement, hemoptysis signifying bronchial involvement, dysphagia signaling esophageal involvement, or hoarseness involving vocal cord paralysis. There can be a 20-point difference in blood pressure readings between the two arms, but this does not necessarily rule in a dissection.[5]

Aortic dissection is more common in patients with a history of hypertension, prior thoracic surgery, and bicuspid aortic valve, all of which this patient had. Diagnosis of dissection is often missed and found while working up other issues, such as in this case. The migrating complaints of flank, abdominal and chest pain, nausea, and hematuria, combined with a normal chest x-ray and renal stone CT, did not put the aortic dissection diagnosis on the top of my list. That being said, CT with IV contrast is the mainstay of diagnosing aortic dissection, as the false lumen has slower flow (better illustrated in CT). MRI can also be used but this patient has a pacemaker, prohibiting MRI.[5]

This patient was very fortunate in that he had an uncomplicated surgical repair and was discharged home without any further sequelae. Future learning points for me include the understanding that while uncommon, dissection occurs in 3 per 100,000 persons annually and it carries a 1% mortality rate per hour if left untreated.[6,7]

In conclusion, clinical presentations of aortic dissection may vary and some presentations are atypical such as found in this patient. Thus, due to its critical nature acute aortic dissection should be kept near the top of a differential diagnosis in a patient with similar symptoms. Rapid identification and treatment of acute aortic dissection significantly reduces the morbidity and mortality of this diagnosis. Once this patient has been treated and discharged, he will need close follow-up for blood pressure control and annual imaging using CT with contrast.

References

1. Meisel J, Cottrell D. Differential of chest pain in an adult. http://www.uptodate.com/contents/differential-diagnosis-of-chest-pain-in-adults. Updated February 25, 2015.

2. Fishman M, Aronson M. Differential of abdominal pain in an adult. UpToDate. 2014. http://www.uptodate.com/contents/differential-diagnosis-of-abdominal-pain-in-adults.

3. Kendall J, Moreira M. Evaluation of the adult with abdominal pain in the emergency department. http://www.uptodate.com/contents/evaluation-of-the-adult-with-abdominal-pain-in-the-emergency-department. Updated October 14, 2015.

4. Brusch J, Bronze M. Medscape. Urinary tract infection in males; emedicine. April 1, 2014. http://emedicine.medscape.com/article/231574-treatment.

5. Wiesenfarth J. Acute aortic dissection. Medscape. http://emedicine.medscape.com/article/756835-overview. Updated August 19, 2015.

6. Aldeen A, Rosiere L. Focus On: Acute Aortic Dissection. ACEP News. July 2009. http://www.acep.org/Clinical---Practice-Management/Focus-On--Acute-Aortic-Dissection/.

7. Mancini M. Medscape, emedicine. Aortic dissection treatment and management. http://emedicine.medscape.com/article/2062452-treatment. Updated December 2, 2015.

CASE 9

Helen-Marie Molnar

Helen-Marie Molnar is an ACNP and a FNP with over 25 years of experience in cardiology, both inpatient and outpatient. She currently works in an outpatient cardiology practice at the University of Virginia Health System.

CASE INFORMATION

Chief Complaint
A 72-year-old man (FT) is brought to the emergency room by the rescue squad after he passed out at home.

❓ What is the potential cause?

Case Analysis: Syncope has a long list of etiologies, many of which can be life threatening. I need to start by evaluating the causes which are the most life threatening, then consider more common causes, then entertain less likely possibilities if needed.

Comprehensive Differential Diagnoses for Patient with Syncope[1,2]

Life-threatening conditions requiring immediate treatment:
1. Cardiac syncope: arrhythmia, myocardial ischemia/infarction, structural/valvular abnormalities (eg, aortic stenosis), cardiac tamponade, and pacemaker malfunction
2. Blood loss from trauma, gastrointestinal bleeding, ruptured aortic aneurysm, ruptured spleen, in women—ruptured ovarian cyst, ruptured ectopic pregnancy
3. Pulmonary embolism (PE)
4. Subarachnoid hemorrhage (if the patient had severe headache and then syncope)
5. Seizure (technically not true syncope but should be considered)
6. Stroke (technically not true syncope but should be considered)

Common causes:
1. Neurocardiogenic syncope (also known as vasovagal syncope or reflex syncope): vasovagal response from emotional distress such as fear, instrumentation, blood phobia; carotid sinus syncope; situational

(cough, sneeze, GI stimulation such as swallowing, defecation, visceral pain, micturition, postexercise, postprandial, and others such as laughter, playing brass instruments, weightlifting); and atypical forms without apparent triggers or with an atypical presentation

2. Orthostatic syncope from loss of intravascular volume or failure/instability of the autonomic nervous system
3. Medications causing orthostasis or cardiotoxicity including diuretics, vasodilators, calcium channel blockers, β-blockers, α-blockers, medications that affect the QTC (antipsychotics, antiemetics), muscle relaxants, tricyclic antidepressants
4. Neurologic: subarachnoid hemorrhage, transient ischemic attack, subclavian steal syndrome, complex migraine headache
5. Metabolic (hypoglycemia, hypoxemia)
6. Psychiatric (psychogenic pseudosyncope)

Rare causes: atrial myxoma, Takayasu arteritis, systemic mastocytosis, carcinoid

CASE INFORMATION

General Survey and History of Present Illness

As soon as I walk in the room, I can tell a lot just by looking at the patient. He is lying comfortably on the bed at a 30° angle, his skin is pink, he does not appear to be short of breath or in pain, he is conversing normally with his wife and son, his face is symmetric, and he is using both upper extremities equally. I start by asking the patient if he can tell me what happened. He tells me he has been feeling a little lightheaded when he stands up, but this time it was much worse and everything started to get dark like he was in a tunnel. That was the last thing he remembers until he woke up on the floor looking up at his family. He denies injury except for a sore right knee and elbow. He says this is the first time he has passed out. He denies having chest pain, but he does admit to having some shortness of breath when walking up stairs or inclines over the past 6 months. He denies waking up at night short of breath, using more pillows to sleep, sleeping in a recliner, or having lower extremity edema. I seek confirmation from his family at the bedside, and they nod in agreement. I ask them how long he was unconscious, and his son replies, "He was out for maybe 5 seconds. He didn't hit his head. I was right there." I ask them if they saw any shaking of his limbs, any loss of bowel or bladder function, or any confusion after he woke up, and they reply, "No." I then ask them if they have noticed anything else or have anything else to add. His wife states, "He has seemed a little more short of breath recently and has not been as active as he used to be. I told him he should see his cardiologist but he wanted to wait until his next appointment next month."

At the same time I am questioning the patient, the nurses are placing him on the cardiac monitor, obtaining vital signs and an ECG. I note that he is in normal sinus rhythm (NSR) without ectopy at a rate of 66 beats per minute. Right arm blood pressure 108/70 mm Hg, left arm blood pressure 104/68 mm Hg, respiratory rate 18/min, T 36.8°C oral, SaO$_2$ 97% on room air. His ECG shows NSR with increased QRS voltage consistent with left ventricular hypertrophy. It does not show ST elevation and looks the same as the previous ECG stored in the electronic medical record 1 year ago. I ask his family if he was speaking normally when he woke up, and if he was able to move all of his extremities without difficulty. They reply affirmatively. I then ask the patient if he has been eating and drinking normally or if he has been sick recently. He states he has been in his usual state of health until today. I also ask him if he has started any new medications recently. "Yeah, my primary care physician said my blood pressure was too high a month ago. I think it was about 148/80, so he started me on… (looking at his wife) What's the name of that new pill?" She replies "it starts with 'H,'…'HC'…. Oh, I don't know. Here, I have a list of your medications in my purse." She pulls out the list. He is on aspirin 81 mg/day, lisinopril 40 mg/day, metoprolol XL 50 mg/day, and the new pill is hydrochlorothiazide 25 mg/day.

Past Medical History

I ask him about his past medical history. He states he sees his PCP and his cardiologist on a regular basis. His cardiologist, he says, has been following his heart murmur closely over the last 5 years. He also says he has a history of hypertension (HTN), "mild" diabetes which is diet controlled, kidney stones (last one 20 years ago), and arthritis. When I review the hospital's electronic medical record, I see that the patient has been followed for aortic stenosis by his cardiologist. The last echocardiogram, performed 6 months ago, showed moderate aortic stenosis and normal left ventricular systolic function, ejection fraction 65%, and mild left ventricular hypertrophy. He is scheduled to see his cardiologist next month for his routine 6-month appointment.

❓ What are the pertinent positives from the information given so far?

- A history of moderate aortic stenosis
- Recent onset of orthostatic lightheadedness with prodromal symptoms before passing out
- Mild dyspnea on exertion
- Recently started on a diuretic

? What are the significant negatives from the information given so far?

- No chest pain or ECG changes to suggest ischemia or infarction
- No arrhythmias on telemetry
- No history of pacemaker
- No heart failure symptoms
- No unilateral leg edema or sudden onset shortness of breath to suggest pulmonary embolism
- No seizure-like activity or confusion after the event
- No facial droop or slurred speech
- No recent illness
- No melena or other bleeding
- No apparent significant injury from the fall

? Can the information gathered so far be restated in a single sentence highlighting the pieces that narrow down the cause? Putting the information gathered so far in a single statement—a problem representation—sets the state for gathering more information and determining the cause.

Given the information acquired so far, the problem representation in this case might be "a 72-year-old man with known moderate aortic stenosis by echo 6 months ago presents with a witnessed syncopal episode preceded by lightheadedness after being started recently on a diuretic."

? How does this information affect the list of possible causes?

Case Analysis: So far, I am strongly considering that the recently added diuretic may have caused volume depletion and orthostatic hypotension and that he did not tolerate this due to his aortic stenosis. There are some diagnoses that can be established quickly, but to do this, I have lowered my index of suspicion for many other diagnoses and continue to keep an open mind while gathering more data.

The lack of chest pain and absence of ECG changes argue against myocardial ischemia or infarction. The absence of acute shortness of breath, the normal SaO2, and the lack of ECG changes of right heart strain argue against a large pulmonary embolism. The prodromal symptoms of lightheadedness argue against an arrhythmic cause since there are often no warning symptoms prior to an arrhythmia severe enough to cause syncope.

He had a syncopal episode which was witnessed, and this is very helpful. His loss of consciousness was very brief, there was no seizure-like activity, and he did not hit his head. He is also conversing and moving his extremities normally, which makes stroke very unlikely. I will do a full neurologic examination very shortly, but I do not suspect a stroke based on the information gathered so far.

He has not been sick, has been eating and drinking normally, and has had no melena or bleeding, which argue against additional causes of volume depletion.

CASE INFORMATION

Review of Systems

- Constitutional: Denies fevers or chills, appetite has been good.
- Cardiovascular: + for syncope and orthostatic lightheadedness when changing from a sitting to standing position. The patient denies chest pain, pressure, tightness, or achiness as well as arm, neck, or jaw pain. He also denies orthopnea, paroxysmal nocturnal dyspnea, edema, and palpitations.
- Pulmonary: + for mild dyspnea on exertion, denies sudden onset of shortness of breath
- Gastrointestinal: Denies nausea, vomiting, diarrhea, melena, bright red blood per rectum. Last BM yesterday morning.
- Genitourinary: + for nocturia two times/night, which is stable over many years. Denies dysuria, hematuria, and odoriferous urine.
- Neurologic: Denies unilateral weakness, diplopia, difficulty with expressive or receptive language, and states he does not feel off balance when walking. Reports a rare headache which is easily controlled with acetaminophen, which is unchanged over "many years." Last headache was 3 to 4 months ago and described as fairly mild.
- Endocrine: Denies polyuria, polyphagia, and polydipsia.

Physical Examination

- Vital signs: Right arm blood pressure 108/70 mm Hg, left arm blood pressure 104/68 mm Hg, no pulsus paradoxus, heart rate 66 beats per minute and regular, respiratory rate 18/min, temperature 36.8°C oral, SaO$_2$ 97% on room air. BMI 28. Fingerstick blood glucose is 118.
- Constitutional: The patient is a well-appearing white male in no acute distress.

- Head/eyes/ears/nose/throat: Normocephalic, atraumatic. Pupils are equal, round, and reactive to light and accommodation.
- Neck: Delayed and diminished bilateral carotid upstrokes with bruits vs referred murmur from aortic valve. Jugular venous pressure (JVP) 5 cm.
- Cardiovascular: S1, S2 regular with a 3/6 harsh late peaking crescendo-decrescendo systolic murmur at the base of the heart with radiation to the carotids but also heard throughout the precordium. Absent A2 (absent aortic component of the second heart sound). Normal point of maximal impulse (PMI) located in the fifth intercostal space, midclavicular line (ICS MCL). No left ventricular (LV) heave. No rubs or gallops. Radial, femoral, and pedal pulses 3+ palpable and equal bilaterally. No femoral bruits.
- Pulmonary: Lungs clear to auscultation with good air movement throughout. No rhonchi, rales, or wheezes.
- Gastrointestinal: Soft and nontender with active bowel sounds. No hepatosplenomegaly. No abdominal bruit.
- Integumentary: Pink, warm, and dry. Brisk capillary refill. No cyanosis or edema. Normal skin turgor. Superficial scrapes with mild erythema noted on the right elbow and knee without edema.
- Neurological: Alert, oriented ×3. Moves all extremities with 5/5 strength bilaterally. Cranial nerves II-XII intact. Speech is fluent.

❓ What elements of the review of systems and physical examination should be added to the list of pertinent positives?

- 3/6 harsh late peaking crescendo-decrescendo systolic murmur at the base of the heart with radiation to the carotids
- Delayed and diminished carotid upstrokes
- Absent A2

❓ What elements of the review of systems and physical examination should be added to the significant negatives list?

- No jugular venous distention (JVD)
- Heart sounds are clearly audible, no pulsus paradoxus
- No leg swelling (or any swelling)
- Normal neuro examination

❓ How does this information affect the list of possible causes?

Case Analysis: The cardiac examination is consistent with severe aortic stenosis, worse than what was described by the last echocardiogram, so I am strongly considering this as the most likely etiology of the patient's syncope. The rest of the physical examination and review of systems do not point to an alternative diagnosis. The prodromal symptom of lightheadedness prior to syncope helps preclude a sudden onset arrhythmia such as ventricular tachycardia or ventricular fibrillation, which often has no warning symptoms prior to syncope. The lack of anginal symptoms and ischemic changes on the ECG makes myocardial ischemia or infarction unlikely. The lack of JVD, low QRS voltage on the ECG, and pulsus paradoxus, as well as the clearly audible heart sounds, argue against a significant pericardial effusion or cardiac tamponade. The pink skin and absence of recent trauma or known bleeding argue against significant anemia, but I will get a complete blood count (CBC) to confirm this. The normal oxygen saturation, lack of unilateral leg swelling, and absence of acute onset shortness of breath argue against a large pulmonary embolism. The absence of neurologic signs or symptoms helps rule out a stroke. The patient did not complain of a severe headache and then have syncope, so a subarachnoid hemorrhage is unlikely. The witnessed event with the absence of tonic-clonic activity or postevent confusion makes seizure highly unlikely.

? What diagnostic testing should be done and in what order?

The vital signs and ECG have already been done since they should be obtained immediately upon arrival to the emergency department. I would not do orthostatic blood pressures on this patient who has an examination consistent with severe aortic stenosis because I do not want to precipitate another episode of syncope. The patient is on continuous telemetry, which shows normal sinus rhythm without ectopy. Laboratory evaluation should include a comprehensive chemistry, which is normal except for a mildly low sodium of 133 mEq/L from the hydrochlorothiazide (not significant), mildly elevated BUN of 28 mg/dL with a normal creatinine of 1.2 mg/dL consistent with very mild dehydration from the hydrochlorothiazide, and a mildly elevated glucose of 115 mg/dL due to his diabetes mellitus. Labs should also include a CBC with platelets (all normal with a WBC of 6000, hemoglobin of 14, hematocrit of 43, and platelet count 198,000), which rules out anemia as a cause of his syncope, troponins (negative ×3) confirming lack of myocardial injury, and brain natriuretic peptide (negative) which confirms that his recent dyspnea on exertion is not due to heart failure. Chest x-ray shows normal heart size and no acute cardiopulmonary process. A head CT is not needed since stroke and subarachnoid hemorrhage are highly unlikely, and the family confirmed no head injury when he fell.

Based on the data I have so far, I order a transthoracic echocardiogram to be done in the emergency room to evaluate the severity of his aortic stenosis. This demonstrates severe aortic stenosis with a mean aortic valve gradient of 60 mm Hg, aortic valve area of 0.8 cm^2, normal left ventricular function with normal wall motion, and mild left ventricular hypertrophy. The echocardiogram confirms my physical examination findings. I believe the patient has severe aortic stenosis and developed orthostatic hypotension leading to syncope today due to the recent addition of hydrochlorothiazide. Severe aortic stenosis becomes my primary diagnosis.

Diagnosis and Management of Aortic Stenosis

Clinical suspicion for significant aortic stenosis is based on the cardiac examination. A mid or late peaking harsh crescendo-decrescendo systolic murmur should raise a red flag and needs to be evaluated by a transthoracic echocardiogram whether or not the patient is symptomatic. Classic examination findings of severe aortic stenosis include a harsh, late peaking crescendo-decrescendo systolic murmur best heard in the right second intercostal space with radiation to the carotids. The murmur is often also heard throughout the precordium including the apex. The intensity of the murmur does not correlate with the severity of stenosis; a soft murmur is sometimes heard even when severe disease is present. Other examination findings of severe aortic stenosis include a diminished and delayed carotid upstroke and a diminished or absent A2 (aortic component of the second heart sound). If the patient has severe left ventricular hypertrophy from pumping against a stenotic aortic valve over time, a sustained apical impulse may be felt in the fifth intercostal space midclavicular line. An apical impulse that has shifted downward and laterally is indicative of a dilated heart. This would occur if the severe aortic stenosis was unrecognized and untreated for many years causing a cardiomyopathy or if the patient had developed a cardiomyopathy from a different cause.

Classic symptoms of severe aortic stenosis include chest pain, shortness of breath, and syncope (lightheadedness, presyncope, or syncope) and indicate hemodynamically significant aortic stenosis. Decreased exercise tolerance is an early symptom that is often overlooked but may also indicate hemodynamically significant aortic stenosis. Precipitating factors should be eliminated if possible (such as reducing blood pressure medications if the blood pressure is too low, avoiding all medications that significantly reduce preload such as nitroglycerin, and using diuretics with extreme caution). I strongly advise my patients to wear a medical alert bracelet or neck chain to alert emergency health workers of the severe aortic stenosis and the need to avoid nitroglycerin (ie, "severe aortic stenosis—no NTG"). Once symptoms develop in a patient with severe aortic stenosis, the event-free survival rate is only 30% to 50% at 2 years,[3] and very strong consideration should be given to immediate aortic valve replacement.

There are two main options for aortic valve replacement (AVR). The traditional surgical open-heart AVR replaces the diseased valve with either a mechanical valve or a bioprosthetic valve. A minimally invasive approach is possible in some patients, which limits the size of the incision and typically the length of the recovery period. A newer option, the transcatheter aortic valve replacement (TAVR), also known as the transcatheter aortic valve implantation (TAVI), is a bioprosthetic valve inserted percutaneously into the orifice of the native aortic valve using either a transfemoral or a transapical approach. The heart valve team considers a patient's surgical risk to determine which approach is the best for the patient. The 2014 guidelines recommend surgical AVR for patients who have a low or intermediate surgical risk and recommend TAVR for patients who have a high or prohibitive surgical risk.[3] The guidelines recommend patients be treated at a Heart Valve Center of Excellence for optimal outcomes.

Case Follow-up

Our patient (FT) was admitted to the acute cardiology service for 2 days, and his regular cardiologist was notified of his admission. He was taken off the hydrochlorothiazide but continued on lisinopril, metoprolol, and aspirin. His blood pressure came up to 135/70 mm Hg without any other interventions, and he had no further orthostatic symptoms. However, he continued to have symptomatic severe aortic stenosis with dyspnea on exertion, which was felt to be due to the valve, so he was referred to the heart valve team for consideration of surgical AVR versus TAVR. After their evaluation and discussion with the patient and his family, he was discharged in stable condition and returned in 5 days for a minimally invasive surgical AVR without complications.

References

1. McDermott D, Quinn J. Approach to the adult patient with syncope in the emergency department. *UpToDate*. Waltham, MA. http://www.uptodate.com/contents/approach-to-the-adult-patient-with-syncope-in-the-emergency-department. Accessed July 25, 2014.
2. Olshansky B. Pathogenesis and etiology of syncope. In: Ganz LI, Yeon SB, eds. *UpToDate*. Waltham, MA. Accessed July 25, 2014.
3. Nishimura RA, Otto CM, Bonow RO, et al. 2014 AHA/ACC guideline for the management of patients with valvular heart disease: a report of the American College of Cardiology/American Heart Association Task Force on Practice Guidelines. *J Am Coll Cardiol*. 2014;63(22):e57-e185. doi:10.1016/j.jacc.2014.02.536.

CASE 10

Shawn Floyd

Shawn Floyd is a Transplant NP with the Cardiopulmonary Transplant Team at the University of Virginia Health System. He manages patients from postoperative ICU to the outpatient clinic and all stages of posttransplant care.

CASE INFORMATION

Chief Complaint

Rob, a 34-year-old male, who underwent a bilateral lung transplant for cystic fibrosis 20 months ago, now presents to an emergency department (ED) in his hometown after coughing up approximately ¼ cup of blood over the course of a few hours.

General Survey and History of Present Illness

The patient's episode of hemoptysis is preceded by a 2-month history of intermittent mild cough that is not consistently productive. He denies any fevers, chills, nausea, and vomiting, but does report shortness of breath with exertion and malaise, which is similar to his baseline since undergoing lung transplantation 20 months ago. Because he is hemodynamically stable and the only sign of infection is a slight elevation in WBC to 11,000 with a left shift, he is not admitted to his local hospital from the ED. Instead, the ED doctor notifies the transplant center and Rob is scheduled to be seen in the lung transplant clinic the following the day.

Rob presents to the transplant clinic and is seen by me as I am the nurse practitioner who follows him for his posttransplant care. He is unchanged since his last visit to the transplant clinic except for the new onset of hemoptysis. Since his ED visit on the previous day, he has continued to cough up approximately ½ cup of old blood clots and mucous plugs.

❓ What is the potential cause?

Case Analysis: Hemoptysis in a lung transplant patient is a significant danger. If the hemoptysis represents a vascular complication of the transplant surgery, it could be immediately life threatening. If the hemoptysis is due to an infection, there is time to do a more extensive workup, but delays in treatment will be detrimental and are to be avoided. Careful consideration and a comprehensive differential diagnosis list that is specific to the patient's history of lung transplantation are essential to identifying the cause of Rob's hemoptysis.

Differential Diagnoses of Hemoptysis

- Airway diseases: acute or chronic bronchitis, airway trauma, bronchiectasis, bronchovascular fistulae, Dieulafoy disease (superficial, subepithelial bronchial artery), foreign bodies, neoplasms[1,2]
- Pulmonary parenchymal diseases: genetic defect in connective tissue (Ehlers-Danlos vascular type), infection especially tuberculosis, pneumonia, mycetoma, or lung abscess[1,2]
- Inflammatory or immune disorders: granulomatosis with polyangiitis (Wegener), Goodpasture syndrome, idiopathic pulmonary hemosiderosis, lupus pneumonitis[1,2]
- Pulmonary vascular disorders: left atrial hypertension, pulmonary arteriovenous malformations, pulmonary thromboembolism[1,2]
- Other causes: bevacizumab treatment, catamenial hemoptysis, coagulopathy, cocaine use, cryptogenic, iatrogenic, nitrogen dioxide toxicity[1,2]

CASE INFORMATION

Past Medical History

- Cystic fibrosis
- Cystic fibrosis related diabetes
- Osteopenia
- Immune thrombocytopenia
- Osteopenia

Past Surgical History

- Nasal polypectomy twice, 7 and 10 years ago
- Percutaneous endoscopic gastrostomy tube placement, 7 years ago
- Bilateral lung transplants, 20 months ago

Family History

- Paternal grandmother deceased, positive for colon cancer
- Paternal grandfather alive and well
- Maternal grandmother alive, with chronic obstructive pulmonary disease (COPD)
- Maternal grandfather alive, with hypertension, hyperlipidemia, stroke
- Father alive, with hypertension, and obesity

- Mother alive, with obesity
- Sister alive and well

Social History

Nonsmoker, nondrinker, never been sexually active, denies any substance abuse. Yearly flu shots and currently up to date with vaccinations and health maintenance.

Medication List

- Alendronate (Fosamax) 70 mg by mouth every 7 days
- Ascorbic acid 500 mg by mouth daily
- Azithromycin (Zithromax) 500 mg tablet by mouth three times a week
- Calcium carbonate-vitamin D (calcium + D) 600–200 mg-unit tabs 1 tablet daily
- Cholecalciferol (vitamin D) 2000 units caps 1 capsule by mouth two times daily
- Creon 24000 units capsules, 8 capsules with meals and 4 with snacks
- Cyclobenzaprine (Flexeril) 5 mg tablet by mouth three times daily as needed for muscle spasms
- Dapsone 100 mg tablet by mouth daily
- Docusate sodium (Colace) 100 mg capsule by mouth two times daily
- Duloxetine (Cymbalta) 30 mg capsule by mouth daily
- Esomeprazole (Nexium) 40 mg capsule by mouth every morning
- Insulin aspart (NovoLog FlexPen) 100 unit/mL, 10 units subcutaneously three times daily (before meals)
- Insulin glargine (Lantus SoloSTAR) 100 unit/mL injection 11 units subcutaneously daily
- Loratadine (Claritin) 10 mg one tablet daily
- Magnesium oxide (Mag-Ox) 400 mg by mouth two times daily
- Multiple vitamin (multivitamins) by mouth daily
- Mycophenolate (CellCept) 250 mg capsule by mouth twice daily
- Prednisone (Deltasone) 5 mg tablet by mouth daily
- Tacrolimus (Prograf) 0.5 mg capsule, 3 capsules by mouth two times daily
- Ursodiol (Actigall) 300 mg capsule by mouth daily

Review of Systems

- General: States he has been well with the exception of the recent cough and bloody sputum. Denies fevers, night sweats, or recent weight loss.
- Head/eyes/ears/nose/throat: Complains of sinus congestion and a small amount of old blood with daily sinus rinses, no hearing problems, wears corrective glasses (no changes in over a year), no changes in vision.

- Cardiovascular: Denies chest pain, palpitations, and orthopnea.
- Pulmonary: Denies shortness of breath and wheezing. Denies smoking, use of any inhalants (recreational or environmental). Endorses hemoptysis as noted in chief complaint.
- Gastrointestinal: No nausea, vomiting or constipation. Occasional diarrhea, occasional reflux symptoms.
- Genitourinary: Denies dysuria and hematuria.
- Integumentary: Notes that his skin is fragile.
- Musculoskeletal: Generalized myalgia and arthralgia for the last 2 months.
- Neurological: Occasional headaches.
- Lymphatic: Denies presence of any nodes.
- Hematologic: Easy bruising, nose bleeds.
- Endocrine: High blood sugars with diet changes. Denies thirst and frequent urination. Denies sweating or hot/cold intolerance.

Physical Assessment

- Vital signs: heart rate 98 beats per minute, blood pressure 145/88, respirations 16 breaths per minute, oxygen saturation 96% on room air, height 5'6", weight 124 lb, body mass index 19.3
- General: well-developed, well-nourished, white male in no acute distress
- Head/eyes/ears/nose/throat: head normocephalic, atraumatic, pupils equal, round, and reactive to light and accommodation, ears no gross abnormalities, nose with bilateral non-occlusive polyps, oropharynx clear with adult dentation, no cervical adenopathy.
- Cardiovascular: regular rate, no murmurs, gallops, rubs, normal S1 and S2. Carotids: strong bilateral pulses, no bruits heard. Peripheral pulses 4+ bilaterally
- Pulmonary: symmetrical chest rise, no crepitus or areas that elicit pain, on percussion, normal resonance in all fields except right upper lobe and left lower lobe dullness, clear to auscultation bilaterally with diminished sounds in right upper lobe.
- Gastrointestinal: percutaneous gastrostomy button in place in right lower quadrant, bowel sounds present, abdomen soft, nontender, nondistended.
- Rectum: deferred
- Genitalia/pelvic: deferred
- Neurologic: cranial nerve II thru XII grossly intact, normal mood and affect, mild bilateral fine motor hand tremors
- Lymphatic: no lymphadenopathy

❓ What are the pertinent positives from the information given so far?

Vitals stable, coughing ½ cup of blood and clots, dullness to percussion, and decreased breath sounds in right lower lobe

❓ What are the significant negatives from the information given so far?

No palpable nodes, afebrile, no night sweats, no weight loss, normal activity tolerance

Case Analysis: The fact that this patient underwent lung transplant only 20 months ago means that the differential for hemoptysis will be very broad and inclusive of diagnoses that are more likely in an immunocompromised patient, such as infections with opportunistic organisms. But I am able to quickly eliminate a number of potential diagnoses including cocaine use, nitrogen dioxide toxicity, and Dieulafoy disease because he denies drug use, exposures to any inhalants, and his pulmonary vasculature was reconstructed at time of transplant. He is also not on any drugs that may potentially increase bleeding such as bevacizumab. However, all the others on the differential must still be considered and I will keep them in mind as I continue my evaluation of the patient. The first diagnostic test I need to review is the patient's chest film to determine if it has changed since his last chest film. Until I do so, it is difficult to eliminate any other potential causes of hemoptysis. His last chest x-ray is shown in Figure 10-1.

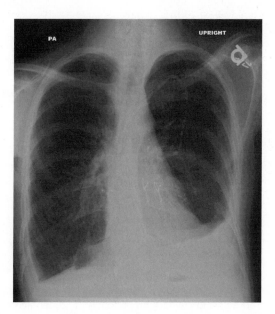

Figure 10-1   Chest x-ray 1 year posttransplant.

❓ What other diagnostic tests are necessary at this time?

Case Analysis: His 1-year posttransplant film is clear with only an elevated left hemidiaphragm, which represents atelectasis or vagus nerve injury. I order a repeat chest x-ray on his visit today to look for potential causes of the new hemoptysis. A PA and lateral chest x-ray is one of the most effective strategies to look for abnormalities when ruling out conditions on the hemoptysis differential diagnoses. The x-ray is noninvasive, and quickly available and can rule out major infiltrates, some airway disruptions, and interstitial and alveolar processes.

Additional diagnostic data to obtain include a complete blood count (CBC) with differential, platelets, coagulation studies, metabolic profile, and immunosuppressive drug levels.

📱 CASE INFORMATION

Laboratory values and new x-ray (*Figures 10-2A and B*) below:

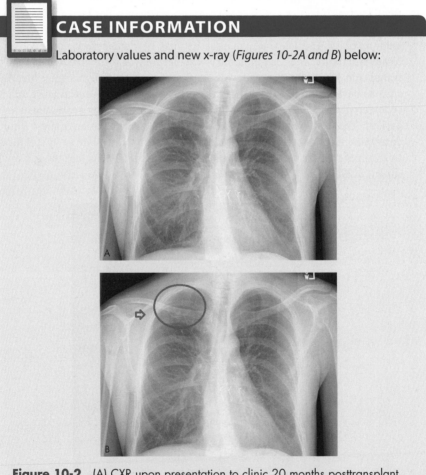

Figure 10-2 (A) CXR upon presentation to clinic 20 months posttransplant. (B) Circled area points to cavitary lesion found on 20-month posttransplant film.

Lab	Normal Range	Patient Value
WBC	4,000–11,000 cells/µL	7.999
Bands	0%–9%	14 (H)
RBC	4.60–6.20 M/µL	4.29 (L)
Hemoglobin	14.0–18.0 g/dL	13.0 (L)
Hematocrit	40.0%–52.0%	37.5 (L)
MCV	83.0–95.0 fL	87.4
MCH	28.0–32.0 pg	30.3
MCHC	32.0–36.0 g/dL	34.7
RDW	11.0%–14.0%	13.2
Platelets	150–450 K/µL	163
MPV		11.1
Sodium	136–145 mmol/L	140
Potassium	3.5–4.5 mmol/L	4.5
Chloride	98–107 mmol/L	109 (H)
CO_2	22–29 mmol/L	24
BUN	8.9–20.6 mg/dL	22 (H)
Creatinine	0.7–1.3 mg/dL	0.8
Glucose	74–99 mg/dL	108 (H)
Calcium	8.4–10.2 mg/dL	8.5
Calculated GFR (mL/min/1.73 m^2)		>60
ProTime	11.9–15.2 s	13.8
ProTime INR	0.9–1.2	1.0
PTT, average	24.1–35.8 s	33.3
Magnesium	1.6–2.6 mg/dL	1.9
Phosphorus	2.3–4.7 mg/dL	4.0
Tacrolimus	5–17 ng/dL	7.2

❓ What elements of the review of systems and physical examination should be added to the list of pertinent positives?

Clinically stable, cavitary lesion in right upper lobe on chest x-ray, resolved elevated left hemidiaphragm, normal white cell count with shift to the left, slight anemia, elevated BUN no abnormal coagulation values, no electrolyte abnormalities, therapeutic tacrolimus immunosuppression level

---

❓ What elements of the review of systems and physical examination should be added to the significant negatives list?

Significant negatives: no abnormal coagulation values, no electrolyte abnormalities, therapeutic Tacrolimus immunosuppression level

---

❓ How does the new information from the diagnostic tests affect your differential?

Case Analysis: Comparing his current lab values to values obtained previously in the clinic confirms that they are stable. There are no red flags to suggest the need for urgent treatment such as a profound anemia due to bleeding or abnormal coagulation studies. The metabolic profile is also normal for a posttransplant patient and while his BUN is slightly elevated, this is likely due to dehydration. His white count is normal although there is a slight shift to the left. Because he is immunocompromised, he will not mount a normal white blood cell response, so I am cautious about this seemingly normal finding. I cannot rule out an active infection at this point. To determine the cause of his hemoptysis, further imaging studies are essential.

Upon review of his film I note a large cavitary lesion in the right upper lobe (circled on x-ray [Figure 10-2B]) that was not present on prior radiologic studies. The finding of a new cavitary lesion in his right upper lobe narrows my differential diagnosis significantly. I am now thinking that this lesion is the cause of the hemoptysis. My first step to further evaluate this lesion is to obtain a computed tomography (CT) scan. I have to weigh the risks of using contrast, including kidney injury, with the benefit of better visualization of his pulmonary vasculature. A CT scan with contrast will also help guide treatment if an invasive procedure is required.

Given the data accumulated so far, I can start to eliminate some of the differential diagnoses on my list and focus on others that are more likely. Knowing that he has a lesion on his chest x-ray, and relatively normal lab values, we can definitely eliminate foreign bodies, which would likely cause an increase in WBCs, catamenial hemoptysis (a rare condition that is associated with the presence of intrapulmonary or endobronchial endometrial tissue, but which is not cavitary), coagulopathy (his PT/PTT are normal), cocaine use (this effects the entire lung field not one area). Other conditions we can rule out at this time are cryptogenic, iatrogenic, and nitrogen dioxide toxicity (these generally all affect the entire lung parenchyma not one area).

To complete this workup in a timely manner, admission to the hospital is essential. The patient initially objects to the hospital admission, but once I explain that the minor cough with hemoptysis could become massive hemoptysis, he agrees to stay and undergo the necessary workup to determine the cause of the lesion and to ensure we can vigilantly monitor him for excessive bleeding. Because the patient is immunocompromised, I need to obtain multiple studies quickly to determine the next course of action. His white blood cell count did have a slight shift to the left, so infection remains high on the differential and I cannot exclude other diagnoses that could result in hemopty-sis and/or infection at this point.

The following potential diagnoses remain on my differential:

Airway diseases: bronchovascular fistulae, neoplasms[1,2]

Pulmonary parenchymal diseases: infection especially tuberculosis, pneumonia, mycetoma, or lung abscess[1,2]

Inflammatory or immune disorders: granulomatosis with polyangiitis (Wegener), Goodpasture syndrome, idiopathic pulmonary hemosiderosis[1,2]

Pulmonary vascular disorders: left atrial hypertension, pulmonary arteriovenous malformations, pulmonary thromboembolism[1,2]

CASE INFORMATION

Diagnostic Tests and Results

Many of the diagnoses remaining on the differential put the patient at high risk for massive hemoptysis. The first test I order upon admission to the hospital is a CT (with contrast) (Figure 10-3). The CT scan shows that the lesion is in the lung parenchyma and does not appear to have any large blood vessels in it or around it.

The CT findings tell me that Rob has a large cavitary lesion that appears to have fluid in it, but due to the inflammatory changes noted in the right upper lobe, a neoplasm cannot be excluded at this time. A bronchoscopy with brushings of the area is performed and the pulmonologist weighs the risks versus benefits of performing a needle biopsy. A CT-guided biopsy of the lesion is considered, but because the lesion does not communicate with the pleura, the procedure puts the patient at high risk for pneumothorax.

A bronchoscopic biopsy of the area is obtained without complication. The lesion extends into the right middle lobe but tissue analysis shows only focal hemorrhage and hemosiderin-laden macrophages. All the cultures for bacteria, fungal, viral, and acid-fast bacteria are negative for several days. The bronchial brushings and biopsy for cytopathology do not show any signs of malignancy, but tissue samples are poor quality so neoplasm can not be excluded at this point. Unfortunately, after the bronchoscopy Rob began to cough up more blood and to have decreasing oxygen saturations with activity.

At this point, I consult thoracic surgery for evaluation and possible open lung biopsy. These options present significant challenges for two main reasons. First, the bilateral lung transplants 20 months ago produce a significant surgical challenge now in terms of gaining access to the lesion. The second is that the patient is maintained on oral corticosteroids and tacrolimus to prevent rejection. The use of chronic oral corticosteroids results

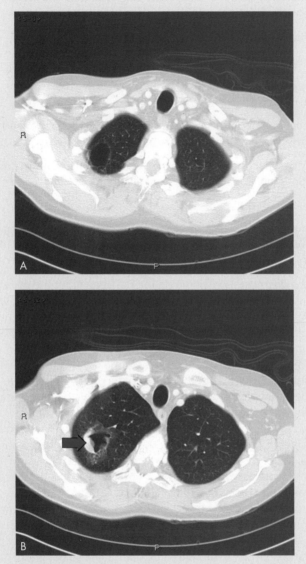

Figure 10-3   (A) CT of thorax on admission. Both CT views demonstrate the cavitary lesion in the RUL. (B) The arrow points to blood in the cavitation.

in very friable tissues and even with a small needle insertion through the chest wall, the chance of causing a pneumothorax is significantly high. At the same time, any open procedure that causes an airway disruption will take a very long time to heal.

After consultation with the thoracic surgery team it is decided that CT-guided biopsy is the best option. Though the inherent risks are high, other options are even more risky. To ensure Rob's safety, thoracic surgery is on standby for urgent chest tube placement and possible thoracoscopy if needed. Fortunately, the CT-guided biopsy and fine needle aspiration (FNA) of this lesion is completed without major complications and this core sampling was sent for analysis.

The results from the FNA are negative for malignancy but positive for fungal changes on cytopathology. When the fungal changes are noted, a series of serum fungal markers are ordered including a galactomannan antigen test (which detects aspergillosis) and this comes back grossly positive. At this point, Rob is started on broad spectrum antifungal coverage to cover potential spillage of material outside of the lesion. The culture returns 3 days later with a final result identifying the presence of *Aspergillus fumigatus*. *Aspergillus* species are the second most common invasive fungal infections in solid organ transplant patients.[3] At this point the diagnosis is clear: the patient's lesion is caused by invasive aspergillosis that has resulted in hemoptysis.

Diagnosis and Management of Aspergillosis

This large lung lesion is recognized as a chronic aspergilloma; resection is necessary to prevent dissemination in this immunocompromised patient. Given the size and location of this lesion it is not possible to treat it with intravenous antifungals alone. Rob is young and in good physical shape at the time of the diagnosis, so resection is the preferred and appropriate definitive therapy. After long discussions with Rob, his family, the transplant infectious disease team, and the surgical team, Rob decides to undergo a right upper lobe resection of the aspergilloma on hospital day 5. He is managed after the operation in the cardiothoracic intensive care unit (ICU).

Rob will be treated with long-term intravenous fungal therapy for at least 3 months and closely monitored for changes in renal function throughout the treatment. His postoperative course is complicated only by small bilateral infiltrates but he recovers quickly and is transferred from the ICU to the surgical floor on postoperative day 2. Rob's hemoptysis resolves following the right upper lobe resection and he tolerates the intravenous antifungals well. He is discharged home on hospital day 19.

Long-term antifungal therapy in a patient who is immunocompromised is a standard of care. The choice of antifungal therapy depends on the underlying infection and whether it is invasive or noninvasive. The likelihood of reoccurrence is high if not identified early and treated aggressively. In Rob's case, the outcome of aggressive and evidence-based care is excellent.

References

1. Steven E, Weinberger MD. Etiology and evaluation of hemoptysis in adults. Last updated August 25, 2014. http://www.uptodate.com/contents/etiology-and-evaluation-of-hemoptysis-in-adults.
2. Baughman RP, Lower EE. Diagnosis of pneumonia in immunocompromised patient. In: Baughman RP, Lower EE, Agusti C, Torres A, eds. *Pulmonary Infection in the Immunocompromised Patient: Strategies for Management*. Hoboken, NJ: Wiley;2009:53-80.
3. Neofytos D, Fishman JA, Horn D, et al. Epidemiology and outcome of invasive fungal infections in solid organ transplant recipients. *Transpl Infect Dis*. 2010;12(3):220-229.

CASE 11

Kwame Asante Akuamoah-Boateng

Kwame Asante Akuamoah-Boateng has over 10 years of experience in the surgical trauma setting as a nurse and an ACNP. He precepts ACNP students and is an ACNP in the Division of Trauma, Critical Care, and Emergency Surgery at Virginia Commonwealth University in Richmond, VA.

PART 1

CASE INFORMATION

Chief Complaint

An 86-year-old female is brought to the emergency room by her caregiver son, with complaints of worsening abdominal pain, nausea, and vomiting over the last 36 hours. She is admitted to the acute care surgical ward.

❓ What is the potential cause?

Case Analysis: Acute escalating abdominal pain with nausea and vomiting can be caused by life-threatening conditions such as myocardial infarction or ischemic bowel, or by a less severe condition such as acute gastritis. Rapid assessment including a focused history and physical examination and appropriate diagnostic studies is imperative to identify the presence or absence of the most critical conditions. I begin by developing a comprehensive differential and then identify the diagnoses that are potentially immediately life threatening.

> **Comprehensive Differential Diagnoses for Patient With Acute Abdominal Pain (the Most Life-Threatening Conditions Are Underlined)**
>
> - Neurologic: stroke
> - Pulmonary: pneumonia, pulmonary embolus (PE)
> - Cardiovascular: myocardial infarction (MI), ruptured abdominal aortic aneurysm (AAA), aortic dissection
> - Gastrointestinal: mesenteric ischemic bowel, perforation of gastrointestinal tract such as peptic ulcer, acute bowel obstruction, volvulus, cholecystitis, appendicitis, diverticulitis, constipation, gastritis, colitis, foodborne disease, toxic megacolon, splenic rupture, tumor
> - Genitourinary: urinary tract infection, urinary retention or obstruction, nephrolithiasis, ruptured ovarian cyst
> - Endocrine: diabetic ketoacidosis, adrenal insufficiency, myxedema, thyrotoxicosis

- Metabolic: dehydration, electrolyte imbalance, hyperglycemia, <u>hypoglycemia</u>, <u>hyperkalemia</u>, hepatic encephalopathy
- Exogenous: medication side effect or interaction or withdrawal, <u>drug overdose</u>, cancer

CASE INFORMATION

General Survey and History of Present Illness

I begin my evaluation with a general survey of the patient. The patient is a frail elderly lady laying on the stretcher in the fetal position. She is well groomed, but appears very uncomfortable. She is alert and cooperative, but moaning as she speaks. I ask the patient, "What brought you in to see us in the emergency room today." With a soft voice the patient states: "My belly hurts and I can't take it no more." I ask her about the onset, duration, and characteristic of the pain. She states: "it's been going on for almost two days, I woke up in the morning feeling very nauseated, I thought it was the cheeseburger I ate; however, my belly started to hurt and I started vomiting. I have been vomiting green liquid since it started." She denies seeing any blood in her vomit, and she denies any diarrhea. She states the pain began with intermittent cramping and that it covers all of her abdomen, and has become more consistent over the past few hours. She also notes that her abdomen feels distended and tender when touched. She denies chest pain, back pain, and any history of abdominal trauma. She says that her vomiting has gotten worse in the last few hours, as she has vomited almost a cup of liquid every hour. The patient rates her pain as a 12 on a scale where 10 is the worst pain, and she notes that nothing makes it worse or better. She tried ibuprofen but it did not help.

As I ask additional questions about her past medical history, the patient becomes less interactive and defers to the son. The son states: "She has had high blood pressure for a long time, and the doctors also said she has a big heart. She quickly gets very tired and short of breath because of her heart." He also adds that the patient regularly takes all her medications but that for the past 2 days, starting when her belly started hurting, she has been unable to take them.

Medication List (Taken From Patient's Son)

- Lisinopril 5 mg by mouth once a day
- Metoprolol XL (Toprol) 25 mg by mouth twice a day
- Furosemide 40 mg by mouth once a day
- Amlodipine 10 mg by mouth once a day

Past Surgical History

- Abdominal hernia repair, 5 years ago, without any complications

❓ **What are the pertinent positives from the information given so far?**

- The patient's abdominal pain is acute and has been progressively getting worse over the last 48 hours.
- Her pain is associated with nausea and vomiting.
- Her pain is now diffuse over the abdomen but does not radiate to chest or back.
- Her self-rated pain intensity is a 12 on a 10-point scale with 10 being the worst pain.
- She has a history of hypertension and congestive heart failure (HF).
- She had abdominal surgery 5 years ago for a hernia repair.
- She has not been able to take any of her medications for the past 36 hours.
- Her son's report and her medication regimen support a history of hypertension and HF.
- She is alert and appropriate in her responses.

❓ **What are the significant negatives from the information given so far?**

- The patient has not experienced any recent trauma.
- She denies seeing any signs of blood in her emesis.
- She has not had any diarrhea.

❓ **Does the information presented so far change your list of potential causes?**

Case Analysis: The pertinent positives and significant negatives are helpful but not definitive. Excruciating pain in this elderly patient is very concerning as it may be the result of abdominal vascular conditions such as aortic dissection or rupture of a solid organ such as the spleen or appendix. Though the pain does not radiate to the back or chest, it still does not rule out dissection or a myocardial infarction (MI). Gastric bleeding from gastritis or ulcerations caused by chronic use of NSAIDs is common in the elderly, but at this point I have little evidence that she has taken more than a single dose to decrease her stomach pain. Her history of abdominal surgery for a hernia repair 5 years ago is of interest and makes me consider a bowel obstruction due to adhesions as a potential cause of her pain, nausea, and vomiting. But, I need much more data. I proceed with the history and physical and obtain a stat electrocardiogram (ECG) because I have to immediately consider MI as a potential cause. I also order a 50 mg bolus of intravenous fentanyl to make her more comfortable.

CASE INFORMATION

Review of Systems

- Constitutional: denies fever, has had poor appetite for the past few days, unaware of any weight change, denies recent falls or injuries
- Cardiovascular: denies chest pain, leg swelling, or difficulty breathing when lying down, uses two pillows at night for comfort but denies any orthopnea
- Pulmonary: complains of shortness of breath when she ambulates for more than 30 minutes, denies cough and wheezing
- Gastrointestinal: complains of severe nausea and vomiting, denies blood in vomit or stools, no bowel movement for the past 5 days
- Genitourinary: denies blood in her urine, change in urine smell, frequency, or amount
- Musculoskeletal: denies any joint pain
- Neurology: denies any confusion, headache, numbness, or changes in speech
- Endocrine: denies changes in thirst, or urination

Physical Examination

- Vital signs: heart rate 109, blood pressure 95/50, respiratory rate 24, temperature 37.0 axillary, oxygen saturation 96% on room air, blood glucose 95, admission weight 65 kg (BMI 22.4).
- Head/eyes/ears/nose/throat: Skull is normocephalic, atraumatic, pupils are equal, round, reactive to light, buccal mucosa pale, no lesions noted on scalp, moist, has some missing teeth in upper and lower jaw, trachea midline.
- Cardiac: Tachycardia, S4 noted on auscultation, no JVD, and PMI palpated at the fifth intercostal space, nail beds are pale, cool to touch, brisk capillary refill no lower extremity edema.
- Pulmonary: Eupneic respiratory pattern, slightly tachypneic, symmetrical thoracic expansion, lungs resonant to percussion, clear breath sounds throughout lung fields.
- Gastrointestinal: Hyperactive bowel sounds in the right upper quadrant, diffuse generalized tenderness with palpation, worse on the left side of the abdomen, diffuse hyperresonance on percussion without shifting dullness, no ascites, negative psoas sign, negative Rovsing sign, negative Murphy sign, old and healed surgical scar noted at midline of abdomen, no herniation.
- Genitourinary: No CVA tenderness.
- Skin: Intact, no rashes, lesions, sores, or petechiae, decreased skin turgor.

- Neurological: No focal neurologic deficits, face symmetric, speech is clear, upper and lower extremity strength 5/5 throughout, oriented to person, place, and time, follows commands appropriately. Cranial nerves II-XII intact.
- Diagnostic testing: The ECG shows sinus tachycardia at 100 beats per minute and no ST elevation.

❓ What elements of the review of systems and the physical examination should be added to the list of pertinent positives list?

Shortness of breath with prolonged ambulation, hypotension, and tachycardia, diffuse tenderness of the abdomen, worse on the left side of the abdomen, no bowel movement for 5 days, unbearable nausea and vomiting.

❓ What elements of the review of systems and the physical examination should be added to the list of significant negatives?

The review of systems and the physical examination are both negative for focal neurological deficits. No chest pain; ECG reveals sinus tachycardia without arrhythmias or signs of ischemia. No fever, radiating pain, or signs of bleeding in her bowel movement or urine. Negative psoas, Rovsing, and Murphy signs.

❓ How does this information affect the list of possible causes?

Case Analysis: A neurological cause, such acute stroke, is very unlikely given the normal neurological examination. I am eliminating it from my differential. The patient's normal cardiac examination and ECG make arrhythmia or myocardial infarction less likely to be a cause but for now I will keep them on my differential pending additional confirmatory diagnostics. Her hypotension and tachycardia may be signs of a shock state including hypovolemic (ie, blood loss or dehydration) or septic shock, so I will continue to evaluate these signs as they may require immediate emergent interventions.

For now I continue very quickly to further consider potential diagnoses that are the cause of her abdominal pain. Her shortness of breath with prolonged ambulation and her medication history is suggestive of heart failure (HF) but nothing new. Aortic dissection cannot be ruled out yet because of the patient's history of hypertension, but she does not complain of back pain or flank pain, does not describe it as searing or sharp, and while she is uncomfortable, she is relatively stable. Pulmonary embolus (PE) is less likely as well, since there are no changes in her breathing status, she is not experiencing chest pain, her oxygen saturation is normal, and there is no obvious source of potential thrombus formation (such as leg swelling or atrial fibrillation).

The physical examination gives me more information about gastrointestinal and gallbladder causes for her symptoms. Signs of cholecystitis (Murphy sign) and appendicitis (psoas and Rovsing signs) are negative, making these diagnoses less likely though not ruled out. A splenic or other solid organ rupture is unlikely given her negative history of a recent traumatic injury and active bleeding from an ulcer is not supported in the examination or the review of systems. Mesenteric ischemia is less likely but cannot be excluded without additional data. Peptic ulcer generally presents with epigastric pain, and will remain on my differential for now though it is lower on the list. Diverticulitis is less likely as well, as her history does not support it as a cause and her pain is much greater than anticipated with diverticulitis. Urinary tract infection (UTI) in the elderly may be a source of infection and subsequent sepsis without fever but her complaints of pain are much more dramatic than generally seen with UTI.

At this point, while I still have many potentially critical diagnoses to rule out, the constellation of signs and symptoms in concert with her history of abdominal surgery (which potentially can contribute to adhesions and obstruction) makes bowel obstruction the highest on my list. Bowel obstruction often presents with peritoneal pain and shock. She has also not had a bowel movement in 5 days. So my focus is to prioritize my diagnostic information so that I can rapidly rule in this potential diagnosis while eliminating others.

The first diagnostics studies I choose will be ones that can readily be done at the bedside to help eliminate any urgent conditions. I will also proceed with placement of a nasogastric tube due to the severity of the emesis, to try to decompress her abdomen, keep her comfortable, and accurately evaluate amount and nature of the emesis.

❓ What diagnostic testing should be done immediately?

Because bowel obstruction is currently at the top of my differential, I order a stat plain abdominal x-ray to evaluate for the presence or absence of free air or bowel obstruction. I also order a chest x-ray to look for mediastinal widening to help me rule out dissection, an emergent situation. The chest x-ray will also give me additional information about possible pneumonia and the size of her heart. An ultrasound of the abdomen and/or computed tomography (CT) may be necessary depending on the results of the abdominal and chest films.

Laboratory tests that I order include a stat complete blood count (CBC) with differential, basic metabolic profile (BMP), D-dimers, and troponins. The white blood cell (WBC) will reveal if the patient has an infectious process with evidence of leukocytosis and bands (shift to the left). It will also provide information about acute bleeding (ie, drop in hemoglobin and hematocrit). If she is dehydrated from vomiting, however she may have a high hematocrit. If this is the case and she is actively bleeding, it somewhat confounds the picture so I must continue to be vigilant for other signs of bleeding. The BMP will provide information about her metabolic state. Metabolic acidosis would suggest possible sepsis or bowel ischemia. I can also evaluate other electrolytes and her renal status. Although PE is low on my differential, D-dimers are an easy screening tool to obtain and the results will help me consider whether additional diagnostics are necessary. While I do not think the etiology of her pain is cardiac, I am concerned that she is under quite a bit of stress, which may result in an MI. To that end I order troponins and serial ECGs. I also order a urinalysis to rule out UTI. If positive for nitrates, leukoesterase, and white blood cells, I will then add a urine culture as well to evaluate a bacterial source.

CASE INFORMATION

Diagnostic Testing Results

- Abdominal x-ray: Distended loops of small bowel with air-fluid levels and decompression of the bowel distally. No sign of pneumoperitoneum.
- Chest x-ray: Normal mediastinum, enlarged cardiac silhouette and some hilar engorgement, no other sign of cardiopulmonary disease.

Normal Values	Patient Values
CBC	
WBC 4,500–10,000 cells/μL	8K/μL
Hemoglobin 12.1–15.1 g/dL	12 g/dL
Hematocrit 36.1%–44.3%	36%
Platelet 150–350 K/μL	149K/μL
Neutrophils 54%–62%	62.7%
Lymphocytes 25%–33%	26.2%
Monocytes 3%–7%	5.0%
Eosinophils 1%–3%	0.9%
Basophils 0–0.75	0.2%
Band forms (above 8% is shift to left)	5.35%
Lymphocytes 22–44	3.08
Monocytes 3–6	0.79
Eosinophils 0–3	0.10
Basophils 0–1	0.02
Metabolic Profile	
Sodium (135–145)	143 mmol/L
Potassium (3.5–5.2)	4.6 mmol/L
Chloride 101–111 mmol/L	100 mmol/L

Normal Values	Patient Values
Electrolytes	
CO_2 20–29 mmol/L	22 mmol/L
Electrolytes	
BUN 7–20 mg/dL	28 mg/dL
Cr 0.8–1.4 mg/dL	0.8 mg/dL
Glucose 64–128 mg/dL	85 mg/dL
Miscellaneous	
Anion gap 12 +/−4	8 mmol/L
Troponin <0.01 ng/mL	<0.02 ng/mL
D-dimer (>250 ng/mL is positive)	50
Urinalysis	
GFR >60	75
Specific gravity 1.005–1.025	**1.025**
Nitrite	**Negative**
pH 4.5–7	**5.0**
Leukoesterase	**Negative**
Osmolality 50 to 1200 milliosmoles per kilogram (mOsm/kg)	290 mOsm/kg
Creatinine	30
Glucose	Negative
WBC	None

❓ How does this information affect the list of possible causes?

Case Analysis: Based on the abdominal x-ray, small bowel obstruction is likely and is the highest on my differential, however, to ensure I do not miss other concomitant conditions I quickly and systematically review the new information and evaluate my differential.

While I realize heart attacks in women may have atypical signs and symptoms, I can eliminate MI as a diagnosis as the patient has a negative troponin, normal ECG, and absence of chest pain, neck pain, or any other atypical findings that suggest a cardiac etiology. Aortic dissection can be eliminated from the list as the chest x-ray does not show a widened mediastinum and her pain is not in the chest or back. PE is also unlikely as the D-dimer is negative, and no other clinical signs or source of thrombus are evident. Based on the laboratory findings, there are no signs of acute anemia, no leukocytosis, and no nitrates or leukocytes in the urine. At this point I am comfortable eliminating gastrointestinal bleed as there is no physical evidence to support the diagnosis and her hematocrit is stable. Infectious causes may be eliminated from my differential as the CBC shows a normal white count, normal neutrophil count, and no shift to the left and the urinalysis shows no white cells, and negative leukoesterase. Mesenteric ischemia is now less likely with a serum bicarbonate that is normal; however, it still is important to obtain a definite radiographic study such as a CT scan of the abdomen and pelvis, as this will identify areas of decreased or absent blood flow. It will also help definitively rule out diverticulitis and appendicitis. In addition, since bowel obstruction is the highest on my differential, a CT scan will provide better resolution of the bowel obstruction including the location of the bowel obstruction, whether it is in the small or large bowel, and if it is a partial or complete obstruction.

CT With or Without Contrast

Using oral and IV contrast with an abdominal and pelvic CT scan allows for better visualization of the bowel than an x-ray. In addition it can help identify vascular abnormalities such as mesenteric ischemia. However, it is essential to be cautious when using contrast due to the risk of causing contrast-induced nephropathy. My patient is at risk for contrast-induced nephropathy as she is dehydrated due to emesis, is elderly, and has a slightly elevated BUN. Because the patient is at risk, I decide to perform the CT scan without IV contrast. If I were more concerned about the likelihood of the presence of vascular abnormalities I would increase her hydration prior to the scan since I would need to use IV contrast for the study. But for now I can focus on definitively identifying the bowel obstruction and use only oral contrast. Oral contrast is unlikely to cause nephropathy and can provide important information about the obstruction so we can determine treatment. The patient is premedicated with Zofran and then the oral contrast is administered thru the nasogastric tube (NGT).

 CASE INFORMATION

The CT scan demonstrates a distal, small bowel, partial obstruction without any additional abnormalities. At this point we can definitively state that the cause of this patient's clinical presentation is due to small bowel obstruction and other differentials may be eliminated based on radiographic, laboratory, and clinical presentations.

Diagnosis: Small Bowel Obstruction

Management

The initial management for small bowel obstruction (SBO) focuses on alleviating the discomfort the patient is experiencing using an NGT for decompression. Surgical management is considered if symptoms progress despite decompression or the patient develops hemodynamic changes. Once baseline information is obtained, a surgical consult is generally necessary in case the patient's situation worsens and surgical intervention is warranted. I contact the emergency general surgery team and a decision is made to admit the patient to the general surgery unit for further monitoring and care. An intravenous fluid infusion is started at 75 mL/h and 1 L of normal saline is given with careful monitoring given the patient's history of HF. A Foley catheter is placed at this time to ensure an accurate account of the patient's urine output.

PART 2

CASE INFORMATION

Continued

On hospital day 3, despite conservative management of the bowel obstruction and pain medication, the patient continues to experience significant abdominal pain. Over the past 24 hours, her NGT output is 2 L and her urine output is about 0.2 mL/kg/h, using her admission weight of 65 kg. Her total intake from the intravenous fluids is 1.8 L/24 h. The patient now has a new oliguria, which is defined as urine output less than 0.5 mL/kg/h. She is transferred to the intensive care unit (ICU) for further monitoring of her worsening SBO and new onset of oliguria.

With any change in the patient's clinical status, a complete physical assessment is the first step to guide diagnostic testing and management. I examine her again and notable significant changes from previous examinations are found in her vital signs and abdominal examination.

Physical Examination on Admission to ICU

- Current vital signs: HR 125 beats per minute, blood pressure 105/63 mm Hg, respiratory rate 26 breaths per minute with a labored breathing pattern, temperature 37.5°C (99.5°F) axillary, and an oxygen saturation of 96% on room air.
- Constitutional: Appears uncomfortable.
- Head/eyes/ears/nose/throat: Unchanged except for dryness noted in buccal mucosa.
- Cardiovascular: Unchanged.
- Pulmonary: Tachypnea, labored breathing, breath sounds clear to auscultation in all fields.
- Gastrointestinal: Increased abdominal distention compared to previous assessments, hyperactive bowel sounds, hyperresonant percussion, and worsening diffuse tenderness. She also has not had a bowel movement in 7 days according to chart and her NGT output drainage is 750 mL over the last 6 hours, clear bilious (greenish in color) output.
- Integumentary: Skin dry, poor skin turgor.
- Musculoskeletal: Unchanged.
- Neurological: Unchanged.

❓ Given the information obtained so far and the current clinical status of the patient, how will you restate your problem representation?

The new problem representation reads: "an 86-year-old female with history of HF with small bowel obstruction treated conservatively for the last 3 days now presents with worsening acute SBO, new onset oliguria with tachycardia and tachypnea." Her SBO will need to be surgically treated as it is not improving. And, because she now has oliguria, I must evaluate the cause and determine a treatment plan for this new condition prior to the patient going to the operating room.

❓ Of the new information provided so far, what are the pertinent positives?

Worsening distention and diffuse tenderness of the abdomen, hyperactive BS and hyperresonant percussion notes, persistent and increased tachycardia, tachypnea with labored respiratory pattern, dry mucus membranes, poor skin turgor, significant amount of NG output and oliguria, no bowel movement

❓ Of the new information provided so far, what are the significant negatives?

Afebrile, normal blood pressure, no neurologic changes, normal cardiac examination, adequate oxygen saturation on room air, clear breath sounds

❓ Based on what I know now about the patient's condition, what is the differential for her oliguria?

Case Analysis: Acute oliguria suggests underlying acute kidney injury. There are three types of conditions that can cause kidney injury and lead to oliguria and these are pre-renal conditions, intrinsic conditions, and post-renal or obstructive conditions.

1. Pre-renal causes: dehydration, abdominal compartment syndrome, HF exacerbation
2. Intrinsic causes: prolonged hypotension, sepsis, exogenous causes such as medications (ie, angiotensin-converting enzyme inhibitors and nonsteroidal anti-inflammatory drugs)
3. Post-renal causes: obstruction such as kidney stone, tumor, or Foley catheter malfunction

What labs, radiographic studies, and findings will also help differentiate the cause of the patient's oliguria?

Cumulative Intake and Output

It is essential to evaluate the patient's intake and output. She has a total of 5 L intake since admission 3 days ago and 4.5 L of NGT drainage. This is significant especially given the fact that her prehospitalization intake was low as well.

Laboratory Tests

I order a CBC with differential to evaluate for any leukocytosis and a left shift to determine if sepsis is a cause. I also order a basic metabolic panel, urine electrolytes, and a urinalysis to evaluate for increases in her blood urea nitrogen and her creatinine, metabolic acidosis, or electrolyte abnormalities especially hyperkalemia. The urinalysis and urine electrolytes will aid in reviewing any microscopic findings. With these lab results, I can calculate a fractional excretion of sodium (FENa), which helps identify whether oliguria is pre-renal, intrinsic, or post-renal failure. The kidneys generally excrete or reabsorb sodium as needed to ensure intravascular homeostasis. In pre-renal causes of acute kidney injury, such as dehydration and hypovolemia, the kidneys reabsorb sodium as a compensatory mechanism to increase the intravascular oncotic pressure and retain fluid. Thus the FENa will be low because sodium is not excreted in the urine (ie, <1%). If the problem is intrinsic (basically injury to the kidneys), the kidneys lose their ability to reabsorb sodium and a higher than normal amount of sodium is excreted in the urine (ie, FENa >1%). When diuretics such as the commonly used loop diuretics have been used, the FENa is not accurate. This is because diuretics result in natriuresis (inhibition of sodium reabsorption). Because the fractional excretion of urea (FEUrea) does not rely on urinary sodium to calculate, it is more sensitive and specific in these cases. Since my patient has a history of HF, I will also draw a B-type natriuretic peptide (BNP). The BNP is an enzyme released from the ventricles of the heart when the myocardium is stretched. In an acute HF exacerbation, BNP will be elevated, which may be the cause of a pre-renal failure.

Imaging Tests

Along with the BNP, an echocardiogram is a useful noninvasive test to evaluate the patient's cardiac function. This study will give me the patient's ejection fraction (EF) so that I know her baseline cardiac function. I also plan to obtain any prior echocardiogram results done in the last 5 years.

I will also order a renal ultrasound. This study is useful to rule out hydronephrosis or renal stones that could cause an obstruction leading to a post-renal oliguria acute kidney injury (AKI).

CASE INFORMATION

Results of Diagnostic Testing

Normal Values	Patient Values
CBC	
WBC 4,500–10,000 cells/μL	11 K/μL
Hemoglobin 12.1–15.1 g/dL	11 g/dL
Hematocrit 36.1%–44.3%	34%
Platelet 150–350 K/μL	14 K/μL
Neutrophils 54%–62%	61.8%
Lymphocytes 25%–33%	28.2%
Monocytes 3%–7%	6.1%
Eosinophils 1%–3%	0.9%
Basophils 0%–0.75%	0.2%
Band forms	6.85
Lymphocytes 22–44	3.18
Monocytes 3–6	0.79
Eosinophils 0–3	0.10
Basophils 0–1	0.02
Metabolic profile	
Sodium (135–145)	140 mmol/L
Potassium (3.5–5.2)	4.7 mmol/L
Chloride 101–111 mmol/L	105 mmol/L
CO_2 20–29 mmol/L	25 mmol/L
BUN 7–20 mg/dL	35 mg/dL
Cr 0.8–1.4 mg/dL	1.7 mg/dL
Glucose 64–128 mg/dL	75
Anion gap	8 mmol/L
Urinalysis	
GFR >60	42
Sodium	14 mmol/L
Specific gravity 1.005–1.025	**1.028**
Nitrite	**Negative**
pH 4.5–7	**5.0**
Leukocytes	**Negative**

Normal Values	Patient Values
Osmolality	550 mOsm/kg
Creatinine	30
Glucose	Negative
WBC	None
Urine sediment	Hyaline casts

BNP

Patient value—300 pg/ml
<100 pg/mL—HF unlikely
>400 pg/mL-HF likely

Calculating the Fractional Excretion of Sodium (FENa)

$$FE_{Na} = \frac{U_{Na} \times P_{Cr}}{P_{Na} \times U_{Cr}} \times 100$$

Pre-renal failure-FENa is <1% or Urine Na <20
Intrinsic Renal failure- FENa is >1% or Urine Na >40
Post-renal failure-FENa is >4% or Urine Na >40
Calculation of FENa for this patient: (14 × 1.7)/ (140 × 30) × 100 = 0.6

- Echocardiogram: EF of 45%, no change from previous echocardiogram done 2 years ago, no valve regurgitation noted, no wall motion abnormality, low filling pressures, inferior vena cava collapse on inspiration
- Renal ultrasound: no hydronephrosis or kidney stones

❓ What are the pertinent positives from the additional information?

Diagnostic testing shows increasing creatinine and blood urea nitrogen, mild leukocytosis, urine sodium <20, hyaline casts noted in urine, inferior vena cava collapse on inspiration on echocardiogram, FENa <1%.

❓ What are the significant negatives from the additional information?

BNP is normal, no hydronephrosis or signs of obstruction on renal ultrasound, serum bicarbonate is normal ruling out metabolic acidosis, no significant electrolyte imbalance. Her WBC is only mildly elevated, making sepsis unlikely.

? Given this new information, how does it affect your differential diagnosis for oliguria?

Case Analysis: At this time I am ready to diagnose the patient's oliguria as a pre-renal AKI due to volume depletion.

Diagnosis and Management: Acute Kidney Injury

AKI is defined by an abrupt decrease in kidney function that includes, but is not limited to, acute renal failure (ARF). It is a broad clinical syndrome encompassing various etiologies, including specific kidney diseases (eg, acute interstitial nephritis, acute glomerulonephritis, and renal vascular diseases); nonspecific conditions (eg, ischemia, toxic injury); as well as extrarenal pathology (eg, pre-renal azotemia, and acute post-renal obstructive nephropathy).[2]

The Kidney Disease Improving Global Outcomes (KDIGO) guidelines define AKI as:

- Increase in serum creatinine by >0.3 mg/dL (>26.5 lmol/L) within 48 hours; or
- Increase in serum creatinine to >1.5 times baseline, which is known or presumed to have occurred within the prior 7 days; or
- Urine volume < 0.5 mL/kg/h for 6 hours.[2]

Acute kidney injury is one of the common complications in the acute hospital population, and contributes to hospital morbidity and mortality. A delay in treating or correction of the cause of AKI puts the patient at risk for other complications. When AKI is diagnosed, the next step is to identify the possible cause of the AKI and the type. As briefly discussed earlier, AKI is categorized into three groups: prerenal, renal, and post-renal. In pre-renal, the cause is due to decreased flow to the kidneys or an alteration in renal blood perfusion due to volume depletion, deceased cardiac output, or reduced arterial blood volume such as found in sepsis, burns, or hepatorenal syndrome. Findings on urinalysis will include a high specific gravity and normal microscopic findings with normal sediment, while laboratory results will reveal a BUN and creatinine ratio >20:1; urine electrolytes will show a sodium of less than 20 mEq/L; and the calculated FENa will be less than 1%.

In post-renal kidney failure one of the main causes is obstruction of urine. Examples include stones in the ureters or in the urinary flow outlets, tumors, enlarged prostate, or obstructed Foley catheters. In post-renal failure the presentation on the urinalysis can vary due to the site of the obstruction thus the most efficient way to establish this diagnosis is with a renal ultrasound. The presence of hydronephrosis on ultrasound confirms the presence of an obstruction causing urine to fill the kidney instead of draining into the bladder.

Intrinsic renal injury occurs when the renal glomeruli or tubules are affected. In the hospitalized patient, profound hypotension, sepsis, or exposure to nephrotoxic agents such as drugs or dyes can all contribute to intrinsic kidney injury. A urine specimen from a patient with intrinsic renal failure shows urine sodium greater than 20 mEq/L due to the failure of the kidneys to reabsorb sodium, the presence of protein and muddy brown granular casts on microscopic evaluation.

The FENa will be greater than 1%. BUN and creatinine will both be elevated, but the ratio is often less than 20:1.

The patient described in this case has a history of CHF, vomiting at home for almost 2 days prior to admission, and continuous high output from her NGT due to worsening progression of a small bowel obstruction—all factors that predispose her to AKI due to pre-renal causes. On examination, she has signs of dehydration such as dry mucous membranes and decreased skin turgor. She also had exposure to NSAIDs, a potentially nephrotoxic agent, and though she reports only taking a few doses, she was also on an angiotensin-converting enzyme inhibitor for blood pressure control. This combination poses a significant risk of kidney injury, particularly in the setting of dehydration. "NSAIDs inhibit renal prostaglandin production, limiting renal afferent vasodilatation—necessary to increase renal blood flow in times of volume depletion. ACE inhibitors and angiotensin receptor blockers (ARBs) limit renal efferent vasoconstriction needed to maintain perfusion pressure inside the glomerulus in times of low renal blood flow. The combined use of NSAID and ACE inhibitors or ARBs poses a particularly high risk of developing pre-renal azotemia."[3] In addition to the patient's history, the results of her laboratory studies including the basic metabolic panel, urine electrolytes, and urinalysis all suggest pre-renal kidney injury. She has experienced an abrupt increase in serum creatinine and BUN, increased serum sodium, a decrease in GFR, and a FENa <1%.

The treatment plan for pre-renal AKI is focused on correcting the underlying issue by optimizing renal perfusion. In this case, her significant fluid depletion caused by her NG output and pre-hospital dehydration required correction. To that end, I order 2 L of crystalloid fluid (normal saline) over 2 hours. The surgical team orders preoperative evaluation and schedules the patient to go to the operating room to repair her SBO. Addressing the patient's AKI prior to going to the operating room is essential. Serum electrolytes are closely monitored and adequate fluid management assured. The patient started voiding between 30 and 60 mL/h during the interval of aggressive fluid challenge. After stabilizing the patient for 12 hours and assuring an adequate urine output, the patient was taken to the operating room. Intraoperatively, the patient underwent a small bowel resection with extensive lysis of adhesions around the old surgical site.

❓ What essential information is necessary to obtain from the OR handoff of care to manage the patient postoperatively?

Case Analysis: Because the patient has pre-renal AKI, I focus on obtaining the following intraoperative information:

1. Fluid status: Fluid repletion, estimated blood loss, and urine output.
2. Intraoperative vital signs: Any periods of hemodynamic instability such as hypotension may contribute to further kidney injury so I need to know how this was managed.
3. Procedure: What was done and how long did it take.

CASE INFORMATION

Transfer From OR to Surgical ICU

The handoff from the operating room includes the following information: the procedure took 7 hours due to the extensive lysis of adhesions, the estimated blood loss was 600 mL, the total fluids given were 3.5 L, total urine output was 350 mL, no blood products were given, and intermittent periods of hypotension required a brief infusion of Levophed. The patient returns to the surgical intensive care unit for further monitoring and remains intubated.

Postoperatively, the patient again demonstrates a significant decrease in urine output, voiding 10 mL/h. In addition she is hypotensive, with systolic blood pressures in the low 90s. I order an additional 2 L of crystalloid intravenous fluid but there is no improvement in urine output. Because she is not responding to fluid challenge, I begin a norepinephrine infusion for blood pressure support and consult nephrology. At this point I need further diagnostics to determine her renal status and whether her AKI is now progressing to intrinsic renal failure.

I order a stat BMP and urine electrolytes to evaluate for an increase in creatinine and BUN, and electrolyte abnormalities such as hyperkalemia, and acidosis. The urine electrolytes will also help me calculate the current FENa. Urine microscopy is sent to evaluate for any casts or sediment. I order a CBC to help determine if AKI is pre-renal due to hypovolemia and blood loss.

CASE INFORMATION

Laboratory Results

Normal Values	Patient Values
CBC	
WBC 4,500–10,000 cells/μL	11 K/μL
Hemoglobin 12.1–15.1 g/dL	11 g/dL
Hematocrit 36.1%–44.3%	34%
Platelet 150–350 K/μL	14 K/μL
Neutrophils 54%–62%	61.8%
Lymphocytes 25%–33%	26.2%
Monocytes 3%–7%	6.1%
Eosinophils 1%–3%	0.6%
Basophils 0%–0.75%	0.3%
Band forms	6.05

Normal Values	Patient Values
Lymphocytes 22–44	3.02
Monocytes 3–6	0.75
Eosinophils 0–3	0.15
Basophils 0–1	0.04
GFR	32
Urinalysis	
Sodium	42 mmol/L
Specific gravity 1.005–1.025	1.028
Nitrite	Negative
pH 4.5–7	5.0
Leukocytes	Negative
Osmolality	1205 mOsm/kg
Creatinine	30
Glucose	Negative
WBC	none
Urine sediment	Muddy brown casts

❓ How does the new information affect your problem representation?

The new problem representation reads: "an 86-year-old female with a history of CHF presents with pre-renal AKI and SBO and following surgical management has postoperative intrinsic kidney injury and hypotension unresponsive to fluids."

Case Analysis: Based on the above labs, her CBC is stable without significant changes from previous labs; her relatively normal hematocrit despite blood loss most likely represents dehydration. The patients estimated blood loss was 600 mL, she received 3.5 L of crystalloid without receiving blood transfusion thus I can assume that there should be a decrease in her hematocrit. I calculate another FENa and it is greater than 1%, and there are muddy brown granular casts on microscopic evaluation as well as urine sediment and increased urine sodium. All these findings suggest an intrinsic kidney injury. With the information at hand I conclude that the patient's AKI has transitioned from a pre-renal state to intrinsic AKI (acute tubular necrosis). Reclassifying the type of AKI I am dealing with helps guide me in the appropriate management. In my patient her intrinsic renal failure was likely due to a combination of her unresolved pre-renal condition and intraoperative and postoperative hypotension.

An important predictor of AKI is volume depletion. Adequate preoperative fluid resuscitation is a significant factor in preventing AKI related to postoperative hypotension following surgery.

Nephrology is consulted and initiates continuous renal replacement therapy (CRRT). General indications for dialysis are based on these criteria: development of refractory acidosis, electrolyte imbalances (most often hyperkalemia), harmful toxic ingestions (lithium, salicylates, etc), refractory volume overload and symptoms of severe uremia. In the case of my patient, she is acidotic with serum bicarbonate of 13 and also has hyperkalemia, and significant uremia. The patient tolerates CRRT very well, and over the course of 24 hours, is weaned off vasopressors, and shows significant improvement in her urine output. After 4 days on CRRT, nephrology determines that her urine output, greater than 0.5 mL/kg/h, and improved serum creatinine, BUN, bicarbonate, and potassium levels all indicate that her AKI is resolving. The CRRT is discontinued and she is transferred to the acute care ward for further recovery. The patient was discharged home with her son 10 days after surgery.

References

1. Kendall J, Moreira M. Evaluation of the adult with abdominal pain in the emergency department. www.uptodate.com. Accessed August 26, 2014.
2. Acute Kidney Injury Work Group, ed. Kidney disease: improving global outcomes (KDIGO). *Kidney Int*. 2012;2:1-138.
3. Sushrut Waikar JB. Acute kidney injury. In: Longo DL, Fauci AS, Kasper DL, Hauser SL, eds. *Harrison's Principles of Internal Medicine*. Vol 2. 18th ed. New York, NY: McGraw-Hill; 2012:2293-2308.

CASE 12

Angela Nelson

Angela Nelson works as an ACNP for the Department of Neurosurgery at New York University Langone Medical Center.

CASE INFORMATION

Chief Complaint

A 67-year-old male presents to the neurology clinic with word-finding difficulty for the last 6 months and increasing transient episodes of "blanking out," moderate intermittent left temporal headaches, and memory loss over the last few months.

❓ What is the potential cause?

Case Analysis: This patient is exhibiting mental status changes of unknown etiology. Causes could include infectious etiologies, dementia, thyroid disease, drugs, stroke, epilepsy, or structural lesions.

CASE INFORMATION

General Survey and History of Present Illness

This is a 67-year-old right-handed male who works as a sports psychologist with several college teams. The patient appears very anxious, contending that he is in good physical and mental health, has not experienced any recent illnesses, takes care of himself, and works out regularly. He states that he is a "positive" person and will "beat" this. He seems very concerned about getting back to work quickly as he states that people are depending on him. The patient reports experiencing word-finding difficulty during the last 6 months, but his wife reports that she has only noticed word substitutions and word-finding difficulty during the last 6 weeks, becoming more frequent in the last 2 weeks, which prompted the neurology visit. The patient's wife also reports witnessing several episodes of "blanking out" where he does not respond or acts like he does not hear. The episodes last about 1 to 2 minutes and have increased in frequency over the last 2 weeks. She goes on to say that previously, when deep in thought, he typically might not respond but this appears different to her. She reports that he has been forgetful over the last 6 months but more so in the last 2 weeks. The patient reports moderate temporal headaches occurring on a daily basis but states that they are tolerable. He occasionally takes acetaminophen (Tylenol) with inconsistent response. The patient reports that he has not been able to read for the last week or so. As I watch the patient and ask additional questions, I note mixed receptive and expressive aphasia, and some trouble following complex commands.

Case Analysis: The constellation of symptoms experienced by this patient can be classified as dementia. Dementia is a broad term referring to a decline in cognitive abilities involving one or more areas including learning and memory, language, executive functioning, complex attention, perceptual-motor, and social cognition.[1] The more common forms of dementia typically have both memory and language dysfunction. These dysfunctions typically have an insidious onset and progress over time. This patient's symptoms are more acute in onset. There are many potential causes of dementia, a minority of which respond to early intervention.

The patient's episodes of "blanking out" are also concerning because they may represent a complex partial seizure where one appears to be awake but does not interact with his/her environment. The postictal state that follows a seizure includes symptoms of confusion, sleepiness, and a decreased level of alertness, which this patient is experiencing. Less than one-half of seizures have an identifiable cause and the causes can be vast including head trauma, stroke, brain tumors, intracranial infection, cerebral degeneration, or congenital brain malformations.[2] I will start with a broad differential for dementia as all the potential differential diagnoses for the condition may be causal.

Comprehensive Differential Diagnoses for Dementia

- Neurologic: different types of dementia syndromes include Alzheimer's disease, dementia with Lewy Bodies, frontotemporal dementia, vascular (multi-infarct) dementia, Parkinson disease dementia, progressive supranuclear palsy (PSP), Huntington disease, epilepsy, alcohol-related dementia, chronic traumatic encephalopathy, brain abscess, meningitis, embolic or hemorrhagic stroke, brain tumor, diseases of CNS caused by prions such as kuru, Creutzfeldt-Jakob disease (CJD), variant Creutzfeldt-Jakob disease (vCJD), Gerstmann-Sträussler-Scheinker syndrome (GSS), and fatal familiar insomnia (FFI)
- Cardiovascular: carotid artery disease, hypertensive encephalopathy
- Pulmonary: hypoxia
- Gastrointestinal: B_{12} deficiency, folate deficiency
- Genitourinary: urinary tract infection

- Musculoskeletal: none
- Endocrine: hypothyroidism
- Psychiatric disorder: major depressive disorder, schizophrenia
- Metabolic: hypernatremia, hyponatremia, hepatic encephalopathy
- Exogenous: medication side effects, alcohol withdrawal

CASE INFORMATION

- Past medical history: Hyperlipidemia.
- Past surgical history: Laparoscopic cholecystectomy.
- Family history: Significant for stroke and colon cancer.
- Social history: As per HPI, no recent travel out of the country, nonsmoker, denies alcohol or illicit drug use.
- Medications: Crestor 10 mg once daily, daily multivitamin, Tylenol or acet-aminophen as needed for headache.
- No known allergies, immunizations up to date (flu, Pneumovax, shingles).

Review of systems

- Review of systems is conducted with both the patient and wife. Although the patient does have both receptive and expressive aphasia he is able to communicate some information, and his wife assists when necessary.
- Constitutional: Denies weight loss, fatigue, fever, chills or night sweats. He denies any recent travel out of the country.
- Head/eyes/ears/nose/throat: Denies head trauma, change in vision or hearing. Denies nasal stuffiness or discharge, sore throat, swollen nodes.
- Cardiovascular: Denies chest pain, palpitations, dyspnea on exertion, or leg swelling.
- Pulmonary: Denies shortness of breath or cough.
- Gastrointestinal: Denies nausea, vomiting, blood in stools, heartburn and reports daily bowel movements.
- Genitourinary: Denies urinary frequency or urgency, foul odor or blood in urine.
- Musculoskeletal: Denies painful joints or joint swelling.
- Neurological: Reports headaches, episodes of unresponsiveness, aphasia, memory problems, and difficulty reading. Denies any visual abnormalities, falls, coordination problems, and alteration in sensation. Reports feeling very anxious concerning his worsening of symptoms.
- Integumentary: Denies rashes, itching, bug bites.
- Psychiatric: Denies depression or mood changes, states concern about current condition.

Physical Examination

- Vital signs: Pulse is 78 beats per minute, blood pressure is 128/77 mm Hg, respiratory rate is 18 breaths per minute, and temperature is 98.3°F orally, oxygen saturation by pulse oximetry is 98% on room air, and a fingerstick blood glucose is 100.
- Constitutional: Well groomed, appears stated age, appears anxious when speaking about remaining positive and returning to work as soon as possible.
- Head/eyes/ears/nose/throat: Head atraumatic, pupils are equal, round, and reactive to light. Buccal mucosa is moist and uvula is midline.
- Neck: No jugular venous distention, and no carotid bruits.
- Cardiac: Heart rate and rhythm are regular, normal S1 and S2, with no murmurs or gallops. 2+ capillary refill, no pedal edema, and hands and feet warm to touch, with equal pulses throughout.
- Pulmonary: Respirations unlabored, with no use of accessory muscles. Lungs clear to auscultation bilaterally.
- Gastrointestinal: Bowel sounds active in all four quadrants. Abdomen soft and nontender.
- Neurological: Awake, alert, and oriented to person, place, and time. Cranial nerves II–VII grossly intact. V1–V3 facial sensation intact. Extraocular movements intact. Tongue midline. No dysmetria. Negative Hoffman sign bilaterally. Toes bilaterally downgoing. No pronator drift. Full strength throughout, symmetric. Predominantly expressive aphasia, however, naming and repetition intact. Sensation intact to light touch and proprioception. No extinction to double simultaneous stimuli. Right lower extremity with three beat clonus. Reflexes nonpathologic. Mini-Mental Status examination: positive for moderate cognitive impairment and Mini-Cog examination: positive for cognitive impairment.[3,4]
- Skin: Intact, no rashes, lesions, or open areas. Normal skin turgor.
- Lymphatics: No lymphadenopathy.

? What are the pertinent positives from the information given thus far?

- Progressive, increasing neurological dysfunction occurring over a relatively short period of time including aphasia, memory loss, word finding difficulty, "blanking out" (possibly seizure), difficulty following complex commands, and difficulty reading
- Headaches
- Mini-Mental Status and Mini-Cog examinations: positive for cognitive impairment

❓ What are the significant negatives from the information given so far?

• No reports of recent illnesses or trauma

• No chronic health problems

• Physical examination normal with exception of neurological findings

❓ Can the information gathered so far be restated in a single sentence highlighting the pieces that narrow down the cause?

Putting information obtained so far in a single statement—a problem representation—sets the stage for gathering more information and determining the cause.

At this point the problem representation is as follows: a 67-year-old male in good health presents with new onset dementia, receptive and expressive aphasia, and possible seizures, beginning 6 months ago and worsening over the last 2 weeks.

❓ How does this information affect the list of possible causes?

Case Analysis: At this point, I am able to eliminate many causes of dementia listed in my differential. The patient is neither hypertensive nor hypoxic, and I doubt he has an infection such as meningitis, brain abscess, or urinary tract infection given the long duration of symptoms, the absence of fever, normal vital signs and general appearance of good health. In addition, the duration of symptoms and the normal motor and sensory findings on his neurological examination make embolic or hemorrhagic stroke unlikely to be the cause of his symptoms. The absence of motor symptoms effectively rules out dementia due to Parkinson disease and Huntington disease. He has no psychiatric history and he and his wife deny significant exposures, thus psychiatric and exogenous causes are unlikely.

The remaining items on my differential list include neurological causes such as dementia syndromes, tumor, genetic conditions; metabolic causes including hypothyroidism and electrolyte disturbances; or carotid artery stenosis. If my findings so far were more suggestive of an emergent life-threating stroke, or infection such as meningitis, my diagnostics would include an immediate CT scan, possibly a lumbar puncture, and stat antibiotics. However, this patient is otherwise healthy and is without deficits that suggest a stroke or infection so I am more inclined to think that a less urgent disorder is causing his symptoms. The most common form of dementia, particularly in a patient of this age, is Alzheimer disease. This is generally a clinical diagnosis, made after other less common causes of dementia are ruled out. Some of the pieces of this patient's story fit with an Alzheimer diagnosis, particularly the gradually worsening memory and language deficits. However, the periodic "blank periods" and sudden worsening of symptoms over the past 2 weeks are less consistent with Alzheimer disease. I will need further information, particularly imaging of the patient's brain, to further rule out or in the items on my differential.

❓ What diagnostic testing is needed, and in what order?

Case Analysis: First, to detect a thyroid disorder, vitamin deficiency, or electrolyte disturbance, I order the following: thyroid testing (TSH, and total T3, T4), folate and B_{12} levels, and a comprehensive metabolic panel with calcium and magnesium levels. Though infection is low on my list of possible causes at this point, I need to specifically rule this out before I can diagnose the patient with another dementia syndrome such as Alzheimer. Therefore, I also order a urinalysis, an erythrocyte sedimentation rate (ESR), a rapid plasma reagin (RPR), a serum lyme, and a complete blood count.

I also order cardiac imaging to include an echocardiogram and a carotid duplex. The echocardiogram will reveal any clots that could have become emboli causing transient ischemic attacks or contributing to multi-infarct dementia. The echocardiogram also gives an estimate of the patient's heart function, which may be useful when I need to select therapy to treat the cause of neurological symptoms. The carotid duplex will determine whether carotid artery disease is present.

To address my concern for a structural disorder such as a tumor, I order a magnetic resonance imaging (MRI) of the head, and a positron emission tomography (PET) scan to reveal areas of heightened metabolic activity. These images will help determine if the patient has a tumor, vascular (multi-infarct) dementia, or Lewy body dementia. Given the increasingly frequent episodes of blanking out, an electroencephalogram (EEG) is useful to determine if the patient has any seizure activity. If these tests are unrevealing, I may consider proceeding to a lumbar puncture.

CASE INFORMATION

Diagnostic Testing Results

The following tests were completed over a period of 3 days:
- Electrolyte and liver function tests are all within normal limits.
- Thyroid workup negative: T3 = 1.06 ng/dL (normal is 1.00–2.00 ng/dL), T4 = 8.2 μg/dL (normal is 4.5–12.5 μg/dL), TSH 1.440 μIU/mL (0.5–4.70 μIU/mL).
- Nutritional workup negative with folate greater than 20 (normal is 7–38 nmol/L) and B_{12} level of 219 (normal is 130–700 ng/L).
- Infectious disease workup is negative as follows: Urine analysis is within normal limits. ESR 6 (normal ≤30 mm/h), RPR nonreactive, white blood cell

count on CBC is 8.3 cells/mL (normal = 4–10 cells/mL) and Lyme disease titers are negative.

- Cardiac workup is also negative. Normal ECG. Carotid duplex with no plaque seen in the carotid bulb, no stenosis in extracranial portion of carotid arteries on either side, and vertebral arteries patent with antegrade flow. Echocardiogram with normal ejection fraction and with no significant valvular disease.
- MRI with and without contrast shows a large necrotic mass in left temporal lobe (52 × 34.5 mm) with surrounding edema, and mass effect with midline shift toward the right and compression of left lateral ventricle as well as left uncal herniation. Edema extends to left frontoparietal white matter as well as left basal ganglionic, internal capsule region.
- PET scan confirms a centrally necrotic mass in left anterior/mid temporal lobe.
- Electroencephalography (EEG) with no evidence of active seizures.

Case Analysis: The MRI and PET scan identified the source of the patient's symptoms. He has a large necrotic left temporal lobe mass, likely either a glioblastoma or a metastatic lesion, with significant vasogenic edema and early uncal herniation (see Figure 12-1).

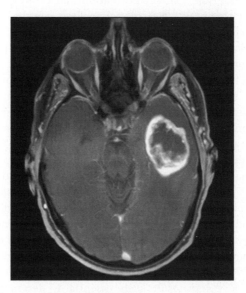

Figure 12-1   Left temporal lobe glioblastoma.

After discussing the test results with the patient and his wife, I instruct the patient to go to the emergency department at the local university medical center. He is subsequently admitted to the neurosurgical ICU. He is started on dexamethasone (Decadron) for brain edema and levetiracetam (Keppra) for seizure prophylaxis and taken to the operating room 2 days later for the resection of the left temporal lesion. Tissue biopsy confirms that the lesion was a glioblastoma.

Diagnosis: Left Temporal Brain Tumor

This patient's assessment led me to suspect that he had a left temporal lobe lesion. His right handedness makes him left-sided hemisphere dominant. The symptoms of any brain lesion are related to the location of the mass and edema in surrounding areas. The left temporal lobe includes Wernicke area. A dysfunction in this area includes words being heard but not understood, sometimes referred to as receptive aphasia. The temporal lobe is also an interpretative area for visual, auditory, olfactory perception, learning, and memory. A dysfunction in this area can cause significant cognitive dysfunction.[5] The temporal lobe is also most closely linked to the development of seizures.

The frontal lobe is responsible for high-level cognitive functioning, memory, control of voluntary eye movements, and the somatic motor control of respirations, gastrointestinal, and blood pressure. When lesions are in the frontal lobe dominant hemisphere, deficits in the motor control of speech are seen, commonly known as expressive aphasia.

The parietal lobe is a cortical sensory processing area where sensation is localized and awareness of body position and location are recognized. The nondominant lobe processes visual-spatial information and disorders in the dominant lobe lead to ideomotor apraxia, a disconnection between the language and visual center involved in following a motor command.[5] Types of dysfunction that might be found include lack of stereognosis, which is the ability to recognize an object by touch or lack of graphesthesia, which is the ability to recognize numbers or letters written on the skin. The ability to differentiate one-point from two-point skin stimulation is referred to as two-point discrimination, which represents another dysfunction seen in patients with parietal lobe dysfunction. Lastly, a sensory extinction can be seen where there is an inability to sense two stimuli when touched at the same time.

All of this patient's symptoms correlate with the left temporal lesion and the surrounding edema in the frontoparietal areas. Temporal lobe dysfunction is demonstrated by the receptive aphasia, memory impairment, possible seizure activity in the "blanking out" episodes, and not being able to read (alexia). The frontal lobe involvement can additionally be seen with the memory impairment and expressive aphasia. The parietal lobe involvement is demonstrated in the difficulty following complex motor commands especially as the lesion is in the dominant hemisphere. However, one could also argue that this difficulty is also due to his receptive aphasia.[5]

The MRI and PET scan results were essential to determining this patient's diagnosis, and the patient's focal neurologic deficits convinced me that this kind of testing was warranted. A negative MRI scan and a PET scan showing low levels of metabolic activity suggests dementia and a very different course of action including referral for neuropsychiatric evaluation. This kind of evaluation is helpful in identifying which dementia syndrome a person has, which in turn directs treatment.

Management of Glioblastoma

A diagnosis of World Health Organization (WHO) Grade IV Glioblastoma is confirmed on biopsy after gross total resection of the lesion. Histological grading is a means of predicting biological behavior. Such grading is also known as the WHO Classification System.[6] Histological grading is as follows:

   a. Grade I: relatively circumscribed, noninfiltrating, low proliferative potential

   b. Grade II: atypical cells, well differentiated, infiltrating, low proliferative potential

   c. Grade III: (anaplastic) diffusely infiltrating, nuclear atypia, significant proliferation

   d. Grade IV: (glioblastoma) poorly differentiated, presence of necrosis and/or microvascular proliferation.

The incidence of primary brain tumors in adults is 19.89 per 100,000 with the incidence increasing with age. The most common malignant gliomas are glioblastomas that are 1.6 times more common in women and twice as common in whites than blacks. Glioblastoma has a 4.7% 5-year survival rate and 2.32% 10-year survival rate. The histological grading is a means to predict biological behavior of the tumor worsening with higher grades. The only cause known at this point is exposure to ionized radiation. The median rate of survival with an aggressive glioblastoma with resection, radiation, and chemotherapy is 14.6 months. The gold standard for diagnosis is MRI with and without IV contrast. This allows for identification of tumor location, characteristics, and presence of mass effect. The National Comprehensive Cancer Center (NCCN) guidelines recommend a gross total resection when possible or a stereotactic biopsy to provide sufficient tissue for pathology identification. For high-grade gliomas, radiation and chemotherapy is standard following resection. Temozolomide (Temodar) is the standard chemotherapy for a newly diagnosed glioma.[7]

Case Follow-Up

The patient underwent a total gross resection of the left temporal lesion without complications. He was discharged to home 3 days after surgery. Two weeks later, he began a 3-week course of radiation and a 42-day course of chemotherapy with 145 mg temozolomide. He subsequently had regrowth of his tumor and was started on another chemotherapeutic agent as part of a clinical study. At the time of writing this case, he is 5 months into his initial diagnosis.

References

1. American Psychiatric Association. *Diagnostic and Statistical Manual of Mental Disorders.* 5th ed. Arlington VA: American Psychiatric Association, DSM-5; 2013.
2. Schacter SC, Pedley TA, Eichler AF, et al. Evaluation of the first seizure in adults. 2015 UpToDate. www.uptodate.com. Last updated May 21, 2014. Accessed March 3, 2015.
3. Mini Mental Exam. Standardised Mini-Mental State Examination (SMMSE). http://www.ihpa. gov.au/internet/ihpa/publishing.nsf/Content/4E22FCBF77981A7BCA257D09000AA8CD/$File/ smmse-guidelines-v2.pdf. Accessed April 11, 2015.
4. Mini Cog Exam. Mental status assessment of older adults: the Mini-Cog. http://consultgerirn.org/ uploads/File/trythis/try_this_3.pdf. Accessed April 11, 2015.
5. Hickey JV. *The Clinical Practice of Neurological and Neurosurgical Nursing.* 7th ed. Philadelphia, PA: Wolters/Kluwer/Lippincott Williams and Wilkins; 2014.
6. Louis DN, Ohgaki H, Wiestler OD, et al., eds. *WHO Classification of Tumours of the Central Nervous System.* 4th ed. Geneva, Switzerland: International Agency for Research on Cancer; 2007.
7. Lovely MP, Stewart-Amidea C, Arzbaecher J, et al. *Care of the Adult Patient with a Brain Tumor.* Chicago, IL: AANN; 2014. *AANN Clinical Practice Guidelines Series.*

CASE 13

Shawn Floyd

Shawn Floyd is a Transplant NP with the Cardiopulmonary Transplant Team at the University of Virginia Health System. He manages patients from postoperative ICU to the outpatient clinic and all stages of posttransplant care.

CASE INFORMATION

Chief Complaint

Georgia is a 71-year-old female with a history of idiopathic pulmonary fibrosis (IPF) who underwent single left lung transplant 6 years ago and now presents to the emergency department with right upper quadrant abdominal pain.

❓ What is the potential cause?

Case Analysis: I immediately begin to think that this is related to the gallbladder but acute abdominal pain can be localized or diffuse in nature. While this patient is specific about the location of the pain, I need more information about the nature of the pain and related history before I eliminate diagnoses from my differential. Because the patient is a lung transplant patient, and subsequently immunocompromised, I need to quickly and comprehensively gather data to help me determine the cause. I start with a general survey of the patient and the history of present illness.

CASE INFORMATION

General Survey and History of Present Illness

The patient reports that the pain began about 2 months ago. Around 4 weeks ago she felt a small knot in her right lower quadrant. Last night she developed severe right lower quadrant abdominal pain and presented to her community emergency department (ED). During the ED workup for acute abdomen, a CT scan revealed an abdominal mass in her right lower quadrant (*Figure 13-1*). The emergency room providers told her she would need to follow up at with her transplant center as soon as possible. She immediately came to her transplant center emergency department to have the mass evaluated.

When she arrives at the transplant center ED she reports that the pain is intermittent and ranges from a 4/10 to a 10/10. At the time of my assessment, she rated the pain as 4–5/10. She reports she took two Tylenol and two Percocet prior to arrival to help relieve the pain and says that this helped. She

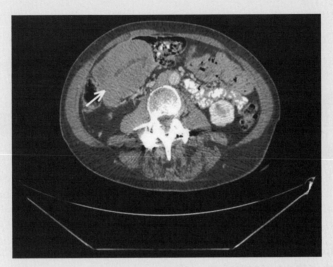

Figure 13-1 Arrow points to abdominal mass in right lower quadrant.

states the pain is worse with movement and improves with rest and does not radiate. She denies any nausea or vomiting but states she may have had some blood mixed in her stool for the last few days. She is drinking fluids but has not eaten since early this morning. She is immediately admitted to the transplant service and I begin my workup to determine the etiology of this mass.

Differential Diagnose for Abdominal Mass[1,2]

- Infectious disorders: pelvic actinomycosis, tuberculosis, ileocecal, actinomycosis
- Infected organ: abscesses, appendicitis, pelvic inflammatory disease, diverticulitis, colon, ovarian abscess/tubo-ovarian abscess, diverticulitis/phlegmon/abscess, omentum abscess, pelvic abscess, left-sided acute appendicitis
- Neoplastic disorders: metastasis to peritoneum, adenocarcinoma, ovarian adenoma, ovarian cancer/carcinoma, uterine fibroid/leiomyomas, infarcted/twisted uterine fibroid, hydatidiform mole, metastasis/carcinoma to ovary, ovarian cystadenoma, ovarian teratocarcinoma, ovary teratoma, solid/cystic, prostate rhabdomyosarcoma/sarcoma, pseudomyxoma, peritonei, teratoma of ovary, carcinoid, ovarian, carcinoma, small intestine, uterine leiomyosarcoma, carcinoma jejunum
- Allergic, collagen, autoimmune disorders: Crohn disease (regional enteritis)
- Congenital, developmental disorders: urachus, cyst, wandering spleen

- Anatomic, foreign body, structural disorders: diverticulitis, ectopic pregnancy, ectopic pregnancy hemorrhage, obstipation, impacted feces, ovarian cyst/hemorrhagic cyst, cecum diverticulum/diverticulitis, cecum, volvulus, colon/sigmoid perforation, omentum torsion, ovarian cyst/torsion pedicle, abdominal pregnancy, hernia, spigelian, hydrosalpinx, pelvic hematoma, ovarian pregnancy
- Arteriosclerotic, vascular, venous disorders: infarct/epiploic/mesoappendix, or omentum infarction
- Functional, physiologic variant disorders: constipation, pregnancy
- Endocrine disorders: bladder, neurogenic atonic, polycystic ovaries/Stein-Leventhal syndrome

? What are the pertinent positives from the information given so far?

- Able to keep orals down
- Intermittent abdominal pain that is worse with movement and improves with rest
- Imunocompromised patient
- Mass on CT
- Blood in stool

? What are the significant negatives from the information given so far?

- Afebrile
- No sign of active abdominal infection
- No nausea or vomiting

Case Analysis: Because the outside emergency department already did a CT scan of the patient's abdomen, this information will help me rule out some of the immediate life-threatening conditions that may cause abdominal pain. For instance mesenteric ischemia, perforation, acute bowel obstruction, volvulus, and splenic rupture can all cause abdominal pain but these conditions are less likely as they were not identified on the scan at the outside hospital. All of these would generally make the patient acutely ill, hemodynamically unstable, and in severe pain.[1] Given the information so far I am ready to state the problem representation of the patient. This is a 71-year-old patient with a history of idiopathic pulmonary fibrosis (IPF) who underwent single left lung transplant 6 years ago and now presents with the complaint of right upper quadrant abdominal pain and a right upper abdominal mass of unknown etiology.

CASE INFORMATION

Past Medical History

- IPF
- Osteoporosis
- Uterine cancer 15 years prior
- Hyperlipidemia
- Hypertension
- Gastroesophageal reflux disease
- Colon polyps

Past Surgical History

- Total abdominal hysterectomy 14 years ago
- Left lung transplant 7 years ago

Family and Social History

- Mother died of old age
- Father died of colon cancer, positive for hypertension
- Three adult children all alive and well
- Retired as a nurse at age 62 after diagnosis of IPF, former smoker 60 pack-year, social alcohol use

Medication List

- Acetaminophen (Tylenol) 500 mg tablet: take 1000 mg by mouth every 6 hours as needed
- Acyclovir (Zovirax) 200 mg capsule: 2 capsules by mouth 2 times daily
- Ascorbic acid (vitamin C) 500 mg tablet by mouth 2 times daily
- Aspirin 81 mg chewable tablet by mouth daily
- Atovaquone (Mepron) 750 mg/5 mL suspension, 750 mg by mouth daily
- Bupropion (Wellbutrin SR) 150 mg 12 hour tablet, 1 tablet by mouth 2 times daily
- Calcium-vitamin D (calcium 500 +D), 1 tablet by mouth 2 times daily
- Clotrimazole (Mycelex) 10 mg troche by mouth 3 times daily
- Diphenoxylate-atropine (Lomotil) 2.5–0.025 mg/5 mL liquid, 5 mL by mouth 4 times daily as needed for diarrhea
- Famotidine (Pepcid) 20 mg tablet by mouth 2 times daily
- Furosemide (Lasix) 20 mg tablet by mouth daily
- Loperamide (Imodium) 2 mg capsule by mouth 4 times daily as needed for diarrhea
- Multiple Vitamin (multivitamins) tabs: take 1 tablet by mouth daily
- Mycophenolate mofetil (CellCept) 250 mg capsule by mouth every 12 hours

- Ondansetron (Zofran) 8 mg tablet by mouth every 8 hours as needed for nausea
- Oxybutynin (Ditropan XL) 5 mg 24 hour tablet by mouth daily
- Prednisone (Deltasone) 10 mg tablet by mouth daily
- Psyllium (Metamucil) 58.6% packet by mouth daily
- Sirolimus (Rapamune) 1 mg tablet, 2 tablets by mouth daily
- Sulfamethoxazole-trimethoprim (Bactrim DS) 800–160 mg tablet by mouth on Monday, Wednesday, and Friday

Review of Systems

- General: not feeling well, denies fevers or chills
- Head/eyes/ears/nose/throat: wears corrective glasses
- Cardiovascular: denies chest pain, peripheral edema, and orthopnea
- Pulmonary: some shortness of breath with exertion, none at rest
- Gastrointestinal: as per chief complaint, no diarrhea, nausea, or vomiting. Noted a "knot" in right lower quadrant, denies constipation, has daily bowel movement. Recently some blood
- Genitourinary: denies pain with urination, blood in urine, or change in urine output
- Skin: normal
- Musculoskeletal: normal
- Neurological: negative
- Lymphatic: has not noted enlarged nodes
- Hematologic: bruises easily
- Endocrine: normal
- Mental health: normal

Physical Assessment

- Vital signs: Heart rate 68 beats per minute, blood pressure 110/58 mm Hg, respirations 22 breaths per minute, oxygen saturation 93% on room air, height 5'1", weight 115 lb, body mass index 21.7.
- General: Well-nourished and groomed elderly white female in no acute distress.
- Head/eyes/ears/nose/throat: pupils equal, round, reactive to light and accommodation, normocephalic, normal dentation, no thrush noted. Thyroid midline with no palpable nodules noted. No carotid bruits noted.
- Cardiovascular: Regular rate, S1 and S2, PMI auscultated at the fifth rib space mid clavicular, no murmurs, rubs, or gallops. +3 palpable peripheral pulses throughout.
- Pulmonary: Eupneic respiratory pattern, crackles in right lower lobe and diminished breath sounds on the right, left lung is clear to auscultation.

- Gastrointestinal: Normal appearing abdominal area, active bowel sounds throughout all quadrants, palpable mass in lower right quadrant, painful to deep palpation. No hepatomegaly or splenomegaly.
- Rectum: No masses or lesions palpable in vault.
- Musculoskeletal: Equal strength in upper and lower extremities.
- Neurologic: Alert and oriented, cranial nerves II thru X grossly intact, no focal deficits noted.
- Lymphatic: No lymphadenopathy.

? What elements of the review of systems and physical examination should be added to the list of pertinent positives?

- Feels fatigued
- Abdominal pain
- Bruises easily
- Palpable mass in lower right quadrant
- Regular bowel movements

? What elements of the review of systems and physical examination should be added to the significant negatives list?

- Vital signs stable
- No nausea, vomiting, or diarrhea
- No palpable nodes
- No signs of infection
- Normal cardiovascular and neurological examinations

Case Analysis: The review of systems and the physical examination help me rule out a number of items on the differential. At this point, given the patient's age, past medical history and the fact that she is a transplant patient, the presence of a mass does place neoplasm at the top of my list. She also has a past medical history of uterine cancer so this has to be considered as a potential source of metastases and a cause of the mass. However, a gastrointestinal cancer is also a possibility. I am also thinking that this mass may be a transplant-related cancer such as a posttransplant lymphoproliferative disorder or a cancer that has metastasized from a different organ system. Because my first concern is for malignancy, I start by consulting gastroenterology and hematology-oncology to assist me in determining the best way to define this mass. At the same time I consider diagnostics that will yield information quickly, and identify specific tumor markers.

While I have not detected any potential signs of infection as of yet, I cannot rule out infectious causes and/or abscesses (intraperitoneal or pelvic) and will need to consider imaging and diagnostics to further evaluate for this. She is at high risk for infection due to her immunocompromised state and transplant patients often present with atypical symptoms of infection. Due to her age and her history of regular bowel movements, I can eliminate pregnancy and pregnancy-related conditions as well as fecal impaction, obstipation, and constipation from the differential. While she feels poorly, she does not appear or feel ill enough to have mesenteric ischemia. Her normal genitourinary history makes disorders of the bladder and urinary tract less likely.

? What additional diagnostic tests would you order at this time?

Labs that I order include a complete blood count with differential and a complete metabolic profile with hepatic profile. I order the following tumor markers: α-fetoprotein (AFP), a marker for hepatocellular carcinoma; carcinoembryonic antigen (CEA), a marker for colorectal cancer; CA 125, a marker for ovarian cancer; and CA 19, a marker for pancreatic cancer.[3] Also I order a total abdominal ultrasound to further evaluate the mass identified on the previous abdominal CT.

CASE INFORMATION
Results of Diagnostic Testing

Component	Ref Range	Result
Sodium	136–145 mmol/L	132
Potassium	3.4–4.8 mmol/L	3.7
Chloride	98–107 mmol/L	96
CO_2	23–31 mmol/L	23
BUN	9.8–20.1 mg/dL	26
Creatinine	0.6–1.1 mg/dL	1.1
Glucose	74–99 mg/dL	104
Calcium	8.5–10.5 mg/dL	9.2
Total protein	5.8–8.1 g/dL	7.0
Albumin	3.2–5.2 g/dL	4.0
Total bilirubin	0.3–1.2 mg/dL	0.4
Alkaline phosphatase	40–150 U/L	80
AST	<35 U/L	35
ALT	<55 U/L	22

Component	Ref Range	Result
CALC GFR (mL/min/1.73 m²)		51
WBC	4.0–11.0 cells/μL	9.50
RBC	4.20–5.20 M/μL	3.82
Hemoglobin	12.0–16.0 g/dL	13.0
Hematocrit	35.0%–47.0%	36.1
MCV	83.0–95.0 fL	94.5
MCH	28.0–32.0 pg	34.0
MCHC	32.0–36.0 g/dL	36.0
RDW	11.0%–14.0%	13.3
Platelets	150–450 K/μL	228
MPV	9.0–12.0 fL	9.5
CA 125 ovarian cancer antigen		5
CEA		3.7

Case Analysis: The lab evaluation does not reveal any significant findings that point to a specific etiology of this mass. Of note, all the tumor markers are within the normal reference ranges, which helps rule out specific neoplasm diagnoses such as ovarian and colon cancer, but they do not rule out all malignancies.[3] To determine if the mass is malignant or some other type of mass, a procedure is necessary. I consult the gastroenterology service to help determine how best to accomplish this. After reviewing the patient's history, examination, and diagnostics, the consultant notes that while the mass can be biopsied via colonoscopy, the risk of perforation of the colon is very high. This is because Georgia is on chronic prednisone therapy to prevent rejection. Because of this very real concern, I next consult a colorectal surgeon to establish a plan for management should the colon perforate during the endoscopy procedure. The surgeon states that if the bowel perforates during the endoscopy, Georgia will be taken to the operating room for an emergent exploratory laparotomy and resection of the mass. The team and the patient agree to this approach and she is taken to the endoscopy suite the following day for the procedure.

CASE INFORMATION

The colonoscopy shows that the mass is invading the proximal right colon and distal portion of the cecum. A biopsy of the mass is sent to pathology for tissue diagnosis. This information helps determine my next steps in managing Georgia's care. Because of the invasive nature of the mass, and the high risk that the tumor would lead to bowel perforation, surgery is considered the appropriate and necessary next step; however, Georgia's age and immuno-compromised put her at risk for surgical complications. I recognize the need to weigh the risks and benefits of surgical intervention carefully. Georgia's wishes related to undergoing surgery are a key consideration in how we might proceed and I thoroughly discuss all potential outcomes with her.

In response to the team's inquiries, the patient asks for a 24-hour period to discuss her treatment options with her husband and family. During this interval, the pathology results from the biopsy taken during the colonos-copy confirm that she has atypical intramucosal lymphoid infiltrates con-sistent with a posttransplant lymphoproliferative disorder. Because this is a fast-growing malignancy, I recognize the urgent need for surgery to prevent perforation. Given her very high risk for surgical complications, I plan for a postoperative stay in the surgical intensive care unit.

Georgia is taken to the operating room and undergoes an exploratory laparotomy with tumor debulking and total colectomy with ostomy place-ment. She tolerates the procedure well and all tissue is sent for pathology to evaluate the stage of the disease. She is placed in the surgical intensive care unit overnight and is then transferred to a surgical floor the following day. Unfortunately multiple lymph nodes come back positive for lymphop-roliferative disease and she requires several rounds of chemotherapy and radiation therapy. The hematology and oncology team works with Georgia to ensure that her treatments are the least invasive and time consuming possible. Inevitably she develops multiple areas of metastasis, decides to end treatment, and passed away a few months later.

Diagnosis and Management: Posttransplant Lymphoproliferative Disorder

Transplant patients like Georgia are at higher risk for malignancy due to the chronic immunosuppression used to prevent rejection. The antirejection medi-cations that are used are the best prevention for the rejection of solid organ transplants but they come with a price. The immunosuppressed state allows can-cers to multiply quickly and develop in an unregulated fashion. With the use of immunosuppression, common viral infections can cause specific malignancies including posttransplant lymphoma, squamous cell cancers, and hepatoma.[4] These cancers require rapid and aggressive identification and treatment by the transplant team and oncology service. Increasingly, transplant programs are looking at different models of immunosuppression to hopefully reduce the num-ber of posttransplant infections and malignancies. In this case the abdominal mass was found late in Georgia's course and her wish to avoid overly aggres-sive treatment, which would negatively affect her quality of life, was honored. Georgia lived another 6 months after diagnosis and she died at home with her husband and family at her side.

References

1. Mcquaid K. Approach to the patient with gastrointestinal disease. In: Goldman L, Schafer AI, eds. *Cecil Medicine*. 24th ed. Philadelphia, PA: Saunders Elsevier; 2011:chap 134.
2. Penner RM, Majumdar SR. Diagnostic approach to abdominal pain in adults. UptoDate. http://www.uptodate.com/contents/diagnostic-approach-to-abdominal-pain-in-adults. Last updated April 11, 2013.
3. Perkins GL, Slater ED, Sanders GK, Prichard JG. Serum tumor markers. *Am Fam Physician*. 2003 Sep 15;68(6):1075-1082.
4. McGill RL, Ko TY. Transplantation and the primary care physician. *Adv Chronic Kidney Dis*. 2011;18(6):433-438.

CASE 14

Janie Heath

Janie Heath is Dean and the Warwick Professor of Nursing at the University of Kentucky in Lexington. For the past 30 years Janie has been a national leader for tobacco control and advanced practice nursing where she has directed academic programs and practiced as an ACNP in South Carolina, Washington DC, Georgia, and Virginia.

CASE INFORMATION

Chief Complaint

A 30-year-old Caucasian male is brought to the emergency room (ER) by friends with the complaint of new onset chest pain that occurred while grilling at picnic in a screened-in porch area.

❓ What is the potential cause?

Case Analysis: Chest pain, particularly in a young adult male, can be a non-specific symptom and the list of potential etiologies is long. I first think about prioritizing those conditions that are most serious and immediate. Thus in the case of this patient, the priority is to quickly determine if his chest pain might be caused by a myocardial infarction, pulmonary emboli, pneumothorax, or dissecting aortic aneurysm, which are unlikely causes but require immediate intervention.

> ### Comprehensive Differential Diagnoses for Patient With Chest Pain[1]
>
> - Cardiac: acute coronary syndrome, myocardial infarction including ST elevation and non-ST elevation, unstable angina, Prinzmetal angina, pericarditis, mitral valve prolapse, aortic aneurysm, cardiac arrhythmia, heart failure exacerbation
> - Pulmonary: pulmonary emboli, pneumonia, pleuritis, pneumothorax, pulmonary hypertension, hypoxia, chronic obstructive pulmonary disease (COPD) exacerbation, tracheobronchitis
> - Gastrointestinal: esophageal spasm, esophageal reflux, esophageal tear, esophagitis, peptic ulcer disease, gastritis, cholecystitis, pancreatitis
> - Musculoskeletal: chest wall injury or strain, rib fracture, cervical or thoracic disk disease, shoulder arthroscopy, costochondritis, trauma
> - Neurological: neuropathy from herpes zoster, nerve root compression

- Psychiatric: anxiety, panic disorders
- Hematological: anemia
- Exogenous: medication side effect or interaction or withdrawal, drug overdose, carbon monoxide inhalation

CASE INFORMATION

General Survey and History of Present Illness

In this case, as in all cases, I begin with a general survey of the patient: he is a well-nourished, well-developed, appropriately groomed male who appears anxious but in no acute distress. He has an odor of smoke and alcohol on his breath. He is without pallor, cyanosis, diaphoresis, or dyspnea. His appearance is not suggestive of a life-threatening process. When asked what happened, he states, "I'm not sure; we were all having a good time at the picnic barbeque when I started feeling tightness in my chest but I'm okay now; I think I just pulled a muscle moving the grill onto the porch." The patient's friend quickly responds, "I think you should explain how much fun you were having because you were really drinking a lot of beers today, more so than what you usually do, and there was 100 degree heat index today, especially since your dad died of a heart attack." The patient looks at his friend and says clearly, "What do you know, you had as many beers, if not more than I did and besides this is between me and my doctor so you can wait in the lobby now." The friend stomps out of the room and the patient explains that he is under a lot stress recently in his job as a marketing manager for a national clothing manufacturer and was looking forward to relaxing and having a good time. He states he drank four to six beers and that he was fine with that; in fact he was the one cooking the burgers and was smart enough to pull that heavy grill to the porch to save the party from a sudden rainstorm.

He describes the pain as substernal without radiation and lasting about 20 minutes. He stated it felt like an "elephant sitting on him." He denies nausea, vomiting, or dyspnea. He also denies pain with inspiration or movement. He did complain of diaphoresis during the 20 minutes of chest pain. He reports the chest pain went away when he got into a cool car and it was gone by the time he got to the ER. He denies taking an aspirin during the chest pain episode.

Past Medical History

When asked about his past medical history he states he has been told he has high blood pressure, but that with lifestyle modification he could avoid the need for medication. He denies a history of heart disease, stroke, lung disease, gastrointestinal disorders, neurological disorders, diabetes, cancer, or recent injury/physical trauma or mental health conditions.

Review of the electronic medical record reveals that he has never been admitted to this hospital before. There is a note from a primary care appointment 2 years ago, which confirms the history given by the patient.

Social History

He admits to daily alcohol use, tobacco use for 10 years, currently less than 1 pack per day, occasionally smokes marijuana, but does not use any other illicit substances. He is active physically, works out at the gym every day, eats healthy, and is seeing someone to help him quit smoking and manage his stress. He is single, lives alone, has no children, and is employed as a marketing manager for a large clothing company in Seattle.

Medications

He has no allergies and denies taking any medication except for a vitamin supplement.

Family History

Both parents deceased and were former smokers and both took medication for hypertension. Father died from myocardial infarction; mother died from complications of diabetes. Two living sisters in good health, nonsmokers.

❓ What are the pertinent positives from the information given so far?

- The pain is described as a heavy pressure (elephant sitting on him).
- The patient was in the heat and consuming alcohol.
- The patient was diaphoretic with chest pain.
- The patient pulled a heavy grill before the chest pain started.
- The patient was grilling in a poorly ventilated area before the chest pain started.
- The patient was diagnosed with hypertension and treated with lifestyle modification only.
- The patient is a smoker and seeing someone to help quit.
- The patient is seeing someone to help manage stress.
- At the time of the chest pain, the patient was relaxing and having a good time.
- The patient has a family history of heart disease.

❓ What are the significant negatives from the information given so far?

- The patient is in no distress.
- The patient has no chest pain currently.

- The patient has no chronic health problems such as heart disease, pulmonary disease, or diabetes.
- There is an absence of GI disorders, neurological disorders, or musculoskeletal disorders.
- There is an absence of recent injury or trauma.
- No pallor, cyanosis, dyspnea, pain with inspiration, or nausea/vomiting.

CASE INFORMATION

Problem Representation

Given the information acquired so far the problem representation is: "A 30-year-old male with hypertension and substance use presents with one 20-minute episode of chest pain that began while grilling in an enclosed area and resolved when he was transported to the hospital."

❓ How does this information affect the list of possible causes and what do you need to do now?

Case Analysis: The nature of the patient's chest pain, a heavy pressure, and his two cardiac risk factors, hypertension and smoking, lead to concern for myocardial infarction, so a stat ECG is ordered and the patient is placed on cardiac monitor and pulse oximeter. A stat bedside carbon monoxide (CO) measurement and a portable chest x-ray are also ordered. He is placed on oxygen by 100% nonrebreather mask to obtain an O_2 saturation of 100%.

While I suspect that CO poisoning secondary to his exposure to smoke in an enclosed space may be the etiology of his chest pain, other life-threatening etiologies must also be ruled out including aortic dissection, pneumothorax, and pulmonary embolus (PE). These are less likely as his overall condition is stable and he no longer has chest pain. Regardless I will obtain a portable chest x-ray to rule out a pneumothorax and to look for potential signs of a dissection such as mediastinal widening. A focused review of systems and physical examination will help me further sort my differential.

CASE INFORMATION

Review of Systems

The patient appears to be a good historian although his alcohol use prior to ER admission is taken into consideration.

- Constitutional: denies fever and chills, denies upper respiratory infection symptoms, reports diaphoresis during chest pain episode, weight stable, his appetite is good but admits not eating at the barbeque party, no recent falls, no trauma

- Cardiovascular: denies palpitations, edema, or orthopnea
- Pulmonary: denies dyspnea or cough
- Gastrointestinal: denies nausea/vomiting, denies pain with eating or drinking, reports regular bowel movements that are soft and formed, denies blood in stools, denies abdominal pain or reflux disease
- Genitourinary: noncontributory
- Musculoskeletal: denies chest tenderness or pain with movement, occasional left knee pain from past surgery and exercise that is relieved with Advil, denies cervical or thoracic disk pain
- Neurological: denies shingles, headaches, vertigo, syncope, falls, history of seizure disorder or stroke, numbness, tingling or extremity weakness, change in speech or motor activity
- Endocrine: denies diabetes, thyroid disorder, change in appetite, excessive thirst or urination
- Hematological: denies blood dyscrasias, infections, or cancer
- Psychiatric: denies suicidal ideation, depression, or panic disorders, states, "I am under a lot of work stress because we are ramping up our marketing division and I am up for promotion. But, I generally manage that with a few smokes a day and relax with a few beers or mixed drinks at night and I exercise every day."

Physical Examination

- Vital signs: pulse 104 beats per minute, blood pressure 154/98 mm Hg, respiratory rate 28 breaths per minute, and oral temperature 98.5°F
- Bedside monitoring: oxygen saturation by pulse oximeter 100% on oxygen at 100% nonrebreather mask, breath carbon monoxide (CO) 120 parts per million, continuous cardiac monitoring—sinus tachycardia no ST elevation or depression
- Constitutional: 30-year-old Caucasian male, well developed and appears stated age, well groomed, no acute distress but appears anxious, maintains eye contact, and communicates effectively
- Cardiovascular: no heaves, lifts or thrills; S_1 and S_2 tachycardic with regular rhythm; no murmurs, gallops, or rubs; no edema; peripheral pulses intact 2+ symmetrical, no carotid or abdominal bruits, nail beds pink without clubbing, brisk capillary refill
- Pulmonary: tachypnea without use of accessory muscles, lungs clear to auscultation and resonant to percussion
- Head/eyes/ears/nose/throat: head symmetrical without lesions or pain, pupils equal, round, reactive to light and accommodation, ear canals with

small amount dry cerumen, no nasal deviation or polyps, buccal mucosa moist, oropharynx moist without lesions
- Neck: trachea midline and freely movable, thyroid without masses or enlargement, no palpable lymph nodes, no jugular venous distension
- Gastrointestinal: nondistended, normoactive bowel sounds, tympanic on percussion, abdomen soft without tenderness, no organomegaly
- Integumentary: intact, no rashes at the site of the pain, no lesions, normal skin turgor, pink flushed face
- Musculoskeletal: no chest point tenderness or pain with palpation. Active range of motion of all extremities unlimited by pain
- Neurological: no focal neurologic deficits, face symmetric, speech clear, upper and lower extremity strength 5/5 throughout, oriented to person, place and time. Cranial nerves II-XII intact

What elements of the review of systems and physical examination should be added to the list of pertinent positives?

- Subjective—history of alcohol use, tobacco use, and stressful work environment; positive family history of cardiovascular disease. Objective—tachycardia, elevated blood pressure, elevated breath carbon monoxide level, pink flushed face

What elements of the review of systems and physical examination should be added to the significant negatives list?

- The review of systems and the physical examination are both consistent with an adult male in good health. Subjective—the review of systems reveals no localizing complaints such as substernal pain, radiation of pain, nausea, and vomiting; the review of systems for other pertinent systems such as pulmonary, GI, musculoskeletal, and neuro are normal. Objective—the physical examination is essentially normal with the exception of sinus tachycardia (however, no additional signs of ischemia are noted) and there is no chest wall tenderness or pain with palpation.

How does this information affect the list of possible causes?

Case Analysis: The review of systems and physical examination help me further sort my differential. The high carbon monoxide level makes me suspicious that this is the etiology of the chest pain. But to confirm this I order an arterial blood sample for co-oximeter analysis. Bedside monitoring demonstrates a tachycardia but no signs of ischemia. Regardless, more definitive testing is essential to rule out a myocardial infarction (MI). I order serial ECGs and troponins. The elevated blood pressure will require monitoring and may be a contributing factor to the tachycardia. An aortic dissection is less likely now, given the patient's stable condition, and essentially normal physical examination;

however, the portable chest x-ray may demonstrate mediastinal widening and prompt additional testing. The chest x-ray will also determine if the patient has a pneumothorax. The patient's physical examination does not demonstrate any signs of deep vein thrombosis, such as swelling or tenderness in his extremities that might be a source of a PE. In addition, he appears well hydrated and has no history of inactivity or recent trauma to his extremities. Pneumonia can cause chest pain but he has no complaints of fever, chills, cough, or sputum production and the x-ray will rule this in or out. Other potential etiologies include a chest muscle strain but this is not supported by the patient's review of systems or physical examination findings; he has no tenderness or pain with movement or localization with palpation.

An adverse reaction to substance use or gastroesophageal reflux with esophageal spasm is low on the differential since he denies use of ingested medications or substances other than beer at the party, has no history of gastroesophageal reflux disease, and did not eat prior to the onset of the pain. Heat exhaustion may have contributed but is very unlikely as he has few if any signs that are typical for this condition such as confusion, dizziness, fainting, headache muscle cramps, nausea, and vomiting. The thought of herpes zoster causing the chest pain is also ruled out because of the intact skin and absence of regional lymph nodes.

❓ At this point do you need to reexamine and restate the problem representation?

After reviewing the data as described above I will keep my problem representation as per my last notation following the history of present illness: "A 30-year-old male with hypertension and substance use presents with new onset chest pain that began while grilling in an enclosed area that resolved when he was transported to the hospital."

The patient's carbon monoxide level, 120 parts per million, is a key finding. This level is quite high and means that his pulse oximetry reading of 100% actually reflects a carboxyhemoglobin (COHb) of 21% and an oxyhemoglobin of only 79% (a PaO_2 of ~ 40 mm Hg). While very low, this is likely a higher oxygen level than at the time he experienced his chest pain. While this puts carbon monoxide poisoning at the top of my differential, I still need to assure that I have ruled out other conditions that may be causing his chest pain.

❓ What additional diagnostic testing should be done and in what order?

As mentioned above, an ECG, a troponin level, and a stat portable chest x-ray are ordered upon admission and completed prior to the history and physical. I also order a comprehensive metabolic panel (CMP), and a complete blood count (CBC). These tests will help me determine if the patient has a metabolic disorder, anemia, or infection, which are contributing to his chest pain. I also order a urine drug screen and a blood alcohol level as I am concerned that substance use may have contributed to his symptoms.

CASE INFORMATION

Results of Diagnostic Testing

The ECG is normal except for a tachycardia. Cardiac troponin drawn at the same time as the initial ECG is normal, and repeat ECGs and troponin levels have been ordered for every 6 hours × 3. The portable CXR is normal with no signs of acute processes such as pneumothorax, pneumonia, or mediastinal widening. An ultrasound and CT would be necessary next steps if any changes suggestive of dissection should occur such as tearing chest pain. But given the findings to this point I will not order these tests now. I place aortic dissection much lower on my differential and eliminate pneumonia.

The comprehensive metabolic panel is drawn and is normal, except for a mildly elevated blood urea nitrogen (BUN) at 25mg/dL. The complete blood count shows a normal white blood cell count, red blood cell count, hemoglobin and hematocrit, and platelet count and an absence of abnormal or lysed cells. Anemia and hemolysis are ruled out, as is infection. His urine drug screen is positive for a tetrahydrocannabinol (THC) level of 10 ng/mL . His blood alcohol level is 0.15 mg/dL.

The results of the testing confirm a diagnosis of carbon monoxide poisoning, with mild dehydration, evidenced by the elevated BUN. Further discussion with the patient reveals that over a 4-hour period approximately 10 cigarettes were smoked and one marijuana joint was smoked while grilling hamburgers over an open flame in an enclosed space. The new diagnosis of carbon monoxide poisoning–induced chest pain is made and falls in the category of "exogenous etiology," which was at the top of my differential list.

Diagnosis: Carbon Monoxide Poisoning

Diagnosis and Management

A diagnosis of carbon monoxide (CO) poisoning can be made with the presence of symptoms and significantly elevated CO levels. Carbon monoxide is a gas produced by the combustion of carbon-containing fuels such as cigarettes, marijuana, and grilling or inadequate ventilation of natural gas. In this case, the combination of multiple combustible fuels plus limited ventilation presented a constellation of symptoms that resulted in hypoxia and mimicked a coronary event. CO has approximately 240 times the affinity of oxygen for binding to hemoglobin, and forms the COHb complex which impairs tissue oxygen delivery, inhibits mitochondrial oxidative phosphorylation, and inactivates cytochrome oxidase.[2] There is a spectrum of clinical features from headache, nausea, and flu-like symptoms to coma with hyperventilation, seizures, pulmonary edema, myocardial infarction/ischemia, and cherry red skin coloring. Levels of COHb correlate poorly with clinical features, but it is generally accepted that an initial level greater than 15% suggests significant toxicity.[1,3]

Recognizing that a normal COHb level for nonsmokers is <1.5% and the average for smokers can be 3% to 15% COHb, the combined effects of a combustible fuel environment consisting of cigarette and marijuana smoke and grill smoke may result in a significant CO exposure and poisoning. One marijuana joint is the equivalent of smoking four cigarettes[3,4] so for this patient, the CO level quickly elevated to very toxic levels with exposure to the accumulating CO resulting from grilling in an enclosed area. This patient demonstrated moderate, but still potentially lethal, CO poisoning with a COHb of 21%.[2,3] While the breath CO detector value and the COHB do not correlate precisely, they are close and indicate a seriously impaired oxygen-carrying capacity, and a high possibility that tissue hypoxia may ensue.

Although the exact duration of his CO exposure is unknown, it can be estimated at approximately 4 hours based on the patient's self-report. The half-life of CO is 4 to 6 hours while breathing room air, and 40 to 60 minutes when breathing 100% oxygen, thus, the patient's peak CO exposure occurred at the time of his chest pain. When the patient arrived in the ER his oxygen saturation was 97% and he was started on oxygen by mask (100% nonrebreather) bringing his O_2 saturation to 100%. It is essential to start O_2 in patients immediately when CO exposure is suspected. Even with a saturation of 100%, if the COHb is 21%, the patient's oxyhemoglobin is only 79%. As described previously this is the equivalent to a PaO_2 of ~40 or less dependent on his metabolic state. When the patient first experienced the chest pain, his CO level was likely higher and caused further hypoxemia and cardiac ischemia leading to chest pain.

CO poisoning should be suspected in any individual exposed to potentially high CO such as grilling in an enclosed space or in situations such as those experienced by firefighters. However, an understanding of how the patient may present is key to appropriate and life-saving treatment. Most standard pulse oximeters, such as used in the ER, display the saturation as a total of bound Hg but do not discriminate between the types (ie, oxyhemoglobin, methemoglobin, carboxyhemoglobin). Thus the O_2 saturation readings obtained by standard pulse oximeters are inaccurate when CO is bound to Hg and not a true reflection of oxygen bound to Hg (oxyhemoglobin). In addition, though the patient may be experiencing significant hypoxemia and tissue hypoxia, s/he may look pink. Normally cyanosis is what we expect with tissue hypoxia. However, when the hemoglobin is saturated with any bound form, it appears pink. Thus a high index of suspicion is key to making an accurate diagnosis of CO poisoning. Immediately administering oxygen to these patients is essential.

While treatment guidelines suggest 100% oxygen by mask, high flow device, or hyperbaric therapy, treatment is guided by the severity of the clinical manifestations of the carboxyhemoglobinemia.[3] Fortunately, in this patient CO poisoning was managed with short-term O_2 by mask and 24-hour observation for any neuropsychiatric and/or abnormal cardiac sequelae.

Case Follow-Up

Additional interventions provided in this case included substance abuse counseling for his tobacco, marijuana, and alcohol use, as well as a review of the hazards of using combustible products over an open flame grill in a confined space. The importance of quitting smoking for his health was emphasized. Questioning his level of readiness to quit on a scale of 0 to 10 with "0" representing not ready and "10" representing highly ready, the patient reported a "10." As with most teachable moments in acute care settings, smokers are highly motivated to quit after a near-death episode.[5] Thus, the five Rs (relevance, risks, rewards, roadblocks, and repetition) were reviewed.[6]

Further exploration of his smoking history revealed a moderate Fagerström test for nicotine dependence level of 6/10 with "10" representing highly dependent. A recommendation for a 24-hour release nicotine replacement therapy (NRT) patch 21 mg with NRT gum/lozenge 2 mg every 2 to 4 hours for breakthrough cravings.[6]

A CAGE (cut down, annoy, guilty, eye opening) assessment was also obtained to determine the degree of concern about alcohol use. His CAGE screening indicated low alcohol dependence with only "one" item out of four he responded with "yes" when asked "do you ever feel like you should cut down."

During the patient's observation unit admission his heart rate returned to normal (70 beats per minute) and serial ECGs and cardiac biomarkers were negative. His blood pressure remained elevated at 140/92 and his O_2 saturation was 98% on room air with a COHb of 2% (thus his real oxyhemoglobin was 96%). The patient was discharged from the observation unit 1 day after admission. He was provided a prescription for low-dose hydrochlorothiazide and a follow-up appointment with his primary care provider. A note was dictated to the PCP and the tobacco cessation specialist.

References

1. Chest pain of recent onset: assessment and diagnosis. National Institute for Heath and Care Excellence: NICE guidelines [CG95] Published on March 2010. https://www.nice.org.uk/guidance/cg95/chapter/guidance.

2. U.S. Department of Health and Human Services. Agency for Toxic Substances and Disease Registry Division of Toxicology and Human Health Sciences/Environmental Toxicology Branch. Toxicology profile for carbon monoxide. Published June 2012. http://www.atsdr.cdc.gov/toxprofiles/tp201-c3.pdf. Accessed June 5, 2014.

3. Clardy PF, Manaker S, Perry H. Carbon monoxide poisoning. UpToDate. http://www.uptodate.com/contents/carbon-monoxide-poisoning. Accessed January 11, 2015.

4. Moir D, Rickett WS, Genevieve L, et al. A comparison of mainstream and sidestream marijuana and tobacco cigarette smoke produced under two machine smoking conditions. *Chem Res Toxicol.* 2008;21(2):494-502.

5. Katz DA, Vander MW, Holman J, et al. The Emergency Department Action in Smoking Cessation (EDASC) trial: impact on delivery of smoking cessation counseling. *Acad Emerg Med.* 2012;19(4):409-420.

6. Fiore MC, Jaén CR, Baker TB, et al. *Treating Tobacco Use and Dependence: 2008 Update. Clinical Practice Guideline.* Rockville, MD: U.S. Department of Health and Human Services. Public Health Service; 2008.

CASE 15

Janet H. Johnson

Janet H. Johnson practices in a Cardiology Telemetry Service that admits over 9000 patients a year and manages patients with acute coronary syndrome, congestive heart failure, and cardiac arrhythmias. She is also preceptor for ACNP students.

CASE INFORMATION

Chief Complaint

A 57-year-old female is admitted to a local hospital with the complaint of chest discomfort and "fullness" lasting several hours. After the initial workup in her local emergency department (ED), she is transferred to a tertiary care facility for further evaluation.

? What is the potential cause?

Case Analysis: The complaint of chest discomfort needs to be triaged quickly as the etiology can range from benign musculoskeletal problems to a life-threatening cardiac disease. The differential diagnoses are extensive. Along with a focused cardiac history and physical assessment, a rapid interpretation of a 12-lead electrocardiogram (ECG) should be completed. Six of the potential diagnoses are life threatening: acute coronary syndrome, aortic dissection, effort rupture of esophagus, perforating peptic ulcer, pulmonary embolus, and tension pneumothorax. And the standard of care for a patient experiencing an ST-elevation myocardial infarction (STEMI) is to reach the cardiac catheterization lab within 90 minutes of ER admission.[1]

Comprehensive Differential Diagnoses for Chest Pain[2]

- Chest wall pain: musculoskeletal pain, rheumatic disease, non-rheumatic disease; neuropathic pain
- Cardiovascular: ischemic chest pain syndrome related to coronary disease, coronary vasospasm, cardiac syndrome X; valvular heart disease; nonischemic cardiac chest pain syndrome related to pericarditis, myocarditis, acute aortic syndrome, cardiac amyloid
- Hyperadrenergic states: stress-induced cardiomyopathy, cocaine intoxication, methamphetamine intoxication, pheochromocytoma
- Gastrointestinal: gastroesophageal reflux disease; esophageal hypersensitivity; abnormal motility patterns and achalasia; esophageal rupture, perforation, and foreign bodies; esophagitis

- Pulmonary: acute pulmonary embolism, pulmonary hypertension, cor pulmonale, pneumonia, cancer, sarcoidosis, asthma, COPD, pneumothorax, pleuritis, pleural effusion
- Mediastinal: mediastinitis, sternal wound post CABG, sternal wound infection
- Psychogenic/psychosomatic: panic disorder, anxiety

CASE INFORMATION

General Survey and History of Present Illness

Information gathered from the patient and from the outside ER records tells the following: Over the past month, the patient has had episodes of chest discomfort. The episodes were associated with a fainting-like feeling, flushing, and diaphoresis. These symptoms occurred several times a week, lasting a few minutes to ½ hour, and always occurred with activity. The symptoms resolved either spontaneously or with rest. She has also noticed dyspnea on exertion, increased fatigue and heaviness in her legs, all worse with stair climbing. These symptoms all improve with rest. She saw her primary care provider and was referred for a cardiac nuclear stress test that showed abnormal perfusion with a small area of lateral ischemia. No anterior infarction was noted. She was scheduled to undergo cardiac catheterization at our facility as an outpatient but today she had chest pain and "fullness" that lasted for several hours, so she went to her local ED. Workup at that ED included a troponin level of 0.04, an ECG showing normal sinus rhythm with no acute changes, a normal chest x-ray, a negative D-dimer, and normal oxygen saturation on room air. Because an outpatient cardiac catheterization was planned previously, she was transferred to this facility for further workup. She is normotensive at 92/60 mm Hg, with a heart rate of 60 beats per minute, and room air oxygen saturation of 98%.

Past Medical History

The patient has a history of monoclonal gammopathy (MGUS), congenital single kidney, hyperthyroidism, and carpal tunnel syndrome. The patient is followed at a cancer specialty hospital for her diagnosis of MGUS and states it is under control without symptoms. She denies any history of coronary artery disease, denies diabetes, denies high cholesterol, reports eating a healthy diet, and performs regular exercise. She is postmenopausal.

- Family history: Denies family history of coronary heart disease.
- Medications: Her regular medications are loratadine 10 mg daily and a therapeutic multivitamin. It was suggested she start on a low-dose β-blocker

because of her abnormal stress test, but after taking it two or three times, she discontinued it because she felt light-headed.

• Social history: She denies smoking history and illicit substance use. She is a stay-at-home mother of two children, married for 25 years. She describes her home and family as supportive, with the "normal stresses" but not anything unusual. Her husband accompanied her on transfer and remains at her bedside.

? What are the pertinent positives obtained from the information so far?

• Symptoms of chest fullness that were relieved with rest, but are now progressively worse

• Dyspnea on exertion, fatigue, light-headedness

• Abnormal nuclear stress test obtained prior to admission

? What are the significant negatives obtained from the information so far?

• No past medical history of heart disease, COPD, or asthma

• No acute distress at time of transfer

• Negative risk factors for coronary heart disease: nonsmoker, not diabetic, normal blood pressure, no family history

• Troponin I negative × 1

• ECG without ischemic changes

Case Analysis: In my initial analysis, I focus first on the six most life-threatening concerns. Thus far, while I cannot definitively rule out coronary heart disease (CHD) without proceeding to cardiac catheterization, the diagnosis of acute myocardial infarction seems less likely based on her lack of risk factors and test results from the outside hospital. The ECG does not show ST-segment elevation, Q waves, or a conduction defect such as a new left bundle branch block that would suggest an acute myocardial infarction. The first Troponin I was negative and this was drawn several hours after the onset chest discomfort. In addition, her Framingham risk score is less than 1% though I still plan to check a fasting lipid profile to confirm that she does not have hyperlipidemia. The progressive worsening of her symptoms with activity concerns me, however, and her recent stress test was positive. Her chest pain can be described as "atypical angina" because it has two of three characteristics, provoked by exertion and relieved by rest.[3] The third characteristic of angina is substernal location and in this patient's case the pain is actually diffuse across her anterior chest and abdomen. In addition, she is female and women sometimes have atypical symptoms with CHD. I plan to order another Troponin I and ECG to definitively rule out an acute coronary syndrome, as well as a beta-natriuretic peptide (BNP) to evaluate for heart failure. Additional admission lab work includes metabolic profile, complete blood count, and coagulation times. I will call the cardiac catheterization lab to schedule her for a catheterization to rule out CHD.

The normal chest x-ray findings from the local hospital helps rule out two potential life-threatening diagnoses: tension pneumothorax and aortic dissection. A pneumothorax would be seen on plain chest film, and, I would expect to see widening of the mediastinum on a plain chest if she had an aortic dissection, which classically causes severe pain with a ripping or tearing sensation. While this is not always the case, her symptoms also do not correlate well with dissection. I am less inclined to think this is a pulmonary embolism based on her negative D-dimer, normal oxygen saturation, and the fact that her pain has resolved and she is not currently in any distress. When I complete a review of systems and physical examination, I will check for a potential source of a deep vein thrombosis (DVT), which usually precedes a pulmonary embolism; however, this diagnosis remains unlikely. Esophageal rupture and perforated peptic ulcer cannot be definitely ruled out at this point but are unlikely given the chronic recurrent nature of the pain and lack of distress on current presentation. To further evaluate this, I will collect more information about gastrointestinal symptoms when I do my complete review of systems.

CASE INFORMATION

Review of Systems

- Constitutional: denies fever, chills, night sweats, or weight loss, no recent travel or prolonged immobility
- Head/eyes/ears/nose/throat: + episodes of dizziness, light-headedness, denies headache
- Cardiovascular: + intermittent chest discomfort/burning/fullness, anterior diffuse. No radiation to upper extremities, back. + dyspnea on exertion, with exercise intolerance. + Intermittent palpitations. Denies swelling to lower extremities, denies lower extremity pain with ambulation
- Pulmonary: denies shortness of breath but endorses dyspnea on exertion. Denies cough wheezes, pain on inspiration
- Gastrointestinal: denies nausea, vomiting, dysphagia, constipation or diarrhea. Denies heartburn, indigestion. No change in appetite
- Genitourinary: + urinary frequency
- Neurological: + tingling and weakness in lower extremities on exertion
- Psychological: Denies anxiety

Physical Examination

- Vital signs: blood pressure 92/61, heart rate 62 beats per minute, respiratory rate 16/min, oxygen saturation 98%.
- Orthostatic blood pressure values:
  - Lying: blood pressure 115/62 mm Hg, heart rate 63 beats per minute
  - Sitting: blood pressure 103/63 mm Hg, heart rate 50 beats per minute
  - Standing: blood pressure 88/52 mm Hg, heart rate 52 beats per minute
- Constitutional: Middle-aged, well-nourished white female. Appears in good state of health, and stated age, in no acute distress.
- Head/eyes/ears/nose/throat: Pupils equal, round, react to light, no jugular venous distention.
- Cardiovascular: S1, S2 heart rate and rhythm regular. No murmurs, rubs, or grades. No lower extremities edema or discoloration.
- Extremities: warm to touch, no erythema, no edema.
- Pulmonary: Breathing unlabored, no use of accessory muscles. Denies any chest pain with palpation. Breath sounds clear to auscultation, anterior and posterior. No cyanosis or clubbing.
- Gastrointestinal: Abdomen soft, slightly distended, not tender. + bowel sounds in all four quadrants.
- Neurological: Alert and oriented × 3, no focal deficits noted.
- Psychological: Normal effect.

? What elements of the review of systems and physical examination should be added to the list of pertinent positives?

Dysnea on exertion, presyncopal episodes, + intermittent chest discomfort/burning/fullness, anterior diffuse, palpitations, lower extremity weakness/tingling, unusual fatigue. On examination, she is bradycardic, orthostatic, hypotensive with standing BP 88/52 mm Hg.

? What elements of the review of systems and physical examination should be added to the significant negatives list?

Cardiac and pulmonary examination are normal, no signs of fluid overload, negative gastrointestinal symptoms, chest pain not reproducible, no lower extremity swelling, pain, or redness.

? How does the information affect your problem representation and your list of potential causes?

Case Analysis: She does not have any of the clinical findings associated with a pulmonary embolism (Wells criteria) such as leg swelling or pain, tachycardia, or hemoptysis, and she has no risk factors such as history of DVT or PE, malignancy, or recent period of immobility. The D-dimer assay obtained at the local hospital was negative so I am ruling out pulmonary embolus. The diagnosis of esophageal rupture is unlikely because the patient has no history of forceful vomiting, trauma, or ingestion of corrosive material. The patient's clinical picture does not fit a diagnosis of perforated peptic ulcer. Her symptoms are not described as sudden, agonizing, intense, severe, or persistent. Movement, jostling, or touching does not worsen her chest/abdominal fullness. The chest pain is not reproducible on palpitation, so is unlikely to be due to musculoskeletal etiology. I need to review the diagnostic tests done to date and sort the information to hone in on the potential cause of my patient's symptoms.

CASE INFORMATION

Results of Diagnostic Testing

Labs (Done on Transfer)
- Troponin I 0.06, (N = 0.0–0.5)
- CBC, chem panel, and coags are all within normal limits
- Total cholesterol 202 (N = <200). Triglycerides 115, HDL 45 (Normal = <60), LDL 134 (Normal = <100 mg/dL)
- BNP 505 (Normal < 100 pg/mL)
- TSH 3.88, (Normal = 0.5–4.70 μIU/mL), free T4 1.04 (Normal = 0.8–2.8 ng/dL)

Admission ECG (see Figure 15-1)
- Sinus bradycardia with sinus arrhythmia. HR 52 beats per minute.
- RSR' pattern or QR pattern in lead V1 suggests right ventricular conduction delay.
- Low voltage.
- Left anterior fascicular block.
- Septal infarct.
- Prolonged QTc—486 ms.

Myocardial Perfusion Study Previously Done as an Outpatient
Exercise and rest sestamibi perfusion scan: good exercise capacity. Occasional premature ventricular contractions. Abnormal sestamibi perfusion with a small area of lateral ischemia changes and no antecedent infarction noted.

Echocardiogram previously done as an outpatient:

Left ventricle shows normal dimensions with no wall motion abnormality and an ejection fraction of 60% (normal), no left ventricle hypertrophy, decreased E/A ratio consistent with grade 2 diastolic dysfunction. Right ventricle—normal size with normal contractility. No aortic regurgitation or stenosis.

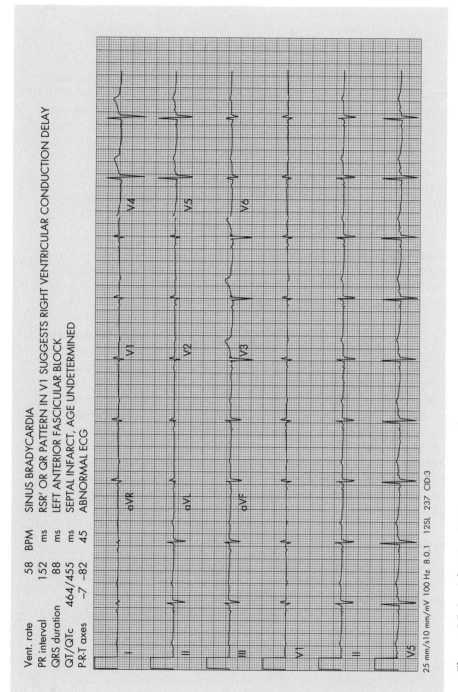

Vent. rate	58	BPM	SINUS BRADYCARDIA
PR interval	152	ms	RSR' OR QR PATTERN IN V1 SUGGESTS RIGHT VENTRICULAR CONDUCTION DELAY
QRS duration	88	ms	LEFT ANTERIOR FASCICULAR BLOCK
QT/QTc	464/455	ms	SEPTAL INFARCT, AGE UNDETERMINED
P-R-T axes	-7 -82	45	ABNORMAL ECG

25 mm/s 10 mm/mV 100 Hz 8.0.1   12SL 237 CID:3

Figure 15-1 Admission ECG

Cardiac Catheterization:

The evening of the patient's admission, she experiences two separate runs of nonsustained ventricular tachycardia (NSVT), a 12 beat and a 13 beat, and is started on a low-dose β-blocker, metoprolol immediate release 12.5 bid, for the antiarrhythmic effect. She experiences symptoms of palpitations during these episodes and is sent for cardiac catheterization. The catheterization reveals normal coronaries, normal systolic function, and no aortic stenosis.

❓ The normal cardiac catheterization rules out coronary artery disease. So the question remains what is the cause of this patient's chest discomfort?

Case Analysis: At this point, I review the patient's history and pertinent findings with my team. It is notable that the patient has a history of monoclonal gammopathy (MGUS). This condition was detected through routine lab work done during an annual physical and the patient states that she has not experienced any symptoms with this diagnosis. However, patients with MGUS are more likely to have complications such as amyloidosis and multiple myeloma. In addition, the patient does report leg numbness and peripheral neuropathy, which is a common complaint among patients with systemic amyloidosis. Cardiac amyloidosis can produce clinical features of postural hypotension, arrhythmias, weakness, dyspnea, peripheral edema, and presyncope—all of which are present in this patient.[3] Patients with cardiac amyloid also have angina due to deposits of proteins in the coronary arteries, usually the smaller intracardiac arterioles, which are not visualized on cardiac catheterization. In addition, patients with cardiac amyloid often have low voltage ECG and findings consistent with pseudoinfarction, both of which were evident on this patient's admission ECG. At this point, cardiac amyloid seems a likely diagnosis for this patient and further imaging is ordered to confirm this.

CASE INFORMATION

Further Diagnostic Test Results

An inpatient cardiac magnetic resonance imaging (MRI) study is ordered. Results of the study are:

1. Normal LV size and systolic function with mild concentric increase in wall thickness. Normal RV size, wall thickness, and systolic function.

2. Diffuse myocardial enhancement predominately involving the intramyocardial to subendocardial regions and abnormal contrast kinetics between blood and myocardium.

These findings are suggestive of infiltrative heart disease, such as Fabry disease, sarcoidosis, or amyloid disease. This result, in conjunction with the patient's ECG findings, confirms a diagnosis of cardiac amyloidosis.

Diagnosis and Management: Cardiac Amyloidosis

The most common clinical presentation of cardiac amyloid is heart failure, with symptoms of dyspnea and edema. An elevated BNP in patients with amyloid without overt signs of CHF and symptoms of angina is a marker for cardiac involvement. BNP and cardiac troponin are widely used to assess the severity of cardiac involvement and to determine a prognosis. The Mayo Clinic staging system is based on a BNP of 100 ng/L and cardiac troponin of 0.035 µg/L, and stratifies patients into three group: stage III, a high risk for cardiac involvement with both biomarkers elevated; stage II, an intermediate risk, with at least one biomarker elevated; and stage I, a low risk where both biomarkers are below the established limit. Amyloid-induced regional myocardial stress, caused by local myocyte deformities, is likely the cause of BNP elevation. In addition, amyloid-induced small-vessel disease may cause purpura, claudication, or angina. Syncope or presyncope in a patient with cardiac amyloidosis represents a low cardiac output. Peripheral neuropathy such as numbness, paresthesia, pain, and orthostatic hypotension along with carpal tunnel syndrome are common systemic symptoms of amyloidosis.[4]

In noninvasive testing for cardiac amyloid, an echocardiogram is the initial test. The earliest echo abnormalities include increased left ventricular LV wall thickness with evidence of diastolic dysfunction. These findings are more commonly caused by hypertensive heart disease, which sometimes delays the diagnosis of cardiac amyloid. More advanced disease is evident on echocardiogram as progressive LV wall thickening resulting in a nondilated or small LV cavity with systolic impairment and restrictive disease. LV wall thickening is generally symmetric.[4] My patient had evidence of grade 2 diastolic dysfunction, which is consistent with amyloid.

Low voltage and a pseudoinfarct pattern are the most common ECG abnormalities on ECG for cardiac amyloid. Other findings include first-degree AV block, nonspecific intraventricular conduction delay, second- or third-degree AV block, atrial fibrillation/atrial flutter, and ventricular tachycardia.[5] On ECG, my patient has low voltage, pseudo-septal infarct pattern, conduction delay and she had two runs of NSVT while on telemetry.

Amyloidosis is a severe systemic disease and patients who have cardiac involvement have a poor prognosis. New treatment strategies involving chemotherapy, management of heart failure, and organ transplant are improving survival, and depend in part on what type of amyloid the patient has, monoclonal light chain, familial, or senile.[6] Endomyocardial biopsy of the cardiac tissue is the gold standard for diagnosing cardiac amyloidosis and determining which form of amyloidosis is causing the disease. While all forms of cardiac amyloidosis carry a poor prognosis, there are some treatment options and these are best selected once the type of disease is confirmed.

Case Follow-up

The patient was discharged after the cardiac MRI and referred to the outpatient heart failure team for cardiac biopsy and follow-up. To treat her arrhythmia, she was continued on a low-dose β-blocker, and advised to take magnesium and potassium supplements. Loop diuretics and ACE inhibitors were avoided because of her baseline hypotension and orthostasis.

References

1. O'Gara P, Kushner F, Asheim D, et al. (2013). ACCF/AHA Guidelines for the management of ST-elevation myocardial infarction: executive summary. http://circ.ahajournals.org/content/127/4/529.full. Accessed August 17, 2014.
2. UpToDate 2014. Diagnostic approach to chest pain in adults. http://www.uptodate.com. Accessed July 10, 2014.
3. Cayley W. Diagnosing the cause of chest pain. November 15, 2005;72(10): 2012-2021. http://www.aafp.org/afp/2005/1115/p2012.html.
4. Mohty D, Damy T, Cosnay P, et al. Cardiac amyloidosis: updates in diagnosis and management. *Arch Cardiovasc Dis.* 2013;106:528-540.
5. UpToDate 2014. Cardiac amyloidosis. http://www.uptodate.com. Accessed July 15, 2014.
6. Firkrle M, Palecek T, Kuchynka P, et al. Cardiac amyloidosis: a comprehensive review. *Cor et Vasa.* December 3, 2012, 55; e60-e75. www.elsevier.com/locate/crvasa. Accessed July 15, 2014.

CASE 16

Rachel Anderson

Rachel Anderson is an ACNP with the Lung Transplant Program at the University of Virginia Medical Center. She has previous experience in both cardiac surgery intensive care unit and coronary care unit.

CASE INFORMATION

Chief Complaint

A 75-year-old male is brought to the cardiac surgery intensive care unit 4 hours following coronary artery bypass graft surgery (CABG). He remains intubated and is noted to be increasingly tachypneic with a respiratory rate in the 30s.

? What is the potential cause?

Case Analysis: Tachypnea is a nonspecific symptom that can be attributed to several conditions in the immediate cardiac surgery postoperative period. While it may be related to pain or anxiety, it may also be an early, subtle sign, of more life-threatening conditions such as cardiac tamponade or pneumothorax. Using a system-based approach, beginning with the cardiac and pulmonary systems, will allow me to develop a differential with the most emergent conditions identified first while still being inclusive of less serious, but still urgent, considerations in this postoperative patient.

> **Comprehensive Differential Diagnoses for Tachypnea Immediately Following Cardiac Surgery**
> - Cardiac: acute myocardial infarction, myocardial stunning, cardiac tamponade, pericarditis, volume overload
> - Pulmonary: hemothorax, pneumothorax, pulmonary embolism, inadequate ventilator support, airway occlusion, respiratory insufficiency related to underlying pulmonary disease, pulmonary artery infarct, pulmonary artery injury, pulmonary edema, paralyzed diaphragm
> - Neurologic: acute embolic or hemorrhagic stroke
> - Gastrointestinal: ischemic bowel
> - Genitourinary: bladder distention, urethral trauma related to urinary catheter placement
> - Musculoskeletal: rib fracture, joint displacement
> - Psychiatric: anxiety, pain, exacerbation of psychiatric disorder, postoperative delirium

- Metabolic: acid-base imbalance
- Exogenous: side effects of anesthesia medications, withdrawal from alcohol or drugs. Anaphylaxis to medications

Since the patient is intubated, he can only answer by shaking his head or nodding. I have to consider that he has had narcotics and anesthesia, which may cloud his ability to give meaningful answers. As a result, I will rely on his bedside nurse for a timeline and data from the chart and his family, to obtain his medical history. I will also gather data from the OR handoff, a verbal report given by the surgeons or anesthesiologist which includes the history of present illness and any events that occurred in the OR.

CASE INFORMATION

General Survey and History of Present Illness

The patient had a positive stress test last month while being worked up for his increasing chest pain and shortness of breath. After his stress test, he was taken to the cardiac catheterization lab and found to have multi-vessel disease, involving his right coronary artery as well as his left circumflex artery. Grafts from his CABG 15 years ago were patent. Neither of the identified lesions was amenable to stenting. Today, a week after his catheterization, the surgeons preformed a bypass using a saphenous vein graft to his right coronary artery lesion and his left internal mammary artery to bypass the left circumflex lesion. Other than the prior CABG, he has no surgical history. His medical history is significant for type 2 diabetes, high cholesterol, chronic obstructive pulmonary disease (COPD), and peripheral vascular disease (PVD). His medication list includes metformin, simvastatin, budesonide/formoterol fumarate dihydrate inhaler, and clopidogrel bisulfate in addition to his herbal medication list of garlic and fish oil. He stopped taking the clopidogrel bisulfate 7 days prior to surgery and he stopped the metformin 3 days before. The operation was uneventful; however, the surgeons did note more generalized bleeding during the case than is typical.

My initial assessment of the patient focuses on evaluating the degree of his distress. This will determine how I move through my review of systems and physical examination. It is obvious when I walk into the room that the patient is not only tachypneic, but also diaphoretic and struggling to breathe with nasal flaring and subcostal retractions. His eyes are closed but he is still lying in the bed. This degree of respiratory distress must be quickly addressed. I first establish a timeline to look for cause and effect relationships and obtain additional information. I ask the bedside nurse about the duration of the tachypnea, and she reports it started 30 minutes ago. I also ask about trends in hemodynamic status and I learn that the epinephrine has been increased in response to the hypotension and that only 1 L of crystalloid has been given since admission to the postoperative unit. Also, his cardiac index (CI) this hour has dropped from 3 to 2.1 (N = 2.5–4.0 L/min/m^2). His pulmonary artery diastolic pressure (PAD) and central venous pressure (CVP) have both slowly increased and stabilized at 20 mm Hg. Additional information from the nurse indicates that his chest tube drainage has declined from 200 to 250 mL/h to 10 mL in the last hour.

I now ask the respiratory therapist about his respiratory status over the past hour. "His blood gases have never looked bad, though this hour he does have a mild respiratory alkalosis. He breathes better on pressure support so I changed his setting about 15 minutes ago. His settings are: 5 of PEEP, 10 of pressure support, and he has been on 40% FIO$_2$ since his first blood gas following admission to the ICU." I note that on pressure support ventilation, he is achieving tidal volumes of 350 to 400 mL. His last arterial blood gas (ABG) drawn on this setting is: pH 7.49, CO$_2$ 28 mm Hg, PaO$_2$ 80 mm Hg, and HCO$_3^-$ 23 mm Hg. The patient shakes his head no when asked if he is in pain but affirms that he is short of breath by nodding yes when asked.

Since no family is immediately available, I scan his chart quickly for any additional medications or pertinent history that anesthesia may have not mentioned. I note he is a former smoker with a 30 pack-year history, though he did stop smoking 5 years ago. He drinks socially, and does not use any prescription narcotics, anxiolytics, or street drugs. He has no known drug allergies.

What are the pertinent positives from the information given so far?

- This surgery is a CABG via a "redo" sternotomy.
- There was increased generalized bleeding noted during the case.
- He is in acute respiratory distress, starting about 30 minutes ago.
- He was on clopidogrel bisulfate up until 7 days before surgery but he continued to take two herbs (garlic and fish oil) that are known to cause increased bleeding risk.
- He has a history of COPD.
- He has a history of PVD.
- In the past hour the nurse has noted his vasopressors have increased, along with a decrease in the cardiac index.
- His CVP and PAD have both increased and are now approximately equal to each other.
- The chest tube output went from a moderately high amount of 200 to 250 cc/h to a sudden decrease of 10 cc this hour.
- His ventilator requirements for support have decreased since he has become more tachypneic.

- His blood gasses reflect respiratory alkalosis with adequate oxygenation.
- He is able to answer questions and respond appropriately despite his dyspnea.

❓ What are the significant negatives from the information given so far?

- No acute or unexpected events were noted during the surgery.
- He appears calm in bed despite tachypnea.
- He denies pain.
- No history of blood clots or hypercoagulable diseases.
- No history of alcohol or drug abuse.
- No psychiatric history.
- No use of anxiolytics.

❓ How does this information affect the list of possible causes?

The problem representation could be stated as, "This is a 75-year male, 4 hours s/p CABG via redo sternotomy who now presents with new sudden onset tachypnea with coinciding decline in hemodynamic stability and chest tube output."

Case Analysis: The tachypnea coupled with the hemodynamic instability affirms my concern that the cause of tachypnea is most likely cardiac or pulmonary. Therefore, as I focus on the information I have from these two systems, the drop in cardiac index and blood pressure are key signs. To fully understand this I need to review the changes in his infusions and what other fluids have been given in the last 4 hours since these things can also affect hemodynamics. The fall in his cardiac index has occurred despite increased administration of inotropes, and his central venous pressure (CVP) and pulmonary artery diastolic (PAD) pressure have increased without the administration of large volumes of fluid. Equalization of the CVP and PAD is not typical and is suggestive of tamponade. Typically, in cardiac surgery, the target CVP is lower than the PAD by a margin of about 5 mm Hg. Complicating my assessment is the fact that he was on a β-blocker (metoprolol) until the day before surgery, thus his heart rate may not increase in response to a decreased cardiac output. I note that the nurses have appropriately increased his temporary pacer to a set rate of 100 beats per minute and that he is capturing with 100% pacing. His underlying rhythm is a sinus rhythm at a rate of 68 beats per minute.

An acute pulmonary embolism increases pulmonary vascular resistance, and mean pulmonary artery pressure. Right-sided heart failure ensues and the CVP increases. But, in the case of PE the left ventricular filling pressure often falls and both the pulmonary artery systolic pressure and diastolic rise together, which is not the case in this patient. Large pulmonary embolism, tension pneumothorax, and acute tamponade can all look very similar and be very difficult to differentiate with hemodynamics alone (see Table 16-1).

Table 16-1   Effect of Large Pulmonary Embolism, Cardiac Tamponade, and Tension Pneumothorax on Hemodynamic Values

	Heart Rate	Blood Pressure	Cardiac Output	Pulmonary Artery Pressures	Central Venous Pressure	Pulmonary Artery Occlusion Pressure
Large pulmonary embolism	Increased	Decreased	Decreased	Increased	Increased	Normal or low
Cardiac tamponade	Increased	Decreased	Decreased	Increased	Increased	Increased and close to central venous pressure values
Tension pneumo-thorax	Increased	Decreased	Decreased	Increased	Increased	Increased

Because of how intertwined the cardiac and pulmonary systems are, there may be a primary pulmonary diagnosis that is causing the changes in hemo-dynamics. For instance, if the change in hemodynamics is due to a pneumo-thorax, pulmonary edema, paralyzed diaphragm, or airway occlusion, I would expect his blood gases to be worse, his ventilator requirements to be more, or at a minimum to see a drop in the patient's spontaneous tidal volume. Because he is oxygenating well on 40% FIO_2 and achieving tidal volumes of 375 cc, my suspicion for an acute pulmonary process is much lower. Considering compli-cations from his COPD as a potential cause, he may be tachypneic related to CO_2 retention from bronchospasm or he may be tachypneic from auto-PEEP on the ventilator. Since his ABG shows adequate gas exchange with a CO_2 of 28 mm Hg and PaO_2 of 80 mm Hg, complications related to his COPD are a less likely cause; however, a good physical examination will be necessary to fully exclude these as a cause.

The decrease in chest tube output may at first seem to be a positive sign. However, in cardiac surgery patients, abrupt decreases in output may be an ominous sign that the chest tube drains have become occluded and blood is therefore accumulating in the chest. Based on that concern, I will need to know the patient's admission coagulation labs and if any blood products or any prothrombotics have recently been given, which may result in a sudden decrease in bleeding. In addition to traditional anticoagulants, herbal agents may result in changes in bleeding and must be considered. This patient was taking garlic and fish oil before surgery.

Seeing how unstable his cardiac numbers look and knowing his history do not suggest any drug or alcohol use or medications from which he could be withdrawing. I eliminate psychological or medication causes from my differen-tial list. Also his appropriate responses and interactions with the nurses and me lessen my concerns for an acute neurologic event.

CASE INFORMATION

Review of Systems

Because the patient is intubated, his review of systems is limited to yes and no answers. Also, he has received intravenous pain medications within the last 30 minutes. Therefore, several areas will be deferred.
- Constitutional: deferred
- Head/eyes/ears/nose/throat: deferred
- Cardiovascular: denies chest pain, incisional pain, tightness, or pressure
- Pulmonary: nods yes to feeling short of breath
- Gastrointestinal: denies abdominal pain
- Genitourinary: deferred
- Musculoskeletal: denies muscle or joint pain
- Neurologic: denies numbness or tingling in any extremities
- Endocrine: deferred

Physical Examination

- Vital signs: Pulse is 100 beats per minute by pacemaker (full capture). Blood pressure is 90/65 mm Hg. Respiratory rate is 35/min. Temperature is 96.8°F (36°C) via cardiac output catheter.
- Constitutional: Well-developed, well-nourished, pale appearing male, who is in acute respiratory distress, intubated, and under a warming blanket.
- Head/eyes/ears/nose/throat: Pupils round, equal, and reactive to light. Endotracheal tube in place 25 cm at the lip.
- Cardiovascular: Heart rate is 100% paced with 100% capture at 100 beats per minute, without ectopy. Rub present throughout all cardiac auscultation points. Heart tones distant. Jugular venous distension present to approximately 8 cm above the clavicle. Radial pulse weak and both posterior tibial and dorsalis pedis pulses unable to palpate but detectable with Doppler. Capillary refill >3 seconds.
- Pulmonary: Respiratory rate even, rapid, and shallow. Use of accessory muscles and nasal flaring present. Secretions from in-line suction clear and thin without hemoptysis. Diminished breath sounds in bilateral bases otherwise clear to auscultation. Percussion deferred.
- Gastrointestinal: Absent bowel sounds. Mild distention. No grimace to deep palpation.
- Genitourinary: Foley catheter in place draining dark, yellow urine. No kinks or obvious occlusions in catheter or drainage tubing.
- Integumentary: Midsternal and chest tube dressing in place with scant amount of blood present on dressing. All extremities cool and clammy. Without rashes or erythema.

- Musculoskeletal: Able to move bilateral upper and lower extremities to command.
- Neurologic: Able to nod his head yes and no to basic questions. Face symmetric, able to move all four extremities to command. No focal neurologic deficits.
- Lymph nodes: Deferred.
- Lines and drains: Right internal jugular central venous catheter present with pulmonary artery catheter in place at 55 cm. Right radial arterial line in place. Wave forms for pulmonary artery catheter as well as the arterial line are both appropriate. Two mediastinal chest tubes and two pleural chest tubes in place, both attached to collection device with bright red blood collected in the chambers. The chest tubes have clotted blood that does not appear to be occluding the tubes. Temporary pacing wires exit on both sides of the sternum and are intact and attached to a pacer box.
- Hemodynamics:
  - Central venous pressure (CVP): 20 mm Hg
  - Cardiac index (CI) : 2.1 L/min/m²
  - Pulmonary artery pressures (PAP)—systolic/diastolic (S/D): 35/20 mm Hg
  - Pulmonary artery occlusion pressure (PAOP): 19 mm Hg

❓ What elements of the review of systems and the physical examination should be added to the list of pertinent positives?

- Hypothermic
- Distant heart tones
- Rub present on cardiac examination
- Jugular venous distension present
- Weak peripheral pulses
- Capillary refill >3 seconds
- Nasal flaring
- Accessory muscle use
- Rapid, shallow breathing
- Endorses feeling short of breath
- Absent bowel sounds with mild distention
- Foley draining dark yellow urine

- Cool and clammy skin over entire body
- Chest tubes have clotted blood along the drain that do not appear to be fully occluding tubes

? What elements of the review of systems and physical examination should be added to the significant negatives list?

- No neuromuscular deficits
- No musculoskeletal pain
- No chest pain
- No abdominal pain
- Breath sounds are present and symmetrical
- No bladder distention
- No hemoptysis

? How does this information affect the list of possible problems?

Case Analysis: Because he is intubated and on sedative medication, the review of systems for this patient does not contribute much to the diagnosis. But his physical examination findings are supportive of tamponade. He is hypotensive, and has signs of low cardiac output including cool and clammy skin, diminished capillary refill, and weak pulses. These coupled with his respiratory distress highlight the urgency to identify the cause of his condition so that interventions can be initiated quickly.

The most telling findings on his examination are the low blood pressure, the distended neck veins, and the muffled heart tones. These are known collectively as Beck's triad and are associated with acute tamponade.[1] The cardiac rub does not contribute much to sorting through his diagnosis as the chest tubes cause a rub in most patients after cardiac surgery, making it a nonspecific finding for this population. While tachycardia is expected with tamponade he was on a β -blocker prior to surgery, explaining his blunted response and need for pacing. His hypothermia makes him at risk for continued bleeding despite the infusion of fresh frozen plasma (FFP).

His neurologic examination is grossly intact, which helps exclude primary neurologic pathology and assures me that he has maintained adequate perfusion to the brain during his shock state.

The absence of bowel sounds is not unexpected after surgery as anesthesia affects the sympathetic nervous system. His distended abdomen, however, is not a normal finding after surgery; therefore, bowel ischemia as either a primary or secondary diagnosis cannot be excluded at this point. Given his shock state, less serious causes such as bladder distension or joint pain can be excluded for now.

There is a possibility that he could have an acute myocardial infarction or myocardial stunning, as each of these could produce hypotension, elevated jugular venous distention (JVD), and elevated filling pressures, PAOP and CVP. However, an acute MI would normally affect only one of these pressures, not both. In this patient, both the PAOP and CVP are elevated to a nearly equal number, therefore suggesting that whatever process is going on is affecting the patient on both the right and left side of the heart simultaneously (see Table 16-1). Pericarditis is excluded since the hemodynamic compromise would not be present with this diagnosis.

If this were a pulmonary embolism that was large enough to affect the patient's hemodynamics, I would expect to see the CVP rise, pulmonary artery mean pressure increase, pulmonary resistance increase but the PAOP pressure to fall, which again is not the case in this patient. Since the patient has essentially clear bilateral breath sounds, aside from his diminished basilar hypoventilation that is most likely related to his low tidal volumes, hemothorax and pneumothorax are less likely to be the cause, though they cannot be eliminated from the differential list without further diagnostic studies. Additionally, since he does not have hemoptysis, pulmonary artery infarct or injury is much less likely to be the cause of his tachypnea.

❓ What diagnostic testing should be done and in what order?

Case Analysis: The order of testing will depend on the conditions Testing should be prioritized so that the most life threatening diagnoses are worked up first. I will then consider what resources are readily available at the medical center. I call for a stat echocardiogram (ECHO) because my primary concern, based on the patient's hemodynamic changes, is cardiac tamponade. Since it will be at least 15 minutes before the ECHO tech can arrive, I also order a stat chest x-ray. The chest x-ray will not definitely rule in a cardiac tamponade but there is often evidence of cardiac tamponade that can be seen on a plain film. I also order stat labs, including a complete blood count (CBC), comprehensive metabolic profile (CMP), a prothrombin time (PT), partial thromboplastin time (PTT), international normalized ratio (INR), and a lactic acid. The CBC helps determine if the patient has had significant bleeding, and the CMP and lactic acid will help me evaluate the impact of his hemodynamic instability on his organs, if poor perfusion has caused end-organ damage. I need to determine his clotting times if he requires further surgery. In addition I contact the surgeon to discuss my findings and alert necessary staff for what may be an emergent reoperation.

Diagnosis and Management: Acute Cardiac Tamponade

An echocardiogram (ECHO) is the gold standard for diagnosing cardiac tamponade, and the most recent American Heart Associated and American College of Cardiology guidelines highly recommend ECHO for patients who are believed to

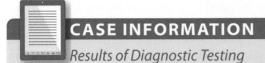

CASE INFORMATION
Results of Diagnostic Testing

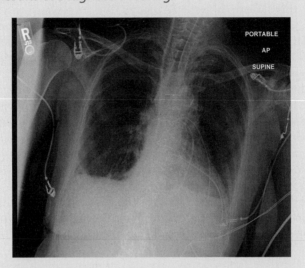

Figure 16-1 Immediate post-operative chest x-ray.

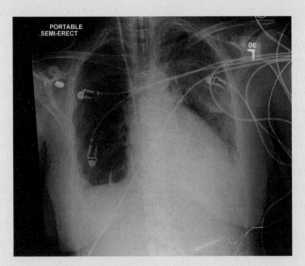

Figure 16-2 Progression of mediastinal widening on chest x-ray.

The chest film shows mediastinal widening of approximately 4 cm greater than his last film, without pulmonary edema or diaphragm abnormalities (see Figures 16-1 and 16-2). Labs are drawn and yield a hemoglobin of 6.5 (g/dL) and hematocrit of 20%; therefore, I order two units of packed red blood cells. His platelets are 60,000, also prompting me to order a unit of platelets. A comprehensive metabolic panel shows that his creatinine, glomerular filtration rate (GFR), aspartate transaminase (AST), and alanine transaminase (ALT) are all normal as follows: creatinine of 0.9 mg/dL (N = 0.5–1.4), GFR >60, AST of 25 (Normal: 5–35 IU/dL), and ALT of 18 (N = 40–120 U/L). With liver ischemia, AST and ALT would be drastically elevated, usually up to 20 times the normal limits. With poor kidney perfusion and ischemia, creatinine will be elevated and the GFR will fall. Lab work also shows that this patient's lactic acid is elevated at 4.5 (N = 1.0–1.8 mmol/L). This elevation indicates that there is circulatory compromise leading to cellular hypoperfusion, though this result does not help me specify the cause of that compromise. An ionized calcium of 3.8 (N = 4.64–5.28 mg/dL) should be repleted because hypocalcaemia can contribute to his coagulopathy and if blood products are given, the citrate will further lower his calcium level. In talking with the nurse, I learn the patient was given two units of fresh frozen plasma approximately 2 hours ago. PT and INR as well as a fibrinogen are within normal limits; therefore, he will not require further transfusions of fresh frozen plasma or cryoprecipitate blood products. The PTT is normal as well, which tells me he does not need more protamine to reverse the heparin he received while on cardiopulmonary bypass. An ABG confirms he is not acidotic, which can also contribute to coagulopathy. The echocardiogram findings are cardiac tamponade with large pericardial effusion estimated at 500 cc and inferior vena cava dilatation. Left and right ventricular function and size were difficult to visualize (see Figure 16-3).

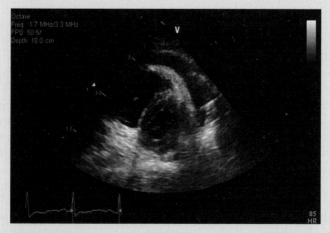

Figure 16-3   Post-operative echocardgram showing cardiac tamponade with pericardial effusion.

have a cardiac tamponade.[2] However, despite its high sensitivity and specificity for detecting tamponade, if air is present in the mediastinum following cardiac surgery, the echocardiogram may be less definitive. When the myocardium is able to be visualized, classic tamponade findings on ECHO are decreased left ventricular filling on inspiration, increased pulmonary venous diastolic forward flow on expiration, right atrial compression during late diastole, right ventricular collapse during early diastole, abnormalities of mitral valve motion, and dilated inferior vena cava with lack of inspiratory collapse.[3] Each of these findings should be taken seriously as in some patients with large pericardial effusions, chamber collapse may not be seen, yet the patients are still at high risk for adverse outcomes such as death.[4]

A chest x-ray is also helpful in determining the presence of cardiac tamponade and is often available sooner than the echocardiogram. On this patient's chest x-ray, I look for several things. First, if this is cardiac tamponade, I may see a widened mediastinum. However, I must be careful in interpreting this finding. If the mediastinum is not widened, I will still proceed with the ECHO, as it usually takes a large volume of blood before mediastinal widening appears on a chest film. Also, if the mediastinum is widened, a comparison of the degree of widening is made to the previous postoperative x-ray, as blood accumulation during surgery does make mild mediastinal widening a normal finding after surgery.

Before deciding to reexplore a patient for a cardiac tamponade, other interventions are necessary. Correction of coagulation defects is necessary to reduce undesired bleeding. This patient is still cold, and both his calcium and platelet levels are low. These are corrected as a timeline for potential surgical reexploration is determined. Chest tube stripping is also a consideration. There has been much debate about the efficacy of stripping chest tubes after cardiac surgery because during the process of stripping the chest tube, exorbitant amounts of negative pressure are transmitted to the chest cavity, potentially exacerbating air leaks and causing bleeding. A recent Cochrane Review found that there is insufficient literature to either support or refute the practice of stripping chest tubes to improve blood clearance.[5] Therefore, the decision to strip the chest tube is up to the individual practitioner. Because this patient has reasons other than the surgical error to have unanticipated bleeding, and his chest tube contains clotted blood, it is worthwhile to attempt stripping the chest tube. After 5 minutes of stripping the patient's chest tubes, there is no change in output and the patient's vasopressor requirements have slightly increased. Since the ECHO shows a clear tamponade physiology with continued hemodynamic instability, the decision is made to return the patient to the operating room. The surgeons confirm the ECHO findings of tamponade. They find that there is only generalized low-level bleeding throughout the chest cavity with approximately 300 cc of blood present at the time of chest opening. Also, the pericardial drains in the chest were completely occluded with clotted blood. Once the patient was returned to the intensive care unit, he was rewarmed, blood products were administered based on his CBC and bleeding times, and his calcium was repleted. His bleeding resolved and pressors were weaned over the next 24 hours. He was sent to the step-down unit on hospital day 4 and was discharged home after an 8-day hospital stay without further complication.

References

1. Sabatine M. *Poket Medicine*. 4th ed. Philadelphia, PA: Lippincott Williams & Wilkins; 2011.
2. ACC/AHA/ASE 2003 guideline update for the clinical application of echocardiography: summary article. http://circ.ahajournals.org/content/108/9/1146.full. Accessed July 30, 2014.
3. Tsang TS, Oh JK, Seward JB. Diagnosis and management of cardiac tamponade in the era of echocardiography. *Clin Cardiol*. 1999;22(7):446-452.
4. Argulian E, Messerli F. Misconceptions and facts about pericardial effusion and tamponade. *Am J Med*. 2013;126(10):858-861. doi: 10.1016/j.amjmed.2013.03.022.
5. Wallen M, Morrison A, Gillies D, O'Riordan E, Bridge C, Stoddart F. Mediastinal chest drain clearance for cardiac surgery. *Cochrane Database Syst Rev*. 2002;(2):CD003042. doi: CD003042 [pii].

CASE 17

Joshua Squiers

Joshua Squiers is dual board certified as an ACNP with specialization in surgical critical care. Dr Squiers holds a faculty appointment within the Oregon Health & Science University, School of Nursing, where he serves as the Director of the AG-ACNP Program, and an appointment within the school of medicine where he serves as Assistant Professor in the Department of Anesthesiology/Perioperative Medicine and the Division of Cardiac and Surgical Subspecialty Critical Care.

CASE INFORMATION

Chief Complaint

I am called to the bedside of a 75-year-old male on the cardiovascular step-down floor for acute confusion and mental status changes.

? What is the potential cause?

Case Analysis: There are many etiologies for acute confusion, so the list of possible diagnoses is long. When responding to acute physiologic changes, identifying life-threatening differentials is the highest priority. Acute confusion is nonspecific and has a variety of causes, including hypoglycemia, malperfusion, sepsis, stroke, and delirium. Additional but less urgent causes include depression and dementia.

> **Comprehensive Differential Diagnoses for Acute Confusion**
> - Immediate life-threatening causes
>   - Malperfusion
>   - Cerebrovascular accident (hemorrhagic or thrombotic)
> - Hypoglycemia
> - Hypothermia/hyperthermia
> - Infection/sepsis
> - Hyponatremia
> - Seizure
> - Nonconvulsive status epilepticus

- Drug overdose/reaction
- Other causes to consider
  - Delirium
  - Dementia
  - Primary psychiatric illness
  - Azotemia
  - Encephalopathy
  - Heart failure
  - Fecal impaction
  - Urinary retention

CASE INFORMATION
General Survey and History of Present Illness

A 75-year-old Caucasian male with a past medical history of hypertension and hyperlipidemia was admitted with dyspnea on exertion and chest pain worsening over the past 6 months. Initially, his dyspnea and pain resolved with rest. Yesterday he presented to the emergency room with dyspnea and chest pain that was sustained despite rest. The emergency department ruled in ST-elevation myocardial infarction (STEMI) and he was treated medically until undergoing cardiac catheterization. During his catheterization, percutaneous coronary intervention (PCI) was performed including drug-eluding stents to a 99% stenosis of the first diagonal branch of the left anterior descending artery. The catheterization findings were also significant for diffuse coronary disease, but no other focal lesions were identified or treated. Following the procedure he was admitted to the intermediate cardiac care floor for observation.

Over the past 3 hours the bedside nurse notes that he is less interactive and intermittently confused. The confusion appears to be worsening, with the patient in great emotional distress at times. On arrival to the bedside I note a confused elderly male in apparent emotional distress. His son is at the bedside and reports the patient has no history of dementia, and has never behaved this way before. The nursing staff is attempting to reassure and reorient the patient.

Past Medical History/Past Surgical History (Based on Medical Records and His Son)
- Hyperlipidemia: controlled with diet and exercise
- Hypertension: managed with hydrochlorothiazide
- Osteoarthritis
- Seasonal allergic rhinitis

Social History
- Retired car salesman
- Currently lives with wife
- Smoked occasional cigars as young man, quit 40 years ago
- Social alcohol intake at one to two drinks per week
- No illicit drug use

Family History
- Adopted as child, does not know family medical history

Home Medication List
- Aspirin 81 mg once daily
- Hydrochlorothiazide 25 mg twice a day
- Ibuprofen as needed for osteoarthritic pain

Current Medication List
- Aspirin 81 mg daily
- Plavix 75 mg daily
- Hydrochlorothiazide 25 mg twice a day
- Ibuprofen as needed for osteoarthritic pain

Allergies
- No known drug or food allergies

? **What are the pertinent positives from the information given so far?**
- STEMI with emergency PCI for revascularization within the past 24 hours
- Confirmed atherosclerotic disease via cardiac angiography
- hypertension and hyperlipidemia

❓ What are the significant negatives from the information given so far?

• No past medical history of dementia or confusional states
• No previous history of neurologic disorder including stroke or seizure

❓ Can the information gathered so far be restated in a single sentence highlighting the pieces that narrow down the cause?

The problem representation in this case might be: "a 75-year-old gentleman with sudden onset of acute confusion who is several hours postadmission for STEMI with percutaneous coronary revascularization."

❓ How does this information affect the list of possible causes?

Case Analysis: Inexperienced clinicians often forget to obtain/review a clear history of the presenting illness when responding to sudden changes in the patient status. Often during the course of an emergency response, the HPI and combined subjective information are not adequately collected. In emergencies, this information is often key to sorting the differential rapidly and providing focused intervention.

Confusion is an important sign and symptom that often is dismissed in elderly patients. Unfortunately many clinicians perceive confusion as part of the normal aging process. Confusion is always a sign of pathology, regardless of age or context. The brain is one of the most sensitive organs to perfusion and substrate (glucose) availability, and minor changes in these parameters can cause drastic changes in mental status. Confusion, in particular acute onset confusion, is often a sign of malperfusion and/or lack of metabolic substrate availability.

At this point I am able to do a little sorting of the differential list based on what I know about the patient's history so far. The patient does not appear to have a history of dementia that might present as confusion. The lack of seizure history also suggests, but does not completely rule out, that this is not some form of postictal confusion. Overall, this increases my suspicion of some acute etiology of his confusion, rather than a manifestation or exacerbation of a long-term disease process. This still does not rule out the possibility of stroke, or other acute disease. Stroke in particular is concerning as some patients present with confusion as part of their initial signs and symptoms of stroke. The patient obviously has atherosclerotic disease and has probably had it for a while, and this likely affects all his blood vessels, including the small intracerebral vessels where a thrombotic stroke might occur. Delirium is also a likely differential diagnosis in this patient, and his age, multiple medications during his procedure and hospitalization all put him at risk. At this point, I am also curious about a potential relationship between sudden onset confusion and his recent STEMI, as a worsening of his cardiac status may present as acute confusion secondary to malperfusion.

CASE INFORMATION

Review of Systems

- The patient is unable to provide a history. Review of systems is obtained from the patient's hospital records and son at the bedside.
- Constitutional: Denies fever, appetite or weight change, no recent falls or trauma. Patient does not like to see his primary care provider, and often has "avoidant" health behaviors as noted by his spouse.
- Head/eyes/ears/nose/throat: Denies history of enlarged thyroid, vision changes, or hearing loss. Denies headache, neck pain, tinnitus, glaucoma, nosebleed, or seasonal allergies. The patient wears reading glasses.
- Pulmonary: Denies history of wheezing, cough, night sweats, or smoking. Denies coughing up blood or sputum. Endorses dyspnea on exertion as noted in the history of present illness.
- Cardiovascular: Denies leg swelling, or difficulty breathing when lying down. Denies palpitations and orthopnea. Chest pain noted on exertion over the past 6 months, which has progressively increased in duration and intensity.
- Gastrointestinal: Denies nausea/vomiting, blood in stools, diarrhea, constipation.
- Genitourinary: Denies blood in urine, denies inappropriate urinary frequency and nocturia.
- Musculoskeletal: Denies muscle weakness, joint or back pain. Notes that he may have arthritis, but has never been diagnosed.
- Neurological: Denies dizziness, stroke, transient ischemic attack (TIA), fainting, seizures, numbness, tingling or tremors of the extremities.
- Psychosocial: Denies nervousness, stress, depression, or memory loss. Denies any previous history of confusion, dementia, or neuropsychiatric disorders.
- Endocrine: Denies increased hunger, thirst, or urination.

Physical Examination

- Vital signs: Pulse is 110 beats per minute, blood pressure is 105/65 mm Hg (MAP 78), respiratory rate is 24/min and temperature is 98.9°F oral, oxygen saturation by pulse oximeter is 99% on room air, and finger stick blood glucose is 105 mg/dL.
- Neurological: The patient is orientated to person, but not to place or time. He states that the health care team members are intruders in his home. Not combative or agitated. Inattentive during examination. CAM (confusion assessment method) positive due to inattention and disorganized thinking. Strength and sensation are grossly intact in bilateral extremities. Face is symmetric. No facial droop noted.

- Head/eyes/ears/nose/throat: Head: Normocephalic and atraumatic. Pupils are equal and reactive.
- Cardiovascular: Heart rate and rhythm regular, no murmurs, no gallops. Jugular venous distension is present at 45° head elevation.
- Pulmonary: Tachypnea present but synchronous respiratory pattern. Clear to auscultation from apexes to bases.
- Gastrointestinal: Hypoactive bowel sounds, tympanic on percussion, abdomen soft without masses and nontender.
- Extremities: Nail beds are pale, extremities are cool to touch, capillary refill 3 seconds. Mottling of the bilateral lower extremities is noted.

? What elements of the review of systems and the physical examination should be added to the list of pertinent positives?

- Mild hypotension, tachycardia, jugular venous distension, confusion, cool extremities, mottling of the legs

? What elements of the review of systems and physical examination should be added to the significant negatives list?

- No prior history of confusion or dementia, nonfocal neurologic examination

? How does this information affect the list of possible causes?

Case Analysis: The differential can now be rapidly sorted based on the physical examination of the patient. First and foremost, hypoglycemia can be ruled out since blood glucose measurement is normal. This is an important first step for an acute confusion workup, as hypoglycemia is a direct cause of confusion and can be easily treated in the acute setting. In addition, the neurologic examination, while brief, does provide information that helps sort the differential. In this case, the patient has no focal neurological deficits. While a nonfocal neurologic examination does not completely rule out the presence of an ischemic or hemorrhagic stroke, it does decrease the likelihood that this presentation represents an acute stroke.

The positive findings on his physical examination, specifically, cool extremities, cap refill >2 seconds, and mottling over the knees are highly predictive of a low cardiac output.[1] This is somewhat counterintuitive as many would expect the cardiac examination to be the key indicator of an early malperfusion state. However, these peripheral vascular findings evaluate perfusion at sites distant from the heart, so these abnormalities often occur earlier in a state of malperfusion than central cardiac examination findings.

Beyond the malperfusion identified in the periphery, elevated jugular venous distention is suggestive of elevated left heart filling pressures, a sign of loss of cardiac stroke volume and reduced ejection fraction.[2] In this case, tachycardia also suggests early compensatory effort for malperfusion and could indicate reduced cardiac stroke volume.

Most importantly, the combination of findings found in the physical examination combined with the history of presenting illness is highly suggestive of cardiogenic shock. Most patients suffering from a myocardial infarction do not present with cardiogenic shock, but typically develop it after hospital admission. This case represents a classic presentation of cardiogenic shock postadmission for myocardial infarction. Once the diagnosis of cardiogenic shock has been made, further workup is necessary to determine the etiology and identify any reversible causes. In the case above, further evaluation of stent reocclusion is warranted.

❓ What diagnostic testing should be done and in what order?

Several different approaches can be used to confirm the diagnosis of cardiogenic shock. In most institutions, bedside echocardiography is available for emergency cardiac evaluation. This can be completed via cardiology consultation, or by bedside critical care ultrasound evaluation. Echo will like reveal myocardial wall motion abnormalities, with reduced stroke volume and reduced ejection fraction.[3] If imaging is not available, further evaluation of cardiac output, hemodynamics, and mixed venous saturations can be accomplished via central line placement.[4]

Diagnosis and Management: Cardiogenic Shock

Cardiogenic shock syndrome is "a state of inadequate tissue perfusion due to cardiac dysfunction."[5] Caution should be taken in conceptualizing this definition in light of heart failure (HF) syndrome, which can be defined as a "syndrome that results from any structural or functional impairment of ventricular filling or ejection of blood."[6] At first glance these definitions appear similar, but operationally represent different clinical pictures on the same continuum. The symptoms of HF can be wide ranging from no symptoms to classic HF symptoms, to fulminant cardiogenic shock. Therefore, cardiogenic shock is really severe HF, when the signs and symptoms demonstrate that the heart is not maintaining adequate perfusion of tissues to sustain life. While all cardiogenic shock is essentially severe HF, HF is not always cardiogenic shock.

Cardiogenic shock usually results from a reduction in cardiac output secondary to ventricular dysfunction, and the resulting loss of the systemic mechanism for nutrient and oxygen delivery to tissues. This loss of cardiac output occurs from two different mechanisms: (1) myocardium's inability to adequately fill and/or pump blood and/or (2) a reduction of venous return to the heart. In essence the heart loses its muscular abilities that affect filling and ejection of blood, or there is inadequate blood returning to the heart to "prime" the pump. These factors reduce cardiac output and eventually lead to inadequate delivery of oxygen and nutrients, loss of cellular waste removal, and eventual tissue death.

Several organs are highly sensitive to malperfusion including the brain. The brain is highly sensitive to glucose availability. As the primary, and essentially only metabolic substrate utilized by the brain, reduced levels of circulating glucose can have a dramatic effect on cognition, including the acute development of confusion. The loss of blood flow, and the concomitant serum glucose supply, can result in various levels of symptoms from minor confusion to coma. Any patient with acute changes in cognition must be aggressively evaluated for malperfusion, and hypoglycemia.

While cardiogenic shock can have a number of etiologies, it is most commonly found following myocardial infarction. In 1967, Killip and Kimball wrote the seminal work on the morbidity and mortality associated with myocardial infarction.[7] This study followed 434 patients admitted to a coronary care unit (CCU) over the course of 2 years. Of the 265 patients who had "definite myocardial infarction," 19% of them were found to be in cardiogenic shock during their hospital stay and had a mortality rate of 81%. Of the patients in shock 94% developed life-threatening dysrhythmias, of which ventricular dysrhythmia was the most common. During the course of care for these patients, subsequent shock and death were noted to have variable timing from admission to as late as 65 days following the event.

The rate of cardiogenic shock found among patients with STEMI is 8.6% according the National Registry of Myocardial Infarction from 1994 to 2005.[8] Substantial improvements in the clinical care of these patients has reduced the mortality rate from 81% in 1967[7] to 47.9% in 2004.[8] This drastic improvement in mortality is largely a result of the increased utilization of emergent coronary revascularization in the setting of MI and cardiogenic shock.[9]

Frequently cardiogenic shock develops hours after a myocardial infarction, even with adequate coronary revascularization. The SHOCK trial registry found that of patients who develop MI-related cardiogenic shock, 75% of them occurred up to 24 hours after initial presentation, with a median delay of 7 hours.[10] Similar results were found in the GUSTO clinical trial, which found that of patients developing cardiogenic shock, 89% developed it after admission, and only 11% of patients were diagnosed at admission.[11] This is important clinically, as it indicates that the majority of patients who develop cardiogenic shock do not have it on admission, but develop it during their hospitalization.

Conclusion

This case demonstrates several key points for clinicians caring for the patients at risk of cardiogenic shock. First, that for patients with acute changes in cognition a number of differentials should be considered with the focus initially on life-threatening etiologies. In particular malperfusion and hypoglycemia should always be included and ruled out. The patient history, including the past medical history, often provides strong clues to help sort the initial differential to reveal the most probable etiologies. Second, the physical examination is important in identifying patients with cardiogenic shock. The cluster of symptoms found during the peripheral examination, including cool extremities, cap refill >2 seconds, and mottling over the knees can be very sensitive for clinical malperfusion. And finally, that cardiogenic shock is often late sequelae of myocardial infarction with presentation often occurring during the course of hospitalization. Clinicians should be sensitive to early signs of malperfusion, such as acute cognitive changes, in any patient with myocardial infarction.

References

1. Grissom CK, Morris AH, Lanken PN, et al. Association of physical examination with pulmonary artery catheter parameters in acute lung injury. *Crit Care Med.* 2009;37(10):2720-2726.
2. Butman SM, Ewy GA, Standen JR, Kern KB, Hahn E. Bedside cardiovascular examination in patients with severe chronic heart failure: importance of rest or inducible jugular venous distension. *J Am Coll Cardiol.* 1993;22(4):968-974.
3. Perera P, Mailhot T, Riley D, Mandavia D. The RUSH exam: Rapid Ultrasound in SHock in the evaluation of the critically ill. *Emerg Med Clin North Am.* 2010;28(1):29-56.
4. Parrillo JE, Dellinger RP. *Critical Care Medicine: Principles of Diagnosis and Management in the Adult (Expert Consult-Online and Print).* Elsevier Health Sciences; 2013.
5. Hollenberg SM, Kavinsky CJ, Parrillo JE. Cardiogenic shock. *Ann Intern Med.* 1999;131(1):47-59.
6. Yancy CW, Jessup M, Bozkurt B, et al. 2013 ACCF/AHA guideline for the management of heart failure: a report of the American College of Cardiology Foundation/American Heart Association Task Force on practice guidelines. *Circulation.* 2013;128:e240-e327.
7. Killip T, Kimball JT. Treatment of myocardial infarction in a coronary care unit: a two year experience with 250 patients. *Am J Cardiol.* 1967;20(4):457-464.
8. Babaev A, Frederick PD, Pasta DJ, Every N, Sichrovsky T, Hochman JS. Trends in management and outcomes of patients with acute myocardial infarction complicated by cardiogenic shock. *JAMA.* 2005;294(4):448-454.
9. Webb JG, Sanborn TA, Sleeper LA, et al. Percutaneous coronary intervention for cardiogenic shock in the SHOCK Trial Registry. *Am Heart J.* 2001;141(6):964-970.
10. Hochman JS, Boland J, Sleeper LA, et al. Current spectrum of cardiogenic shock and effect of early revascularization on mortality. Results of an International Registry. *Circulation.* 1995;91(3):873-881.
11. Holmes DR, Bates ER, Kleiman NS, et al. Contemporary reperfusion therapy for cardiogenic shock: the GUSTO-I trial experience. *J Am Coll Cardiol.* 1995;26(3):668-674.

CASE 18

Mary Ann Whelan-Gales

Mary Ann Whelan-Gales is a House Officer/team member on an inpatient cardiology service which admits over 9000 patients/year. Dr Whelan-Gales has more than 20 years of critical care experience as a clinical nurse.

CASE INFORMATION

Chief Complaint

A 57-year-old man presents to the emergency room having experienced a syncopal episode the evening before.

? What is the potential cause?

Syncope can be a symptom of a life-threatening condition that requires immediate intervention. There are a myriad of etiologies for syncope. They can be classified into cardiac, noncardiac, and unknown causes.

Differential Diagnoses for Syncope

Cardiac Arrhythmias
- Ventricular arrhythmias
- Sinus node dysfunction (including bradycardia/tachycardia)
- Atrioventricular conduction system blocks
- Paroxysmal supraventricular tachycardia
- Implanted device malfunction: pacemaker, implantable cardioverter defibrillator
- Drug-induced proarrhythmias: sotalol, flecainide, quinidine, procainamide, disopyramide

Structural Cardiac and Cardiopulmonary Disease
- Cardiac valvular diseases: most commonly aortic stenosis
- Hypertropic obstructive cardiomyopathy
- Atrial myxoma
- Acute aortic dissection
- Pulmonary embolism and pulmonary hypertension
- Cardiac tamponade

Noncardiac Causes

Neurologically mediated or vasovagal
- Neurocardiogenic syncope or reflex syncope
- Situational: cough, sneeze, swallowing, defecation, micturition, post-prandial, postexercise, weightlifting
- Carotid sinus sensitivity
- Glossopharyngeal

Orthostatic and dysautonomia
- Catecholamine disorders: baroreflex, dopamine-β-hydroxylase defi-ciency, pheochromocytoma, neuroblastoma, familial paraganglioma syndrome, tetrahydrobiopterin deficiency
- Central autonomic disorders: multiple system atrophy (Shy-Drager syndrome), Parkinson disease with autonomic failure
- Orthostatic intolerance syndrome: postural tachycardia syndrome, mitral valve prolapse, idiopathic hypovolemia
- Paroxysmal autonomic syncopes: neurocardiogenic syncope
- Peripheral autonomic disorders: acute idiopathic polyneuropathy (Guillain-Barré syndrome, Chagas disease, diabetic autonomic failure, familial dysautonomia, pure autonomic failure (Bradbury-Eggleston syndrome)

Neurologic
- Migraine or transient ischemic attacks (TIA)
- Seizure

Toxic or metabolic
- Drug toxicities such as antiarrhythmic agents causing proarrhythmic effects and antihypertensive agents causing proarrhythmic effects, and antihypertensive agents causing orthostatic hypotension; hypoglyce-mia; hypoxia; hyperventilation with hypocapnia

Other
- Hypovolemia: diarrhea, hemorrhage, Addison disease; postexercise; postprandial
- Drug induced: the most common cause of orthostatic hypotension
- Anatomic: subclavian steal syndrome
- Psychiatric
- Idiopathic

CASE INFORMATION

I begin with a general survey of the patient: he is a well-nourished, well-developed man in no distress who is able to give all the details of the event and his past medical history.

History of Present Illness

The night prior to admission, he was sitting down when he began feeling very tired and weak. This lasted for a couple of minutes. Then he went to the bathroom to brush his teeth, felt weaker, left the bathroom and was walking when suddenly he lost consciousness. He reports having some recollection of falling, but was not able to catch himself and he reports having lost consciousness for what he thinks is just a brief amount of time. He sustained a laceration to the right side of his lower lip. When he awoke, he still felt weak. In addition he noticed that he was incontinent of urine. No tongue biting or focal deficits were noted. He went to bed and felt better in the morning. He denies having any chest pain, shortness of breath, palpitations, nausea, vomiting, diarrhea, or diaphoresis before or after the event. He denies any recent illness. He has never had an episode like this before but he does note that in the past 2 to 3 weeks, he has had a few episodes where he would suddenly feel short of breath and look a bit pale, sometimes after just a mild amount of exertion, and these symptoms would subside after a couple of minutes without any treatment. Since the episode, he has felt back to his normal self, without any residual symptoms, but he later decided to go to the hospital to be checked out.

Medical History

The patient reports a previous diagnosis of cardiomyopathy and denies prior myocardial infarction, stroke, diabetes, cancer, or lung disease. He has never had surgery or procedures to implant a cardiac device.

When I review the hospital electronic medical record, I learn that the patient underwent a voluntary workup 2 years ago after a sibling died from cardiomyopathy. This work up included:

- Cardiac magnetic resonance image (MRI) showing asymmetric hypertrophic cardiomyopathy with dynamic left ventricular outflow tract (LVOT) obstruction at rest and maximal wall thickness of 2.2 cm. Normal biventricular size and systolic function. Intramyocardial scarring, probably moderate mitral regurgitation; severity may be overestimated.
- Computed tomography angiogram of the chest showed nonobstructive disease.
- Holter monitoring that showed no arrhythmias.

Social History

The patient reports that he does not smoke, has a glass of wine with dinner each evening, and denies use of illicit substances.

Family History

- He reports that his brother and sister "dropped dead" at young ages, 45 and 37, respectively. There is a family history of hypertrophic obstructive cardiomyopathy (HOCM) and premature sudden cardiac death (SCD).
- Allergies: Penicillin.
- Medications: The patient denies taking any medications, prescribed or over the counter.

❓ What are the pertinent positives from the information given so far?

- Syncope of unclear cause.
- Two-week history of episodes of shortness of breath and pallor after just a mild amount of exertion and lasting several minutes.
- Urinary incontinence at the time of syncope.
- There is a family history of HOCM/premature SCD cardiac in two siblings.
- The patient's cardiac MRI 2 years ago shows HOCM.

❓ What are the significant negatives from the information given so far?

- The patient is in no distress at the time of my examination.
- There is no previous history of syncope.
- His Holter monitor in the past showed no arrhythmia.
- He takes no prescription medications.
- He has no implanted cardiac devices.

❓ Can the information gathered so far be restated in a single sentence highlighting the pieces that narrow down the cause?

The problem representation in this case is: a 57-year-old male with cardiomyopathy presenting after a single syncopal episode.

Case Analysis: In reviewing the differential diagnosis and the information I have so far about this patient, I can immediately rule out medication-related causes of his syncope, since he takes no medications. In addition, pulmonary embolism, aortic dissection, and cardiac tamponade are all conditions that do not resolve spontaneously. The fact that the patient recovered from the episode and feels fine now makes these diagnoses very unlikely. The most likely cause of his syncope is hypovolemia, simply because this occurs very commonly. There is nothing in his history so far to suggest he became hypovolemic, he denies vomiting and diarrhea, or recent illness. Based on the fact that he has had prior episodes, albeit much more mild than this one, a structural cardiac disease, such as a valve disorder, is a possible diagnosis. I am less inclined to think the cause is a cardiac arrhythmia, because this is uncommon and he had a normal Holter monitor 2 years ago. I am still considering neurological disorders, such as a transient ischemic attack (TIA), which if it occurs from a vertebrobasilar origin may cause loss of consciousness, but this too is unusual. A seizure, which seems possible given his urinary incontinence, is less likely in the absence of a postictal period of extreme fatigue or confusion.

In approaching this patient, I acknowledge the American Heart Association recommendations regarding syncope evaluation.[1] Current guidelines recognize that the majority of adults with syncope do not have structural heart disease or significant arrhythmia. So, extensive medical workup is rarely needed. A careful physical examination including blood pressure and heart rate measured lying and standing is generally the only evaluation required. In other cases an electrocardiogram is used to test for abnormal heart rhythms such as long QT syndrome, a genetic heart condition that can cause sudden cardiac death. Other tests, such as exercise stress test to evaluate for cardiac ischemia, a Holter monitor to record changes in the heart rhythm, or an echocardiogram to examine the structure of the cardiac muscle may be needed to rule out cardiac causes of syncope. Recognizing this, I proceed with my history and physical examination of this patient.

CASE INFORMATION

Review of Systems

- The patient is a good historian.
- Constitutional: Negative for fever and chills; no changes in appetite, weight, activity level, or fluid intake.
- Head/ears/nose/throat: Negative for neck stiffness.
- Eyes: Negative for visual disturbance.
- Pulmonary: Negative for cough, shortness of breath, and wheezing.
- Cardiovascular: Negative for chest pain, palpitations, and leg swelling.
- Gastrointestinal: Negative for bowel incontinence, nausea, vomiting, and diarrhea, denies blood in stool.
- Genitourinary: Positive for urine incontinence, denies pain with urination or blood in urine.
- Skin: Positive for wound (lip laceration). Negative for rash.
- Musculoskeletal: Negative for back pain.
- Neurological: Positive for syncope. Negative for dizziness, light-headedness, and headaches.

Physical Examination

- Blood pressure: 152/83 mm Hg (sitting), 150/88 (standing).
- Pulse: 66 (sitting), 72 (standing).

- Temp: 36°C (96.8°F).
- Respirations: 16.
- Oxygen saturation: 99%.
- Height: 5' 6" (167.6 cm); weight: 156 lb.
- Constitutional: He appears well developed and well nourished and in no distress.
- Head/eyes/ears/nose/throat: Normocephalic, conjunctivae and extraocular movements are normal. Pupils are equal, round, and reactive to light. No scleral icterus.
- Oropharynx is clear and moist; 4 cm laceration through the vermilion border of the lower right lip, neck with normal range of motion. Neck supple. No jugular venous distention present.
- Cardiovascular: Normal rate, regular rhythm, normal S1, S2, with a 2-3/6 mid-sternal systolic ejection murmur loudest by the left sternal border and apex, no gallops, no friction rub. Distal pulses intact and equal bilaterally, no edema.
- Pulmonary: Effort normal, no respiratory distress. Lungs are clear to auscultation bilaterally. He has no rales or wheezes.
- Gastrointestinal: Bowel sounds present in all four quadrants. Abdomen soft, nontender, and nondistended.
- Musculoskeletal: Normal range of motion.
- Neurological: He is alert and oriented to person, place, and time. Cranial nerves II-XII intact. Sensory and motor examinations show no focal deficits.
- Integumentary: Skin is warm and dry. Normal skin turgor. No rash noted. He is not diaphoretic. No erythema.
- No pallor.
- ECG: Normal sinus rhythm with nonspecific T-wave changes; QT 0.434 / QTc 0.545 (normally <0.4), no arrhythmia, no sign of ischemia; not significantly changed from 2012.

❓ What additional pertinent positives are found on review of systems and physical examination?

- Lip laceration from fall, suggests loss of consciousness, with no effort to break his fall.
- He has a murmur heard on left sternal border.
- Nonspecific T-wave changes on ECG, with prolonged QT interval.

? What additional significant are found on review of systems and physical examination?

• Normal orthostatic vital signs.

• Review of systems and physical examination show no neurological deficits, no history of volume loss such as diarrhea or vomiting, and no signs of hypovolemia (dry mouth or poor skin turgor).

• There are no signs or symptoms of heart failure such as weight gain, crackles on lung auscultation, or edema. He is not hypoxic.

• His pulmonary and gastrointestinal examinations are normal.

? How does the information change the problem statement?

The problem statement now reads: "a 57-year-old male with a history of HOCM presents following a syncopal event."

Case Analysis: Looking back at my differential diagnosis list, I consider each possible category in turn. A cardiac arrhythmia is possible even with a normal admission ECG; he could easily have a transient arrhythmia that is not captured on this single study. By placing the patient on a telemetry monitor and observing him over the course of a hospital stay, I can further evaluate him for any arrhythmias. This patient is particularly at risk for ventricular arrhythmias given his history of HOCM. Sinus node dysfunction (including bradycardia or tachycardia), atrioventricular conduction system blocks, and paroxysmal supraventricular tachycardia are additional arrhythmias I will observe for with ongoing telemetry monitoring. Inherited syndromes such as long QT syndromes and Brugada syndrome are still a possibility, particularly given the mildly prolonged QT interval on his admission ECG. I will do further ECGs to evaluate this. I am not concerned about implanted device malfunction or drug-induced arrhythmia because the patient has no implanted devices and does not take any medications, herbals, or supplements.

Structural cardiac and cardiopulmonary diseases also need to be considered as possible causes of this patient's syncope. This patient's echocardiogram within the last 2 years shows no evidence of valve disease or atrial myxoma so these diagnoses are very unlikely. Acute aortic dissection, cardiac tamponade, pulmonary embolism, and pulmonary hypertension are eliminated given that he presents without any distress and his physical examination shows no sign of these conditions. The patient's past workup including an echocardiogram confirms hypertropic obstructive cardiomyopathy so there is high likelihood that this is contributing to his syncope.

Syncope can also result from a neurally mediated or vasovagal event. Neurocardiogenic syncope or reflex syncope includes a number of disorders where coughing, sneezing, swallowing, defecation, and/or micturition may result in a transitory reduction in cerebral blood flow due to a centrally mediated or "reflex fall" in blood pressure. The onset of reflex syncope is sudden, usually occurring after a specific triggering event, and this patient's history of present illness is not consistent with that pattern. He experienced a period of generalized weakness and was actually walking immediately prior to losing consciousness. So while I cannot definitively rule out this diagnosis, I highly doubt this as the cause. Similarly, the patient's history rules out postprandial, postexercise, and post-weight lifting syncope.

Dysautonomia, while not ruled out by the current information, is less likely as it is less common and given that he has structural cardiac disease, this is likely to be contributing to his presenting complaint of syncope. On the other hand, hypovolemia is a very common cause of syncope and needs to be considered. He is not orthostatic on this examination and this suggests that he is not hypovolemic. I will order a comprehensive metabolic panel and look at his sodium, blood urea nitrogen, and creatinine to gather more data in regard to his fluid balance.

At this point, a neurological event is less likely based on the absence of residual neurological signs or symptoms and the presence of HCOM, which makes a cardiac disorder more likely. While a TIA is difficult to rule out as it causes only transient symptoms, it is rare that a TIA would be the cause of a syncopal event. I will hold off on consulting neurology or ordering an MRI of the brain and pursue further cardiac evaluation.

Based on the information I have so far, I believe the patient's syncope is due to hypertrophic cardiomyopathy, though I need to do some further evaluation to rule out more common causes, such as acute coronary syndrome, dehydration, and orthostatis. I plan to admit the patient, place him on a telemetry monitor, and do serial ECGs and cardiac enzymes to rule out an acute coronary event and monitor his QT interval. I will also order a metabolic panel to determine if he is hypovolemic, a thyroid stimulating hormone level (TSH) to determine if thyroid dysfunction is contributing to a cardiac arrhythmia, and a hemoglobin A1C to determine if the patient has diabetes as this would place him at higher risk for metabolic disturbance. Given the high likelihood that this is cardiac syncope, based on the patient's prior diagnosis of HOCM and his family history, I also order echocardiogram, stress test, and cardiac catheterization. Depending on the results, I may also need to order electrophysiology studies to further evaluate for cardiac arrhythmia.

CASE INFORMATION

Diagnostic Test Results

- Labs: Comprehensive metabolic panel, TSH, and hemoglobin A1C are all within normal limits. His troponin is normal; serial ECGs show normal sinus rhythm with no significant change in QT interval.
- Echocardiogram with hemodynamics completed on this admission: Findings are consistent with HOCM including small left ventricular size, localized left ventricular hypertrophy, hyperdynamic left ventricular systolic

function, left ventricular outflow tract (LVOT) obstruction. Additional findings:

- Severe LVOT gradient with standing and Valsalva with a flow velocity of 5 m/s, which corresponds to a gradient of 100 mm Hg. LVOT obstruction in HCM is defined as a resting LVOT gradient ≥30 mm Hg, with severe obstruction defined as ≥50 mm Hg.[1]
- Basal septal hypertrophy = 19 mm. The normal septal thickness in an adult is <12 mm.[1]
- Moderate to severe systolic anterior motion of mitral chordae with septal contact.
- Abnormal left ventricular diastolic filling pattern (may be due to age or left ventricular hypertrophy).
- Normal right ventricular function.
- Mild mitral regurgitation.
- Stress test:
  - With exercise, right-sided pressures are increased, mild pulmonary hypertension, pulmonary vascular resistance index is mildly increased, pulmonary capillary wedge pressure is normal, left ventricular end-diastolic pressure is normal, decreased cardiac output. Duration: 5 minutes.
- Cardiac catheterization:
  - Hemodynamics: Baseline normal right-sided pressures, pulmonary vascular resistance index is mildly increased, pulmonary wedge pressure is normal, left ventricular end-diastolic pressure is normal, decreased cardiac output. Resting left ventricular outlet tract (LVOT) gradient is 60 mm Hg (LVOT obstruction in HCM is defined as a resting LVOT gradient ≥30 mm Hg, with severe obstruction defined as ≥50 mm Hg.[1])
- Post-premature ventricular contraction, the left ventricular end-diastolic pressure is normal, there is marked rise (160 mm Hg) in LVOT gradient.
- Coronary anatomy: Two-vessel coronary artery disease; 80% to 90% proximal right coronary artery (RCA) and 70% to 80% proximal left anterior descending artery, second diagonal (LAD-D2).
  - Left ventricular function/aorta : hyperkinetic systolic left ventricular function
  - Valves : no mitral stenosis, HOCM with resting and provocable gradient

Diagnosis and Management of HOCM

At this point, the echocardiogram and cardiac catheterization results confirm HOCM as the cause of this patient's syncope. I will plan to start the patient on aspirin, β-blocker, and a statin to treat his coronary artery disease and he will be referred to cardiac surgery for coronary bypass graft and a transaortic radical ventricular septal myectomy. In addition, an AICD will be placed for the ongoing risk for cardiac arrhythmia/sudden cardiac death that the diagnosis of HOCM carries.

Septal myectomy is a surgical intervention for patients with symptomatic hypertrophic cardiomyopathy (HCM) and for patients with resting left ventricular outflow tract (LVOT) gradients of more than 30 mm Hg. The surgery entails removing a portion of the septum that is obstructing the flow of blood from the left ventricle to the aorta. After the induction of general anesthesia, a transesophageal echocardiogram (TEE) is performed to confirm the cardiac anatomy and assess the mitral valve function and the appearance and thickness of the ventricular septum.[2] With surgery, 90% of patients improve by at least one New York Heart Association class, and improvements persist in most individuals on late follow-up.[2]

In this case, a transverse aortotomy was made to view the aortic leaflets and the septum beneath them. The thickened septum was resected to the level of the papillary muscles. The aortotomy was closed. The TEE confirmed normal left ventricular function and no residual LVOT obstruction. Peak gradient was reduced from 60% to 17%.

The patient's right lower lip and cheek lacerations were treated with excisional debridement and multiple layered wound closure performed by a plastic surgeon. He was discharged home on post-op day 6 with scheduled follow-up appointments with his primary cardiologist, cardiothoracic surgeon, and an electrophysiologist.

References

1. Gersh BJ, Maron BJ, Bonow RO, et al. 2011 ACCF/AHA guideline for the diagnosis and treatment of hypertrophic cardiomyopathy: a report of the American College of Cardiology Foundation/American Heart Association Task Force on Practice Guidelines. *Circulation.* 2011;124:e783-e831.
2. Schaff HV, Dearani JA, Ommen SR, et al. Expanding the indications for septal myectomy in patients with hypertrophic cardiomyopathy: results of operation in patients with latent obstruction. *J Thorac Cardiovasc Surg.* 2012;143:303-308.

CASE 19

Mary M. Brennan

Mary Brennan is an ACNP on a cardiology service in a major teaching hospital in New York City. Dr Brennan is the Coordinator of the ACNP Program at New York University College of Nursing.

CASE INFORMATION

Chief Complaint

A 66-year-old African American male presents to the emergency room with progressive shortness of breath over 2 weeks, a 15-lb weight gain in the last month, and swelling of his bilateral lower extremities.

Case Analysis: Performing a quick assessment of the patient's overall appearance is a priority when a patient presents with shortness of breath. Assessing the quality and rate of the respirations, and checking for the presence of accompanying respiratory symptoms such as audible wheezing, stridor, coughing, or choking, will provide important information as to the acuity and potential etiology of the patient's condition. Reviewing the patient's vital signs is the next step in the initial evaluation. Counting the patient's respiratory rate, an often overlooked and underassessed vital sign, is imperative. A respiratory rate less than eight breaths per minute, or more than 30 breaths per minute, constitutes respiratory failure. Evaluating the oxygen saturation via pulse oximetry gives information about the effectiveness of the patient's breathing. If the spontaneous respirations are ineffective, or if the patient is hypoxemic, immediate resuscitative measures should be implemented, such as the application of oxygen, administration of positive pressure ventilation, and/or insertion of an endotracheal tube with mechanical ventilation. Evaluating the patient's heart rate and cardiac rhythm may identify the presence of a tachycardia, bradycardia, or conduction abnormalities and may require the administration of pharmacologic therapy, cardioversion, or a temporary pacemaker. Checking the blood pressure for hypotension and hypertension helps determine the hemodynamic stability of the patient.

❓ What is the potential cause?

Comprehensive list of differential diagnoses: shortness of breath

- Neurologic: Guillain-Barré, myasthenia gravis, anxiety
- Cardiovascular: myocardial infarction, aortic stenosis, mitral regurgitation, pericardial effusion, pericardial effusion, heart failure, cardiomyopathy

- Pulmonary: asthma, chronic obstructive lung disease, pneumothorax, pulmonary emboli, pneumonia, lung cancer, sarcoidosis, pleural effusion, choking, aspiration of a foreign object, epiglottitis
- Gastrointestinal: obesity, ascites
- Hematological: anemia
- Metabolic: diabetic ketoacidosis
- Exogenous: cocaine, alcoholic

CASE INFORMATION

General Survey

The patient looks uncomfortable but not in distress, alert, and able to answer questions. His respiratory rate at rest is 32 breaths per minute, even and regular without stridor, or audible wheezing, diminishing the possibility of an obstruction by a foreign body, or epiglottitis. His blood pressure is 184/110 in both arms and the pulse rate is 110 beats per minute, sinus tachycardia, with occasional premature ventricular contractions on telemetry. The patient's oxygen saturation is 88% on room air; immediately, a non-rebreather oxygen mask delivering 100% oxygen is applied and his oxygen saturation improves to 95%. His weight is 195 lb and with a reported height of 5'8", he has a body mass index (BMI) of 29.6 consistent with obesity.

History of Present Illness

The patient reports progressive shortness of breath over the last 2 to 3 weeks, initially associated with exertion, but now occurring at rest. Last evening, he was unable to sleep due to shortness of breath and asked his wife to call 911. He denies accompanying chest pain, palpitations, dizziness, light-headedness, headache, cough, fever, chills, nausea, or vomiting. He notes a 15-lb weight gain in the last month and a 20-lb weight gain since his heart attack 1 year ago. He also notes progressive swelling of his bilateral lower extremities and scrotum. The patient previously worked as an executive vice president of a prominent corporation but retired following his heart attack. He notes that since his cardiac event, he has felt fatigued, and attributes this to the medications he takes. He reports compliance with his medications but does mention that he stopped taking his lisinopril due to a persistent cough. Initially he kept appointments with his cardiologist but missed his appointment last month and thus has not been evaluated for the last 6 months. Additionally, he finds it difficult to adhere to a low-sodium, low-fat diet.

A review of the electronic medical record reveals the following information:

Past Medical History

The patient's medical history includes obesity, hypertension (HTN), hyperlipidemia, type II diabetes mellitus, and Stage 3 chronic kidney disease (CKD) with a glomerular filtration rate (GFR) of 45 mL/minute, anemia of chronic disease, and gout.

He also has coronary artery disease and had a myocardial infarction 13 months ago. He underwent cardiac catheterization that revealed a 70% occlusion of the mid-left anterior descending artery with a successful implantation of a drug-eluting stent (DES). He took dual antiplatelet therapy, aspirin, and clopidogrel for 1 year and remains on aspirin.

An echocardiogram done at the time of his myocardial infarction showed an ejection fraction of 45% with a mildly enlarged left ventricle.

Social History

- 20 pack-year history of smoking, quit 20 years ago
- Occasional alcohol
- Lives with spouse, retired

Medication list

- Ibuprofen (Motrin) 400 by mouth twice a day
- Aspirin 81 mg by mouth once a day
- Metoprolol, extended release (Toprol XL) 100 mg by mouth once a day
- Metformin (Glucophage) 500 mg by mouth once a day
- Lisinopril 10 mg by mouth once a day (stopped 8 months ago due to a cough)
- Atorvastatin (Lipitor) 20 mg by mouth at bedtime

? **What are the pertinent positives and significant negatives from the information at this point in the diagnostic workup?**

Pertinent Positives

- Unexplained fatigue for 1 year
- Progressive shortness of breath over 2 to 3 weeks
- 15 lb weight gain in last month
- 20 lb weight gain in 1 year (following MI)
- Hypoxemia on room air
- Tachypnea, tachycardia, and hypertension on this examination

- History of an acute myocardial infarction 1 year ago, treated with DES implantation
- Multiple risk factors for CAD including hypertension, hyperlipidemia, and type II diabetes.
- Discontinued taking lisinopril (angiotensin-converting enzyme inhibitor)
- Difficulty adhering to a low-fat, low-sodium diet
- History of 20 pack-year smoking 20 years ago

Significant Negatives

- The patient is not complaining of chest pain.
- The patient is not confused, and answers questions appropriately.
- The patient is afebrile.
- There is no history of cancer, or chronic obstructive pulmonary disease.
- The patient is not on any diuretic medications.
- The patient is not currently smoking.

❓ Can the information gathered so far be restated in a single sentence highlighting the pieces that narrow down the cause?

The problem representation may be stated as: A 66-year-old African American male with multiple risk factors for CAD, MI 1 year ago with DES to mid-LAD, ejection fraction of 45% with 2- to 3-week history of progressive shortness of breath, now occurring at rest, and accompanied by significant lower extremity edema.

Case Analysis: The patient's accompanying symptoms including a 15-lb weight gain and significant swelling of his lower extremities suggest fluid accumulation and make a neurologic or pulmonary cause for his shortness of breath less likely. While worsening renal function or liver failure can both cause fluid accumulation, this patient's cardiac history makes heart failure the most likely cause. Heart failure following myocardial infarction occurs frequently, particularly in older male patients with a history of hypertension.[1] Other factors that contribute to the development of heart failure after a myocardial infarction include the size and location of the myocardial infarction and the presence of mitral regurgitation.[1]

With a history of an MI, diabetes, hypertension, and hyperlipidemia, a recurrent myocardial infarction is also a leading differential. Ischemic cardiomyopathy, described as a severely reduced left ventricular function resulting from coronary artery disease, is a likely consideration given his previous history of a MI. A history of diabetes mellitus increases the risk of coronary artery disease as well as the risk of heart failure. I also need to consider the possibility of diabetic cardiomyopathy. I will need to gather more information, including a complete review of systems and physical examination, to help me further sort the differential diagnosis but at the moment, MI and heart failure are the top considerations.

CASE INFORMATION

Review of Systems

- Constitutional: complains of fatigue since his heart attack 1 year ago; denies fever; endorses exercise intolerance—reports he is unable to walk more than two blocks due to shortness of breath and fatigue
- Cardiovascular: denies chest pain, neck or jaw discomfort, palpitations, dizziness, light-headedness, fainting
- Pulmonary: progressive shortness of breath over the last 3 weeks; notes congested cough, but nonproductive; sleeps with two to three pillows at night; endorses paroxysmal nocturnal dyspnea
- Gastrointestinal: complains of indigestion following meals; early satiety; notes frequent belching, normal brown stool yesterday; has a history of constipation; denies blood in stools
- Genitourinary: denies burning, urinary hesitancy or urgency
- Musculoskeletal: notes occasional back pain for the last 10 years, worse when getting up in the morning; also notes pain in knees with walking
- Neurological: denies headache, paresthesias, and weakness; denies difficulty with speech

Physical Examination

- Head/eyes/ears/nose/throat: His head is normocephalic. Eyes: extraocular movements intact, pupils are equal and reactive to light and accommodation. An examination of his oral cavity reveals no buccal lesion, but multiple missing teeth (a common finding associated with smoking and diabetes). The internal jugular pulsation is elevated at 7 cm above the sternal angle.
- Cardiovascular: Tachycardia with regular rhythm. S1 and S2 are clearly heard, with a S3 noted at the beginning of diastole and best heard at the cardiac apex, over the mitral component (a sign associated with increased left ventricular filling and highly suggestive of heart failure). A displaced point of maximal impulse is noted at the left anterior axillary line. Peripheral pulses palpable and equal bilaterally, 3-4+ pitting edema of his bilateral lower extremities.
- Pulmonary: Tachypneic at rest, but no accessory muscle use. Breath sounds reveal crackles throughout (consistent with alveolar and/or interstitial fluid).
- Gastrointestinal: The abdominal examination reveals an enlarged, non-tender abdomen, with a fluid wave consistent with ascites. The patient's liver is enlarged, and smooth, estimated at a size of 15 cm (exceeds normal liver size of 10 cm in males).
- Genitourinary: Scrotal edema.
- Neurological: The patient is awake and oriented to time, person, and place. The cranial nerves II-XII are intact. The patient is able to move all extremities without difficulty.

❓ After conducting the history and physical, what additional pertinent positives and significant negatives can be added to the list?

Pertinent Positives

• Paroxysmal nocturnal dyspnea

• Cough

• Jugular venous distention is noted

• S3, an extra heart sound is appreciated

• Crackles on lung examination

• Enlarged, soft, nonnodular liver

• Distended abdomen

• Edema of his lower extremities and scrotum

Significant Negatives

• Heart rhythm is regular

• Cough is without purulent sputum

• No rhonchi or wheezing on lung examination

• Nontender abdomen

• No rebound tenderness

❓ How does the additional information obtained from the history and physical influence the list of differential diagnoses?

Case Analysis: The history of progressive weight gain, and sob, along with the physical examination findings of jugular venous distention, a displaced point of maximal impulse, a third heart sound, inspiratory crackles, and lower extremity edema strongly suggest heart failure in a patient with a history of coronary heart disease, and multiple comorbidities. An S3 extra heart sound is highly specific for heart failure. The patient's report of paroxysmal nocturnal dyspnea is also strongly suggestive of heart failure. In light of the additional information obtained from the history and physical examination, a diagnosis of heart failure is the leading explanation for the symptoms; however, the etiology of the heart failure remains to be elucidated.

Chronic obstructive pulmonary disease (COPD) remains a consideration in light of the patient's remote 20 pack-year smoking history. COPD patients with cor pulmonale display symptoms of venous congestion; however, the patient's other physical examination findings do not reflect cor pulmonale or COPD. An S3 gallop may be heard in COPD; yet, this sign is usually heard best along the lower sternal border, overlying the pulmonic component of S2, and is associated with increased filling of the right ventricle. Additionally, the patient does not have the typical barrel chest, decreased breath sounds, wheezing, and prolonged expiration that occur with advanced COPD.

Other possibilities, such as acute or chronic pulmonary emboli and pulmonary hypertension, may cause signs and symptoms of venous congestion; however, these conditions are more likely to present with a low blood pressure rather than a high blood pressure. A pericardial effusion may also cause heart failure symptoms; however, the heart sounds are usually diminished as fluid accumulates within the pericardial space and that is not the case in this patient. With the absence of a fever, and a productive cough, clinical suspicion of a pneumonia is less likely; however, diabetic patients are considered immune compromised and may not present with the typical symptoms of purulent sputum, cough, chest pain associated with respirations, chills, or fever.

? What diagnostic testing should be done and in what order?

The initial evaluation of a patient who presents with shortness of breath includes a 12-lead electrocardiogram and chest radiograph, performed within 5 minutes of the admission. These two noninvasive studies can quickly rule in or out several diagnoses on my list including acute ST elevation myocardial infarction, pneumothorax, pleural effusion, and pneumonia. Heart size and the appearance of the lungs on chest x-ray will give further evidence of his underlying chronic health problems. Because myocardial infarction is a concern, I also order serial troponin levels, a sensitive and specific measure of myocardial damage. Brain natriuretic peptide (BNP) and N-terminal propeptide of BNP (NT-proBNP) are biomarker assays used to establish and support the diagnosis of heart failure. Both are peptide hormones synthesized and released by cardiomyocytes in response to myocardial stretch, expansion of the ventricular walls due to volume overload. In a meta-analysis, both tests revealed a high accuracy for the diagnosis of acute and chronic heart failure.[2] Serial monitoring of BNPs may be helpful in trending the response to treatment measures, with reductions in the level of BNP associated with an improvement in symptoms. Using BNPs for the diagnosis of heart failure may be complicated by the fact that BNPs may be elevated in the setting of a number of noncardiac conditions including chronic obstructive pulmonary disease, anemia, renal failure, and critical illness. Additional laboratory tests include a comprehensive metabolic panel to assess the patient's renal function and electrolytes and a complete blood count to assess for anemia, a predictor of increased mortality in heart failure patients.

CASE INFORMATION
Preliminary Diagnostic Results

- The 12-lead ECG reveals a sinus tachycardia, with a heart rate of 110 beats per minute, a PR interval of 140 milliseconds (ms), a QRS interval of 120 ms, and QT interval of 400 ms—all of which are within normal limits. The patient has a left bundle branch block as evidenced by a QS wave in lead V1, and an RSR prime in lead V6, indicating delayed conduction in the left bundle, and may reflect an enlarged left ventricle. This finding is unchanged since the patient's last ECG.

- The chest radiograph reveals an enlarged cardiac silhouette, or cardiomegaly, with pulmonary vascular congestion. There is no pleural effusion, no pneumothorax, and no hyperinflation or a flattened diaphragm, which are often signs of COPD. The patient does not have an enlarged right ventricle or pulmonary artery, findings which would suggest advanced COPD or cor pulmonale.
- Serial troponin levels peak at an elevation of 3.0, reflecting myocardial necrosis.
- The patient's BNP level is 2953 pg/mL, consistent with severe heart failure.
- The comprehensive metabolic panel shows a GFR of 35 mL/min according to the Cockcroft-Gault formula, indicating Stage 3B chronic kidney disease, or moderately reduced renal function.
- Urinalysis reveals +100 protein. Further testing will be necessary to evaluate the degree of proteinuria including an albumin/creatinine ratio or a protein/creatinine ratio. Chronic kidney disease increases the risk of adverse cardiovascular events.
- Results reveal an anemia of chronic disease, with a serum ferritin of 110 ng/mL, and a serum iron level of 22 µg/mL.
- A lipid profile shows the patient's low-density lipoprotein (LDL) of 136 mg/dL (normal is 65–180 mg/dL), which is above the target goal of less than 70 mg/dL for a patient with a history of an MI and diabetes.

LAB (normal range)	Value
Troponin (<0.1 ng/mL)	3.0 ng/mL
Na (136–145 mEq/L)	Na 136 mEq/L
K (3.5–5.0 mEq/L)	K 4.4 mEq/L
Cl (98–106 mEq/L)	Cl 107 mEq/L
CO_2 (23–28 mEq/L)	CO_2 22 mEq/L
Total cholesterol (<200 mg/dL)	Total cholesterol 231 mg/dL
LDL (65–180 mg/dL)	LDL 136 mg/dL
HDL (>35 mg/dL)	HDL 35 mg/dL
Triglycerides (<150 mg/dL)	Triglycerides: 302 mg/dL
BUN (8–20 mg/dL)	BUN 23 mg/dL
Creatinine (0.7–1.3 mg/dL)	Creatinine 2.6 mg/dL
WBC (3,900–11,000 cells/µL)	WBC 7,600 cells/µL
Hgb (13.5–16.5 g/dL)	Hgb 13.8 g/dL
Hct (41%–50%)	Hct 38.5%

LAB (normal range)	Value
Glucose (60–110 mg/dL)	Glucose 205 mg/dL
Hgb a1c (<5.4%)	Hgb a1c 8.6%
C-reactive protein (<0.5mg/dL)	C-reactive protein 26 mg/L
Ferritin (15–200 ng/mL)	Ferritin 110 ng/mL
Iron (60–160 U/L)	Iron 22 µg/mL
Glomerular filtration rate (GFR) (>60 mL/min)	Glomerular filtration rate (GFR) = 35 mL/min
BNP (less than 100 pg/mL)	BNP 2953 pg/mL

Urinalysis: Specific gravity 1.010, pH 5.0, color clear, protein 100mg/dL; leukocyte esterase negative; nitrite negative, ketones negative, red blood cells negative.

Diagnosis

At this juncture, the leading differential to explain the progressive shortness of breath is acute decompensated left ventricular heart failure (ADHF). The troponin elevation reveals that the patient has myocardial damage. Additional diagnostic testing is necessary to reveal the extent of the coronary disease and determine the etiology of the heart failure. The American College of Cardiology Foundation/ American Heart Association (ACCF/AHA) 2013 Heart Failure Guidelines recommend performance of cardiac arteriography to investigate the cause of unexplained heart failure in patients who are suspected of having ischemic heart disease and who are candidates for revascularization.[3] The management of the patient includes the following additional diagnostic studies:

- Cardiac catheterization: Patent intervention site of LAD: occlusion of the mid-left circumflex; successful drug-eluting stent (DES) to the left circumflex. Severely reduced left ventricular ejection fraction of 28%. Increased pulmonary artery pressure of 48/30 mm Hg and a pulmonary capillary wedge pressure of 32 mm Hg.

- Two-dimensional echocardiogram: Severe left ventricular dilatation, overall decreased left ventricular systolic function; ejection fraction (EF) of 28%; mild mitral regurgitation,

- Abdominal ultrasound: Impression: hepatomegaly; no biliary dilatation; moderate amount of abdominal ascites, increased compared to the previous examination. Additional findings include mild echogenic kidneys, compatible with medical renal disease; no hydronephrosis.

Management of Ischemic Cardiomyopathy; Coronary Artery Disease; Stage D, Class IV Systolic Heart Failure

There are many diverse causes of heart failure, but the most common cause, occurring in up to 70% of patients, is coronary artery disease.[4] When the left ventricular ejection fraction is less than 35% in the setting of ischemic coronary artery disease, the diagnosis of ischemic cardiomyopathy can be established. Heart failure following a myocardial infarction may be caused by inflammatory factors, the presence of significant mitral regurgitation, or the area and location of the necrosis.[4] The patient's C-reactive protein is elevated to 26 mg/dL, revealing an inflammatory component. Could diabetes mellitus have affected the progression of the systolic dysfunction? Emerging evidence indicates that diabetes causes both diastolic and systolic dysfunction by increasing the level of interstitial and perivascular fibrosis.[5] While it is difficult to differentiate the contribution of diabetic cardiomyopathy from ischemic cardiomyopathy in this case, tissue Doppler imaging is being used to document slight reductions in left ventricular function attributable to diabetes that occurs early in the disease and is underdiagnosed in most cases.[5]

Hypertrophic cardiomyopathy (HCM) is the most common cause of genetically induced cardiomyopathy, and contrary to popular misconceptions, may be diagnosed at any point during the lifespan. A three-generation family history is indicated if HCM is strongly suspected. Usually, the echocardiogram reveals substantial hypertrophy of the ventricular septum with left ventricular wall thickness greater than 50 mm.[6] Changes in wall thickness do not occur with systolic heart failure.

Heart failure occurring in the absence of coronary artery disease may be due to a number of conditions including alcohol use, acquired immunodeficiency syndrome, peripartum state, or Takotsubo cardiomyopathy. Other causes include myocarditis, Chagas disease, and endocrine disorders such as hyperthyroidism, acromegaly, and growth hormone deficiency. Less commonly, conditions such as amyloidosis or hemochromatosis, a condition of iron overload, can result in heart failure.

Evidence-Based Treatment of Ischemic Cardiomyopathy

Regardless of whether the cause of the systolic heart failure is ischemic or nonischemic, the treatments are similar. Immediate pharmacologic treatment is indicated including the gold standard regimen of diuretic therapy, angiotensin-converting enzyme inhibitors, and β-blockers. Intravenous nitroglycerin will be started if the response to the diuretics is not sufficient.

Diuretic therapy may be initially ordered for the patient who presents with lower extremity edema and pulmonary crackles. Since this patient is naïve to diuretics, an initial dose of furosemide (Lasix) 40 mg intravenously, a loop diuretic, is administered in accordance with the ACCF/AHA Heart Failure Guidelines.[3] Careful and serial monitoring of serum electrolytes will be undertaken as loop diuretics inhibit the body's reabsorption of sodium, potassium, chloride, calcium, magnesium, and phosphorus, leading to possible electrolyte abnormalities. Potentially, these abnormalities may contribute to the development of cardiac arrhythmias, an increased concern in patients with an enlarged left ventricle and a reduced ejection fraction.

For this patient, parenteral vasodilator agents are necessary because his blood pressure remained refractory to the initial therapy. A number of pharmacologic agents may be considered including nitroglycerin and nitroprusside, both of which release nitric oxide contributing to vasodilation. Intravenous nitroglycerin works almost immediately to increase venous capacitance, decrease venous return, and decrease preload, lessening the symptoms of venous congestion. In larger doses, arterial vasodilation may occur; however, the venous actions predominate. These pharmacodynamic actions help reduce the oxygen demands on the heart. The half-life of nitroglycerin is 5 minutes, allowing for careful and dynamic titration of blood pressure to a goal of less than 140/90.

Angiotensin-converting enzyme inhibitors (ACEIs), a Class I level of evidence (LOE) AHA recommendation are a mainstay of pharmacologic treatment for patients with heart failure, particularly those patients with reduced EF (rEF).[3] The patient's medical history reveals that lisinopril was discontinued due to the development of a persistent cough. Additionally, the patient's Stage 3B renal failure is a concern. The guidelines recommend that ACEI and angiotensin receptor blockers (ARBs) be held when the GFR is below 30 mL/min. In this case, a low-dose ARB will be started within 24 hours of admission and the patient's renal function will be closely monitored. ARBs work directly at the cell's receptor site and do not cause an accumulation of bradykinin, the proposed mechanism responsible for the cough. An ARB, such as valsartan (Diovan), will inhibit angiotensin II, and aldosterone, reducing circulating blood volume and increasing vasodilatation. Aldosterone inhibition reduces sodium and water reabsorption in exchange for the retention of potassium. As a result, monitoring for hyperkalemia is important since the combination of an ARB and a low GFR both increase the risk of hyperkalemia. Careful monitoring of the patient's renal function while on the ARB is also necessary, as both ACEIs and ARBs lower the glomerular filtration pressure and can further impair the GFR.

Recent research reveals that three β-blockers are superior in decreasing the progression of cardiovascular disease and overall mortality. The three pharmacologic agents are carvedilol, bisoprolol, and sustained-release metoprolol, representing an AHA/ACA Class I level of evidence (A) recommendation.[3] In the setting of acute decompensated heart failure, with significant volume overload, consideration will be given toward holding the β-blocker until the patient's volume status equilibrates and returns to near normal range. Metoprolol is a selective-B1-receptor antagonist that slows the conduction and contractile forces of the heart, reducing the amount of work performed by the heart and lessening the oxygen demands of the heart. In the setting of acute volume overload, these β-1-antagonist effects may further impair the function of the left ventricle with a resultant decrease in cardiac output and worsening fluid volume accumulation. Once the patient's fluid volume status returns to near normal, the β-blockers will be resumed.

Case Follow-Up

Once the patient is stabilized with initial and immediate treatment, I take the opportunity to review the patient's treatment regimen to ensure that the patient is receiving high-quality, guideline-directed treatment (GDT) to reduce cardiovascular events, rehospitalization, and mortality. Aggressive efforts to reduce risk factors and prevent further episodes of ischemia are central to the care of this patient.

A review of the medication regimen reveals that the patient is taking ibuprofen (Motrin) for osteoarthritis of his knees. Ibuprofen a nonsteroidal anti-inflammatory agent, is contraindicated in patients with coronary artery disease, and carries a black box warning indicating an increased risk of cardiovascular thrombotic events. In addition, regular use of ibuprofen is likely to worsen his chronic kidney disease. Acetaminophen represents an option for mild pain; however, if the pain and stiffness persist, injections of hyaluronic acid or steroids may be necessary. Reviewing the patient laboratory results reveals that the LDL is not at goal level of less than 70 mg/dL. The patient is on a relatively low dose of atorvastatin, and this will be increased to a moderate- to high-intensity dose of 80 mg in the patient with CAD and in accordance with the newly revised guidelines.[7]

The patient's uncontrolled diabetes mellitus poses an additional risk factor and portends an increased risk of cardiovascular mortality. With a serum creatinine of 2.6 mg/dL and a GFR of 37 mL/min, metformin is contraindicated. The patient will be started on a basal Lantus insulin as well as preprandial lispro.

The patient has acknowledged difficulty with adherence to the nutritional recommendations of a heart healthy lifestyle including avoidance of concentrated sweets. A few dietary options were discussed with the patient and his wife such as substituting whole grains for white breads, and adding increased fiber to his diet. A referral to a nutritionist was made as obesity is a predictor of worse cardiovascular outcomes.

Lifestyle recommendations are central to the treatment plan. Weight loss, diet, and exercise are key recommendations. Physical rehabilitation will be recommended for this patient.

References

1. Hellermann JP, Jacobsen SJ, Redfield MM, et al. Heart failure after myocardial infarction: clinical presentation and survival. *Eur J Heart Fail*. 2005;7:119.
2. Clerico A, Fontana M, Zyw L. Comparison of the diagnostic accuracy of brain natriuretic peptide (BNP) and the N-Terminal part of the propeptide of BNP immunoassays in chronic and acute heart failure: a systemic review. *Clin Chem*. 2007;53(5):813-822.
3. Yancy CW, Jessup M, Bozkurt B, et al. ACCF/AHA guideline for the management of heart failure: executive summary. A report of the American College of Cardiology Foundation/American Heart Association Task Force on practice guidelines. *Circulation*. 2013;128:1810.
4. Fang JC, Aranki S. Diagnosis and management of ischemic cardiomyopathy. *UpToDate*. 2014. http://www.uptodate.com/contents/diagnosis-and-management-of-ischemic-cardiomyopathy.
5. Miki T, Yuda S, Kouzu H, Miura T. Diabetic cardiomyopathy pathophysiology and clinical features. *Heart Fail Rev*. 2012;18(2):149-166.
6. Maron BJ. Hypertrophic cardiomyopathy. A systemic review. *JAMA*. 2002;28(10):1308-1320.
7. Stone NJ, Robinson J, Lichtenstein AH. 2013 ACC/AHA guideline on the treatment of blood cholesterol to reduce atherosclerotic cardiovascular risk in adults: a report of the American College of Cardiology/American Heart Association Task Force on Practice Guidelines. *Circulation*. 2013;1-84.

CASE 20

Eliza Ajero Granflor

Eliza Ajero Granflor is an ACNP in the surgical ICU at The Queen's Medical Center in Honolulu, Hawaii. She collaborates with a team of fellows, residents, interns, and intensivists to provide care to adults presenting with trauma and general surgery conditions.

CASE INFORMATION

Chief Complaint

A 64-year-old male restrained passenger status post motor vehicle crash traveling at 60 mph, complaining of chest pain, difficulty breathing, and right leg pain.

? What is the potential cause?

Respiratory distress following blunt chest trauma may indicate a number of life-threatening injuries that require immediate intervention. The mechanism of injury directs my thought process toward common injuries associated with thoracic trauma. Rather than focusing on a single symptom, my assessment of any trauma patient follows a stepwise process, which the American College of Surgeons outlines in the Advanced Trauma Life Support (ATLS) course.[1] The primary survey begins with an assessment of the airway, then breathing, followed by circulation. Life-threatening conditions are identified and promptly treated during the primary survey.

The secondary survey focuses on identifying potential life-threatening thoracic injuries through further in-depth physical examination, diagnostic imaging, and labs. Rather than completing a list of possible causes of respiratory distress by body system and checking off each potential diagnosis, I organize diagnoses into categories of primary survey and secondary survey. This ensures that the most life-threatening injuries are prioritized first.

Differential Diagnoses for a Patient With Respiratory Distress Following Chest Trauma[1]

Primary survey

- Airway: foreign-body obstruction, laryngeal injury, upper chest injury, facial fractures, neck trauma, sternoclavicular dislocation
- Breathing: tension pneumothorax, open pneumothorax (sucking chest wound), flail chest, pulmonary contusion, massive hemothorax

Secondary survey

- Simple pneumothorax, hemothorax, pulmonary contusion, tracheo-bronchial tree injury, blunt cardiac injury, traumatic aortic disruption, traumatic diaphragmatic injury, blunt esophageal rupture, rib fracture, scapula fracture, clavicle fracture

CASE INFORMATION

History of Present Illness

Trauma patient evaluations differ from the usual inpatient or outpatient encounters in that a review of systems and history are often not feasible, nor the initial priority. Measurement of vital signs and assessment of level of consciousness are the first step of the primary survey.

The initial primary, secondary, and tertiary surveys are done in emergency department (ED). As the patient is transferred to the surgical intensive care unit (ICU), the trauma intern gives me the following history and ED course summary: the patient is a 64-year-old male, restrained passenger, involved in a motor vehicle crash traveling 60 mph, requiring extraction from the vehicle. He had loss of consciousness on the scene, but arrived to the ED awake, alert, and talking. He presented to the ED on a backboard, with an Aspen collar, and a nonrebreather mask at 15 liters of oxygen. His chief complaints were chest pain, difficulty breathing, and right leg pain. He was able to protect his airway but complaining of dyspnea. His chest wall had crepitus and there were palpable rib fractures on the left. After procedural fentanyl and versed intravenous boluses were given, a left-sided chest tube was placed with evacuation of air and an initial 100 cc of blood. He was hemodynamically stable. The focused assessment sonography in trauma (FAST) evaluation was positive only for a left-sided pneumothorax. X-ray and CT imaging revealed left-sided hemopneumothorax, flail chest, sternal fracture, pneumomediastinum, and a right femoral diaphyseal fracture. The trauma team ordered an orthopedic consult and transferred the patient to the ICU.

When the patient arrives in the surgical ICU, I start with a new primary survey. Trauma patients must be continuously reevaluated for intact airway, breathing, and circulation. If there is any change in a patient's status, assessment starts over with primary survey until life-threatening issues are resolved.

The patient is a well-nourished, well-developed male. He is still awake and alert with a Glasgow coma scale (GCS) of 15. He is maintaining his airway but is in obvious respiratory distress with uncontrolled pain. He is having difficulty speaking in full sentences due to pain on inspiration. Despite a chest tube and fentanyl, he is still dyspneic and complaining of severe chest and right leg pain. He is in too much distress to provide an extensive medical history or review of systems, but does give a history of hypertension and denies any use of any anticoagulants. He denies any other significant cardiac history and any chronic respiratory diseases such as chronic obstructive pulmonary disease (COPD), asthma, or lung cancer.

❓ What are the pertinent positives from the information given so far?

- Blunt chest trauma
- Obvious respiratory distress
- Uncontrolled chest pain worse with inspiration
- Positive loss of consciousness at the scene
- Imaging confirmed left-sided rib fractures, left pulmonary contusion, sternal fracture, pneumomediastinum, and hemopneumothorax

❓ What are the significant negatives from the information given so far?

- Denies history of chronic respiratory disease such as COPD, asthma, or cancer
- Patent airway
- Imaging negative for aortic injury or other thoracic great vessel injury

❓ Can the information gathered so far be restated in a single sentence highlighting the pieces that narrow down the cause?

Putting the information obtained so far in a single statement—a problem representation—sets the stage for gathering more information and determining the cause.

The problem representation in this case might be: "a 64-year-old male with hypertension status post motor vehicle crash who presents with dyspnea and chest pain following blunt chest trauma."

❓ How does this information affect the list of possible causes?

Case Analysis: At this point, I'm still addressing possible life-threatening injuries in the airway and breathing categories. His ability to speak gives the impression of an intact airway, but I need to inspect for facial and chest trauma. Imaging already confirmed left-sided rib fractures with a flail chest, pulmonary contusion, hemopneumothorax, and sternal fracture. His loss of consciousness in the field concerns me as there is a possibility of an aspiration and subsequent pneumonitis. The presence of a left pneumothorax, mediastinal air, sternal injury, and severe pain raise the suspicion of a possible esophageal rupture. The patient denies chronic pulmonary disease, so his dyspnea is most likely an acute result of his chest trauma. There is history of hypertension, but no coronary artery disease or congestive heart failure. Imaging is negative for thoracic great vessel injury. Cardiogenic causes of respiratory distress are still a concern given the mechanism of blunt chest trauma, but I will address this later and do a complete examination once I establish airway and breathing.

CASE INFORMATION

Review of Systems

A review of systems is unable to be performed due to the patient's high acuity. He is only able to give a brief history of hypertension, deny other medical problems or allergies to medications.

Physical Examination (Starting With Airway and Breathing)

- Airway: He is awake; his speech is appropriate though with labored verbal responses, indicating an intact airway. C-collar in place. Tachypneic. No stridor or dysphonia. Trachea midline. No visible facial or neck trauma, and no open chest wounds.
- Breathing: Paradoxical chest wall movements on the left side. Audible clicking with inspiration on left and diminished bilateral breath sounds in bases with clear upper lobes. Palpable chest wall crepitus, tenderness, and rib fractures on left. The left-sided chest tube is patent on 20 cm suction without air leak; only 100 mL blood in the chest tube drainage system. The patient complains of pain with deep inspiration. His breathing is rapid and shallow.
- Vital signs: Pulse is 96 beats per minute, blood pressure is 108/65 mm Hg, respiratory rate is 30 breaths per minute, temperature is 98.6°F tympanic; oxygen saturation is 96% on 15 L 100% nonrebreather mask.
- Constitutional: Well-nourished, well-developed, pale, obvious respiratory distress on 100% nonrebreather. His mood is anxious, and he is agitated. He is cooperative.
- Head/eyes/ears/nose/throat: 6 mm laceration to right temple, and multiple 1 to 2 cm lacerations on forehead and scalp. There is a 2-cm partial scalp avulsion to left forehead. No periorbital edema or erythema; no Battle sign.
- Cardiovascular: Heart rate and rhythm regular, S1 and S2, point of maximal impulse over his fifth intercostal on his left side, no murmurs, rubs, or gallops. Extremities: nail beds are warm, brisk capillary refill.
- Pulmonary: As per "breathing" above.
- Gastrointestinal: Abdominal distension with tenderness. Normal bowel sounds.
- Genitourinary: Foley catheter in place, yellow clear urine. Normal genitalia.
- Integumentary: His skin is warm and pale. Abrasions are noted scattered over face.
- Neurological: Pupils 3 mm, equal, round, reactive. There are no focal neurologic deficits. The face is symmetric; his speech is clear and appropriate. He is awake and alert, following commands, opening his eyes spontaneously, with a Glasgow coma scale of 15.

❓ What elements of the review of systems and the physical examination should be added to the list of pertinent positives? Which items should be added to the list of significant negatives?

- **Pertinent positives:** Paradoxical chest wall movements on left; pain with deep inspiration; crepitus and tenderness to palpation on left chest; anxious and agitated.
- **Significant negatives:** Vital signs are stable, normal cardiac examination, no neurological deficits. Breath sounds are equally diminished at bases but present, indicating some lung reexpansion on left.

❓ How does this information affect the list of possible causes?

Although I have the full physical assessment listed above, I have already determined signs and symptoms of inadequate oxygenation and ventilation by assessing the patient's level of mentation. The patient's uncontrolled pain from his consecutive rib fractures is causing splinting, asymmetrical movement of the chest wall, and impaired ventilation. Called a flail chest, the associated breathing pattern, pendelluft breathing (swinging like a pendulum), is further compromising his oxygenation and ventilation. Pendelluft breathing is thought to cause deoxygenated air to shunt back and forth from the healthy lung and the injured lung. Treatment is aimed at correcting the paradoxical movement through either external fixation or internal fixation. Mechanical ventilation with positive pressure is thought to provide internal fixation of the collapsed broken rib segments.[2]

CASE INFORMATION

I hold further physical examination until issues with oxygenation and ventilation are resolved. Anesthesia is called to the bedside to place an epidural catheter and provide fentanyl and bupivacaine for pain relief. But despite the medications, the oxygen saturation drops to 88% on 100% oxygen via a nonrebreather mask and the patient becomes confused. I draw an arterial blood gas. The results are pH: 7.26, $PaCO_2$: 51 mm Hg, PaO_2: 84 mm Hg, base excess: −5, bicarbonate: 22 mEq/L, and O_2 saturation of 93 on 100% nonrebreather. The blood gas shows a combined respiratory and metabolic acidosis with a fully corrected hypoxemia. But the PaO_2/FiO_2 ratio is 84, indicating that the baseline hypoxemia is severe. Generally this index is used to stratify the severity of ARDS but it is also used to evaluate oxygenation problems in critically ill patients. The patient is emergently intubated and placed on assist control pressure mode, 100% FiO_2 with positive end-expiratory pressure (PEEP) of 12 cm H_2O, set rate 18 breaths per minute, and pressure support of 18 cm H_2O. With these settings, his tidal volume is 488 mL and minute ventilation is 8.8 L/min.

What diagnostic testing should be done and in what order?

After intubation, I order a stat portable chest x-ray to confirm endotracheal tube placement. While waiting, I order a 12-lead ECG. The following stat labs were drawn earlier with the ABG: CBC with differential, complete metabolic profile, coagulation studies, and troponin I.

CASE INFORMATION
Results of Diagnostic Testing

- ECG: reveals normal sinus rhythm without ST changes or evidence of ischemia.
- Chest x-ray: the endotracheal tube is in correct position 2 to 4 cm above the carina. The left chest tube is in correct position, but there is a new right lobar collapse and persisting right mediastinal shift. I am concerned that the left chest tube has not adequately evacuated the left pneumothorax, so I contact the trauma resident who emergently places a new left chest tube superior to the original. There is no output from the second chest tube, suggesting that the right lobar collapse may be a mucus plug rather than as a result of an unresolved left pneumothorax. I order a bronchoscopy cart to the unit.
- Laboratory results: His labs reveal a creatinine of 1.2 mg/dL (normal range 0.5–1.4 mg/dL), which is elevated from a baseline of 0.8 mg/dL, suggesting acute kidney injury. His chemistry panel is otherwise normal. The complete blood count with differential reveals a leukocytosis of 20 cells/µL, which is likely due to acute trauma. His hemoglobin and hematocrit are normal. His coagulation panel is normal, but he has a mildly elevated lactic acid at 2.2 mEq/L (normal range 0.5–2.2 mmol/L), and an elevated troponin of 0.56 (normal is less than 0.01 ng/mL). I will follow additional troponins but this elevation is likely due to trauma, and his normal ECG makes myocardial infarction less likely. I also order a formal echocardiogram in the morning to evaluate for myocardial injury from a cardiac contusion. I do not need an emergent echocardiogram because the patient is hemodynamically stable with no ECG changes.
- As the bronchoscopy cart arrives, I still have in mind that I need to rule out tracheobronchial tree injury and blunt esophageal rupture due to radiographic evidence of pneumomediastinum. The trauma surgeon and resident perform the bronchoscopy, which reveals intact large airways, and thick mucus plugging of the right main-stem bronchus. This area is lavaged and a bronchial alveolar lavage sample sent for Gram stain and culture. After the mucus plugs are cleared, the distal bronchial segments are visualized and are negative for injury.
- I order a repeat CT scan of the chest the next day, which reveals resolved pneumomediastinum, ruling out esophageal injury. The echocardiogram the next day reveals a normal ejection fraction of 65% to 70%.

Diagnosis and Treatment: Flail Chest

Flail chest is diagnosed when there is radiographic evidence of multiple rib fractures with two or more adjacent ribs fractured in two or more places, thereby causing a segment of the chest wall to lose bony continuity with the rest of the thoracic cage.[1] The main complicating injury that accompanies flail chest in severe blunt chest wall trauma is actually pulmonary contusion.[2]

Initial treatment of flail chest with pulmonary contusion includes humidified oxygenation, adequate ventilation, fluid resuscitation, and pain control. Noninvasive positive pressure ventilation can be considered in alert patients with marginal respiratory status in combination with adequate analgesia, but obligatory mechanical ventilation in the absence of respiratory failure is not recommended.[2] Pain control can be achieved with intravenous narcotics or local anesthetic administration. Options for local anesthetic administration include intermittent intercostal nerve blocks, intrapleural, extrapleural, or epidural anesthesia. Epidural catheter is the preferred mode of analgesia delivery in severe flail chest.[2] Surgical fixation can be considered in severe flail chest, but it has not been shown to definitively improve outcomes.

In this patient's case, I follow the usual diagnostic and treatment algorithm per the Eastern Association for the Surgery of Trauma (EAST) guidelines for management of flail chest and pulmonary contusion.[2] Following epidural placement, intubation, ventilation, and bronchoscopy, I resuscitate the patient with crystalloid to treat his acute kidney injury.

Case Follow-Up

By the patient's second ICU day, he develops aspiration pneumonia in addition to his left flail chest with pulmonary contusion, which quickly progresses to adult respiratory distress syndrome (ARDS) as defined by the Berlin criteria.[3] I already obtained sputum cultures from his bronchoscopy, so I initiate empiric coverage with vancomycin and piperacillin-tazobactam to cover for gram-positive and intra-abdominal organisms. He becomes hypotensive, requiring aggressive fluid resuscitation. Guidelines state that adequate fluid resuscitation is essential even in patients with flail chest and pulmonary contusions. I place a pulmonary artery catheter to guide fluid resuscitation. His pulmonary artery occlusion pressure (PAOP) is high at 22 mm Hg suggesting adequate fluid resuscitation, so I initiate diuresis with intermittent IV boluses of loop diuretics to a target PAOP of 14 to 16 mm Hg.

The patient has a long and complicated 18-day ICU stay that includes rotational bed therapy and the use of ARDS lung protective strategies. These strategies include low tidal volumes with 4 to 6 mL/kg predicted body weight, permissive hypercapnia, and maintenance of plateau pressure between 25 and 30 cm H_2O. Permissive hypercapnia is a tolerance of elevated $PaCO_2$ secondary to low-volume ventilation. These protective lung strategies aim to prevent lung overdistention, and cyclic opening and closing of small airways, which are thought to cause further lung injury.[4] Eventually, his sputum cultures reveal *Haemophilus influenzae*, and his antibiotic regimen is narrowed to ceftriaxone. He requires several more bronchoscopies with alveolar lavage due to recurrent mucus plugging. He eventually is weaned to minimal ventilator settings, extubated, and sent to the floor for further monitoring and rehabilitation.

References

1. American College of Surgeons Committee on Trauma. *Advanced Trauma Life Support Student Course Manual*. Chicago, IL: American College of Surgeons; 2012.
2. Simon B, Ebert J, Bokhari F, et al. Management of pulmonary contusion and flail chest: an Eastern Association for the Surgery of Trauma practice management guideline. *J Trauma Acute Care Surg*. 2012:73(5):S351-S361. doi:10.1097/TA.0b013e31827019fd
3. The ARDS Definition Task Force. Acute respiratory distress syndrome: the Berlin definition. *JAMA*. 2012;307(23):2526-2533.
4. Fanelli V, Vlachou A, Ghannadian S, Simonetti U, Slutsky A, Zhang H. Acute respiratory distress syndrome: new definition, current and future therapeutic options. *J Thorac Dis*. 2013:5(3):326-334. doi:10.3978/j.issn.2072-1439.2013.04.05

CASE 21

Michelle A. Weber

Michelle A. Weber works in General Surgery, providing perioperative care for patients undergoing complex abdominal wall reconstructions, foregut operations, and bariatric procedures.

CASE INFORMATION
Chief Complaint
"I had my gallbladder out a week and a half ago and my pain has been worsening for the past 3 days. I haven't been able to keep anything down for the past day either."

Upon first meeting a patient, especially a patient who is new to me, it is important to start with a broad list of differential diagnoses, guided by the patient's chief complaint(s). Given the patient's recent cholecystectomy, it is necessary to think of potential biliary as well as non-biliary causes of her acute, worsening abdominal pain.

Comprehensive Differential Diagnoses for Patient With Abdominal Pain S/P Recent Laparoscopic Cholecystectomy[1,2]

Biliary causes:
- Acute cholangitis
- Choledocholithiasis (retained CBD gallstone)
- Postoperative bile leak/biloma
- Iatrogenic biliary stricture
- Sphincter of Oddi dysfunction

Non-biliary causes:
- Poorly controlled postsurgical pain
- Narcotic-induced postoperative constipation/ileus
- Incisional/port site hernia
- Hepatitis
- Peptic ulcer disease
- Gastritis
- Acute pancreatitis
- Functional or nonulcerative dyspepsia
- GERD
- Gastroenteritis

A significant amount of data is gathered upon first interacting with a patient. The list of differential diagnoses will be modified as additional subjective and objective data are gathered.

CASE INFORMATION

History of Present Illness

Mrs B, a 52-year-old Caucasian female, presents to the general surgery clinic with complaints of a 3-day history of acute onset, worsening abdominal pain. Past medical history is significant for type II diabetes, obesity, gastroesophageal reflux disease (GERD), hypertension, and hyperlipidemia. She is status post laparoscopic cholecystectomy 10 days ago for symptomatic cholelithiasis. Abdominal pain, rated 8/10, is located in epigastrium with radiation to right upper quadrant and also intermittently to right shoulder blade. Says she has not had pain like this before; right upper quadrant pain with gallbladder "attacks" only lasted about 1 hour and was associated with eating high fat foods. The pain is now fairly constant and is not associated with activity. It is somewhat aggravated by oral intake, including water. Pain is described as a "cramping, pressure-like" sensation. Denies alleviating factors. Tried 10 mg oxycodone as well as 650 mg acetaminophen last night without any improvement in pain. Notes associated anorexia for a few days and for the past 24 hours, has developed worsening nausea and vomiting. Denies fever, jaundice, clay-colored stools, or dark urine. Bowel habits have returned to preoperative baseline; last BM was this morning and was soft, nonbloody. Her typical GERD symptoms are well controlled with Ranitidine (Zantac). Overall, she had been feeling pretty well for the first week after surgery; was up and about without difficulty. Reports minimal discomfort associated with port site incisions. Denies redness, drainage from incisions. Her fasting blood sugars have been slightly elevated the past few days, averaging 150 to 160, which is high for her.

Case Analysis: There are a number of key pieces of information that Mrs B shared. Knowing that surgery was 10 days ago slightly lowers the suspicion that her symptoms are related to a bile leak as patients with this complication typically present on average 3 days following surgery.[2] The location of her pain, in the epigastrium and right upper quadrant, duration, as well as its lack of relief from pain medication raises the suspicion for potential biliary causes. Causes for elevated fasting blood sugar levels are multifactorial and include, but are not limited to, recent surgery and subsequent stress response or infection. The fact that she has remained afebrile lowers the likelihood that she has cholangitis or an infection in the biliary tract. Although not noted with this patient, it is important to remember that jaundice, clay-colored stools, and dark urine may be indicative of obstruction of the bile duct as excess bile is reabsorbed into the blood stream and incomplete excretion occurs. Given that her symptoms are new since surgery, suspicion for a potential biliary cause remains high.

CASE INFORMATION

- Past medical history: as listed in history of present illness
- Past surgical history: tubal ligation, umbilical hernia repair without mesh, left ankle open reduction and internal fixation
- Family history: two sisters, mother also had gallbladder removed. No history of other biliary or liver dysfunction. Father and brother are also diabetic.
- Medications: 5 to 10 mg oxycodone every 4 hours as needed for post-surgical pain; 650 mg acetaminophen every 4 hours as needed; Premarin; simvastatin; lisinopril; ranitidine
- Allergies: no known drug allergies

General Survey

With the list of all possible causes in mind, my next step is to begin gathering objective data to assist in ruling out diagnoses and further narrowing in on more likely causes. In this case, I begin with a general survey of the patient: she is an obese, well-developed woman who appears to be uncomfortable, but not in any acute distress. She is sitting on the examination room chair, tapping her foot anxiously.

Further review of the electronic medical records reveals a straight-forward, uneventful laparoscopic cholecystectomy 10 days ago. During dissection and removal of the gallbladder, surgical clips are placed on the cystic duct and cystic artery, which are then divided (see Figure 21-1). An intraoperative cholangiogram, a study in which contrast is injected into the biliary system to look for gallstones in the common bile duct and to help identify the bile duct anatomy, was not performed. There continues to be debate regarding the use of intraoperative cholangiogram at time of laparoscopic cholecystectomy. Those in favor argue that it allows for better delineation of anatomy, therefore reducing the risk of bile duct injuries, and also identifies asymptomatic choledocholithiasis. Opponents to intraoperative cholangiogram argue that it is not always necessary and increases both procedure time and cost.[3]

No complications were noted on the operative report and she was discharged home with her husband from the Day Surgery Center a few hours postoperatively as she was tolerating liquids, had urinated, was ambulating without assistance, all vital signs were stable, she remained afebrile,

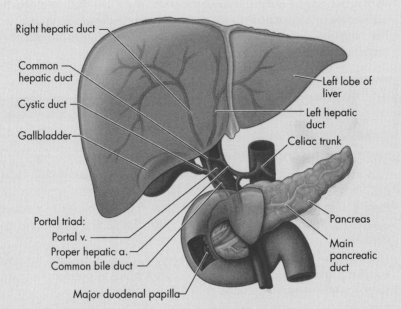

Figure 21-1 Gallbladder, liver, and duodenal anatomy.
Reproduced with permission from Morton, D, Albertine K, and Foreman B. *The Big Picture Gross Anatomy*. New York: McGraw-Hill; 2011.

and pain was well controlled with oral narcotics. She was discharged with a narcotic prescription and was also advised that she may take acetaminophen as well for postoperative pain control.

Review of Systems

The patient provided the majority of below information, but is also assisted by her husband, who is accompanying her today. Review of systems is negative except for the following:

- Constitutional: Fatigue since surgery, but significantly worse in the past few days.
- Pulmonary: Difficult to take a deep breath due to epigastric and right upper quadrant pain, but denies shortness of breath or dyspnea on exertion.
- Gastrointestinal: See history of present illness.

Physical Examination

- Vital signs: blood pressure 152/85 mm Hg, heart rate 94 beats per minute, respiratory rate 16/min, temperature 98.8°F oral, O_2 saturation 97% on room air.
- Constitutional: Appears uncomfortable, but no acute distress. Lying on side on examination table with legs drawn in toward abdomen.
- Head/eyes/ears/nose/throat: Mucous membranes dry, pink, but slightly pale. Sclera anicteric.

- Cardiovascular: Regular rate and rhythm; S1/S2. No peripheral edema.
- Pulmonary: Clear to auscultation bilaterally; unlabored respiratory effort.
- GI: Obese, soft, + hypoactive bowel sounds, tender to palpation of epigastrium and right upper quadrant, nondistended. No rigidity, rebound tenderness, or guarding.
- GU: Normal.
- Integumentary: Slightly pale, but warm and dry. No jaundice.
- Incisions: Abdominal port sites are well approximated, dry, and intact. No signs of erythema, drainage, hernia, or hypergranulation.
- Neurological: Alert, oriented.
- Psychiatric: Pleasant, appropriately interactive.

? Given the information obtained so far, what are the pertinent positives and significant negatives? How do these findings affect the list of potential causes?

Prior to proceeding, it is important to summarize information obtained thus far from the HPI, ROS, and physical examination.

- **Pertinent positives:** Epigastric and right upper quadrant pain—acute onset, worsening, constant in nature, intermittent radiation to right shoulder blade, somewhat aggravated by oral intake; s/p laparoscopic cholecystectomy 10 days ago; anorexia; nausea and vomiting; had soft, nonbloody, brown stool this morning; tender to palpation of epigastrium and right upper quadrant on examination.

- **Significant negatives:** Pain is not associated with activity; afebrile; no acute distress; denies jaundice, clay-colored stools, or dark urine; port sites are without evidence of infection; abdomen without rigidity, rebound tenderness, or guarding.

Case Analysis: Mrs B's physical examination is remarkable for epigastric and right upper quadrant tenderness. A significant negative finding is that she does not demonstrate evidence of jaundice or fever, making cholangitis less likely. Regardless, early recognition of biliary-related complications following cholecystectomy is important for a number of reasons. Complications from choledocholithiasis may include cholangitis, pancreatitis, or obstructive jaundice.[3,5] When a retained stone is obstructing the bile duct, the bile may become infected as a result. Infection resulting from this has the potential to spread quickly. If infection spreads into the liver or ductal system, it can lead to biliary sepsis and become life threatening in a short period of time.

❓ Can the information gathered so far be restated in a single sentence highlighting the pieces that narrow down the cause?

The problem presentation for this case might be: "a 52-year-old woman who presents with a 3-day history of acute onset, progressive epigastric and RUQ pain following laparoscopic cholecystectomy 10 days ago."

❓ What diagnostics and in what order are necessary at this time?

Taking into account Mrs B's recent cholecystectomy, her subjective report, and physical examination, the first diagnostic studies that I obtain include a comprehensive metabolic panel (basic chemistry plus liver function tests) to evaluate current electrolyte status and to look for any elevations in liver enzymes, amylase, and lipase to further evaluate for pancreatitis as a possible cause of her pain, and finally, a complete blood count to evaluate for leukocytosis, which would be expected if she had cholangitis.

When interpreting lab results, the following points should be considered. With biliary obstruction, ALT and AST are often elevated early. Later in the course, serum bilirubin and alkaline phosphatase rise, demonstrating a cholestatic pattern. Previous studies have shown that a rise in serum bilirubin has a sensitivity of 69% and a specificity of 88% for diagnosing choledocholithiasis.[1,3] The positive predictive value of elevated liver tests is poor as liver tests may be elevated for many different reasons, including drug side effects (ie, statins), cirrhosis, obesity, nonalcoholic fatty liver disease, and hepatitis (autoimmune, alcoholic, viral). However, the negative predictive value is high, meaning that normal liver tests play a greater role in ruling out biliary obstruction and choledocholithiasis.[3]

CASE INFORMATION
Laboratory Results

Comprehensive Metabolic Panel	Reference Range	Pre-op	Today
Sodium	136–145 mmol/L	138	140
Potassium	3.4–5.1 mmol/L	4.1	4.2
Calcium	8.6–10.2 mg/dL	9.2	9.0
Chloride	98–107 mmol/L	100	102
Carbon dioxide/bicarbonate	22–32 mmol/L	25	26
Glucose	65–99 mg/dL	100	145
Blood urea nitrogen	6–23 mg/dL	12	20
Creatinine	0.50–1.10 mg/dL	0.76	0.85
Total protein	6.6–8.7 g/dL	6.7	6.4

Comprehensive Metabolic Panel	Reference Range	Pre-op	Today
Albumin	3.5–5.2 g/dL	3.7	3.5
Total bilirubin	0.2–1.2 mg/dL	0.4	2.0
Alkaline phosphatase	35–104 U/L	80	250
Aspartate aminotransferase (AST)/SGOT	10–32 U/L	24	50
Alanine aminotransferase (ALT)/SGPT	8–33 U/L	22	52
Amylase	0–137 U/L	60	44
Lipase	12–70 U/L	48	35

Complete Blood Count	Normal Range	Pre-op	Today
White blood cell count (WBC)	4.0–10.0 10e3 cells/μL	7,600	8,800
Red blood cell count (RBC)	3.9–5.2 10e6/μL	4.0	4.1
Hemoglobin	11.2–15.7 g/dL	12.2	12.9
Hematocrit	34%–45%	36	38
Mean corpuscular volume	80–100 fL	85	84
Mean corpuscular Hgb	25.6–32.2 pg	26.1	27.9
Mean corpuscular Hgb concentration	32–36 g/dL	33	34
Red cell distribution width	11.6%–14.4%	12.1	12.3
Platelet count	163–369 10e3/μL	180	240

Case Analysis: Analysis of laboratory results reveals no evidence of leukocytosis or elevations in pancreatic enzymes, making cholangitis and pancreatitis, respectively, less likely. Of note, there is significant rise in total bilirubin and alkaline phosphatase levels as well as slight rises in both ALT and AST. With these results, I will proceed with biliary obstruction and choledocholithiasis as my working diagnoses as labs demonstrate a cholestatic pattern. Given this fact, as well as her inability to tolerate oral intake, I will arrange for Mrs B to be admitted for further diagnostic testing as this issue needs to be addressed promptly. There are a number of other diagnostic studies that should be considered, which are listed in order from least to most invasive.

❓ What further diagnostic testing should be ordered?

• Abdominal ultrasound: Most useful to evaluate for choledocholithiasis before cholecystectomy. Ultrasound is less helpful in patients who have already had a cholecystectomy because dilatation of the common bile duct (up to 10 mm) may be a normal variance following the surgery itself. False-negative rate may be affected by stones that are small, impacted stones, or ileus that creates a gas pattern that obscures ultrasound imaging.[1,3]

- Magnetic resonance cholangiopancreatography (MRCP): An MRI that focuses on the gallbladder, bile duct system, and pancreatic duct. In terms of detecting stones in the CBD, MRCP has a sensitivity of 82.6% and a specificity of 97.5%.[1-3,4] Contraindications to MRCP are similar to those of other MRI testing and include, but are not limited to, the following: implanted metal (ie, metal clips on an aneurysm, cardiac pacemakers, joint replacements, cochlear implants), claustrophobia, inability to lie still, and obesity that limits the patient from fitting into the opening of imaging equipment.

- Endoscopic ultrasound: An ultrasound study in which a probe is inserted during an upper endoscopy to examine the digestive tract. This procedure typically requires sedation and/or analgesia to perform and is not universally available at all hospitals.

- Endoscopic retrograde cholangiography (ERCP): An invasive procedure requiring intravenous sedation/analgesia that uses a combination of upper endoscopy and x-ray following contrast dye administration to evaluate the bile duct system. Special techniques are available to aid in breaking up and removing retained stones. ERCP may be used as either a diagnostic or therapeutic measure for those with suspected choledocholithiasis. The sensitivity and specificity of ERCP is over 95% in detecting CBD stones.[5] Additional factors to consider are that ERCP requires technical expertise to perform and like an endoscopic ultrasound, is not universally available. Given the procedure's risk for serious complications, including ERCP-induced pancreatitis, bleeding, and perforation,[3] this technique is typically reserved for patients at high risk for choledocholithiasis, if there are clinical findings of cholangitis, or if choledocholithiasis is seen on prior imaging.[3,5,6]

The goal of any test is to exclude or confirm the presence of choledocholithiasis. As with ordering any diagnostic imaging, a provider should consider which tests are least invasive, most accurate, and most cost-effective.[3] Other factors to consider include level of suspicion for etiology, availability at institution, and any specific patient factors that may be contraindications. One specific contraindication to traditional ERCP is patients who have had a previous gastric bypass with Roux-en-Y reconstruction. Given the surgically altered anatomy of the stomach, a transgastric approach, often completed in the operating room, is necessary to gain access to the biliary ductal system.

With all of the information that has been gathered thus far, the next step is to confirm the presence of a retained common bile duct stone. In order to do this, an MRCP has been ordered as it is noninvasive, available at this facility, and does not carry the risks associated with invasive procedures, such as ERCP.

CASE INFORMATION

MRCP Results and Next Steps

It has been estimated that at the time of cholecystectomy, anywhere from 5% to 20% of patients have choledocholithiasis and this incidence increases with age.[3] Choledocholithiasis after cholecystectomy may result from a gallstone that had migrated from the gallbladder or a stone forming de novo in the common bile duct.[1] An MRCP was completed and showed a ductal filling defect as well as choledocholithiasis. Now that the MRCP has confirmed the presence of choledocholithiasis, the patient will proceed with ERCP for stone extraction and possible sphincterotomy in which the muscle surrounding the opening of the duct is cut. The risks associated with ERCP include, but are not limited to, bleeding, postprocedure pancreatitis, and perforation. Administration of prophylactic antibiotics is indicated when biliary obstruction is suspected.[6]

Following ERCP, the patient was observed in the hospital and was released the following day as her liver function tests were trending downward, her abdominal pain subsided, she remained afebrile, and she was again tolerating oral intake. She will return to clinic for follow-up in 1 week with preclinic LFTs to be drawn. One may expect that her enzyme levels will continue to trend toward normal ranges and will eventually normalize.

References

1. American Society for Gastrointestinal Endoscopy (ASGE). Guideline: the role of endoscopy in the evaluation of suspected choledocholithiasis. *Gastrointest Endosc.* 2010;71(1):1-9. doi:10.1016/j.gie.2009.09.041.
2. Macaron C, Qadeer MA, Vargo JJ. Recurrent abdominal pain after laparoscopic cholecystectomy. *Cleve Clin J Med.* 2011;78(3):171-178.
3. Choledocholithiasis: clinical manifestations, diagnosis, and management. UpToDate Web site. http://www.uptodate.com/contents/choledocholithiasis-clinical-manifestations-diagnosis-and-management. Published 2014. Updated February 19, 2014. Accessed June 13, 2014.
4. Cholelithiasis and choledocholithiasis. Elsevier Clinical Key website. https://www.clinicalkey.com/#!/content/medical_topic/21-s2.0-1014767. Revised 2011. Accessed September 23, 2015.
5. American Society for Gastrointestinal Endoscopy (ASGE). ASGE guideline: the role of ERCP in diseases of the biliary tract and the pancreas. *Gastrointest Endosc.* 2005;62(1):1-8. http://www.asge.org/assets/0/71542/71544/123465e3317a42b4a8e4c826ae1b213d.pdf.

CASE 22

Elizabeth W. Good

Elizabeth Good works with hepato-pancreato-biliary surgical oncology patients at the Emily Couric Clinical Cancer Center at the University of Virginia Health System, Charlottesville.

CASE INFORMATION
Chief Complaint

A 73-year-old Caucasian male presents to surgery clinic for clinical evaluation. He called earlier in the day to the nurse triage phone line to report a 1-week history of erythema, tenderness, and protrusion near his right subcostal abdominal incision. He denies fever or chills. He is status post liver resection 8 weeks ago for colorectal metastases.

❓ What is the potential cause?

Cellulitis, fluid collection, and abdominal incisional hernia are my immediate thoughts. I have more questions than answers as of yet. However, I will prioritize my differential diagnosis by considering the timing of his symptoms. The critical element is that he is 8 weeks postoperative from liver surgery.

Although uncommon, potential life-threatening complications following liver resection include bile leak and biloma (an encapsulated collection of bile in the peritoneal cavity), bleeding, pulmonary difficulties, acute kidney injury, and liver failure.[1] He has already surpassed the immediate, acute, and subacute phases of his postoperative recovery and these complications are unlikely to present 8 weeks into his recovery. He is more than a month out from surgery, which categorizes his current symptoms as delayed. Other noninfectious processes that could be causing his symptoms include a hematoma or a peritoneal fluid collection; however, given the duration of time that has passed since surgery these again seem unlikely. The more likely diagnosis is an infection.

A surgical site infection (SSI) is further defined by the terminology of superficial (skin/subcutaneous tissue) incisional, deep (deep soft tissue/fascia and muscle) incisional, or organ/space (intra-abdominal), which represents the deepest level of an abdominal infection.[2] Cellulitis and a deep abdominal abscess represent the most probable causes.[3] Of note, elderly patients may not exhibit fever with infection, and may instead exhibit alternate symptoms such as extreme fatigue or confusion.[4]

My next step is to gather more data and better understand his current presentation to determine if an infectious (abscess) or noninfectious (hematoma, benign peritoneal fluid) process is occurring within his abdomen.

CASE INFORMATION

History of Present Illness

I wonder if he has experienced a complicated recovery course or prior wound infection during these past 8 weeks. I review his electronic medical record and glean that his postoperative course following his liver resection was unremarkable. He returned as scheduled for his postoperative visit 4 weeks ago without complaints, other than "tightness" primarily in the right upper quadrant. His physical examination at the time noted a healed midline and right subcostal surgical incision with some surrounding and resolving swelling/firmness and no erythema, no abdominal pain, no tenderness, no rebound or guarding. He was instructed to contact the office with any clinical changes including worsening tightness, abdominal pain, fever, chills, nausea, vomiting, redness, tenderness, or drainage from the incision.

I start with a thorough and detailed patient history before proceeding with my physical examination. My initial questions include:

Is he a diabetic?

Is he immunocompromised by chemotherapy, medication, malnutrition, or a health condition?

Has he experienced night sweats or episodes of profound coldness requiring him to cover up with blankets and extra clothing?

What other concurrent signs and symptoms is he displaying?

Is his liver compromised?

Here is what I learn from my patient interview:

"My scar is becoming red. There is also this bulge around it that is new and it hurts to touch." He reports a 1-week history of worsening tenderness and swelling to his right subcostal scar. He has not taken pain medication for several weeks though he did take a dose of Tylenol last night to help with the general incisional discomfort. He rates his incisional discomfort at 3 on a 10-point scale. The erythema began in the past 2 days. He denies fevers, night sweats, shaking chills, or any illness since he was seen in clinic 4 weeks ago. He denies previous wound healing problems or wound infection to this scar, and this includes all previous abdominal surgeries. Overall he has been feeling well and denies fatigue. He is active and played 18 holes of golf in the past week. He denies jaundice, pruritus, nausea/vomiting, and tea-colored urine. His appetite is good, and he is without changes in urinary/bowel habits. He recently met with his oncologist and declined adjuvant chemotherapy.

Past Medical History

Colon cancer with metastasis to liver (diagnosed 7 years ago); osteoarthritis; prostate cancer with radiation seed implantation (8 years ago); shingles (3 years ago). No history of diabetes or immunocompromise.

Past Surgical History

Left colectomy and wedge resection for liver metastasis (7 years ago); five previous partial hepatectomy surgeries for liver metastases (in the past 7 years) with the most recent left hepatic lobe resection 8 weeks ago; cholecystectomy (10 years ago); arthroscopic surgeries to bilateral shoulders and knees; exploratory laparotomy for small bowel obstruction (25 years ago); tonsillectomy as a child.

Family History

Lung cancer, diabetes, and coronary artery disease present in his maternal and paternal families.

Social History

He is a retired banker. He is a former smoker of 2 to 3 packs per day for 30 years and quit 25 years ago. He consumes one shot of scotch per night with occasional beer and wine. He has been married for 40 years. He denies current and previous illicit, recreational, or intravenous drug use.

Allergies

No known allergies.

Medications

Tamsulosin hydrochloride 0.4 mg daily; ibuprofen 200 mg daily as needed for arthritic pain; doxylamine 25 mg at bedtime as needed for sleep.

❓ What are the pertinent positives from the information given so far?

- Recent onset of symptoms including:
  - Erythema at right subcostal abdominal scar
  - Tenderness and subacute discomfort/pain at abdominal scar requiring occasional Tylenol
  - Swelling near abdominal scar
- He is 8 weeks postoperative from left hepatic lobe resection for removal of colorectal liver metastases. This represents a total of six surgeries to his liver in the past 7 years. The same abdominal scar has been utilized with each surgery and is the location of his current signs and symptoms.

❓ What are the significant negatives from the information given so far?

- No history of previous wound healing or infection problems at his abdominal incision

- Postoperative recovery up to this point uneventful and followed expected course
- No fever, no night sweats, no shaking chills
- No fatigue. Overall he feels well. He is active daily and able to play golf
- No recent changes in health status
- No history of diabetes
- Not receiving chemotherapy or glucocorticoids
- No changes in appetite or urinary/bowel habits

❓ Can the information gathered so far be restated in a single sentence highlighting the pieces that narrow down the cause?

The problem representation in this case might be: "a 73-year-old male presents with new onset erythema, tenderness, and swelling at right subcostal abdominal incision. He is status post liver resection 8 weeks ago for colorectal metastases."

Case Analysis: An infectious etiology seems the most likely reason for his current symptoms, even without clinical findings of fevers, chills, malaise, or fatigue. I can best rule out a hernia and fluid collection with an abdominal ultrasound (US), and the physical examination will be helpful.

Prior to beginning my complete review of systems and physical examination, I order a complete blood count (CBC), comprehensive metabolic panel (CMP), and clotting times including prothrombin time and international normalized ratio (INR). I am interested in ensuring that his blood counts are stable and liver function is normal or is trending downward toward normal since his liver surgery. Abnormalities with these labs may indicate that his liver is compromised or perhaps he has bled and that is the cause of his symptoms. I am also interested in checking for leukocytosis indicating a possible infection.

CASE INFORMATION

Review of Systems

- Constitutional: Denies fatigue, weight loss, loss of appetite, early satiety, fever, chills, diaphoresis, malaise.
- Head/ears/nose/throat: Endorses mild hearing loss. Denies trouble swallowing, congestion, rhinorrhea. Eyes: Denies itching, pain, redness to eyes, or visual disturbances.
- Cardiovascular: Denies chest pain, leg swelling, or difficulty breathing when lying down.

- Pulmonary: Denies shortness of breath, cough, snoring/apnea when sleeping.
- Gastrointestinal: Endorses abdominal tenderness at surgical scar. Denies nausea, vomiting, changes in bowel habits.
- Genitourinary: Endorses urinary retention takes medication daily. Denies hematuria, dysuria, urgency, incontinence.
- Integumentary: Endorses redness and swelling at abdominal incision/scar. Denies jaundice, itching, rash.
- Musculoskeletal: Endorses generalized arthritis. Denies myalgias or gait difficulties.
- Neurological: Denies weakness, numbness/tingling in extremities, headache, dizziness, change in speech, tremors, seizures.
- Psychiatric: Endorses difficulty sleeping but says this is not new problem. Denies depression, agitation, confusion, nervousness, anxiety.

Physical Examination

- Vital signs: Blood pressure 155/69 mm Hg; temperature 36.7°C (oral); heart rate 72 beats per minute; respirations 18 breaths per minute; oxygen saturation by pulse oximeter is 99% on room air; BMI 27.
- Constitutional: He appears his stated age. He is well developed and well nourished. He is cooperative.
- Head/eyes/ears/nose/throat: Head—Normocephalic and atraumatic. Uvula is midline, oropharynx is clear and moist, and mucous membranes are normal. Eyes—Anicteric sclerae. Conjunctivae, extraocular movements and lids are normal. Pupils are equal, round, and reactive to light. Neck—Normal range of motion and phonation. No tracheal deviation present. No mass and no thyromegaly present. Neck is supple. Carotid bruit is not present.
- Cardiovascular: Normal rate, regular rhythm, normal heart sounds, and intact distal pulses. Examination reveals no gallop or friction rub. No murmur. No pedal edema, capillary refill brisk.
- Pulmonary: Effort normal and breath sounds normal. No respiratory distress. He has no wheezes.
- Gastrointestinal: Well-healed midline and right subcostal incisional scars. Mild redness present at middle aspect of right lateral incision, approximates 1.5 cm circular area. Area of redness is tender to touch. Swelling extends in circular pattern beyond area of redness ~18 cm, firm to touch, no drainage, and no tenderness to this area. No abdominal hernia is present. Rest of the abdomen is soft. There is no rebound, no guarding.
- Genitourinary: He exhibits no CVA tenderness, normal genitalia.
- Integumentary: Skin is warm, and dry. No lesions or rash. No clubbing, no cyanosis.

- Musculoskeletal: Normal range of motion. He exhibits no edema and no tenderness.
- Neurological: He is alert and oriented to person, place, and time. He has normal strength. No cranial nerve or sensory deficits.
- Lymphatic: No cervical or supraclavicular adenopathy. No inguinal adenopathy present.
- Psychiatric: He has a normal mood and affect. His speech is normal and behavior appropriate. Judgment and thought content normal.

Preliminary Lab Work

- Complete blood count: normal white blood cell count of 6 cells/mL (normal is 4–10 cells/mL), normal hemoglobin, hematocrit, and platelet counts
- Comprehensive metabolic panel: all values normal including liver function tests, total bilirubin, and albumin
- Prothrombin time/INR: normal

❓ What elements of the review of systems and the physical examination should be added to the list of pertinent positives? Which items should be added to the list of significant negatives?

- **Pertinent positives:** Abdominal examination abnormal with area of redness, tenderness, swelling, and induration at the middle aspect of the right subcostal abdominal incision and surrounding tissue. These are new and evolving symptoms that began in the last 2 to 7 days.

- **Significant negatives:** Abdominal incision is healed/closed and without drainage. He is not obese or compromised nutritionally. An incisional hernia is not obvious on examination. He denies fever, chills, and diaphoresis. His vital signs are stable, and he is not febrile at the time of presentation to clinic. He is anicteric and without pruritus. There are no laboratory abnormalities, no findings of leukocytosis or elevated liver function. His PT, INR, and albumin are also normal, indicating normal intrinsic liver function.

This additional information adds some key pieces to the puzzle. I reexamine my problem statement and restate it as: "a 73-year-old male presents with localized erythema, tenderness, swelling, and induration at the medial aspect of a right subcostal abdominal incision. He is status post liver resection 8 weeks ago for colorectal metastases. He denies fever or chills. His WBC is not elevated. His LFTs are normal. His symptoms are consistent with a localized infection or fluid collection."

Further diagnostic testing is essential to proceed with confirming or refuting my assumption.

❓ What diagnostic testing should be done and in what order?

The erythema, tenderness, swelling, and induration at the medial aspect of the right subcostal abdominal incision remain the immediate problem. His symptoms have progressed over the past week and are not improving. He is experiencing abdominal discomfort. This is either a localized problem and superficial in nature or involves the deeper abdominal cavity and is an evolving systemic problem. The next step includes an abdominal ultrasound (US) to identify any abnormalities such as a fluid-filled versus solid or dense collection. By starting with an US, he is not exposed to unnecessary radiation until when, and if, it is clinically indicated. A computed tomography (CT) scan would expose him to radiation but this may be warranted depending on the findings of the US. A CT scan is helpful in providing detail and establishing a diagnosis such as an intra-abdominal abscess, hematoma, or other peritoneal fluid collection.

CASE INFORMATION

His abdominal US demonstrates a 13 × 12 × 20 cm complex fluid collection within the abdomen inferior to the liver edge without internal vascularity and more solid components/debris dependently, which may represent a hematoma, biloma, or seroma. The study also notes a smaller second complex collection at the incision and is favored to represent a hematoma, and correlates to the area of visible protrusion. The radiologist pages me with these significant results and we agree that the patient should have a CT scan. The large size of the fluid collection and the extent of the collection will be better evaluated with a CT; this is the imaging modality of choice for intra-abdominal infections.[5]

The contrasted spiral CT scan of the abdomen and pelvis confirms a large oval well-defined fluid collection (in similar dimensions to the US), which is creating a mass effect on the right hepatic lobe. It has a widely enhancing 3-mm smooth wall. While the collection is most likely to represent a hematoma it is also possible that it is a walled off bile leak. A 4 × 3 cm rounded subcutaneous fluid collection is seen in the right upper quadrant anteriorly corresponding with the palpable incisional abnormality, likely a hematoma. Prostate radiation therapy seeds are noted to be present in the pelvis. No other significant findings are noted including free air, intrahepatic or extra-hepatic biliary ductal dilatation, or focal liver lesions. The surrounding vasculature is normal in size and is patent. These findings solidify the diagnosis as a large, deep intra-abdominal fluid collection that represents bile versus hematoma and does not appear to be infected.

The decisive next step includes decompressing the collection and analyzing the fluid/drainage in the laboratory. He will need to be treated with broad-spectrum antibiotics if infection is suspected.

Management of an Abdominal Fluid Collection

After discussion with the patient and the surgical and radiology teams, the patient agrees to have the fluid collection decompressed due to its large size and his current symptoms. He returns the next day to radiology and undergoes US-guided drainage of the subhepatic fluid collection with placement of a percutaneous drain. A clear thin yellow/orange colored fluid, approximating 1.5 L in volume is aspirated. A 14-French locking pigtail catheter/drain is left in place and affixed to the skin. He is instructed to flush the drain with 10 cc of saline three times a day to maintain its patency, and to empty the bag and record drainage volumes and fluid character a few times day, and as needed.

The aspirated fluid is sent to the laboratory for testing including anaerobic, aerobic, and fungal cultures, and Gram stain, to determine the nature of the drainage and decide if further treatment with antibiotics is indicated. Empiric or broad-spectrum antimicrobial treatment includes aerobic, gram-negative enteric bacilli, and anaerobic coverage to cover abdominal or gut organisms. To ensure that my approach is evidence based, I will refer to the "Guidelines by the Surgical Infection Society and the Infectious Diseases Society of America."[5]

The clear aspirate does not suggest an infectious process and the color is also not consistent with bile. I would be concerned, however, if the aspirate was cloudy or purulent or the drainage was bilious (dark green to yellow/brown in color), or he had fever, chills, abdominal pain, nausea/vomiting, or elevated white blood cell count. His fluid aspirate has none of these features, he is afebrile, and his white blood cell count is normal. The smaller subcutaneous fluid collection, the hematoma, identified on US and CT does not require drainage as it is noninfectious and will reabsorb over time.

Case Conclusion

The day after the drain is placed, I speak with him by phone at home and he is feeling much improved. The drain remains intact and is draining pink/dark brown (or old blood appearing) drainage ~200 cc/day. The drain is flushing without difficulty. He declines any pain medication prescription because he is not experiencing any discomfort beyond the percutaneous tube insertion site for which he can take over-the-counter medication. He denies fevers/chills or other complaints.

The goals of the drain are to control and maximally decompress the fluid collection until it has completely resolved. The drain can be removed when the daily output is 20 cc or less for 3 to 5 consecutive days. He will continue to flush the drain with 10 cc normal saline three times a day as previously instructed to maintain drain patency and maximize drainage capability. The fungal culture and smear are negative. The Gram stain identifies no bacteria. The bacterial culture does not identify moderate or heavy concentrations of any organisms, and no anaerobes are isolated. The culture does identify *Enterococcus faecalis* 1+ in the fluid. *Enterococcus faecalis* is commonly found in intestinal flora. This is the most prevalent species cultured from humans, and accounts for more than 90% of clinical isolates.[6]

After conferring with the infectious disease team, I conclude that this finding is likely a contaminant. The patient is clinically free of signs or symptoms of intra-abdominal infection and is not prescribed or treated with antibiotics.

I speculate that he likely developed a combination of bile leak and hematoma in the early days or weeks following surgery that had been resolving for many weeks prior to his presentation with new abdominal tenderness, swelling, and erythema at his incision site. Given the large size of the fluid collection and his recent increase in activity and golfing, the area became irritated and tender. It is possible that the fluid collection may have eventually evolved into an acute intra-abdominal abscess if left unchecked.

At the time of the percutaneous drain placement, he was not actively bleeding or draining bile. Leaving the drain in place allowed for maximal decompression of the fluid collection and for thorough evaluation of its contents. The erythema on the medial aspect of his right subcostal incision correlated on imaging with a separate subcutaneous hematoma, which was also likely aggravated internally by the exerted pressure of the intra-abdominal fluid collection and externally by his increase in physical activity. The erythema was indicative of inflammation and skin irritation, not infection.

I follow the patient's progress by phone and his drainage declines over time and becomes a clear pink/yellow (or serosanginous) color. I schedule him to return for a repeat CT scan 3 weeks following his drain placement. At that time, his daily drainage is 5 to 15 cc/day of clear amber or serosanginous fluid. CT scan demonstrates complete resolution of the large perihepatic fluid collection; his percutaneous drain is removed without difficulty.

Surveillance following hepatic resection includes an MRI scan 3 months after surgery to evaluate for possible recurrence or new metastases. His interval liver MRI is scheduled 6 to 8 weeks after removal of the percutaneous drain to allow for adequate healing. The study demonstrates no evidence of local or recurrent metastatic disease to the liver. Minimal/trace fluid along the anterior aspect was present at the right hepatic lobe at the site of the prior fluid collection drain. He has complete resolution of skin tenderness, erythema, and induration and is without complaints.

Future imaging and follow-up is with his oncologist. The liver is the most common site for metastatic disease from colorectal cancer. Future hepatic surgery is possible but would depend upon the location of any recurrence. Liver resection is the treatment of choice for patients with good performance status and liver metastases that are resectable.

Specific colorectal surveillance guidelines and evidence-based practice guidelines are available at the National Comprehensive Cancer Network (NCCN) and through other oncologic organizations.[7-9]

References

1. Overview of hepatic resection. http://www.uptodate.com/contents/overview-of-hepatic-resection?source=search_result&search=overview+of+hepatic+resection&selectedTitle=1%7E150. Updated November 5, 2014. Accessed February 9, 2015.

2. Complications of abdominal surgical incisions. http://www.uptodate.com/contents/complications-of-abdominal-surgical-incisions?source=search_result&search=complications+of+abdominal+surgical+incisions&selectedTitle=8%7E150. Updated October 1, 2014. Accessed November 16, 2014.

3. Postoperative fever. http://www.uptodate.com/contents/postoperative-fever?source=search_result&search=postoperative+fever&selectedTitle=1%7E27. Updated April 4, 2013. Accessed November 16, 2014.

4. Mouton CP, Bazaldua OV, Pierce B, Espino DV. Common infections in older adults. *Am Fam Physician.* 2001;63(2):257-268. http://www.aafp.org/afp/2001/0115/p257.html.

5. Solomkin JS, Mazuski JE, Bradley JS, et al. Diagnosis and management of complicated intra-abdominal infection in adults and children: guidelines by the Surgical Infection Society and the Infectious Diseases Society of America. *Clin Infect Dis.* 2010;50(2):133-164. doi:10.1086/649554.

6. Fraser SL, Donskey CJ, Salata RA. Enterococcal infections. http://emedicine.medscape.com/article/216993-overview. Updated August 15, 2014.

7. National Comprehensive Cancer Network. NCCN guidelines version 2.2015: colon cancer. http://www.nccn.org/professionals/physician_gls/pdf/colon.pdf. Published October 3, 2014. Accessed February 9, 2015.

8. National Comprehensive Cancer Network. NCCN guidelines version 2.2015: rectal cancer. http://www.nccn.org/professionals/physician_gls/pdf/rectal.pdf. Published December 9, 2014. Accessed February 9, 2015.

9. Meyerhardt JA, Mangu PB, Flynn PJ, et al. Follow-up care, surveillance protocol, and secondary prevention measures for survivors of colorectal cancer: American Society of Clinical Oncology clinical practice guideline endorsement. *J Clin Oncol.* 2013;31(35):4465-4470. doi: 10.1200/JCO.2013.50.7442.

CASE 23

Helen-Marie Molnar

Helen-Marie Molnar is an ACNP and an FNP with over 25 years of experience in cardiology, both inpatient and outpatient. She currently works in an outpatient cardiology practice at the University of Virginia Health System.

CASE INFORMATION

Chief Complaint

A 48-year-old man (DS) presents to the emergency room as a "walk-in" with a complaint of chest pain (CP) lasting 4 hours.

❓ What is the potential cause?

Case Analysis: Chest pain is the most common complaint of patients age 15 and older presenting to the emergency department,[1] and the causes range in severity from benign to life threatening. I start by considering the causes that are most life threatening, then I will focus on the causes most likely for this patient's situation, and finally I will entertain other possibilities.

Comprehensive Differential Diagnoses for Patient With Chest Pain[2]

Life-threatening conditions requiring immediate treatment: myocardial infarction (MI), aortic dissection, pulmonary embolism (PE), tension pneumothorax, pericardial tamponade, esophageal rupture

Common conditions:
- Cardiac: angina (unstable or stable), pericarditis, myocarditis, endocarditis, valvular heart disease, acute heart failure
- Pulmonary/pleural: pneumonia, tracheitis, bronchitis, asthma, pulmonary hypertension, pulmonary malignancy, pleural effusions
- Gastrointestinal: gastroesophageal reflux (GERD), esophageal spasm, hiatal hernia, pancreatitis
- Musculoskeletal: costochondritis, intercostal muscle strain, rib contusions, rib fractures
- Psychiatric: panic attack
- Other: herpes zoster, referred pain, and pain associated with various inflammatory conditions and collagen vascular diseases such as lupus, sarcoid, scleroderma, Kawasaki disease, polyarteritis nodosa, and Takayasu arteritis

Case Analysis: Any time someone presents with chest pain, the health care team must consider it an emergency until data are gathered to prove otherwise. I must act quickly to either rule in or rule out the life-threatening causes, and then I can consider other less serious etiologies.

CASE INFORMATION

General Survey and History of Present Illness

As soon as I walk in the room, I am starting to assess the patient. He is a very fit-looking, muscular man lying in bed at a 30° angle feeling his left chest with his right hand and looking concerned. He says, "My dad had a heart attack at age 50. I don't want to die!" The nursing staff are already hooking him up to the cardiac monitor and getting a blood pressure and an ECG. His skin is pink and dry, and he does not appear to be short of breath. I ask the nurse getting the blood pressure in one arm to also get it in the other arm. Left arm blood pressure 162/82 mm Hg. Right arm blood pressure 164/84 mm Hg. Other vital signs are normal (heart rate 84 beats per min, respiratory rate 20/min, temperature 36.8°C orally, SaO$_2$ 99% on room air). No pulses paradoxus.

When I ask him about his chest pain, he relates that he was at the manufacturing plant about 4 hours ago when he started feeling a sharp pain in his left chest. "It felt sharp, right here ... (pointing to his mid-left chest just to the left of the sternum.) ... but it didn't go away. In fact, it hurts worse." I ask him how bad it is on a scale of 1 to 10, and he replies "6." I ask him if the pain goes anywhere else, and he replies: "No, it's just here." I ask him if he has been having any other symptoms such as shortness of breath, nausea, sweating, racing heart, or light-headedness. He replies: "Well ... I was sweating, but it was hot in the plant. Could this be my heart? Am I having a heart attack?"

As we are talking, the ECG is completed. It shows normal sinus rhythm, rate 84, normal axis, and no ischemic ST-T wave abnormalities. I tell him: "Your ECG tells me that you are not having a big heart attack but it doesn't tell me if you could be having a small heart attack. We'll be doing some blood tests and watching you for a while today to make sure you are okay. Let's talk a little more about your chest pain. What were you doing when it started?" He replies: "I was doing my usual work packing boxes. We manufacture plumbing materials, big pipes, and stuff, but we have machines that move the really big boxes onto the trucks." The patient is not able to identify anything that made the pain better or worse after onset, and answers "no" when asked if he had a sudden onset of shortness of breath when the chest pain started. He also denies fever, chills, and recent illness.

Past Medical History

I ask him about his past medical history. He states he only sees his PCP when he has a problem, and the last time was more than 5 years ago. He had a broken left wrist from a biking accident and right knee reconstructive surgery when he "blew out" his knee playing football 10 years ago. Aside from occasional respiratory infections (last one was over a year ago), he has been well. He denies any known heart problems, hypertension, and diabetes. He is on no daily medications, takes an occasional BC powder for a headache, and does not use illicit drugs. He has no allergies to medications. He smokes 1 pack of cigarettes per day and has done so since he was 24.

Family History

I also ask about his family history. He states that his father died of a heart attack at the age of 50. He smoked and had diabetes and hypertension. His mother is still living, is overweight, and has diabetes and hypertension. His brother who is 2 years older, just had stents put in his heart.

? What are the pertinent positives from the information given so far?

- Localized sharp chest pain along the left sternal border associated with the diaphoresis and mild shortness of breath
- Elevated blood pressure
- The patient is anxious
- Family history of premature coronary artery disease and HTN
- Personal history of smoking (24 pack-years)

? What are the pertinent negatives from the information given so far?

- The patient does not appear ill, pale, short of breath, cyanotic, or diaphoretic.
- No ECG changes of ischemia or infarction.
- No significant difference in the bilateral blood pressures.
- No radiation of the pain to his back. CP is not described as "tearing."
- No recent illness, fever, or chills.
- No recent trauma or medical procedures.

? Can the information gathered so far be restated in a single sentence highlighting the pieces that narrow down the cause?

Putting the information gathered so far in a single statement—a problem representation—sets the stage for gathering more information and determining the cause.

Given the information acquired so far, the problem representation in this case might be: "a 48-year-old man with a significant history of smoking and a strong family history of premature coronary artery disease presents with left-sided sharp chest pain without radiation, with elevated blood pressure, and a normal ECG."

Case Analysis: At this point, I know based on his EKG he is not having an ST-elevation myocardial infarction (STEMI), but I do not know if he could be having a non-ST elevation MI (NSTEMI), so we will continue to gather more data. His chest pain is sharp, but not described as tearing or radiating to his back, his blood pressures are essentially equal in both arms, and he does not have the appearance of a patient with Marfan syndrome, so I am doubtful he is having an aortic dissection. I do not think he is having a pulmonary embolus (PE) or tension pneumothorax since he did not have an acute onset of shortness of breath with the chest pain, has a normal SaO_2, does not look acutely ill, and does not have conditions that predispose him to either of these conditions, such as prolonged inactivity or cancer that are associated with PE, or trauma or recent respiratory infection that might cause a tension pneumothorax. Pericardial tamponade is unlikely based on the available evidence so far since he does not have a pulses paradoxus when his BP is taken, I did not see a variation in the QRS amplitude on the ECG, and he is not tachycardic. Esophageal rupture is also highly unlikely since he has no risk factors for it such as recent esophageal procedures or trauma secondary to violent vomiting.

In addition to considering NSTEMI in the differential, I am also considering other less serious causes, and I will continue to gather more data as I go through the review of systems and physical examination.

CASE INFORMATION

Review of Systems

- Constitutional: Denies fevers, chills, and recent illnesses.
- Cardiovascular: + for sharp chest pain adjacent to the left sternum without radiation. Denies symptoms with exertion such as chest pain, pressure, tightness, or achiness, neck, jaw, or arm pain, shortness of breath on exertion, orthopnea, paroxysmal nocturnal dyspnea, edema, palpitations, presyncope, and syncope. Usual activity includes the ability to climb four flights of stairs without stopping and climbing steep mountains while hunting.
- Pulmonary: + for mild left-sided chest pain with deep inspiration. Denies shortness of breath, cough, and wheezing.
- Gastrointestinal: Denies indigestion, difficulty swallowing, nausea, vomiting, diarrhea, constipation, and melena. Last bowel movement this morning.

- Genitourinary: Denies dysuria and hematuria.
- Neurologic: + for occasional headaches relieved easily by BC Powder. Denies unilateral numbness or weakness, diplopia, and difficulty with expressive or receptive language.
- Endocrine: Denies polyuria, polyphagia, and polydipsia.

Physical Examination

- Vital signs: Left arm blood pressure 162/82 mm Hg. Right arm blood pressure 164/84 mm Hg. No pulses paradoxus. Heart rate 84 beats per minute, respiratory rate 20/min, temperature 36.8°C oral, SaO_2 99%. Height 72 in, weight 250 lb, BMI 34 kg/m².
- Constitutional: The patient is a muscular, well-appearing white man in no acute distress.
- Head/eyes/ears/nose/throat: Normocephalic, atraumatic. Pupils are equal, round, and reactive to light and accommodation. Neck: Normal carotid upstrokes without bruits. No jugular venous distention.
- Cardiovascular: S1, S2 regular without murmurs, rubs, or gallops. Normal PMI (point of maximal impulse) located in the fifth ICS MCL (intercostal space, mid-clavicular line). No LV (left ventricular) heave. Radial, femoral, and pedal pulses 3+ palpable and equal bilaterally. No radial-femoral delay. No femoral bruits.
- Pulmonary: Lungs clear to auscultation with good air movement throughout. No rhonchi, rales, or wheezes.
- Abdomen: Soft and nontender with active bowel sounds. No hepatosplenomegaly. No abdominal bruit.
- Integumentary: Pink, warm, and dry with brisk capillary refill. No cyanosis or edema. No rashes.
- Musculoskeletal: + tenderness to palpation over the third and fourth costochondral joints. Pain also reproduced in the same area with movement of the left arm. No pain with palpation of other areas of the thorax, spine, or clavicles.
- Neurologic: Alert, oriented × 3. Cranial nerves II-XII intact. Moves all extremities with 5/5 strength bilaterally.
- Psychiatric: Initially very anxious, now fairly calm.

❓ What elements of the review of systems and physical examination should be added to the list of pertinent positives?

- + tenderness to palpation over the third and fourth costochondral joints.
- Pain is reproduced in the same area with movement of the left arm.

? What elements of the review of systems and physical examination should be added to the significant negatives list?

- Equal pulses and blood pressures bilaterally
- No jugular venous distention
- Normal cardiac examination
- Normal physical examination except for that noted above
- No symptoms of esophageal reflux

? How does this information affect the list of possible causes?

The tenderness to palpation over the third and fourth costochondral joints, the same pain for which he presented, is very suggestive of musculoskeletal pain, most likely costochondritis. It could also be an intercostal muscle strain. Therefore, musculoskeletal pain is now very high on my list of differential diagnoses. He does, though, have several risk factors for coronary artery disease including a very strong family history of premature coronary artery disease (father and brother), smoking, and elevated blood pressure (he may have hypertension, but I am unable to make this diagnosis based on a single ED visit). Consequently, we still need to watch him in the ED for a while and rule out a myocardial infarction.

There is nothing else on the review of systems or on the physical examination that point to any other cause of his chest pain such as heart failure, valvular heart disease, or inflammatory heart conditions. I believe his chest pain with deep inspiration is due to a musculoskeletal problem instead of bronchitis, pneumonia, or asthma because he has no pulmonary symptoms and has a normal pulmonary examination. Gastroesophageal reflux is a very common cause of noncardiac chest pain, but his physical examination is highly suggestive of a musculoskeletal etiology, so reflux is much lower on my list of differential diagnoses.

? What diagnostic testing should be done and in what order?

The vital signs and ECG have already been done since they should be obtained immediately upon arrival to the emergency department and serially per ED protocol after that. The patient is on continuous telemetry showing normal sinus rhythm without ectopy. Laboratory evaluation includes a comprehensive chemistry and CBC with differential, which are normal except for a glucose of 120 (nonfasting), elevated but nondiagnostic since it was not a fasting sample. The most important laboratory evaluation in this patient is the troponin I, which needs to be done to rule out a myocardial infarction. These were drawn every 4 hours × 3, and all were <0.02 ng/mL (normal). A chest x-ray shows normal heart size, normal mediastinum, and no acute cardiopulmonary process.

Diagnosis and Management: Musculoskeletal Chest Pain/ Costochondritis

DS's discharge diagnosis is "musculoskeletal chest pain." It could also be listed as "noncardiac chest pain most likely due to costochondritis." Patients presenting with musculoskeletal chest pain often describe it as lasting hours to days, and it is often positional or exacerbated by twisting, moving the arms, or deep breathing. It is frequently described as sharp and localized to one specific area (patients will often use one finger to point to the area), but it may be more diffuse. Palpation of the chest wall or maneuvers such as a "crowing rooster" may reproduce the patient's pain. However, the presence of tenderness to palpation, even if it reproduces the patient's chest pain, does not exclude ischemic chest pain.[2] In a prospective study of 122 consecutive patients in the emergency department, 30% were thought to have costochondritis with almost half having reproducible pain to palpation of the chest wall. Of the patients who had reproducible chest pain, 6% were having an acute myocardial infarction.[3] Therefore, before making the diagnosis of musculoskeletal chest pain, a thorough history and physical examination are needed to exclude other causes of chest pain. Diagnostic tests are used to rule in or rule out possible etiologies of chest pain based on the likelihood of that condition.

Treatment of musculoskeletal chest pain consists of patient education and reassurance, avoidance of activities that could cause further injury (heavy lifting), and pain relief with nonnarcotic analgesics such as acetaminophen up to 3 g/day in divided doses, over-the-counter nonsteroidal anti-inflammatories such as ibuprofen 600 mg every 6 hours if no contraindication, or topical agents such as capsaicin cream. It is important to tell the patient that musculoskeletal pain can take weeks to months to resolve.

In addition to treating the musculoskeletal pain, we cannot overlook the fact that he is at high risk of developing coronary heart disease in the future based on his risk factors. We should discuss the importance of regular medical care due to his family history of premature coronary artery disease (father and brother), current smoking, obesity, possible insulin resistance, and possible hypertension. I schedule him to see his primary care physician within 1 to 2 weeks to address all of these and to check his lipids, fasting blood sugar, and HbA1c. He will need intensive education on lifestyle modification and will benefit greatly from a cardiology prevention clinic if one is available in his area. I will not start medication for his blood pressure during this ED visit since his discharge blood pressure was better at 148/80 mm Hg. Treating mild to moderately elevated blood pressures while someone is in pain may lead to hypotension, presyncope, or syncope when the pain has resolved. However, his blood pressure should be followed closely by his primary care physician.

While his presentation to the ED was for musculoskeletal pain, the biggest benefit for this young man was identifying his risk factors for coronary heart disease and getting him back into the health care system.

References

1. Pitts SR, Niska RW, Xu J, Burt CW. National Hospital Ambulatory Medical Care Survey: 2006 emergency department summary. *Natl Health Stat Reports*. 2008;7. www.cdc.gov/nchs/data/nhsr/nhsr007.pdf.
2. Jesse RL, Kontos MC. Evaluation of chest pain in the emergency department. *Curr Probl Cardiol*. Apr 1997;22(4):149-236. http://www.ncbi.nlm.nih.gov/pubmed/9107535
3. Wise CM. Major causes of musculoskeletal chest pain. In: UpToDate. Goldenberg DL, Shefner JM, eds. *UpToDate*. Waltham, MA: UpToDate; 2014. http://www.uptodate.com/contents/major-causes-of-musculoskeletal-chest-pain-in-adults. Accessed July 31, 2014.

CASE 24

Tonja M. Hartjes

Dr Hartjes is an Associate Clinical Professor at the University of Florida, College of Nursing in the AG-ACNP Program. She has extensive work experience in surgical critical care.

CASE INFORMATION

Chief Complaint

Ms W is a 28-year-old woman, postoperative day 1 following a trans-sphenoidal resection of a pituitary tumor (TSRPT) with new onset confusion, increased thirst, and increased urinary output.[1] The nurse calls me to her bedside in the intensive care unit (ICU).

❓ What is the potential cause?

My first thought for this patient is that her symptoms result from a complication of her recent surgery. While I consider all her symptoms in my evaluation, I begin with a focus on confusion. Surgical complications such as water and electrolyte imbalances, cerebrospinal fluid (CSF) leak, swelling or bleeding at the surgical site, and diabetes insipidus are associated with pituitary tumor resection.[1,2] These will be first on my list. Of course her confusion may also result from a condition unrelated to her recent surgery. Confusion is a vague and nonspecific symptom, and can result from disorders of any body system, and can range from life threatening to relatively benign. Below is a list of other potential causes of confusion.

Differential Diagnoses for Confusion

- Neurologic: acute stroke (embolic or hemorrhagic), vasospasm, cerebral edema, traumatic head injury, seizure with postictal state, seizure, brain tumor, meningitis, delirium
- Cardiovascular: myocardial infarction, cardiac dysrhythmias, congestive heart failure exacerbation, hypertensive encephalopathy, hypotension
- Pulmonary: hypoxia, hypoventilation resulting in hypercapnia, carbon monoxide poisoning, pulmonary embolism, pneumonia, chronic obstructive pulmonary disease exacerbation
- Gastrointestinal: ischemic bowel, cholecystitis, appendicitis, diverticulitis, constipation, gastritis, colitis

- Genitourinary: renal failure, urinary tract infection, urinary retention or obstruction
- Hematologic: anemia, infection/sepsis
- Musculoskeletal: fracture, rhabdomyolysis
- Endocrine: adrenal insufficiency, myxedema, thyrotoxicosis, hypoglycemia, diabetes insipidus
- Psychiatric disorder: depression, new onset or exacerbation of bipolar disorder, psychosis
- Metabolic: dehydration, electrolyte imbalance, hyperglycemia, hypoglycemia, hypernatremia, hyponatremia, hepatic encephalopathy, metabolic acidosis or alkalosis
- Exogenous: medication side effect or interaction or withdrawal, drug overdose, alcohol withdrawal, pain[2-5]

CASE INFORMATION

History of Present Illness

When I receive the call from the bedside nurse, I know I need more information. I start by asking the nurse additional questions such as: "When did the symptoms appear" and "what was she like prior to the onset of the symptoms?" I want to determine if the situation is life threatening, emergent, or urgent, and rule out or initiate immediate treatment for life-threatening etiologies. I visit the patient to obtain a general survey. Ms W looks at me as I walk into the room, she appears mildly anxious; however, her breathing is quiet and unlabored and she does not appear to be in any acute distress. I ask her: "How are you feeling?" and she answers: "My head hurts". I note she is on room air with an oxygen saturation of 100%, and the bedside monitor shows a sinus tachycardia. The initial neurologic examinations were normal; however, over the last 6 to 8 hours, she has become mildly confused, and is now only oriented to herself. She is complaining of increased thirst, and the nurse states the patient's urine output (UOP) increased quickly from 100 to 200 mL/h to 700 mL/h over the past 2 hours.

? What are the pertinent positives and significant negatives so far?

Pertinent Positives
- Postoperative day 1 following TSRPT
- Currently experiencing mild confusion
- Patient complains of increased thirst

• Increased urinary output
• Tachycardia

Significant Negatives
• No acute distress
• No postoperative complications
• Normal oxygen saturation on room air

Case Analysis: Based on the information obtained in my initial evaluation I determine her overall condition is stable at this time. Because I have determined that Ms W's condition is urgent, but not critical, I can proceed with obtaining more data to help me sort my differential diagnosis. To that end, I will need to review current vital signs, her home and hospital medications, and recent diagnostic tests in addition to conducting my own focused health history and physical examination. However, a key pertinent positive in the information gathered so far is the dramatic increase in her urine output, a symptom which the nurse reported in her call. Even without examining the patient, I am suspicious she may have diabetes insipidus (DI), a common complication of pituitary resection. So I proceed with ordering serum and urinary electrolytes, serum osmolality, and a urine specific gravity, laboratory values that will help me assess for DI.[6,7]

CASE INFORMATION

Past Medical History
Significant for pituitary tumor, no other chronic medical problems

Past Surgical History
Trans-sphenoidal resection of a pituitary tumor 1 day ago, no other surgical procedures

Allergies
No known drug allergies

Home Medications
Tylenol by mouth as needed for headaches, no prescription medications

In-Hospital Medication
• Heparin 5000 mg subcutaneously twice a day

- Famotidine 20 mg by mouth twice a day
- Morphine 2 to 5 mg intravenously every 2 hours as needed for pain—last given 4 hours ago
- Acetaminophen-oxycodone 1 to 2 tabs every 4 to 6 hours as needed for pain—last given 2 hours ago

Psychosocial History

Nonsmoker. Drinks wine occasionally. Denies any illicit drug use.

Review of Systems

- Constitutional: complains of mild headache but no change in intensity with position change, mild weakness, denies fever or chills
- Pulmonary: denies breathing difficulties
- Cardiovascular: denies chest pain or palpitations
- Gastrointestinal: denies abdominal pain, nausea, emesis, diarrhea or constipation, no rectal bleeding
- Genitourinary: denies hematuria, flank pain, or pain or burning upon urination
- Musculoskeletal: denies tremors or involuntary movements
- Neurological: denies syncope, vision or hearing loss, salty taste, loss of consciousness or seizures, per nurse's notes, became confused over past 12-hour shift
- Behavioral/psychiatric: endorses anxiety prior to surgery, denies depression

Physical Examination

- Vital signs: Blood pressure 89/52, heart rate 113 beats per minute, temperature 37.2°C, respiratory rate 22 breaths per minute, oxygen saturation 100% on room air. Height is 63 inches and weight is 73 kg with body mass index 28.3.
- Constitutional: Alert, mildly anxious, difficulty maintaining conversation and train of thought.
- Head/eyes/ears/nose/throat: No obvious deformity or signs of trauma, pupils equal, round, and reactive to light, no nystagmus, extraocular movements intact.
- Neck: Trachea palpable at midline, no jugular venous distension noted, carotid pulses +2 bilaterally, no carotid bruit or thrill noted, no nuchal rigidity.
- Cardiovascular: Point of maximal impulse at fifth intercostal space midclavicular line, S1, S2, regular, no murmur, rubs, or gallops. Extremities are warm, dry, 2+ peripheral pulses in all four extremities.

- Pulmonary: Respirations even, and unlabored with decreased breath sounds bilaterally otherwise clear. No clubbing.
- Gastrointestinal: No visible pulsations, hypoactive bowel sounds in all quadrants, soft, nontender, no hepatosplenomegaly.
- Genitourinary: No costovertebral angle tenderness (CVA) tenderness, urinary catheter in place with light yellow clear urine. Urine output has increased from 100 mL/h to 700 mL/h in last 2 hours.
- Neurological: Awake, oriented only to self, normal language and comprehension, no neglect, follows simple commands, moves all extremities, Glasgow coma scale 15. Cranial nerves 3 to 12 intact, extraocular movements intact, visual fields full to confrontation, smile symmetric, speech clear, shoulder shrug symmetric, tongue midline.
- Motor: 4/5 strength bilateral upper and lower extremities.
- Integumentary: Pale, warm and dry, mild tenting of skin, no masses, rashes, or bruising. Dressing to incision site is clean dry and intact.
- Other: Indwelling urinary catheter for 1 day, no central venous access during hospitalization, no drains present.

Diagnostic Testing Results

Morning Laboratory Results
- Serum sodium level: 138 mEq/L (normal 135–145 mEq/L)
- Serum glucose: 73 mg/dL (normal 70–100 mg/dL)

Current Laboratory Results
- Serum sodium level: 150 mEq/L
- Plasma osmolality: 300 mOsm/kg H_2O (normal 278–300 mOsm/kg H_2O)
- Urine specific gravity: 1.003 g/mL (normal 1.005 to 1.030 g/mL)

? **What elements of the review of systems, physical examination, and diagnostic test results should be added to the pertinent positive and significant negative list?**

Pertinent Positives
- The patient received pain medication orally 2 hours ago, and intravenously 4 hours ago
- Vital signs show she is hypotensive and tachycardic and tachypneic

- Changes in mental status have emerged over the past 6 to 8 hours
- Urine output rapidly increasing in volume (100–200 to 700 mL/h × 2 hours)
- Labs: Elevated serum sodium and plasma osmolality, low urine specific gravity, normal glucose[1]

Significant Negatives

- Normothermic and normal oxygen saturation
- No abnormal neurologic findings with exception of recent mental status change
- Normal pulmonary examination with exception of slightly decrease bilateral breath sounds
- Normal cardiac examination
- Normal gastrointestinal examination

❓ Can the information gathered so far be restated in a single sentence highlighting the pieces that narrow down the cause?

Given the information gathered so far the new problem representation might be: Ms W is a 28-year-old woman, postoperative day one following a transsphenoidal resection of a pituitary tumor (TSRPT) with new onset confusion, increased thirst and urinary output possibly related to the development of postoperative diabetes insipidus.

Case Analysis: The data so far support a diagnosis of diabetes insipidus (DI), a postoperative complication of pituitary tumor surgery. Her confusion emerged over the last 6 to 8 hours and is associated with an increase in urine output and thirst. Ms W has symptoms of volume depletion with a low BP 89/52, elevated heart rate, and mild tenting of the skin. Overnight her urinary output has ranged between 100 and 200 mL/h. But over the last 2 hours she has complained of increased thirst, and her urine output has increased rapidly to 700 mL/h. I know that her sodium this morning was normal at 138 mEq/L and now is elevated at 150 mEq/L. Additionally her plasma osmolality and urine specific gravity were both abnormal. I am highly suspicious that this constellation of findings is consistent with DI and now put DI at the top of my differential.[2,4-7]

Additional analysis is necessary, however, to confirm that she does not have another urgent condition that requires intervention. Fortunately, this patient is young and in relatively good health so I can immediately rule out complications of chronic diseases such as congestive heart failure or chronic obstructive lung disease as contributing factors to her current symptoms. She has a normal gastrointestinal examination, no musculoskeletal complaints, and no psychiatric history so I eliminate disorders in those systems from my differential. In the course of completing the more comprehensive history and physical, I have acquired additional data to rule out other urgent etiologies of confusion, which I do not want to miss.

I am able to rule out CVA[2] as a life-threatening cause because Ms W has an essentially normal neurologic examination with the exception of her new onset confusion. She has no focal deficits, she has normal language, absence of neglect, and can follow simple commands. She has not had any seizures. Complications of pituitary surgery such as cerebral spinal fluid (CSF) leak, cerebral swelling or bleeding at the surgical site are lower on my differential now as Ms W denies syncope, vision changes, metallic or salty taste. She also denies headache that worsens with change in position, nausea, and neck stiffness. Her dressing to her surgical site is clean, dry, and intact. Based on these findings I can rule out a CSF leak. Cerebral swelling or bleeding at the surgical site cannot be ruled out yet, despite the patient's wakeful state and current normal neurologic examination. CSF infection is still a possibility but is lower on my list as she is not febrile and has no other signs of meningitis such as nuchal rigidity or rash, I cannot eliminate it yet.

Acute myocardial infarction is low on my differential as the patient denies chest pain, neck pain, shortness of breath, left arm pain, and diaphoresis. In addition, she is a young woman, 28 years old, and has no risk factors for myocardial infarction, other than her recent surgery. To definitively rule out acute myocardial infarction, I will need to obtain an ECG to compare to prior ECGs, and draw cardiac enzymes. Other cardiopulmonary conditions such as pulmonary edema, pericardial effusion, or tamponade are unlikely due to her normal cardiac and pulmonary findings. A chest x-ray is a noninvasive and easily obtainable study that gives me further information to rule out cardiac or pulmonary pathology.

I am able to rule out hypoxemia based on her normal oxygen saturation. Her pulmonary examination is normal except for mild tachypnea, making a pulmonary disorder unlikely. There is the remote chance that pain medication is causing hypoventilation and she has developed hypercapnia; I will need an arterial blood gas to evaluate for this. Pulmonary embolus (PE) is unlikely as she is on heparin to prevent deep vein thrombosis, moves well in bed, and has no physical examination findings suggesting a source such as swelling in her extremities. Wells criteria for PE prediction include preexisting risk factors for PE: a history of deep vein thrombosis, or PE, age 65 or older, malignancy, signs or symptoms consistent with a deep vein thrombosis or PE, and hemoptysis, all of which are absent in this patient. The only positive Wells criteria in this patient include heart rate greater than 100 and recent surgery. Based on this information, PE is very low on my differential.

Regarding the metabolic conditions on my list, the patient clearly does have metabolic derangement in the form of hypernatremia and volume depletion but her blood glucose is normal so she is not hypoglycemic. In addition, she has no history of diabetes, which would lead to ketoacidosis. A blood gas will determine if she has a metabolic acidosis in addition to DI that is contributing to her symptoms.

Close evaluation of the patient's vital signs shows that she does meet criteria for systemic inflammatory response syndrome; she is both tachycardic and tachypneic with a borderline low blood pressure. Since I have the diagnosis of DI, I can attribute these alterations to volume depletion, but in the presence of infection, these alterations are also consistent with sepsis. Sepsis often presents with confusion and an absence of focal neurological deficits such as this patient is exhibiting. Based on the information I have so far, there is no clear source of infection but I cannot rule out sepsis yet. I will order a complete blood count (CBC) with a differential, to help determine if she has an infection and to rule out blood loss, which could be contributing to her altered vital signs. I will also order a urinalysis as urinary tract infections are common in postoperative patients with urinary catheters, and consider adding blood cultures if she develops a fever, or her altered vital signs do not improve with fluid replacement. I also need to consider the patient's hypotension in the context of her age. While 89/52 is a low blood pressure, she is a young woman and 89/52 may actually be close to her baseline.

❓ What additional diagnostic tests are necessary at this time and in what order?

A 12-lead ECG will help confirm that this change does not represent myocardial ischemia. In addition, on the ECG, signs of right heart strain may be present and consistent with PE. Additional diagnostic testing to be considered include (1) arterial blood gas (ABG), (2) troponins, (3) chest x-ray, (4) basic metabolic panel, (5) current point-of-care glucose level, (6) urinalysis, (7) stat serum sodium, plasma osmolality, and USG and CBC with differential. If her neurologic status and/or condition change, a CT scan of the head with and without contrast may be warranted.

Although I have pending diagnostic tests to rule out the etiology of Ms W's confusion, and to ensure there have been no changes since admission, DI following TSRPT at this point seems to be the most likely etiology.

CASE INFORMATION

Results

The results and continued trend of the serum sodium (151 mEq/L), plasma osmolality (320 mOsm/kg H$_2$O), and USG (1.001 g/mL) confirm my diagnosis of DI. The ECG and first troponin level are negative and the chest x-ray is normal. All other labs including her CBC are normal, thus ruling out my remaining differential diagnoses.[1]

Diagnosis and Management: Diabetes Insipidus

DI is characterized by abrupt polyuria and polydipsia and is the result of a complete or partial failure of antidiuretic hormone (ADH) secretion, in central DI, or from a decrease in the renal response to ADH, in nephrogenic DI. Transient DI occurs in 18% to 31% of patients who undergo a TSRPT, typically within 24 to 48 hours of surgery.[1] Diagnostic testing suggestive for DI includes a serum sodium level >145 mEq/L, serum osmolality >295 mOsm/kg/H_2O, a decreased urine osmolality with high serum osmolality, a decreased USG, and increased BUN/creatinine levels due to hemoconcentration.[2,6,7]

General Management Orders for DI[2,6,7]

- Monitor intake and output every hour

- Draw serum sodium levels every 4 hours (call for Na >145 or <130 mEq/L)

- Check urine specific gravity every 4 hours (call if >1.025 or < 1.005 g/mL— goal is 1.010 g/mL)

- Increase oral intake as tolerated

- Hypotonic intravenous fluids (IVFs): 5% dextrose or 5% dextrose with 0.25% normal saline at 6 to 7 mL/kg per hour and 1:1 urine output replacement every hour

- Desmopressin (DDAVP); many order options exist including the following:

  1 μg intravenously as needed—repeat the DDAVP dose when urine output is 200 to 250 mL/h for 2 hours with urine specific gravity <1.005 g/mL or urine osmolality <200 mOsm/kg H_2O

  DDAVP 2 to 4 μg intravenously scheduled twice a day (hold and call if sodium level 145 mEq/L or less)

As a practical consideration, any patient with postoperative DI should be presumed to have anterior pituitary insufficiency as well, and should receive corticosteroid replacement therapy. In the immediate postoperative setting, hydrocortisone (50–100 mg intravenously every 8 hours) is generally used, which is then rapidly tapered to a maintenance dose (15–25 mg daily) until anterior pituitary function can be definitively evaluated.

In the treatment of patients with DI, it is essential to avoid rapid sodium correction. Ideally, sodium correction occurs no faster than 0.5mEq/L/h or 6mEq/L in a 24-hour period. Rapid correction of serum sodium can cause cerebral edema, seizures, and brain damage. DDAVP, appropriately dosed, will treat DI and effectively reduce sodium levels in most cases.[4,5]

Case Follow-Up

Ms W is treated with oral fluid intake, DDAVP 2 mg twice a day, and monitored with hourly neurologic examinations, intake and output, and every 4 hours laboratory testing, including serum sodium and urine specific gravity. Within 48 hours, the DDAVP is discontinued as her serum sodium, urine specific gravity, and urine output return to normal. She is transferred to the medical-surgical unit within 72 hours and discharged to home within a week.[2,6,7]

References

1. Yuan W. Managing the patient with transsphenoidal pituitary tumor resection. *J Neurosci Nurs.* April 2013;45(2):101-107; quiz E101-102.
2. Boysen T, Drayton-Brooks S, Smith M. Diabetes insipidus. In: Boysen T, Drayton-Brooks S, Smith M, eds. *Acute Care Nurse Practitioner.* Silver Spring, MD: American Nurses Credentialing Center; 2011:183-185.
3. Darby J, Anupam A. Sudden deterioration in neurologic status. In: Vincent J-L, Abraham E, Kochanek P, Moore F, Mitchell P, eds. *Textbook of Critical Care.* 6th ed. Philadelphia, PA: Elsevier Saunders; 2011:3-7.
4. Pokaharel M, Block CA. Dysnatremia in the ICU. *Curr Opin Crit Care.* December 2011;17(6):581-593.
5. Elhassan EA, Schrier RW. Hyponatremia: diagnosis, complications, and management including V2 receptor antagonists. *Curr Opin Nephrol Hy.* 2011;20(2):161-168. doi: 10.1097/MNH.0b013e328 3436f14.
6. Serge B. Diabetes insipidus. In: Vincent J-L, Abraham E, Kochanek P, Moore F, Mitchell P, eds. *Textbook of Critical Care.* 6th ed. Philadelphia, PA: Elsevier Saunders; 2011:1233-1235.
7. Dello Stritto R, Barkley TW. Diabetes insipidus. In: Barkley TW, Myers C, eds. *Practice Consideration for Adult-Gerontology Acute Care Nurse Practitioners.* West Hollywood, CA: Barkley & Associates; 2014:630-635.

CASE 25

Julie A. Grishaw

Julie Grishaw is an ACNP at the Medical ICU at the University of Virginia in Charlottesville. She is also a senior editor for McGraw-Hill Education's ClinicalAccess.

CASE INFORMATION

A Medical Intensive Care Unit (MICU) Acute Care Nurse Practitioner (ACNP) consult was called to request evaluation of a 26-year-old female who presented to the emergency department with altered mental status and hyperglycemia, with a fingerstick blood glucose (BG) of 405 mg/dL. The consulting physician reports the patient has a history of hypertension, type 1 diabetes, and depression.

❓ What is the potential cause?

An acutely altered mental status is a concerning finding in any patient. The differential for altered mental status is broad, and it is vital to quickly determine the etiology in order to avoid treatment delays and resultant adverse outcomes. From the information I have received about this patient's history, I know that she has several potential reasons to have an altered metal status. She may be suffering from an acute stroke given the history of diabetes and hypertension. She may have diabetic ketoacidosis (DKA) given that she is a type 1 diabetic and is also experiencing profound hyperglycemia. She also has a history of depression, so I cannot rule out a potential medication overdose, as a suicide attempt or self-medication. The differential is very broad, so I take a systems-based approach to best hone in on the diagnosis.

> **Comprehensive List of Differential Diagnoses for Patients With Altered Mental Status[1]**
>
> - Neurologic: acute ischemic or embolic stroke, subarachnoid hemorrhage, exposure to a CNS depressant (alcohol, opioids, benzodiazepines, antipsychotics), seizure with a postictal state, meningitis, encephalitis, central sleep apnea
> - Cardiovascular: hypertensive emergency, dysrhythmia, myocardial infarction
> - Pulmonary: pulmonary embolism, untreated obstructive sleep apnea
> - Gastrointestinal: ischemic colitis, intra-abdominal infection leading to sepsis

- Genitourinary: urinary tract infection, acute renal failure
- Metabolic/systemic: lactic acidosis, DKA, hyperglycemic hyperosmolar nonketotic coma (HHNC), hyperglycemia, uremia, electrolytic disturbance, hepatic encephalopathy, severe sepsis, salicylate toxicity, alcoholic ketoacidosis
- Psychiatric disorder: new onset psychosis

CASE INFORMATION

General Survey and History of Present Illness

The patient appears slightly older than her stated age and is somewhat disheveled in appearance. The head of the bed is at 45° and the patient is sitting quietly with her eyes closed and head tilted to the side. She is taking rapid, shallow breaths. I attempt to wake her, and she is able to be aroused, but is groggy. I ask her to tell me her name, but she is unable to do so, and quickly rests her head back on the pillow and closes her eyes. Her boyfriend, with whom she lives, is at the bedside. I ask him to briefly update me on the duration of this current illness, and any factors that he is aware of that may have precipitated the event.

He explains that she has been feeling ill for the past 3 days. She had a "stomach virus" with vomiting that worsened over the last 24 hours. She was unable to go to work for the last 3 days and was so weak she could hardly walk. He explains that she "couldn't keep anything down." He noted that she became much harder to arouse and was sleeping more over the last 12 hours, so he decided to bring her to the emergency department. I ask if she has taken any medications recently or taken any illicit substances, and he reports that he is not aware of her taking anything. He also states that she has no history of substance abuse, or use of illicit drugs or alcohol.

Because of her history of type 1 diabetes and the fingerstick BG of 405 mg/dL, I ask about her insulin regimen. Her boyfriend reports that she had an insulin pump, but "it broke about 6 months ago and she was having a hard time getting a new one." He states that she did see a "diabetes doctor" and that she is now being managed with "a shot at night and then shots before eating." I ask if she was taking her insulin as prescribed prior to admission, and he is not certain. He says she has felt so poorly that she "probably didn't need it because she wasn't eating" and he admits that he did not see her give herself an injection in a couple of days. He notes that he usually sees her inject her insulin right before bed, so this is unusual. He reports that he is not aware that she has any health problems other than diabetes and does not take any prescribed medications other than insulin.

During the time I am speaking with the patient's boyfriend, the nurse obtains another set of vital signs: heart rate (HR) 124 beats per minute, blood pressure (BP) 90/53 mm Hg, respiratory rate (RR) 30/min, SaO_2 95% on room air. The nurse also obtains the patient's weight, which is 65 kg.

❓ What are the pertinent positives from the information given so far?

- Admitted for altered mental status
- History of type 1 diabetes
- Nonadherence to prescribed insulin regimen and unknown recent dosing
- Recent gastrointestinal illness
- Altered mental status followed the gastrointestinal illness
- Hypotensive, tachycardic, and tachypneic

❓ What are the significant negatives from the information given so far?

- Normal cognition prior to the onset of this illness
- No oxygen requirement
- Patient responds to stimuli without gross neurologic deficits
- No history of substance use

❓ Can the information gathered so far be restated in a single sentence highlighting the pieces that narrow down the cause?

Putting the information obtained so far in a single statement—a problem representation—sets the stage for gathering more information and determining the cause.

The problem representation in this case might be: "A 26-year-old female with type 1 diabetes presents to the emergency department with acutely altered mental status and hyperglycemia."

Case Analysis: I am initially concerned that the altered mental status may indicate an acute stroke, given the patient's history of diabetes. However, the altered mental status occurred following a gastrointestinal illness, which makes me think this is more likely to be a metabolic process and not a neurological event. Her age makes an acute coronary syndrome, such as myocardial infarction, less likely. Her oxygen saturation of 95% on room air makes an acute pulmonary etiology much lower on the list. Detailed laboratory data are needed to more accurately hone the differential, as I am quite suspicious that a hyperglycemic crisis is the etiology of her altered mental status.

❓ What laboratory tests would you order given this information?

As the nurse finishes taking the vital signs, I order a stat arterial blood gas (ABG) and a lactic acid. Prior to my arrival, the ED physician ordered a basic metabolic panel (BMP), coagulation studies, and a urinalysis to check for ketones. Because of her age, a urine human chorionic gonadotropin (hCG) is also ordered.

CASE INFORMATION
Laboratory Results

The ABG results are as follows:

Test	Result	Reference Range
pH	7.13	7.35–7.45
Pa_{CO_2}	17 mm Hg	35–45 mm Hg
Pa_{O_2}	96 mm Hg	80–100 mm Hg
HCO_3	10 mEq/L	22–26 mEq/L
Lactic acid	6.1 mmol/L	<2 mmol/L

The metabolic panel results are as follows:

Test	Result	Reference Range[2]
Sodium (Na)	136 mEq/L	136–145 mEq/L
Potassium (K)	5.5 mEq/L	3.5–5 mEq/L
Bicarbonate (serum CO_2)	10 mEq/L	23–28 mEq/L
Chloride (Cl)	100 mEq/L	98–106 mEq/L
Blood urea nitrogen (BUN)	35 mg/dL	8–20 mg/dL
Creatinine (Cr)	2.0 mg/dL	0.7–1.3 mg/dL
Magnesium (Mg)	1.8 mg/dL	1.5–2.4 mg/dL
Phosphorus	5.8 mg/dL	3.0–4.5 mg/dL
Glucose (serum)	435 mg/dL	Fasting 70–105 mg/dL
Albumin	4.1 g/dL	3.5–5 g/dL

• Urinalysis: Her urine dipstick is positive for large amounts of ketones. Urine is hCG negative. Other serum laboratory studies are pending at this point. It is immediately obvious given the additional data that I must stabilize the patient before pursuing any additional diagnostic testing.

Case Analysis: I quickly interpret the ABG and BMP. The pH reveals that the patient has a profound acidosis. The HCO_3^- is very low, suggesting a metabolic acidosis. Her $PaCO_2$ is also low, demonstrating a partial respiratory compensation. In order to fully interpret and understand the ABG, it is helpful to also use the information from the BMP. I calculate the anion gap (AG).[3]

$AG = Na - (Cl + HCO_3)$

$AG = 136 - (100 + 10)$

$AG = 26$ (>10 indicates an anion gap metabolic acidosis)

The formal calculation for calculating the anion gap includes the potassium [ie, AG (Na + K) − (Cl + HCO_3)], but it adds very little to the total cations so conventionally the potassium is dropped when calculating the gap. The measurement of the anion gap is useful in determining the cause of metabolic acidosis. There are certain conditions that cause metabolic acidosis with an anion gap and they include ketoacidosis, salicylates, renal failure, methanol, ethylene glycol, and lactic acidosis. Numerous mnemonics are available to help identify potential causes of an anion gap metabolic acidosis.

The ABG and anion gap reveal that the patient has a large anion gap metabolic acidosis, which is partially compensated by her respiratory system, and which is consistent with the elevated lactic acid, the presence of ketones in the urine, and the probable diagnosis of DKA. Additional calculations can be done to assess the degree of metabolic acidosis and the adequacy of compensation. These include delta-delta gap, delta bicarbonate, and the Winter's formula (see Box 25-1).

BOX 25-1 Calculations to assess complex acid-base disturbances.

The following calculations may be used to assess complex-mixed acid-base disturbances:

First, an *anion gap* is calculated:

$Na - (Cl + HCO_3^-) = $ if > 10 an anion gap acidosis exists

Then, to evaluate *complex metabolic acid-base disturbances*, the delta-delta gap and delta-bicarbonate gap are used. If an anion gap acidosis is the only acid-base abnormality, there should be a one-to-one correlation between the rise in anion gap (delta-delta gap) and the fall in bicarbonate (ie, measured as serum CO_2), called the delta bicarbonate gap. The formulas for these follow:

1. Delta-delta gap: subtract the normal anion gap from the calculated anion gap. Delta gap = calculated AG − 10 (normal anion gap)

2. Delta bicarbonate is calculated by subtracting the serum HCO_3 from 24 (the normal serum HCO_3). Delta bicarbonate = 24 − actual serum HCO_3.

The normal difference between rise in AG and fall in serum CO_2 should be zero. But, if the elevated AG is significantly higher or lower than the bicarbonate gap (positive or negative direction) then the patient has a mixed acid-base disorder. Examples include metabolic alkalosis (+ bicarbonate gap) or hyperchloremic metabolic acidosis (− bicarbonate gap).

To evaluate *respiratory compensation* the *Winter's formula* is calculated to determine if compensation by the respiratory system is adequate given the metabolic acidosis. The formula is:

Measured $PaCO_2 = 1.5 \times [HCO_3{}^-]) + 8 \pm 2 =$ estimated range of $PaCO_2$

If the actual $PaCO_2$ falls within the estimated range, then compensation is adequate and there is no separate respiratory disorder.

How does this information change your problem representation?

The new problem representation is: "A 26-year-old female with type 1 diabetes presents to the emergency department with a severe metabolic acidosis and hyperglycemia in the setting of a recent GI illness."

CASE INFORMATION

Stabilizing the Patient

While drawing the labs, the nurse places two 18-gauge intravenous (IV) lines. I order a dose of sodium bicarbonate (50 mEq) intravenous push to stabilize the pH, although this will only serve as a temporizing measure until the underlying disorder is corrected. I order a stat intravenous bolus of regular insulin 9.75 units (0.15 units/kg) with a continuous infusion rate of 6.5 units/h (0.1 units/kg/h)[3] and two liters of 0.9% normal saline to be given over 1 hour. I also order noninvasive positive pressure ventilation (NIPPV) in an effort to further reduce the $PaCO_2$, support her spontaneous breathing, and prevent fatigue and subsequent hypoventilation, which would further decrease her pH. If she were alert she would spontaneously hyperventilate; however, because she is somnolent, her respiratory compensation is inadequate to correct her pH. Ventilatory support is indicated.

The patient does rouse appropriately with stimulation and has cough and swallow reflexes, thus I am confident she can protect her airway, which is essential for use of non invasive positive pressure ventilation (NIPPV). NIPPV settings on a spontaneous mode of bilevel positive airway pressure (ie, BiPAP) ventilation are ordered at an inspiratory positive airway pressure (IPAP) of 10 cm H_2O (this is pressure support ventilation [PSV]) and an expiratory positive airway pressure (EPAP) of 5 cm H_2O with 21% oxygen, since her oxygenation is normal. This type of NIPPV assists the patient's spontaneous respiratory effort and decreases the work of breathing. I then arrange for transfer to the medical intensive care unit.

Review of Systems

Information is obtained from the patient's significant other as she is on NIPPV and unable to participate.

- Constitutional: Denies fever, increasingly tired and weak. Denies falls or trauma.
- Cardiovascular: Boyfriend is not aware of any cardiac disorders, arrhythmias, or coronary artery disease.
- Pulmonary: Denies cough, but he notes her breathing changed prior to bringing her to the emergency room.
- Gastrointestinal: Reports nausea, vomiting, abdominal pain, and occasional diarrhea which began about 72 hours ago. Minimal oral intake with at least 5 episodes of vomiting in the last 24 hours.
- Genitourinary: Denies blood in her urine, change in urine smell, frequency, or amount.
- Musculoskeletal: Reports weakness following episodes of nausea and vomiting.
- Neurological: Denies headache, falls, history of seizure disorder or stroke, changes in speech, difficulty swallowing.
- Endocrine: Insulin pump stopped working about 6 months ago. Currently being managed with injections at night and with meals.
- Psychiatric: Mood is unchanged from normal. Boyfriend states she has a history of depression but that it is well controlled, he is not aware of any suicidal ideations past or present.

Physical Examination

- Vital signs: Heart rate 125/min, blood pressure 91/46 mm Hg, respiratory rate 25/min, and temperature 37°C, SPO_2 97% on BiPAP with an IPAP of 10 cm H_2O, and an EPAP of 5 cm H_2O with 21% FiO_2.
- Constitutional: 26-year-old female on NIPPV, thin, and appearing slightly older than stated age.
- Head/eyes/ears/neck/throat: Pupils are equal, round, reactive to light, oral examination deferred as the patient is on NIPPV.
- Cardiovascular: Heart rate and rhythm regular, no murmurs, rub, or gallops. No edema noted. Nail beds are pink, cool to touch; capillary refill +3 seconds.
- Pulmonary: Lungs clear to auscultation.
- Gastrointestinal: Hyperactive bowel sounds, tympanic on percussion, abdomen soft, but tender in all quadrants.
- Genitourinary: Unremarkable.
- Skin: intact, no rashes, lesions, or ulcerations; skin turgor +2 seconds.
- Neurological: Unable to fully participate due to lethargy and NIPPV mask. No focal neurologic deficits noted, face symmetric, reflexes intact and symmetric, appropriate blink reflex and response to painful stimuli. Able to shake head yes and no appropriately to questions occasionally.

? What elements of the review of systems and the physical examination should be added to the list of pertinent positives? Which items should be added to the list of significant negatives?

- **Pertinent positives:** history of vomiting, diffuse abdominal tenderness on palpation, nonadherence to insulin regimen, evidence of dehydration on examination, lethargic
- **Significant negatives:** afebrile during the course of the illness, no focal deficits on neurologic examination, normal cardiac and pulmonary examinations, lack of urinary symptoms, absence of suicidal ideations or reported use of illicit substances or alcohol, lack of history of starvation

? How does this information affect the list of possible causes?

The physical examination and review of systems provide further evidence that this not an acute neurologic condition, such as stroke. The neurologic examination does not show focal deficits, and the lethargy occurred following the onset of the gastrointestinal illness. Additionally, the examination and review of systems further assure me that this is not a cardiovascular or pulmonary event. A urinary tract infection cannot be excluded without a urinalysis. Diffuse abdominal tenderness is noted on examination, which is concerning for an abdominal pathology, although the lack of focal pain makes some conditions, such as appendicitis less likely. I have to keep mesenteric ischemia on the list for now, but that does not necessarily fit with the clinical picture, or the patient's history. Other causes of abdominal tenderness include the recent gastrointestinal illness, with associated vomiting and diarrhea, or DKA. Patients with DKA often present with abdominal pain and tenderness.[4]

The most likely cause of the patient's altered mental status is an endocrine emergency, specifically diabetic ketoacidosis. A number of factors support this diagnosis, including the hyperglycemia with a glucose of 405 mg/dL, a partially compensated metabolic acidosis, altered mental status in the setting of hyperglycemia, nonadherence to a prescribed insulin regimen in the setting of type 1 diabetes, presence of urine ketones, and dehydration on physical examination. I am now able to diagnose the patient with DKA.

DKA Diagnosis

DKA is characterized by hyperglycemia, anion gap metabolic acidosis, and urinary ketones in patients with insulin-dependent diabetes mellitus. The American Diabetic Association provides criteria for categorizing DKA severity from mild to severe based on the degree of acidosis and mental status.[4]

The distinction between DKA and hyperosmolar hyperglycemic syndrome (HHS) is important, as the management is different. Patients with HHS typically have a much higher blood glucose (greater than 600mg/dL). While patients with DKA can have serum blood glucoses ranging that high, it is not common. There are a number of other notable differences that distinguish the two disease states. Patients with DKA tend to have a lower pH (<7.30), lower serum bicarbonate, and large ketones in the urine. Patients with HHS most often have a pH >7.30, a higher serum bicarbonate, and small ketones in the urine.[4] For these reasons, I was able to determine that the patient has severe DKA rather than HHS.

DKA Management

The treatment of DKA consists of insulin administration, hydration with intravenous fluids, identification and treatment of the precipitating cause, and management of electrolyte abnormalities. My first priority is to stabilize the patient. As noted earlier, I ordered an insulin infusion and intravenous fluids while the patient was in emergency department. Generally patients with DKA are profoundly volume depleted. Thus multiple liter boluses of 0.9% NS in the first several hours following admission are often required to replete the intravascular fluid stores, maintain blood pressure, and prevent kidney injury. I will continue to order these boluses as needed, but in addition to my stat orders I extend the orders to include:

- Fluids: Maintenance fluids of 0.9%NS at 200 mL/h to be infused until the serum glucose reaches 300 mg/dL. Then, the maintenance fluids are changed to 0.5% dextrose in 0.45% normal saline at 200 mL/h until discontinued.

- Insulin: Continue the rate at 6.5 units/h (0.1 units/kg/h)[3] until serum osmolarity normalizes and the anion gap closes. Goal is to decrease the serum glucose by 50 to75 mg/dL each hour until serum glucose reaches 300 mg/dL.[4] I will double the insulin dose each hour until the desired decline of 50 to 75 mg/h is achieved.[4]

- Electrolyte management: Basic metabolic panel every 2 hours until anion gap closes. I will continue to follow the electrolytes closely, but will hold off on replacing depleted values for now as shifts are common during hydration and correction of DKA.

- As noted earlier I also ordered NIPPV in order to prevent respiratory decompensation given the profound metabolic acidosis.

❓ Given what has been done so far, what additional diagnostics would you order?

I order a stat 12-lead electrocardiogram (ECG), continuous telemetry, hourly vital signs, strict intake and output, abdominal radiographs (flat and side-lying), a repeat BMP, ABG, lactic acid, serum osmolarity, two sets of blood cultures, and a urinalysis with reflex urine culture.

CASE INFORMATION

Upon arrival to the MICU, vital signs were as follows: heart rate 98 beats per minute, blood pressure 95/56 mm Hg, respiratory rate 20/min, SpO$_2$ 96% on NIPPV room air. I order another liter of normal saline bolus, and then review the electronic medical record for more information about the patient. Notes from her outpatient endocrinologist are in the chart. She was prescribed glargine (Lantus) 20 units subcutaneous injection nightly and insulin lispro (Humalog) sliding scale with meals. The notes describe the patient as being compliant with her current regimen over the last 6 months. The notes state that in the past, she has struggled with using an insulin pump. The chart states that she did not manage the injection site, did not input data into the device when eating, and found the device "a hassle." She dropped the device, at which time it ceased to function. Due to these issues, she was started on the above-described regimen. Her last hemoglobin A1c (HbA1c) was 7%. Further evaluation of the EMR reveals that she was given prescriptions for captopril 50 mg every 12 hours for hypertension and fluoxetine 20 mg/day for depression. No other additional medications were prescribed. Her baseline blood pressure is 125/60 mm Hg.

After reviewing the EMR, I review new diagnostic and laboratory results.

Diagnostic Results

- ECG: normal sinus rhythm, no evidence of ischemia, no peaked T waves
- Abdominal radiograph: unremarkable, no signs of bowel obstruction or free air in the abdomen
- Urinalysis: negative for leukocytes or leukesterase, positive for ketones

Laboratory results:

CBC	Result	Reference Range[5]
WBC	5,000 cells/μL	4,000–10,000 cells/μL
Differential:		
• %Neutrophils, bands	• 3%	• 3%–5%
• %Neutrophils, segmented	• 70%	• 37%–73%
• %Lymphocytes	• 42%	• 20%–40%
• %Basophils	• 1%	• 0%–1%
• %Monocytes	• 7%	• 3%–7%
• %Eosinophils	• 1%	• 1%–3%

CBC	Result	Reference Range[5]
Hemoglobin	14.5 g/dL	14.4–16.6 g/dL
Hematocrit	43%	42%–49%
Platelet count	280 10⁹/L	189–287 10⁹/L

Metabolic panel	Result	Reference Range[2]
Sodium (Na)	140 mEq/L	136–145 mEq/L
Potassium (K)	5.0 mEq/L	3.5–5 mEq/L
Serum CO_2 (bicarbonate)	20 mEq/L	23–28 mEq/L
Chloride (Cl)	105 mEq/L	98–106 mEq/L
Blood urea nitrogen (BUN)	35 mg/dL	8–20 mg/dL
Creatinine (Cr)	1.7 mg/dL	0.7–1.3 mg/dL
Magnesium (Mg)	1.4 mg/dL	1.5–2.4 mg/dL
Phosphorus	5.4 mg/dL	3.0–4.5 mg/dL
Glucose (serum)	368 mg/dL	Fasting 70–105 mg/dL

ABG	Result	Reference range
pH	7.25	7.35–7.45
Pa_{CO_2}	25 mm Hg	35–45 mm Hg
Pa_{O_2}	96 mm Hg	80–100 mm Hg
HCO_3	19 mEq/L	22–26 mEq/L
Lactic acid	4 mmol/L	<2 mmol/L

Case Analysis: In DKA serum hyperkalemia is common and may cause T-wave elevation on the ECG, so the negative ECG findings are reassuring. Acidemia causes a shift in serum potassium from the intracellular to extracellular space. The resulting hyperkalemia will correct with resolution of the acidemia and hyperglycemia. Patients with DKA often experience hypokalemia following resolution of the acidemia. Thus, I avoid prescribing potassium-lowering agents to treat her potassium of 5.0 mEq/L given the absence of ECG abnormalities. The BUN and creatinine are elevated, most likely due to dehydration. I will follow this closely to ensure it resolves with the administration of intravenous fluids.

Identifying the cause of the DKA will ensure prompt and appropriate treatment. The absence of neutrophilia, coupled with an absence of fever, suggests that a bacterial infection is not the precipitating factor for the DKA. The slightly elevated lymphocyte and borderline monocyte percentages suggest that a viral etiology may be more likely, which correlates with the patient's clinical history. The decreasing serum lactic acid provides further evidence that a vascular cause, such as mesenteric ischemia, did not precipitate the DKA. The negative urinalysis rules out urinary tract infection as the cause.

The patient continues to display an AG metabolic acidosis, with a gap of 15. This is improved from the initial measured gap of 26. Though the patient is still acidemic with a pH of 7.25, I decide against administration of additional sodium bicarbonate. Studies have failed to demonstrate improved morbidity or mortality associated with the administration of sodium bicarbonate in patients with DKA and a pH greater than 7.14.[4] In addition to the AG metabolic acidosis, the patient continues to display a concomitant respiratory alkalosis (her $PaCO_2$ is 25). While her acidosis is partially compensated, she still has a mixed metabolic acidosis; her bicarbonate is 20 and lactic acid is still high at 4. Both lactic acid and ketoacidosis are present. Patients with DKA may manifest a lactic acidosis in addition to ketoacidosis from an increase in anaerobic metabolism and a decrease in tissue perfusion associated with abnormal glucose metabolism.[6]

After reviewing the laboratory data, I decide against starting antimicrobials at this time. The most likely etiology is that viral gastroenteritis, dehydration, and lack of adherence to the prescribed insulin regimen precipitated the DKA. I will continue to closely watch for results of the blood cultures and will check a daily complete blood count to monitor for leukocytosis. If the blood cultures become positive, the white blood cell count increases to abnormal levels, or the patient displays signs of infection, such as hemodynamic decompensation, I will consider initiation of antibiotics.

Case Follow-up

I make the decision to interrupt the NIPPV, as the patient's DKA is being treated and the patient is more alert. The patient shows no signs of volume overload, and continues to be hypotensive so I order a fourth liter of 0.9% normal saline to be administered over 1 hour.

I closely monitor the patient's vital signs and mental status following interruption of NIPPV. Thirty minutes following interruption of NIPPV vital signs are as follows: heart rate (HR) 96 beats per minute, blood pressure (BP) 97/56 mm Hg, respiratory rate (RR) 21/min, SpO_2 96% on room air. I order a fifth liter of 0.9% normal saline to be administered over 1 hour.

The lactic acid continues to resolve, reaching <2.0 mmol/L within 8 hours of MICU admission. The patient continues to do well without NIPPV. Blood and urine cultures remain negative after 24 hours. Vital signs continue to show hemodynamic stability. Urine output is 35 mL/kg/h. Twenty-four hours after being admitted to the MICU, ABG results are as follows:

Test	Result	Reference Range
pH	7.34	7.35–7.45
Pa_{CO_2}	33 mm Hg	35–45 mm Hg
Pa_{O_2}	96 mm Hg	80–100 mm Hg
HCO_3	22 mEq/L	22–26 mEq/L

The BMP results are as follows:

Test	Result	Reference Range[2]
Sodium (Na)	140 mEq/L	136–145 mEq/L
Potassium (K)	4.3 mEq/L	3.5–5 mEq/L
CO_2	24 mEq/L	23–28 mEq/L
Chloride (Cl)	111 mEq/L	98–106 mEq/L
Blood urea nitrogen (BUN)	20 mg/dL	8–20 mg/dL
Creatinine (Cr)	1.0 mg/dL	0.7–1.3 mg/dL
Magnesium (Mg)	1.8 mg/dL	1.5–2.4 mg/dL
Phosphorus	3.3 mg/dL	3.0–4.5 mg/dL
Glucose (serum)	230 mg/dL	Fasting 70–105 mg/dL

After review of the metabolic panel and ABG, I determined that the metabolic acidosis has resolved.

At this time, the continuous insulin infusion is discontinued, and the patient's home regimen of 20 units of glargine (Lantus) with insulin lispro (Humalog) at meals is reinstated. The patient is then transferred to the general medicine floor to ensure continued stabilization of her blood glucose, close evaluation of electrolytes, and diabetes education for herself and her boyfriend to ensure compliance with her home insulin regimen. I also arrange for a follow-up appointment with her endocrinologist 1 week after discharge.

References

1. Zeiger Roni F. McGraw-Hill's Diagnosaurus 4.0. http://accessmedicine.mhmedical.com/diagnosaurus.aspx.
2. Normal laboratory values. Merck Manual Professional Edition. Merck Sharp & Dohme Corp, a subsidiary of Merck & Co, Inc, Whitehouse Station, NJ. 2014. http://www.merckmanuals.com/professional/appendixes/normal_laboratory_values/blood_tests_normal_values.html#v8508814. Accessed December 19, 2014.
3. Morris JE. Fluid, electrolyte, & acid-base emergencies. In: Stone C, Humphries RL, eds. *CURRENT Diagnosis & Treatment Emergency Medicine*, 7th ed. New York, NY: McGraw-Hill; 2011:chap 44.

http://accessmedicine.mhmedical.com/content.aspx?bookid=385&Sectionid=40357260. Accessed September 30, 2014.

4. Kitabchi AE, Umpierrez GE. Hyperglycemic Crises in Adult Patients with Diabetes: A consensus statement from the American Diabetes Association. *Diabetes Care*. 2006;29:2739-2748. http://care. diabetesjournals.org/content/29/12/2739.full.pdf+html. Accessed November 19, 2015.

5. Gomella LG, Haist SA. Laboratory diagnosis: clinical hematology. In: Gomella LG, Haist SA, eds. *Clinician's Pocket Reference: The Scut Monkey*, 11th ed. New York, NY: McGraw-Hill; 2007: chap 5. http://accessmedicine.mhmedical.com/content.aspx?bookid=365&Sectionid=43074914. Accessed November 19, 2014.

6. Cho KC. Electrolyte & acid-base disorders. In: Papadakis MA, McPhee SJ, Rabow MW, eds. *Current Medical Diagnosis & Treatment 2015*. 2014: http://accessmedicine.mhmedical.com/content.aspx?bookid=1019&Sectionid=57668613. Accessed December 19, 2014

CASE 26

Bonnie Tong

Bonnie Tong works as a cardiology NP at Mount Sinai Hospital in New York, NY. Dr Tong is also adjunct faculty for the ACNP Program at New York University.

CASE INFORMATION

Chief Complaint

A 57-year-old man who is 2 days status post successful pulmonary vein isolation ablation for atrial fibrillation complains of fatigue and "not feeling well" overnight and this morning.

❓ What are the potential causes?

Fatigue is a nonspecific symptom and the list of etiologies is long. In order to narrow down the potential causes, I need to approach all possible differential diagnoses in a systematic way. Going from head to toe, I ask myself, what are the possible causes of this patient's fatigue?

Differential Diagnoses for a Patient With Fatigue[1]

- Neurologic: head injury, sleep disorders, multiple sclerosis, Parkinson disease, stroke
- Cardiovascular: cardiac arrhythmias, heart failure, coronary artery disease, valvular disease
- Pulmonary: hypoxia, pneumonia, chronic obstructive pulmonary disease (COPD), sleep apnea
- Gastrointestinal: celiac disease, primary biliary cirrhosis, gastroenteritis
- Genitourinary: urinary tract infection
- Musculoskeletal: arthritis
- Renal: renal failure
- Endocrine: diabetes mellitus, Addison disease, hypoglycemia, thyroid disease, hypopituitarism, vitamin D deficiency
- Rheumatology: autoimmune diseases (fibromyalgia, rheumatoid arthritis, systemic lupus erythematosus)
- Hematology/oncology: underlying malignancy, hemochromatosis, sickle cell anemia, iron deficiency anemia, iron deficiency without anemia, myelodysplastic syndrome

- Infectious disease: Epstein-Barr virus infection, cytomegalovirus infection, HIV infection, hepatitis, tuberculosis, Lyme disease, brucellosis, toxoplasmosis
- Drugs and toxins: medication-induced fatigue, alcohol dependence, drug dependence
- Physiological: dieting, prolonged exercise, lack of sleep, overworked, sedentary lifestyle
- Psychiatric: depression, stress, anxiety
- Idiopathic: chronic fatigue syndrome, chronic idiopathic fatigue

CASE INFORMATION

General Survey and History of Present Illness

As fatigue is such a nonspecific presentation, I will need to gather more information. While keeping all the possible etiologies in mind, I start with a general survey of the patient, which includes his general state of health, posture, build, motor skills, and any odors from his body or breath. The patient is in no apparent distress but does appear anxious. Asking the patient how he feels, he reports, "I feel tired and I know something is wrong. I don't feel like myself after starting this new medicine. I haven't felt right since last night." He is unable to explain any further as to what he means by feeling "unlike himself." He continues saying, "I know that the new medicine is not good for me. It makes me feel funny and tired." I also ask whether he currently has chest pain or palpitations and he denies both.

I look at his electronic medical record to gather more information and note that the patient was admitted with paroxysmal atrial fibrillation and has a medical history of coronary artery disease (CAD) with stent placement last year, hypertension, and dyslipidemia. Asking the patient why he received an ablation, he reports that several weeks ago, he started having recurrent chest pain that lasted for several hours. He further explained that the chest pain felt like indigestion, and was accompanied by mild shortness of breath. The episodes normally resolved without intervention, but he went to his primary doctor because he had an episode of pain that persisted. His primary doctor performed an ECG in the office, which revealed atrial fibrillation with a rapid ventricular rate of 135 beats per minute and sent the patient to the hospital for an ablation.

When asked about his psychosocial history, the patient denies any history of psychological disorders, and denies any stress factors or depression. He reports no other medical history.

❓ What are the pertinent positives at this time?

- The patient is 2 days status post successful pulmonary vein isolation ablation of atrial fibrillation.
- The patient complains of fatigue and "not feeling well" overnight and this morning.
- The patient appears to have just started a new medication.
- The patient has a significant history of CAD, hypertension, and dyslipidemia.
- The patient thinks his new medication is making him feel bad.

❓ What are the pertinent negatives at this time?

- The patient denies any history of stress or depression.
- The patient denies current chest pain and palpitations.

❓ Does the information gathered so far give you an insight into the possible causes of his fatigue and what other information would be helpful?

Summing up the information gathered so far will help highlight the pertinent information. The summation may look like this:

"A 57- year-old man with a medical history of coronary artery disease s/p percutaneous coronary intervention (PCI) 2 years ago, hypertension, dyslipidemia, who presented with new diagnosis of atrial fibrillation and underwent successful pulmonary vein Isolation ablation 2 days ago, now complains of fatigue and overall not feeling well over the last 12 hours."

More information needs to be gathered to pinpoint a possible cause for the patient's fatigue. The patient's history of atrial fibrillation and recent ablation increases concern for recurrent atrial fibrillation. His cardiac risk factors, which include known CAD, hypertension, and dyslipidemia, also increase the likelihood of an acute coronary syndrome (ACS) as the cause of his fatigue. In addition, medication side effects are a possible cause as the patient associates the onset of the fatigue with starting a new medication. He is clearly anxious about the way he feels and has not felt this way before so I suspect the cause is a new problem, not an exacerbation of a chronic condition, such as COPD, congestive heart failure, or chronic fatigue syndrome.

Due to the patient's recent procedure, I also need to make sure he is not bleeding and rule out anemia as a cause for his fatigue. A workup in a patient with fatigue should also include screening for any psychological causes for fatigue and in this case the patient denies any history of psychological disorders, depression, anxiety, or stress.

CASE INFORMATION

Review of Medical Record

After my brief assessment of the patient, I review his morning ECG performed an hour ago because the likelihood of an arrhythmia or acute coronary syndrome (ACS) is high. The ECG shows sinus bradycardia 40 bpm and a corrected QT interval (QTc) of 498. Although, many ECGs have the QTc measurement listed, I measure the QTc using the Bazett formula: QTc = QT interval/ $\sqrt{}$ [RR interval], which is the gold standard.[2] I now need to compare this recent ECG with his prior one to assess for any significant changes. His prior ECG from the night shows sinus bradycardia 45 bpm and QTc 460 ms. Both QTc levels are above normal (normal QTc < 440 ms). This increase in his QTc level worries me.

I review his medication list and notice that he was started on dofetilide 500 mg by mouth every 12 hours after his ablation to maintain sinus rhythm and this was decreased to 250 mg twice a day overnight secondary to bradycardia. His other medications include aspirin 81 mg daily, metoprolol 25 mg twice a day, rivaroxaban 20 mg daily, and rosuvastatin 5 mg daily. Of note, the patient's metoprolol tartrate was discontinued overnight due to bradycardia.

The morning laboratory results reveal normal blood glucose levels as well as normal complete blood count and negative troponin levels. In addition, the patient's potassium level is 3.7 mEq/L and magnesium level is 1.7 mg/dL. A thyroid stimulating hormone (TSH) level and a cortisol level were drawn on the day of admission and both were normal.

In addition to his ECGs, I look at his telemetry monitor for any current arrhythmias and any events overnight. When analyzing his telemetry readings from the night, I notice his heart rate decreased to a low of 37 bpm. I also notice that he appears to be having some ectopy. The patient's telemetry shows several short runs of premature ventricular beats (PVCs) and then a 2-second pause followed by more PVCs (see Figure 26-1). I immediately obtain another ECG and this time it reveals a QTc of 570 ms (normal QTc < 440 ms).

Review of Systems

The patient is a good historian.

- Constitutional: anxious and fatigued
- Head/eyes/ears/nose/throat: denies sinus drainage or sore throat
- Cardiovascular: denies chest pain or palpitations, denies any lower extremity swelling
- Pulmonary: denies shortness of breath
- Gastrointestinal: denies any changes in bowel movements, last bowel movement was yesterday evening, denies nausea or vomiting, denies any bloating, cramping, or epigastric pain

- Genitourinary: denies urgency, frequency, or painful urination, denies any difficulty urinating.
- Musculoskeletal: denies any joint pain
- Endocrine: denies any heat/cold intolerance, denies any weight gain or loss
- Psych: denies depressed mood, anxiety at this time

Physical Examination

- Constitutional: appears anxious
- Vitals: blood pressure 109/69 mm Hg, heart rate 45 bpm, respiratory rate 14/min, temperature 37.1°C oral, oxygen saturation by pulse oximeter on room air 99%
- Cardiovascular: bradycardic, regular rhythm, no murmurs, no edema, no JVD , brisk capillary refill in all extremities, extremities warm
- Pulmonary: lungs clear to auscultation, resonant to percussion, respiratory rate and rhythm normal, no use of accessory muscles
- Gastrointestinal: normoactive bowel sounds, tympanic on percussion, abdomen soft, no tenderness
- Neurologic: alert and oriented to name, place, and time, no focal neurologic deficits.
- Integumentary: bilateral femoral ablation sites without bleeding, pain, or hematoma, dressings clean, dry, and intact

❓ What are additional pertinent positives that can be added to the list?

- ECGs reveal sinus bradycardia, with increasing prolongation of the QTc.
- The patient was started on dofetilide (Tikosyn) 500 mg by mouth twice a day.
- The patient's laboratory values from this morning reveal hypokalemia and hypomagnesemia.
- Telemetry monitoring reveals ectopy and pauses.

❓ What are additional significant negatives?

- The patient denies chest pain.
- The ECGs show no ST-segment changes.
- The patient's laboratory values reveal negative troponin levels.
- The patient has a normal hemoglobin and hematocrit level and ablation access sites revealed no signs/symptoms of bleeding.
- The patient has normal glucose levels.
- The patient had a normal TSH and cortisol level on admission.

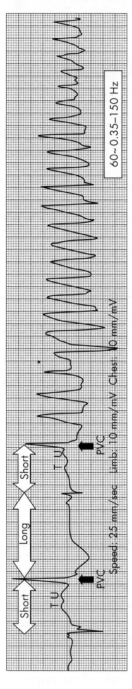

Figure 26-1 Typical of the short-long-short pattern of the R-R cycle seen right before TdP. Reproduced from Drew BJ, Ackerman MJ, Funk M, et al. Prevention of torsades de pointes in hospital settings: a scientific statement from the American Heart Association and the American College of Cardiology foundation. *Circulation*. 2010;121:1048. doi: 10.1161/ CIRCULATIONAHA.109.192704.

❓ Does the information gathered so far give you an insight into the possible causes of his fatigue and what other information would be helpful?

ACS and recurrent atrial fibrillation are unlikely causes of the patient's fatigue given normal troponin levels and lack of ST-segment changes on the ECG. I can also rule out anemia given a normal hemoglobin/hematocrit and no signs/symptoms of bleeding. He does not have a history of trauma, and his review of systems and physical examination show no neurological, gastrointestinal, or genitourinary abnormalities, which makes it unlikely that he has a condition related to these systems. In addition, he has a normal pulmonary examination making COPD or pneumonia unlikely. An endocrine disorder is still possible but his normal TSH, cortisol levels, and normal blood glucose, in addition to a negative history for diabetes, make this less likely. He has no fever and no signs or symptoms of an infectious process. While I cannot rule out an autoimmune disorder or a malignancy based on the data I have so far, the data I do have show a significant cardiac arrhythmia and it is far more likely that this is the cause of his fatigue.

In light of his ECG changes and negative history for other causes of fatigue, I believe his fatigue is most likely due to bradycardia. Some specific changes on my patient's ECG however, are concerning. These include sinus bradycardia and prolonged QTc's, In addition, his telemetry demonstrates some PVCs and pauses. All of these findings are precursors of torsades de pointes (TdP). There are several risk factors of prolonged QT and TdP, which includes antiarrhythmic drugs such as dofetilide (Tikosyn).[3] At this time, I feel comfortable stating that drug-induced prolonged QT is my primary diagnosis.

Now, I reexamine the problem and rewrite a new problem statement which reads: "An anxious 57-year-old man with a medical history of CAD s/p PCI in 2011, HTN, dyslipidemia, atrial fibrillation now s/p successful pulmonary vein ablation 2 days ago complains of fatigue and 'not feeling well' for 12 hours and has ECG changes revealing premonitory signs of TdP."

❓ What should be done at this time?

I will continue the patient on telemetry and have a defibrillator set up and attached to the patient. If the patient progresses into TdP and becomes unstable, I will need to defibrillate. In addition, as the patient is currently on a regular telemetry unit, I obtain an intensive care unit bed. He will need to be monitored more closely.

Drug-Induced Long-QT Syndrome (LQTS) and Prevention of Torsades de Pointe

A diagnosis of fatigue related to bradycardia and drug-induced long-QT syndrome (LQTS) can be made in this case due to his ECG and telemetry findings as well as the presence of dofetilide (Tikosyn) in his treatment plan.

Risk factors for prolonged QT include structural heart disease from myocardial infarction, cardiomyopathy, valvular disease, and heart failure, hypokalemia, consumption of QT prolonging drugs, prolonged baseline QTc ($\geq$450 ms), prior history of drug-induced LQTS, family history of congenital LQTS, bradycardia, atrioventricular block, and hepatic impairment. In addition, females have a higher propensity for LQTS than males as females have been noted to have a longer baseline QTc. A prolonged QTc is normally defined as >480 in females and >470 in males.

LQTS can result in TdP, a form of polymorphic ventricular tachycardia, where the QRS complexes appear to be twisting around the isoelectric line. For every 10 ms increase in the QTc, there is approximately a 5% to 7% increase in risk of TdP.[3] Although TdP is usually short lived, the arrhythmia can progress into ventricular fibrillation and cardiac arrest.

This patient's LQTS was most likely a result of dofetilide (Tikosyn) initiation after his ablation procedure. Tikosyn is a pure class III antiarrhythmic that is a potent I_{kr} blocker and can result in QTc prolongation, which is dose dependent. Dofetilide has a propensity to prolong the QTc. This is thought to be due to a phenomenon called "reverse use dependence." As the heart rate decreases, the QTc increases and vice versa, explaining why drug-induced long QT syndrome and TdP are more common in bradycardia.

Prior to TdP, there are premonitory signs that may be seen on an ECG or telemetry. Episodes of PVCs followed by a pause and more PVCs are typical of the short-long-short pattern of the R-R cycle seen right before TdP. The PVC following a pause is usually right before the peak of the T wave.[4]

The risk factors of TdP must be rectified immediately if possible. In this case, dofetilide (Tikosyn) is discontinued and the electrolyte imbalance is corrected by giving intravenous magnesium sulfate and intravenous potassium chloride.

CASE INFORMATION

ICU Course

Minutes after the patient arrives to the ICU, he progresses to TdP. He complains of palpitations but is otherwise stable. The patient is administered another 2 g of intravenous magnesium and his potassium level is kept in the high normal range (4.5–5 mEq/L), but he continues to have intermittent episodes of TdP. He is started on an isoproterenol drip keeping his heart rate above 90 bpm, which is discontinued after no additional episodes were noted. Due to the medical team's ability to identify the premonitory signs of TdP and rapid treatment, the patient is stable and eventually transfers back to a telemetry unit after several days of monitoring in the ICU.

Treatment of Torsades de Pointe

Both intravenous magnesium and isoproterenol are common treatments of TdP. Magnesium is thought to block sodium and calcium channel currents.[5] Isoproterenol stimulates β-adrenergic receptors, which accelerates AV conduction and increases the heart rate, thereby shortening the QT interval.[2] As such, isoproterenol is effective in drug-induced LQTS and contraindicated in congenital LQTS due to its sympathomimetic effects.[5] TdP in congenital LQTS is initiated by adrenergic stimuli.[5] Oftentimes, intravenous isoproterenol is utilized in the interim awaiting overdrive pacing from a transvenous pacer placement or when the placement of a transvenous pacer is not available. However, isoproterenol can cause hypotension and in cases of a low blood pressure, should be avoided.

Transvenous pacing at 90 to 110 bpm is another effective treatment of TdP by preventing the occurrence of pauses and shortening the QTc interval.[5]

References

1. Evaluation of fatigue. Epocrates Web site. 2014. https://online.epocrates.com/noFrame/showPage. do;jsessionid=0F6107D92FAB4B393D711001572E55AD?method=diseases&MonographId=571 &ActiveSectionId=12. Published 2014. Accessed August 6, 2014.
2. Gupta A, Lawrence AT, Krishnan K, Kavinsky CJ, Trohman RG. Current concepts in the mechanisms and management of drug-induced QT prolongation and torsades de pointes. *Am Heart J.* 2007;153:891-899. doi:10.1016/j.ahj.2007.01.040.
3. Lenz TL, Hilleman DE. Dofetilide, a new class III antiarrhythmic agent. *Pharmacotherapy.* 2000;20:776-786.
4. Drew BJ, Ackerman MJ, Funk M, et al. Prevention of torsades de pointes in hospital settings: a scientific statement from the American Heart Association and the American College of Cardiology foundation. *Circulation.* 2010;121:1047-1060. doi: 10.1161/CIRCULATIONAHA.109.192704.
5. Khan IA. Clinical and therapeutic aspects of congenital and acquired long QT syndrome. *Am J Med.* 2002;112:58-66.

CASE 27

Briana Witherspoon and Joshua Squiers

Briana Witherspoon is an ACNP with specialization in Neurosurgical/Neurological Critical Care. Dr Witherspoon serves on the faculty of the Department of Anesthesiology, Division of Critical Care Medicine, at Vanderbilt University Medical Center.

Joshua Squiers is dual board certified as an ACNP with specialization in surgical critical care. Dr Squiers holds a faculty appointment within the Oregon Health & Science University, School of Nursing where he serves as the Director of the AG-ACNP Program, and an appointment within the school of medicine where he serves as Assistant Professor in the Department of Anesthesiology/Perioperative Medicine and the Division of Cardiac and Surgical Subspecialty Critical Care.

CASE INFORMATION
Chief Complaint/Reason for Admission

An 18-year-old female with no known seizure history presents with acute psychosis leading to refractory seizures.

❓ What is the potential cause?

In patients without a history of epilepsy, seizures are a nonspecific symptom and can arise from a variety of causes including fever, infection, autoimmune abnormalities, metabolic disturbances, medications, overdose or withdrawal, structural abnormalities in the brain, and trauma to the brain. This particular patient's presentation is unique and makes it nearly impossible to quickly identify an etiology. However, regardless of the cause, seizures must be treated immediately as prolonged uncontrolled seizures can lead to hemodynamic instability, respiratory arrest, and permanent neuronal injury.

Comprehensive Differential Diagnoses for a Nonepileptic Patient With Retractable Seizures[1]

- Metabolic abnormalities: acute intermittent porphyria, anoxic injury, hypoglycemia, nonketotic hyperglycemia, hyponatremia, hypocalcemia, hypomagnesaemia, renal failure, hyperthyroidism, carbon monoxide poisoning
- Infection: encephalitis (infectious or autoimmune), primary CNS infection, bacterial/viral meningitis, abscess, secondary effects from another source of infection (UTI, pneumonia, skin)
- Withdrawal: alcohol, opiate, benzodiazepine

- Overdose/intoxication: alcohol, amphetamine, analgesic, antidepressant, antipsychotic medication, antibiotics, insulin
- Seizure imitators (physical and psychological conditions that can be mistaken as seizures): psychiatric disorders, migraines, drop attacks, syncope, transient ischemic attack, paroxysmal movement disorder, transient global amnesia
- Structural abnormality: aneurysm, arteriovenous malformation, brain tumor
- Brain damage: injury to the brain after some type of trauma

CASE INFORMATION

History of Present Illness

An 18-year-old healthy female initially complained of memory difficulties for the past 3 months. During that time abnormal behavior and personality changes were noted by her parents and classmates. Approximately 2 days prior to admission, the patient began to make overt religious verbalizations and experience auditory and visual hallucinations. Manifestations of these symptoms resulted in an altercation with a law enforcement officer, and she was subsequently taken to a community emergency department where she denied anything was wrong and had no recollection of her abnormal behavior. Her head CT was unremarkable at that time, though ED notes indicate slurred speech, delusions, as well as auditory and visual hallucinations. She was treated with antipsychotics and benzodiazepines prior to being transferred to another local hospital.

On admission to the second hospital, an MRI of the brain was obtained and revealed no abnormalities. A lumbar puncture was performed but showed no nucleated cells (thus likely ruling out a bacterial meningitis) and was negative for herpes simplex via polymerase chain reaction (PCR). The patient's clinical status worsened and she began having intractable seizures. Due to these seizures and an inability to protect her airway, the patient was intubated, sedated, and transferred to a tertiary medical center's neurointensive care unit. According to her parents who are at the bedside, the patient has no significant past medical history and did not take any prescription medications. Her parents denied any prior behavioral or amnestic episodes, hallucinations, or religious verbalizations. There is no family history of psychiatric illness. Her parents are unaware of any recent illnesses, fevers, traumas, or falls. They do state that she has been under a large amount of stress lately but she is otherwise in her usual state of health. Upon arrival to the ICU, all sedation is held and an initial examination is obtained. The patient is found to have intact brain reflexes, but is otherwise unresponsive. However, after the sedation is held for several minutes, lip smacking and left nystagmus are observed. Continuous EEG is immediately obtained and reveals an abnormal generalized rhythmic delta activity consistent with nonconvulsive status epilepticus. A chest x-ray is also ordered, which showed appropriate position of the endotracheal tube, clear lung fields but a widened mediastinum.

? What are the pertinent positives from the information given so far?

- The patient has history of memory difficulties 3 months prior to admission.
- The patient had an acute onset of behavioral changes including hallucinations, verbalizations, and personality changes shortly before her seizure activity started.
- Parents state that patient has been under a higher amount of stress than usual.
- Physical examination off sedation reveals seizure-like movements including lip smacking and nystagmus.
- EEG findings are consistent with nonconvulsive status epilepticus.
- Widened mediastinum present on chest x-ray.

? What are the significant negatives from the information given so far?

- No significant past medical history including seizures.
- No recent history of fevers, head trauma, or falls.
- The patient did not take any prescription medication.
- No family history of psychiatric illness.
- No acute abnormalities are noted on CT or MRI of the head.
- Lumbar puncture at outside facility negative for nucleated cells, herpes simplex virus via PCR.

? Can the information gathered so far be restated in a single sentence highlighting the pieces that narrow down the cause?

- The problem representation in this case might be: "an 18-year-old female with no significant past medical history who presents with acute onset of psychosis leading to nonconvulsive status epilepticus."

Case Analysis: EEG tracings revealed nonconvulsive status epilepticus which immediately eliminates any "seizure imitators" from the differential diagnosis list. Given the unremarkable head CT and MRI, structural abnormalities such as lesions, tumors, and vascular abnormalities can also be eliminated. There is no sign of traumatic or anoxic injury on the imaging, which is consistent with the history, so they are also unlikely. The lumbar puncture at the outside hospital was negative only for herpes simplex so infection from other organisms is still possible, but the absence of nucleated cells and the normal glucose in the cerebrospinal fluid make a bacterial infection lower on the differential. Also, her chest x-ray showed clear lung fields and there were no reports of fever, general malaise, or abnormal sputum production, making an infection from another source (bacteremia, urinary tract infection, or pneumonia) unlikely. However, other types of infection such as viral meningitis, encephalitis, or primary CNS infection cannot yet be ruled out. Metabolic abnormalities, overdose, and infection or autoimmune encephalitis are all potential explanations for this patient's unique presentation as well as her seizures. Laboratory data including a comprehensive metabolic panel, liver studies, thyroid studies, urine drug screen, and complete blood count are all obtained to help identify the cause.

CASE INFORMATION

Review of Systems

The patient is unable to provide history. Review of systems is obtained from the patient's parents and outside hospital records.

- Constitutional: Denies fever, any recent changes in the patient's appetite or weight, no recent falls, no trauma.
- Head/eyes/ears/nose/throat: Denies history of enlarged thyroid, vision changes, or hearing loss. The patient does wear glasses and contact lenses.
- Pulmonary: Denies history of wheezing, shortness of breath, cough, night sweats, or smoking.
- Cardiovascular: Denies chest pain, leg swelling, or difficulty breathing when lying down.
- Gastrointestinal: Denies nausea/vomiting, bowel movement documented at outside facility during seizure activity (parents confirm this), denies blood in stools.
- Genitourinary: Denies blood in her urine, change in urine smell, frequency, or amount.
- Musculoskeletal: Denies muscle weakness, joint or back pain.

- Neurological: Parents state the patient had memory problems for approximately 3 months. The patient had difficulty remembering important dates such as family member's birthdays and retaining information when studying. Her parents also state her grades have declined recently as a result of her decreased ability to concentrate. They deny a seizure history prior to recent events. They also deny headache, dizziness, syncope, weakness, or change in speech (except after receiving benzodiazepines at outside facility).
- Psychosocial: Parents state this is the first time the patient has exhibited personality and behavioral changes. They state the patient would be extremely embarrassed by her recent behavior. They state she has been under more stress lately due to an upcoming test, recent decline in grades, and new onset of memory issues. They deny prior history of depression, anxiety, or psychiatric illness.
- Endocrine: Denies increased hunger, thirst, or urination.

Physical Examination

- Vital signs: Pulse is 68 beats per minute, blood pressure is 104/60 mm Hg, respiratory rate is 14 breaths per minute (set rate on ventilator), and temperature is 98.5°F via esophageal probe, oxygen saturation by pulse oximeter is 99% on 40% FiO_2, and finger-stick blood glucose is 89 mg/dL. The patient is intubated, sedated on propofol infusion with EEG in place. Sedation was briefly held for physical examination.
- Neurological: EEG changes indicative of possible seizure activity noted when sedation is paused and the patient is stimulated. Cough, gag, and corneal reflexes all present. Nystagmus noted. No movement to pain in all four extremities. Unable to test cranial nerves given patient's comatose state.
- Head/eyes/ears/nose/throat: EEG headwrap in place, pupils are 2 mm, equal, round, react sluggishly to light, buccal mucosa moist, 7.5-cm endotracheal tube in place at 21 cm at the teeth. Thyroid gland is nonpalpable.
- Cardiovascular: Heart rate and rhythm regular, no murmurs, no gallops. Admission ECG shows normal sinus rhythm. Extremities: nail beds are pale, cool to touch, brisk capillary refill.
- Pulmonary: The patient is intubated on SIMV setting with 40% FiO_2, PEEP of 5 cm H_2O, respiratory rate of 14 breaths per minute (not breathing over the vent), tidal volume 450 mL. Widened mediastinum noted on chest x-ray. No use of accessory muscles, lungs clear to auscultation and resonant to percussion.
- Gastrointestinal: Normoactive bowel sounds, tympanic on percussion, abdomen soft without tenderness on deep palpation.
- Integumentary: Intact, no rashes, lesions or sores, normal skin turgor.

? **What elements of the review of systems and the physical examination should be added to the list of pertinent positives? Which items should be added to the list of significant negatives?**

- **Pertinent positives:** Memory problems for past 3 months, decline in grades, increased level of stress, decreased attention span, nystagmus, and EEG changes concerning for seizure when sedation is paused and the patient is stimulated. Widened mediastinum on CXR (This is bothersome—why would a previously healthy 18-year-old girl have a widened mediastinum?).

- **Significant negatives:** No prior changes in personality or behavior, no history of depression. No signs of lesions or sores on skin indicating recent illicit substance use.

? **How does this information affect the list of possible causes?**

Unfortunately in this scenario, the review of systems and the physical examination provide minimal information to narrow the current list of differentials (infection, autoimmune, metabolic, and overdose). An overdose of an injectable illicit substance such as heroin, methamphetamine, or cocaine is less likely given that the patient has no tract marks or injection sites. However, the urine drug screen should be reviewed prior to completely ruling these substances out. Also of note given the increased amount of stress the patient has been going through, a prescription medication overdose or withdrawal cannot be completely eliminated.

Some metabolic causes of seizures can be ruled out based on the review of systems and physical examination findings. While the decreased attention span and the new behavior changes could be caused by hyperthyroidism, the patient does not show any physical symptoms such as tachycardia, fever, weight loss, and diarrhea. Again, I need to wait until the thyroid studies have returned from the lab to confirm this. Carbon monoxide poisoning can also be ruled out given the patient has not had any nausea or vomiting, and no cardiac or pulmonary signs (arrhythmias, hypotension, pneumonia, pulmonary edema) are noted during the physical examination. A few of the electrolyte abnormalities that can lead to seizures can also be eliminated. The patient's random glucose on arrival to the ICU was 89 mg/dL, and upon chart review the patient has had normal glucose levels since arrival to the first hospital without receiving any insulin or an IV glucose source—thus hypoglycemia and nonketotic hyperglycemia are unlikely to be the cause of the patient's current state. While severe hypomagnesemia or hypocalcemia could cause seizures and nystagmus, these conditions usually also cause tetany and arrhythmias, which are absent in this patient. Both the PR interval and the QRS width were normal on the patient's admission ECG. Lastly, while hyponatremia could definitely cause seizures and altered mental status, again the review of systems and the physical examination do not support the diagnosis. The patient has no history of changes in appetite, nausea, vomiting, muscle weakness, or muscle spasms.

Infectious causes such as a primary CNS infection and encephalitis cannot be ruled out based on the review of system and physical examination findings. Furthermore, although extremely rare and not technically infections, autoimmune diseases can also lead to encephalitis and should be considered once more obvious and common causes of status epilepticus have been ruled out.

❓ What diagnostic testing should be done and in what order?

In this particular case study the patient arrived to the ICU with most of the acute and lethal causes ruled out by imaging. This gave me time to stabilize the patient and perform a thorough workup. The comprehensive metabolic panel is normal, as are the patient's liver and thyroid studies. Her urine drug screen came back positive only for benzodiazepines. While this could indicate a possible prescription medication overdose as the cause, records also indicate that the patient received benzodiazepines at the outside facility in an attempt to treat her seizures. A review of the Tennessee Controlled Substance Monitoring Database confirms that no benzodiazepines have recently prescribed to the patient. The patient's roommate at school confirms that she has not witnessed the patient taking prescription medications of any type.

These findings lead me to believe that an infectious or autoimmune source is the most likely cause of the patient's seizure. Although the patient has remained afebrile with a normal white count, a lumbar puncture is repeated. Again, the CSF has no nucleated cells, the CSF glucose and protein are normal, and once again negative for herpes simplex via PCR. Given that the patient was admitted to the ICU over 48 hours ago and is still seizing, the patient is started on high-dose steroids to help treat any autoimmune encephalitis while the CSF is being sent out for autoimmune testing. A CT of the chest, abdomen, and pelvis is also obtained as part of a neoplastic workup.

CASE INFORMATION

Diagnostic testing results

The CT of the chest reveals a right anterior mediastinal mass measuring approximately 5.3 × 4.2 cm in size (thus explaining the widened mediastinum seen on x-ray). Cardiothoracic surgery is consulted, the mass is removed, and the pathology is consistent with a teratoma. Shortly after, the CSF results come back with anti-*N*-methyl D-aspartate (NMDA) + antibodies. NMDA is a protein found in the brain and is involved in helping control the electrical activity of the neurons. So it is easy to understand why antibodies against these receptors are likely to cause altered mental status and seizures.

Diagnosis: Anti-NMDA Encephalitis

Anti-NMDA receptor encephalitis is a recently discovered diagnosis. It was first described in the early 2000s in a cohort of 12 women with neuropsychiatric symptoms, ovarian teratomas (of the teratomas 11 were ovarian and 1 was mediastinal), and NMDA antibodies.[2] On average, approximately 60% of patients with anti-NMDA receptor encephalitis will have a tumor; however, the probability of an associated neoplasm depends on age and gender.[3] Ovarian teratomas are the most common tumor associated with this condition, although there have been documented cases of mediastinal and testicular teratomas, as well as small cell lung cancer among others.[3]

The overall incidence of anti-NMDA receptor encephalitis is unknown, but one multicenter, prospective study in England found that approximately 4% of 203 encephalopathic patients had anti-NMDA receptor encephalitis.[4] Titulaer et al performed the largest case series to date with 577 patients with anti-NMDA receptor encephalitis. They confirmed the previous findings that women are more commonly affected (81% of the cases were in females), and that the disease onset is usually in younger patients, with a median age onset of 21 years old. Interestingly, the case series also noted that those who are of Asian or Black descent are more likely to have a teratoma when compared to white or Hispanic patients.[5]

Anti-NMDA Encephalitis: Treatment

This case study describes a patient with anti-NMDA receptor encephalitis who went into a coma secondary to nonconvulsive status epilepticus. To date, there are few reports of status epilepticus in association with anti-NMDA encephalitis. Seizures, however, have been noted in several case studies to date.[6-8] Occurring in approximately 75% of patients in a recently published large case series, seizures were found to be one of the most common symptoms of anti-NMDA receptor encephalitis.[8] EEG findings similar to the ones noted in this case study—generalized slow or disorganized delta activity, are commonly seen with this diagnosis.[8]

After a large case review, the clinical picture becomes rather consistent. Some patients will have flu-like symptoms or periods of amnesia days to weeks prior to the onset of acute psychiatric symptoms. Patients frequently appear confused, agitated, with delusional or paranoid thoughts that often result in admission to a psychiatric facility.[9] Most patients will then develop seizures and altered mental status, often requiring admission to an ICU secondary to respiratory failure and autonomic instability.[9] Diagnosis of anti-NMDA receptor encephalitis is confirmed by the presence of antibodies to NR1 subunit of the NMDA receptor in either the serum or the CSF.[9]

Of note, all diagnostic imaging of the head obtained in this particular case was negative for diagnostic lesions or contrast enhancement. However, evidence suggests MRI abnormalities are present in about half of patients, with the EEG irregularities occurring in 90% of patients with the disease.[3] The absence of acute focal lesions and obvious neuronal damage may be secondary to the antibodies causing reversible defects in the number of NMDA receptors.[3]

Despite severity of symptoms, this condition is treatable and potentially even reversible, depending on early recognition, prompt initiation of immunosuppression therapy, and in cases such as this one, complete tumor resection. Evidence suggests that when patients receive first-line therapies including resection of the tumor, administration of glucocorticoids, intravenous immune globulin, and plasma exchange, symptom improvement is typically noted within 4 weeks.[9] In the rare instances symptoms do not improve with first-line therapies, data suggest that rituximab and/or cyclophosphamide should be considered.[9] Patients with anti-NMDA encephalitis may require intensive care support for several weeks or months, and afterward an extensive rehabilitation period that includes both physical therapy and psychiatric management of any prolonged behavioral/cognitive symptoms.[9] Currently about 75% of patents will have positive outcomes, typically with amnesia during the duration of the illness. However, risk of relapse is always a possibility, particularly in cases with tumor recurrence or where the tumor is removed too late, or never found.[2,8,10]

Conclusion

The main purpose of this case study is to increase the index of suspicion for anti-NMDA receptor–related encephalitis as one possible cause of seizures, altered mental status, and psychosis-like symptoms in adults (especially young females). The workup of intractable seizures can be challenging, requiring the clinician to give thoughtful consideration to a wide set of differential diagnoses. While there are many common (high probability) differentials, we are reminded that when these differentials are exhausted, less common culprits should be considered. This case highlights a less common etiology of intractable seizures and reveals the difficulty associated with working up cases with complex differential diagnoses which contain viable but less probable etiologies. The old adage remains true, "When you hear hoof beats think horses, not zebras," but we are reminded that there are cases with zebra diagnoses. Careful consideration should be given to "zebra" diagnoses, when more probably differentials have been excluded.

This case also demonstrates the need to consider a full body scan when searching for the associated neoplasm. While the most common neoplasm associated with anti-NMDA receptor encephalitis is an ovarian teratoma, the condition may also be associated with other tumors, or teratomas in other locations. Multiple case studies have shown that in incidences associated with the presence of a neoplasm, complete tumor removal is crucial to prognosis.

In this particular instance, once the cause of the seizures was identified and treated gradual clinical improvement soon ensued. A few weeks after the surgery and resolution of her seizures, the patient was able to communicate and follow commands. After undergoing several months of rehabilitation, the patient improved almost to baseline cognitive function.

References

1. Schachter, S. Evaluation of the first seizure in adults. UpToDate. 2014. http://www.uptodate.com.
2. Dalmau J, Tuzun E, Wu H, et al. Paraneoplastic anti-N-methyl-D-aspartate receptor encephalitis associated with ovarian teratoma. *Ann Neurol*. 2007;61:25-36.

3. Wandinger K, Saschenbrecker S, Stoecker W, Dalmau J. Anti-NMDA-receptor encephalitis: a severe, multistage, treatable disorder presenting with psychosis. *J Neuroimmunol.* 2011;231:86-91.

4. Granerod J, Ambrose H, Davies N, et al. Causes of encephalitis and differences in their clinical presentations in England: a multicenter, population-based prospective study. *Lancet Infect Dis.* 2010;12:835-844.

5. Titulaer M, McCracken L, Gabilondo I, et al. Treatment and prognostic factors for long-term outcome in patients with anti-NMDA receptor encephalitis: an observational cohort study. *Lancet Neurol.* 2013;12:157-165. doi:10.1016/S1474-4422(12)70310-1.

6. Vitaliani R, Mason W, Ances B, Zwerdling T, Jiang Z, Dalmau J. Paraneoplastic encephalitis, psychiatric symptoms, and hypoventilation in ovarian teratoma. *Ann Neurol.* 2005;58:594-604.

7. Sansing L, Tuzun E, Ko M, Baccon J, Lynch D, Dalmau J. A patient with encephalitis associated with NMDA receptor antibodies. *Nat Clin Pract Neurol.* 2007;3:291-296.

8. Dalmau J, Gleichman A, Hughes E, et al. Anti-NMDA-receptor encephalitis: case series and analysis of the effects of antibodies. *Lancet Neurol.* 2008;7:1091-1098.

9. Dalmau J, Rosenfield M. Paraneoplastic and autoimmune encephalitis. UpToDate. 2014. http://www.uptodate.com.

10. Breese E, Dalmau J, Lennon V, Apiwattanakul M, Sokol D. Anti-N-methyl-D-aspartate receptor encephalitis: early treatment is beneficial. *Pediatr Neurol.* 2010;42:213-214.

CASE 28

Megan M. Shifrin

Megan Shifrin is ACNP faculty at the Vanderbilt School of Nursing in the AG-ACNP program. Dr Shifrin's clinical background is in critical care with an emphasis on trauma and cardiac surgery.

CASE INFORMATION

Chief Complaint

AB is a 37-year-old white male admitted to the inpatient step-down floor with a 6-week history of "fever, chills, muscle soreness, shortness of breath, and weight loss."

? What is the potential cause?

In the adult patient presenting with these particular symptoms, my initial concern is for an active infectious process, particularly given the duration of symptoms. However, there are multiple other pathological processes that need to be considered. The key to determining the potential source of his symptoms is in obtaining a thorough review of systems, history, and physical examination. I start by developing a differential for his constellation of symptoms.

Differential Diagnoses for Fever, Chills, Muscle Soreness, Shortness of Breath, and Weight Loss

Fever, chills, muscle soreness, shortness of breath, and weight loss

Neurological: Meningitis (bacterial or viral)

Cardiovascular: Endocarditis, valvular insufficiency or stenosis, pericarditis (infectious, inflammatory, or autoimmune), heart failure exacerbation

Pulmonary: Pneumonia (bacterial, fungal, or viral), noninfective pneumonitis, tuberculosis, sarcoidosis, pulmonary embolism, pleural effusion, pulmonary tumor

Gastrointestinal: Hepatitis A, B, or C, gastroenteritis

Renal and Genitourinary: Urinary tract infection, pyelonephritis, electrolyte imbalances (hypernatremia, hypokalemia, hyperkalemia)

Musculoskeletal: Fibromyalgia, chronic fatigue syndrome

Endocrine: Hyperthyroidism, diabetes mellitus

Hematologic/Lymphatic/Immunologic: Bacteremia, fungemia, influenza, Lyme disease, valley fever (coccidioidomycosis), Rocky Mountain spotted fever, West Nile virus, mononucleosis, HIV/AIDS, anemia, leukemia, other forms of malignancy

Exogenous: Medication reaction/interaction/side effects

CASE INFORMATION

History of Present Illness (HPI)

In this patient, the HPI will be extremely helpful in determining the etiology of his presenting symptoms. Asking the correct questions and obtaining details and data regarding his health history assists in ruling in, or ruling out, several of the differential diagnoses.

The patient has a history of intravenous (IV) methamphetamine abuse with his last IV drug use being 2 weeks ago. He reports that all of his symptoms (fever, chills, muscle soreness, shortness of breath, and weight loss) began about 6 weeks ago and that his symptoms have continued to steadily progress and intensify over that time period.

He was seen at an outside hospital approximately 1 month ago and was hospitalized for 2 days. Per his report, he was treated for costochondritis but also given a course of antibiotics (outside hospital medical records not available at this time). He reported feeling better for a few days following discharge but states that he now feels that he is "worse than ever." He has been taking acetaminophen as needed for his lower extremity muscle aches, but he states that this has not been effective. He also states that fevers and chills "come and go" but have been occurring more frequently this past week with approximately two to three episodes of chills per day. He has not been measuring his temperature but states that he feels "hot, red, and sweaty" at times.

He denies being exposed to sick contacts or having any known tick or mosquito bites in the past year. He reports being in jail 1 year ago for a total of 90 days. While he was incarcerated, he states that he was tested for HIV, hepatitis C, and tuberculosis and that the results were negative. He denies having any household pets and denies any unusual contact, encounters, or bites from animals or birds. He denies the use of any medications other than acetaminophen as noted previously.

❓ What are the pertinent positives from the current information?

- He has a history of recent IV drug use.
- He was incarcerated for 90 days.
- His symptoms have been progressive and more frequent in nature.
- His symptoms have not been alleviated by the treatment he received for costochondritis or the course of antibiotics he received when hospitalized last month.
- Acetaminophen has not effectively treated his symptoms.

? **What are the significant negatives obtained from the current information?**

- He has not been around any known sick contacts.
- He has not had any known tick or mosquito bites in the past year.
- He does not have any household pets and denies any unusual contact, encounters, or bites from animals or birds.

? **Can the information gathered so far be restated in a single sentence highlighting the pieces that narrow down the cause?**

AB is a 37-year-old white male with a past medical history of incarceration in the past year, recent IV methamphetamine use, and no known sick contacts or animal exposures who now presents with a 6-week history of progressive fever, chills, muscle soreness, shortness of breath, and weight loss.

Case Analysis: The information gathered in the HPI guides my thinking toward a potential viral, bacterial, or fungal etiology to explain his symptom cluster. However, given his shortness of breath, I am still concerned that there is a cardiovascular or respiratory component to his illness. Endocrine conditions should also be considered. A thorough review of systems and blood tests such as hemoglobin A1C, thyroid stimulating hormone and free T4 may be used to determine whether diabetes or thyroid disorders are contributing to his ongoing illness. Although some of his symptoms could be associated with a malignant process, his social history combined with symptoms of fever, chills, and muscle aches makes infection more likely than malignancy.

His history of IV drug use and recent incarceration for a duration of 90 days places him at risk for exposure to communicable diseases such as tuberculosis, hepatitis B, hepatitis C, HIV/AIDS, and septicemia.[1] His reported lack of exposure to mosquitos, ticks, birds, and other mammals makes him less likely to have a disease process arising from these sources. The progression of his symptoms with worsening intensity makes me concerned that his compensatory mechanisms are failing. However, additional questions about his symptoms and further diagnostic testing are necessary to determine a definitive diagnosis.

CASE INFORMATION

Past Medical History

- Current health status: The patient reports that prior to the last 6 weeks, his health was "good."
- Previous medical diagnoses: None.
- Past surgical history: None.

Family History

- Alzheimer disease: father
- COPD: brother, father
- Denies family history of cardiovascular disease, hypertension, kidney disease, liver disease, and obesity
- Current medications: none
- Allergies: none

Social History

- Habits
  - Exercise: Denies.
  - Caffeine intake: Two to three cups of black coffee per day.
  - Alcohol intake: Denies.
  - Illicit substance use: Reports having used marijuana and cocaine previously, but denies use in the past year. States that he has been using IV methamphetamines three to six times per month for the past 2 years.
  - Tobacco use: Denies.
  - Sleep patterns: 4 to 5 hours/night, reports as sufficient.
- Current occupation: Currently unemployed. Previously has worked as a welder in an automobile factory.
- Highest level of education: 10th grade of high school.
- Living situation: Lives with his girlfriend in a trailer in a rural area.

Review of Systems (ROS)

- Constitutional: See HPI regarding history of weakness and fatigue. Also reports having night sweats two to three times/week. States that he has had an unintentional 20 to 25 lb weight loss in the past 6 weeks.
- Head/eyes/ears/nose/throat: Denies history of headaches or recurrent sinus infections. No history of blurred vision, excessive dryness, or tearing. The patient does not wear corrective lenses or contacts. Denies history of recurrent ear infections, hearing loss, tinnitus, or vertigo. No history of nosebleeds, sore throat/tongue, oral lesions, or bleeding gums.
- Cardiovascular: See HPI regarding history of shortness of breath. Denies history of cardiovascular disease, chest pain, and palpitations. Reports having two- to three-pillow orthopnea. States that his shortness of breath is exacerbated by walking greater than 100 feet and partially alleviated by rest. States that he has developed symptoms of lower extremity edema in the past week, but has not noticed any alleviating or exacerbating factors. No history of claudication or thrombophlebitis.
- Pulmonary: See HPI regarding history of shortness of breath. Denies history of respiratory illnesses or disease processes. States that his shortness of breath is exacerbated by walking greater than 100 feet and partially alleviated by rest. Denies wheezing, hemoptysis, and cough.

- Gastrointestinal: See HPI regarding recent weight loss. Reports early satiety when eating and nausea at the sight of food. He denies constipation, diarrhea, melena, hematochezia, and vomiting. No history of dysphagia, gastric reflux symptoms, or jaundice. The patient states he has a bowel movement one time per day.
- Genitourinary: States that his urine has been dark, but denies history of frequency, dysuria, hesitancy, urgency, polyuria, nocturia, hematuria, or incontinence. No history of renal calculi, recurrent UTIs, or flank pain.
- Musculoskeletal: See HPI regarding recent muscle myalgia. The patient states that in the past 5 days his quadriceps have been particularly sore as if he had "been riding a bicycle really hard." Reports taking acetaminophen without much relief. Denies history of muscle trauma or injury, joint pain, swelling, stiffness, or erythema. Denies decreased range of motion.
- Integumentary: Denies history of excessive skin dryness, rashes, lumps, or excessive itching. No history of skin, hair, or scalp scaling.
- Neurological: Denies history of seizures, syncope, numbness, tingling, extremity weakness, or changes in speech. No headaches, memory changes, or forgetfulness.
- Psychiatric: See HPI regarding history of IV methamphetamine use. Denies history of alcohol use, depression, anxiety, suicidal or homicidal ideations.
- Endocrine: Denies history of diabetes, polyphagia, polyuria, polydipsia, heat/cold intolerance, or goiter.
- Hematologic/lymphatic/immunologic: See HPI regarding history of fever and chills. Denies history of cancer, rigors, easy bruising, bleeding, or enlarged/tender lymph nodes. No history of blood product administration. Denies previous history of frequent illness.

Physical Examination

- Vital signs: Temperature 100.2°F oral; Heart rate: 101 beats per minute; respirations 16/breaths per minute; blood pressure 98/52 mm Hg; O_2 saturation on room air 96%, weight 131 lb, 72 inches, BMI 17.8 kg/m^2.
- Constitutional: AB is cachectic, pale, and ill appearing. Appears older than his stated age. He is sitting in the hospital bed upright. He has a disheveled appearance and appears anxious but is alert, cooperative, answers questions appropriately.
- Head/eyes/ears/nose/throat
  - Head: Head is normocephalic and atraumatic with no lesions or masses felt upon palpation. Hair is thin and gray with even distribution. No evidence of hair loss noted. Facial features are symmetrical with no lesions or deformities noted. No tenderness upon palpation of frontal or maxillary sinuses.
  - Eyes: Eyes are symmetrical bilaterally with no drainage or lesions noted. Eyebrows and eyelashes are symmetrical bilaterally with no evidence of hair loss. The sclera appear white without lesions or ulcerations; the

bulbar and palpebral conjunctivae are clear without evidence of ulcerations. The vascular pattern is easily visualized; no opacities or ulcerations noted within the cornea or iris. No tenderness with palpation of the nasal or lacrimal glands.

- Ears: Ears are symmetrical bilaterally with no masses, drainage, or ulcerations. External auditory canals are patent with no exudates or swelling noted. No tenderness upon palpation of pinna.

- Nose: Nose is midline with no drainage; nares patent.

- Mouth/throat: No lesions or ulcerations noted on lips. Buccal and sublingual mucosa intact and patent; pink in color with no ulcerations. Gums are pink with no inflammation, ulcerations, or bleeding present. Evidence of caries and tooth decay in several teeth on both the upper and lower palates. Multiple broken and missing teeth. Hard and soft palate and floor of mouth are intact with no ulcerations. Tongue midline with no lesions; oropharynx without erythema, edema, or exudates. Tonsils present.

- Cardiovascular: Heart rhythm is regular. S1 and S2 present; no S3 or S4 noted. Pansystolic murmur (II/VI) auscultated at the left sternal border, third intercostal space. No rubs, clicks, or gallops. No heaves, thrills, or lifts noted upon palpation. Bilateral jugular venous distension of 4 to 5 cm present with the head of the bed at 45°. Bilateral lower extremity edema (1+). Bilateral carotid pulses easily detected with smooth, regular pulsations; no carotid bruits noted. Capillary refill <3 seconds in upper and lower extremities bilaterally. No varicosities present. Radial, brachial, dorsalis pedis and posterior tibialis pulses 2+ and symmetrical bilaterally. No aortic, renal, iliac, or femoral bruits noted.

- Pulmonary: Regular respiratory rate and rhythm. No use of accessory muscles. Trachea midline. Chest wall expansion symmetrical bilaterally. Breath sounds clear bilaterally in all lung fields. No wheezes, rhonchi, or crackles noted.

- Gastrointestinal: Bowel sounds normoactive in all four quadrants. No abdominal distention, pulsations, heaves, or masses noted. No rebound tenderness or guarding noted. Abdominal contour flat with no scars present. Tympanic percussion note in all quadrants. Liver not palpable.

- Genitourinary: No costovertebral angle tenderness.

- Musculoskeletal: Spine midline without deviation or masses. No tenderness or crepitation upon palpation of upper and lower extremities. Muscle tone equal bilaterally with no masses or tenderness noted upon palpation. Full range of motion noted in neck, shoulders, elbows, wrists, fingers, hips, knees, and ankles.

- Integumentary: Skin dry and intact with no lesions, ulcerations, or rashes noted. Evidence of scarring in left antecubital area, which the patient states is due to his previous IV drug use. Multiple tattoos on neck, back, chest, left leg, and bilateral upper extremities. Skin is warm to the touch with elastic turgor. No infestations, excessive scaling/dryness, or lesions noted.

- Neurological
  - Mental status: The patient is alert and oriented to person, place, and time. Able to answer questions appropriately and respond without difficulty. Short-term memory intact as evidenced by ability to recall three words with no difficulty. Speech tone, volume, and clarity without abnormality.
  - Cranial nerves
    - CN II: No visual deficits noted; the patient able to easily read provider's name badge.
    - CN III, IV, VI: Pupils 2 mm and equal bilaterally, brisk and reactive to light and convergence. Extraocular movements intact with no nystagmus or abnormal movements noted.
    - CN V: The patient able to clench teeth with no difficulties or discomfort; able to appropriately differentiate between sharp versus dull in all three facial dermatomes bilaterally.
    - CN VII: Able to smile, puff out cheeks, wrinkle forehead, and close eyes tightly with no difficulties or discomfort.
    - CN VIII: No hearing deficits noted using the whisper test; the patient able to correctly repeat whispered words.
    - CN IX: Palate noted to rise symmetrically with midline movement of the uvula when patient says "ah."
    - CN X: No hoarseness of voice noted; gag reflex deferred.
    - CN XI: Equal strength of trapezius muscles noted bilaterally when opposing force exerted. Mobility of trapezius muscles symmetrical bilaterally.
    - CN XII: Tongue protrudes midline with no fasciculations or abnormal movements noted.
  - Motor: No involuntary movements noted; muscle tone and bulk equal bilaterally. Muscle strength equal bilaterally in neck, shoulders, elbows, wrists, fingers, hips, knees, and ankles; strength 5/5. No hypotonia/hypertonia present.
  - Sensory: Able to appropriately distinguish sharp versus dull in three dermatomes of upper and lower extremities with eyes closed.
- Psychiatric: The patient reports being anxious about hospitalization and current symptoms. Affect and behavior appropriate for situation. Thought process logical; speech is clear and easily understood. Demonstrates appropriate emotions and cognition.
- Endocrine: Thyroid midline with no masses, goiter, or discomfort noted with palpation.
- Hematologic/lymphatic/immune: No signs of active bleeding. No petechiae, purpura, or ecchymosis noted. No enlarged or tender lymph nodes. Spleen not palpable.

What are the pertinent positives and significant negatives found in the ROS and PE?

Pertinent Positives

- He has had recent and significant weight loss with associated nausea and early satiety.
- In addition to fever and chills, he also has been experiencing night sweats.
- He has developed lower extremity edema in the past week, has a new tricuspid valve murmur, and jugular venous distension.
- He has multiple dental caries, tooth decay, and broken teeth.
- He has evidence of IV drug use on examination of his integumentary system.

Significant Negatives

- He has no past medical history of immunocompromise, malignancy, endocrine disorders, or other chronic disease.
- He has a negative ROS and PE for the genitourinary, neurological, psychiatric, endocrine, and hematologic/lymphatic/immune systems.

Case Analysis: Several aspects of the history and physical allow me to narrow down my list of potential differential diagnoses. First, he denies many of the signs and symptoms associated with common endocrine disorders (polyphagia, polyuria, polydipsia, heat/cold intolerance, and goiter). Although this does not completely eliminate diagnoses such as hyperthyroidism and diabetes mellitus as being final diagnoses, it makes them less likely.

Second, his history of fever, chills, and night sweats again makes me lean toward a pathological process consistent with infection. He denies nuchal rigidity, headache, and has full range of motion in his neck, thus making meningitis an unlikely cause. He denies symptoms of dysuria, hematuria, urinary frequency, and CVA tenderness, making a renal or urinary tract etiology of infection unlikely. He does report having respiratory symptoms of shortness of breath. This could be due to pneumonia; however, he denies having a cough and his lungs are clear to auscultation. He may have been exposed to tuberculosis while incarcerated, but per report, a tuberculosis skin test during his incarceration last year was negative. A chest x-ray or chest computed tomography (CT) scan will be helpful in definitively ruling out these pulmonary etiologies of infection.

His HPI as well as his history and physical findings, particularly that of a new tricuspid valve murmur, lower extremity edema, active tooth decay, and scarring in left antecubital area which the patient attributed to his previous IV drug use make me concerned that the patient may be suffering from infective tricuspid valve endocarditis. Some of the risk factors for infective tricuspid valve endocarditis and/or a bacterial blood stream infection include IV drug use and poor dentition. As the patient explains more about his symptoms, I begin to think about how I should tailor my physical examination to be inclusive of the necessary body systems. For example, in this situation, a confirmed diagnosis of tricuspid valve endocarditis would place the patient at risk of embolic events. Thus, I want to be sure that I thoroughly assess the systems that could be affected by this. I want to pay particular attention to the neurological, respiratory, cardiovascular, musculoskeletal, and gastrointestinal systems as embolic events can be lethal in these body systems.

❓ Given the new information what diagnostic testing should be done and in what order?

When addressing a complex patient presentation, the safest approach is to rule out the most life-threatening issues or diagnoses first. In this situation, the first diagnostic test that needs to be ordered in order to confirm the diagnosis of infective tricuspid valve regurgitation is an echocardiogram (ECHO) and blood cultures.[2] If endocarditis is confirmed by ECHO, a (CT) scan of the head, chest, abdomen, and pelvis is warranted to determine the presence or extent of possible embolic events.[2] The results of these tests can then be used to make the formal diagnosis of infective endocarditis and to evaluate potential embolic sequelae.

A complete blood count, comprehensive metabolic panel, and coagulation studies are also useful in identifying leukocytosis; hemolytic anemia as a result of valvular regurgitation; renal and hepatic dysfunction; and hypocoagulable or hypercoagulable states. Leukocytosis typically appears due to the immunologic response triggered by the infectious process of endocarditis. A low hematocrit is typically the first indication of hemolytic anemia. If suspected, further diagnostic blood tests such as haptoglobin, lactate dehydrogenase, and bilirubin levels may be used to identify if red blood cell components and metabolites are present in systemic circulation. An electrocardiogram (ECG) should be obtained as well, and although an ECG is not diagnostic for endocarditis, it can demonstrate evidence of conduction abnormalities that may be present in endocarditis.

A hemoglobin A1C, thyroid stimulating hormone and free T4 can be used to ultimately rule out endocrine pathophysiology contributing to the patient's weight loss. The HgbA1c will provide us with representation of the patient's blood glucose levels over the past 90 days, thus allowing us to determine if he has diabetes. The TSH and FT4 will provide useful information regarding his thyroid function and if hyperthyroidism is contributing to his symptoms.

CASE INFORMATION

Diagnostic Findings

A transthoracic ECHO is performed with agitated saline. The ECHO demonstrates severe tricuspid valve regurgitation with multiple vegetations on the anterior leaflet and one on the septal leaflet with the largest vegetation measuring 1.3 cm in length (Figure 28-1).

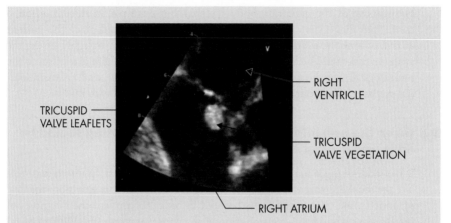

Figure 28-1 ECHO demonstrating tricuspid valve endocarditis. Used with permission from M. Shifrin.

Upon the injection of agitated saline, the ECHO shows an immediate passage of multiple bubbles from the right to left atrium, demonstrating evidence of an atrial septal defect and subsequent shunt. Fortunately, the ECHO also shows normal biventricular systolic function. CT of the chest, abdomen, and pelvis demonstrates no evidence of embolic events but did reveal an enlarged perihilar lymph node. A CT of the head demonstrates no findings of infarct, hemorrhage, or fluid collections. Given these findings, solid tumor malignancy processes can be ruled out as a differential diagnosis. Three sets of blood cultures drawn greater than 12 hours apart are positive with growth of *Streptococcus agalactiae* (Group B). The CBC is notable for leukocytosis (WBC 17.3), and his comprehensive metabolic panel was notable for hyponatremia (Na 129) and hypochloremia (Cl 90). ECG was remarkable for a right bundle branch block. His HgbA1c, TSH, and FT4 levels were unremarkable, indicating that diabetes and hyperthyroidism could be ruled out as differential diagnoses.

Case Analysis: Given these results, the patient is diagnosed with infective endocarditis using the Duke criteria.[3] The Duke Criteria is the gold standard for making a final positive diagnosis of infective endocarditis.[3] The classification considers both major and minor pathological and clinical criteria that are common in the disease process.[3,4] The patient rules in for a definite diagnosis based on meeting the major clinical criteria of persistently positive blood cultures and ECHO findings positive for infective endocarditis. He also meets two of the minor clinical criteria (predisposition to endocarditis and fever) as well. See Table 28-1 for a list of Duke Criteria.

Table 28-1   Duke Criteria for the Diagnosis of Infective Endocarditis[a]

Definite diagnosis

Pathological criteria: microorganisms identified by culture or histologic examination of a vegetation, a vegetation that has embolized, or an intracardiac abscess specimen; or active endocarditis confirmed by histologic examination of vegetation or intracardiac abscess

Clinical criteria: two major, one major and three minor, or five minor criteria

Major clinical criteria

Blood culture positive for infective endocarditis

Microorganisms typically associated with infective endocarditis identified from two separate blood cultures: viridans streptococci, *Streptococcus bovis*, bacteria in the HACEK group, or *Staphylococcus aureus*; or community-acquired enterococci in the absence of a primary focus

Microorganisms consistent with infective endocarditis identified from persistently positive blood cultures: at least two positive cultures of blood samples drawn >12h apart, or positive results of all of three or a majority of four or more separate blood cultures (with first and last samples drawn at least 1h apart)

Single positive blood culture for *Coxiella burnetii* or IgG antibody titer for Q-fever phase 1 antigen >1:800

Evidence of endocardial involvement

Echocardiogram positive for infective endocarditis: pendulum-like intracardiac mass on valve or supporting structures, in the path of regurgitant jets, or on implanted material in the absence of an alternative anatomical explanation; abscess; or new partial dehiscence of prosthetic valve[b]

New valvular regurgitation (worsening or changing of preexisting murmur not a sufficient criterion)

Minor clinical criteria

Predisposition to infective endocarditis, such as a predisposing heart condition, or intravenous drug use

Fever, defined as a temperature >38°C

Vascular phenomena, such as major arterial emboli, septic pulmonary infarcts, mycotic aneurysm, intracranial hemorrhage, conjunctival hemorrhage, and Janeway lesions

Immunologic phenomena, such as glomerulonephritis, Osler nodes, Roth spots, and rheumatoid factor

Microbiologic evidence: positive blood culture but with no major clinical criterion met or serologic evidence of active infection with an organism consistent with infective endocarditis

Possible diagnosis

Clinical criteria (see above): one major criterion and one minor criterion or three minor criteria

Rejected diagnosis

Firmly established alternative diagnosis; resolution of infective endocarditis–like syndrome with antibiotic therapy for ≤4 days; no pathological evidence of infective endocarditis at surgery or autopsy, with antibiotic therapy for ≤4 days; or criteria for possible infective endocarditis not met

[a]HACEK denotes *Haemophilus* species, *Aggregatibacter* (formerly *Actinobacillus*) *actinomycetemcomitans*, *Cardiobacterium hominis*, *Eikenella corrodens*, and *Kingella kingae*.
[b]Transesophageal echocardiography is recommended in patients with prosthetic valves and possible infective endocarditis according to clinical criteria or infective endocarditis complicated by paravalvular abscess; transthoracic echocardiography is recommended as the first test in other patients.
Source: Adapted from Li et al.[3]

Management: Infective Endocarditis

Treatment for infective endocarditis includes targeted antibiotic therapy, and when appropriate, surgical intervention.[5] In patients with a history of intravenous drug use, an oral antibiotic regimen versus IV antibiotics through a peripheral inserted central catheter (PICC) is typically preferred due to the risk of ongoing intravenous substance abuse. However, in situations where oral antibiotics are not sufficient to treat the cultured organism, patients may require inpatient intravenous antibiotic management for the duration of therapy.[2]

Surgical intervention in this case is warranted based on the patient's diagnosis with severe tricuspid valve regurgitation with large tricuspid valve vegetations and a patent atrial septal defect.[6] The type of valve repair or replacement, in this patient, is carefully considered because valve replacement with a mechanical valve requires life-long adherence to anticoagulation therapy. Frequently, a multidisciplinary and collaborative approach to decision making is needed to determine the best surgical option available.

Broad-spectrum antibiotics are started immediately in this case. These consist of antibiotics that target gram-negative and gram-positive bacteria as well as aerobic and anaerobic species. In patients who are able to tolerate β-lactams, amoxicillin-clavulanate and gentamicin are the antibiotics of choice.[7] In this case, broad-spectrum coverage is continued until the blood cultures return positive for *Streptococcus agalactiae* (Group B). Then, the antibiotic regimen is narrowed to a 14-day course of intravenous gentamycin and a 4-week course of intravenous penicillin G. Since several of his teeth are abscessed and pose an additional infective risk, oral and maxiofacial surgery is consulted for teeth extraction prior to cardiac surgery.

A collaborative approach between the infectious disease, cardiology, cardiac surgery, and social work teams is essential in determining the best surgical intervention and medical plan for the patient. After careful review of his ECHO and with consideration of his social history, the team and the patient identified tricuspid valve repair rather than a replacement as the best option.

Case Follow-Up

The patient underwent a successful tricuspid valve repair on his third hospital day of admission. His inpatient postoperative course was unremarkable. He was discharged to an inpatient rehabilitation center for substance abuse treatment and continued intravenous antibiotic therapy.

References

1. Mehta SH, Astemborski J, Kirk GD, et al. Changes in blood-borne infection risk among injection drug users. *J Infect Dis.* 2011;201:587-594. doi: 10.1093/infdis/jiq112.
2. Baddour LM, Wilson WR, Bayer AS, et al. Infective endocarditis: diagnosis, antimicrobial therapy, and management of complications: a statement for healthcare professionals from the Committee on Rheumatic Fever, Endocarditis, and Kawasaki Disease, Council on Cardiovascular Disease in the Young, and the Councils on Clinical Cardiology, Stroke, and Cardiovascular Surgery and Anesthesia, American Heart Association: endorsed by the Infectious Diseases Society of America. *Circulation.* 2005;111:e394-e434.

3. Li JS, Sexton DJ, Mick N, et al. Proposed modifications to the Duke criteria for the diagnosis of infective endocarditis. *Clin Infect Dis*. 2000;30:633-638.
4. Hoen B, Duval X. Infective endocarditis. *N Engl J Med*. 2013;369:1425-1433. doi: 10.1056/NEJMcp1206782.
5. Weymann A, Borst T, Popov AF, et al. Surgical treatment of infective endocarditis in active intravenous drug users: a justified procedure? *J Cardiothorac Surg*. 2014;24:1-8.
6. Taghavi S, Clark R, Jayarajan SN, et al. Surgical management of tricuspid valve endocarditis in systemically infected patients. *J Heart Valve Dis*. 2013;22:578-583.
7. Habib G, Hoen B, Tornos P, et al. Guidelines on the prevention, diagnosis, and treatment of infective endocarditis (new version 2009): the Task Force on the Prevention, Diagnosis, and Treatment of Infective Endocarditis of the European Society of Cardiology (ESC). *Eur Heart J*. 2009;30:2369-2413. doi: 10.1093/eurheartj/ehp285.

CASE 29

Joan E. King

Joan King is the program director for the AG-ACNP Program at Vanderbilt University. Dr King also practices as an ACNP in the Pre-anesthesia Evaluation Clinic at Vanderbilt.

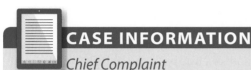

CASE INFORMATION
Chief Complaint

A 52-year-old male states, "I'm having chest pain."

❓ What are the potential causes?

There are many causes of chest pain and some are life threatening. I know that my reasoning must be inclusive of critical conditions and those that are relatively benign.

Differential Diagnoses: Chest Pain

- Cardiovascular: acute coronary syndrome: unstable angina, non–ST-segment elevation MI (NSTEMI), ST-segment MI (STEMI). Aortic aneurysm, mitral valve prolapse, pericarditis, congestive heart failure
- Respiratory: asthma, pneumonia, spontaneous pneumothorax, pulmonary embolism
- Gastrointestinal: gastroesophageal reflux disease (GERD), peptic ulcer disease, cholecystitis, Barrett esophagus, achalasia or esophageal spasms, esophageal dysmotility
- Musculoskeletal: costochondritis, rib fracture, unstable sternum

---

CASE INFORMATION
History of Present Illness (HPI)

This 52-year-old male presents to emergency department with a chief complaint of chest pain. First symptoms of chest pain started 3 months ago, but have increased in intensity over the past 2 weeks. Today the patient states his chest pain started this evening, and did not resolve with over-the-counter antacids. The patient describes the pain as a mid-epigastric burning sensation, which he rates as an 8 out of 10. He denies any radiation of the pain, but he does say he feels short of breath. Up until 3 months ago, the patient had occasional episodes of chest discomfort that he would not really describe as "pain." The discomfort resolved spontaneously and never interfered with any of his normal activities. While he denies any specific pattern to the chest discomfort he does indicate that the pain was more likely to occur at night or after going to bed, and was not related to physical activity or his diet. More recently the discomfort has occurred more frequently and has awakened him twice in the past week. Today the patient describes the symptoms as more intense and more of a true pain, and he feels that he cannot get his breath. Symptoms of shortness of breath started to accompany his symptom of chest discomfort about 1 week ago, and it develops primarily as he is lying down, and resolves if he sits upright. He denies any sense of shortness of breath when engaged in any physical activity such as walking or climbing stairs. Current vital signs are heart rate 89 beats per minute, respiratory rate 12/min blood pressure 150/90 mm Hg, temperature 98.6°F, and SaO$_2$ 98% on room air. Telemetry indicates normal sinus rhythm with no ectopy and no ST-segment changes, pulses are palpable, and the patient is warm and dry.

Past Medical History

• Hypertension × 10 years, denies diabetes
• Hospitalizations: none
• Medications: lisinopril 10 mg once daily
• Allergies: none

Family History

Positive for father who had an MI (age 70)

Social History

30 pack-year history of smoking quit 2 years ago. Alcohol: currently drinks one glass of wine once or twice a week. Denies daily consumption of alcohol. Diet: primarily fast foods. Married, two children, works as a CEO of a major software company. Exercise: walks ½ mile most days of the week.

❓ Given the information obtained so far, what are the pertinent positives and significant negatives?

• **Pertinent positives:** Severe chest pain, woke him from sleep, history of less severe episodes sporadically for a 3-month period, associated with shortness of breath, changes with position, worsening in intensity, history of smoking, history of hypertension, family history of coronary artery disease.

- **Significant negatives:** Pain is not affected by his diet or activity, pain does not radiate, shortness of breath only occurs with pain and not with activity, no history of diabetes, vital signs stable, and no evidence of arrhythmia on telemetry.

Case Analysis: While differential diagnoses are listed system by system, they also need to be prioritized from the most to the least critical. Acute coronary syndrome (ACS) is the first diagnosis to consider, because rapid diagnosis ensures early intervention, which is associated with improved outcomes. ACS is actually a grouping of three differential diagnoses, unstable angina, NSTEMI, or STEMI, with 25% to 40% of myocardial infarctions being STEMI-type infarctions.[1] While telemetry indicates that the patient is in normal sinus rhythm, telemetry only provides one lead (typically Lead II, since it documents P waves well). Obtaining a 12-lead ECG can provide information about the presence of a significant Q wave, ST-segment elevation or depression as well as information about the T wave. These data provide information related to myocardial ischemia or injury. However, it is important to note that a 12-lead ECG cannot fully rule out ACS. Some patients may be experiencing myocardial ischemia and the 12-lead ECG may fail to document these classic changes. Hence serial troponin I enzyme levels are essential for diagnosis.[2] Expected findings if the patient is having an infarction include an initial rise in the troponin I with cardiac injury and a progressive elevation in enzymes as an infarction progresses. Therefore, prior to obtaining a more detailed history and beginning the physical examination, I order a stat 12-lead ECG to look for patterns of ischemia or infarction and a stat troponin I blood level. I also add a complete metabolic profile (CMP) to the blood draw.

As I proceed with the history and physical, I note that this patient has several key pertinent positives that are risk factors for ACS, namely he is having chest pain or chest discomfort, has a history of hypertension and smoking, and a positive family history of coronary artery disease. Factors that make ACS less likely are that his chest discomfort is related to the supine position and not related to exertion or physical activity. The absence of nausea and/or diaphoresis, which may occur with an infarction but are not diagnostic, makes me less inclined to think that his pain is ACS. However, in providing initial care to this patient, I cannot eliminate an NSTEMI or STEMI based on the patient's presentation of chest pain, nor can I eliminate an infarction simply with a 12-lead ECG. Not all patients having ACS have classic signs and symptoms of an infarction, such as "crushing chest pain" or pain radiating down the left arm, nor do all infarctions present with classic ECG changes. While these are important factors to consider that may help confirm an infarction, they cannot be used to rule an infarction out.

As I consider this patient's pattern of pain and the description of his shortness of breath, I recognize that neither is consistent with pulmonary embolism or pneumothorax, so while these conditions are urgent considerations, they are currently lower on my list. His shortness of breath resolves with sitting up, and his oxygen saturation is normal so an urgent pulmonary disorder is less likely. The fact that the shortness of breath occurs only with supine positioning could be a sign of pulmonary edema or congestive heart failure or valve disease, though esophageal diseases may also be aggravated by lying flat. As I proceed to the review of systems and physical examination, my primary concern is a cardiac condition.

CASE INFORMATION

Review of Systems

- Constitutional: Generally in good health, except for the increase in chest discomfort over the past weeks (see HPI).
- Cardiovascular: hypertension × 10 years, well managed with lisinopril. Home blood pressures are 140s/80s. The patient denies history of angina, myocardial infarction, dysrhythmias or palpitations, or heart failure. The patient denies placement of any stents, or any history of mitral valve prolapse (MVP) or thoracic or abdominal aortic aneurysm. The patient indicates that he has never had a stress test or an echocardiogram.
- Pulmonary: shortness of breath × 1 week associated with chest discomfort (see HPI). The patient denies the use of inhalers, and denies any productive or dry cough. The patient denies history of chronic obstructive pulmonary disease, emphysema, asthma, or obstructive sleep apnea. Denies chest pain with inspiration.
- Gastrointestinal: The patient indicates that he periodically takes three to four antacids at night after a "heavy meal," but denies use of any H_2 blockers or proton-pump inhibitors. He indicates he occasionally wakes up with a sour taste in his mouth, and this has increased in frequency over the past 4 weeks. The patient denies any nausea or vomiting, melena, or peptic ulcers. He denies any recent weight loss, and he denies any chest discomfort after a fatty meal, or any radiation of his chest discomfort to his right shoulder. The patient states that he has never had an endoscopy, and he has never been diagnosed with gastroesophageal reflux disease.
- Musculoskeletal: The patient denies any history of costochondritis, or strain or trauma to the chest or ribs.
- Neurological: The patient denies any peripheral neuropathy or cervical or thoracic spinal pain, any history of seizures, stroke, or transient ischemic attacks (TIAs).

Physical Examination Findings

Constitutional: Pleasant male appears comfortable.
- Vital signs: heart rate 89 beats per minute, normal sinus rhythm per telemetry, respiratory rate 12/min, blood pressure 150/90 mm Hg, Temperature 98.6°F, SaO_2 98% on room air.

- Cardiovascular: Heart rate and rhythm regular. No murmurs, rubs, or gallops noted. Point of maximal impulse is the fifth intercostal space midclavicular line, and easily palpable. No jugular venous distension is present, and no carotid, aortic, or femoral bruits noted. Peripheral pulses in upper and lower extremities are 4+, no clubbing noted.
- Pulmonary: Trachea midline. Symmetrical respiratory pattern, no accessory muscle use, breath sounds clear anteriorly and posteriorly in all lobes.
- Gastrointestinal: Active bowel sounds in all four quadrants, tympany on percussion in all four quadrants. No abdominal tenderness with light or deep palpation. Unable to elicit the Murphy sign with deep palpation. Bedside stool guaiac negative.
- Musculoskeletal: No tenderness noted along the ribs bilaterally or along the sternal border.
- Neurological: The patient awake alert and oriented × 4. Pupils are equal and reactive to light. Muscle strength is 4+ in all upper and lower extremities.

12-Lead ECG

No ST- or T-wave abnormalities in any leads, and no PR depression.

Troponin I

0.02 ng/mL (>0.08 µg is considered positive for myocardial injury).

CMP (Drawn With Troponin)

Normal electrolytes and normal liver function tests.

❓ Given this new information, what additional pertinent positives and significant negatives would you add to your list?

- **Pertinent positives:** Sour taste in mouth, heavy antacid use.
- **Significant negatives:** Cardiac history and examination shows no abnormality, respiratory history and examination shows no abnormality, no trauma, no tenderness, ECG indicates no ischemia or infarction and troponin I is within normal limits.

❓ How does this additional information affect your list of possible causes?

The data about the characteristics of the chest pain such as location, radiation, timing, and other associated symptoms were derived from very specific questions asked in the HPI. In this particular case, the chest pain is nonradiating, has occurred previously, but now is associated with shortness of breath. An STEMI or NSTEMI is no longer the top of my differential list because he has no history of an MI or stent placement, and his 12-lead ECG is normal as is his initial troponin I level. However, another diagnosis to consider, which falls in the acute coronary syndrome family, is unstable angina. Unstable angina refers to angina that is either of new onset or has changed in quality or frequency. Unstable angina is pain that results from cardiac ischemia but does not cause ECG changes or an elevation in troponin levels. This patient may be experiencing unstable angina which would be a new diagnosis for him, but before this can be determined a nuclear stress test or a stress echocardiogram must be done.

I asked questions related to a potential dissecting aortic aneurysm such as a tearing or shearing sensation that may have accompanied his chest pain. His vital signs are stable and the patient denies these symptoms but to definitively rule this out an echocardiogram and/or CT scan would need to be done. For now this is very low on my list but cannot be totally eliminated.

When sorting through differential diagnoses, a system by system approach is helpful. Additional cardiovascular diagnoses include mitral valve prolapse, and pericarditis. In order to gain more data related to these two conditions, the cardiac examination needs to include auscultation of the heart specifically listening for a possible systolic murmur or a pericardial friction rub. Also if a stress echocardiogram is ordered to rule out unstable angina or ischemic chest pain, the echocardiogram will also diagnose both mitral valve prolapse and a pericardial effusion, which may be related to pericarditis. The echocardiogram can also note the structure of the aortic valve and if there is any evidence of an aneurysm in the ascending aorta. Hence, I will order a stress echocardiogram in order to gain more specific information about the mitral valve, pericardium, aortic valve, ascending aorta, and to identify the presence of any ischemia.

Once I have considered possible life-threatening cardiovascular differentials, I begin focusing on the pulmonary system. Pulmonary conditions include asthma, pneumonia, or a spontaneous pneumothorax. In reviewing this patient's signs and symptoms, he does not have a prior history of asthma, and his symptom of shortness of breath is a new finding, while his symptoms of chest discomfort have been ongoing. I do consider the possible diagnoses of pneumonia or spontaneous pneumothorax but the patient is afebrile, does not have a cough, and his SaO_2 is 98%. In addition, his stable vital signs do not support either condition, and he is not presenting with any symptoms of being "air hungry." His shortness of breath appears to be an associated symptom, and not his primary chief complaint. In order to definitively rule out pneumonia and pneumothorax, the physical examination needs to evaluate the presence or absence of breath sounds and quality of the breath sounds which in this case are normal. Diagnostics would include a chest x-ray, and white blood cell count.

I believe there are no true neurological diagnoses to consider given his examination and history. But it is still very important to do a brief neurological assessment looking for any comorbidities that may impact his care. For example, assessing specifically for a past history of seizures, stroke, or TIAs is important so that I have an accurate baseline. This will help me anticipate any potential new problems, particularly if this patient's blood pressure were to become unstable.

I have ruled out potentially life-threatening cardiovascular and respiratory disorders, or have placed them very low on my differential. I have confirmed that the patient is stable so now focus on the gastrointestinal (GI) system. Diagnoses that require consideration include gastroesophageal reflux disease (GERD), peptic ulcer disease, cholecystitis, Barrett esophagus, or esophageal motility disorders such as achalasia or esophageal spasms. In sorting through these diagnoses, a key consideration is if the patient is experiencing dysphagia. In order to ensure that the patient truly understands this question, I ask specifically, "Do you have any trouble swallowing or a sense that you are choking? Do you ever have the sense that food is getting stuck or won't go down?" Very few patients will understand the term dysphagia, but they will most likely understand the concept "difficulty swallowing."

Additional data I need to gather at this point include the patient's weight and the relationship of the chest pain/discomfort with eating. Chest discomfort associated with peptic ulcer disease frequently occurs 30 to 60 minutes after eating or when lying down. Another question to ask, "When you lay down at night do you ever have the sense that you have vomited stomach contents?" New onset hoarseness or frequent laryngitis can indicate that the patient is refluxing and the acidic gastric contents are irritating to the vocal cords. Patients with reflux also report occasionally awakening with a cough or a need to "clear my throat."

Patients with cholecystitis often report that the discomfort/pain is worse after a fatty meal, and that the pain radiates to the right shoulder.[3] These specific questions help me reprioritize the gastrointestinal diagnoses on my differential. In exploring this patient's history more thoroughly I find that the patient does have a sense of regurgitating stomach contents when he lies down at night but he denies any hoarseness or laryngitis. He also denies any chest discomfort that radiates to the right shoulder (the Murphy sign). However, because unstable angina is still a viable differential, a stress echocardiogram is ordered and the patient is admitted for 23-hour observation.

Finally the last system to assess is the musculoskeletal system looking primarily for a skeletal problem that could produce chest discomfort. A prior history of chest trauma or a history of costochondritis could explain intermittent chest pain as well as shortness of breath. In the review of systems, the patient indicated that he had never been diagnosed with costochondritis and that he denies any chest trauma.

CASE INFORMATION

Diagnostic Testing Results

• Stress echocardiogram: no ischemic changes with increased heart rate, and no evidence of an infarction. The echocardiogram also shows normal valve function, a normal ejection fraction of 55%, and the absence of a pericardial effusion.

- Chest x-ray: no acute cardiopulmonary disease, heart normal in size, no infiltrates, effusions, or pneumothorax
- Follow up troponin level: less than 10 ng/mL

❓ How does the new additional diagnostic information affect your list of causes?

At this point I can rule out the life-threatening cardiopulmonary differential diagnoses, including NSTEMI, STEMI, pneumothorax, and trauma. My physical examination also rules out cholecystitis. Remaining on my differential list are decreased esophageal motility, esophageal spasm, esophageal or peptic ulcers, Barrett esophagus, and GERD. Narrowing this list of differentials is also very important; given that GERD is the most common of these diagnoses, it is most likely. Reflecting back to the patient's history and review of symptoms he denies symptoms of dysphagia or difficulty swallowing, which makes decreased esophageal motility less likely. To help me sort the remaining differentials, I will order an upper endoscopy as an outpatient test. This test will permit direct visualization of the esophagus including areas of ulceration or changes in the mucosa that indicate Barrett esophagus. Barrett esophagus is particularly important to identify because it can be a precursor to cancer.[4] At this point I am becoming more confident that my patient has GERD.

Diagnosis and Treatment: GERD

In the United States approximately 20% of adults have symptoms related to GERD, and this diagnosis is a reasonable one for this patient as well.[4] Recommendations for treatment focus on decreasing acid production with a proton-pump inhibitor (PPI) such as omeprazole 40 mg once daily. It may take up to 3 months for the symptoms to fully resolve, and patient education is also a key treatment strategy.[4] The American Gastroenterological Association recommends avoiding highly acidic foods such as tomatoes, and foods that may relax the esophageal sphincter such as coffee, chocolate, or peppermints.[5] With GERD now rising to my number one "working diagnosis," I will start the patient on 40 mg omeprazole daily, and refer the patient to a gastroenterologist for an upper endoscopy. While my hope is that omeprazole will control his symptoms, the upper endoscopy will help rule out esophageal ulcers or Barrett esophagus.

If the patient continues to remain symptomatic both esophageal spasm or achalasia should be considered. As noted a detailed history exploring any new symptoms of choking or difficulty swallowing along with weight loss would merit an esophageal motility study. This study will determine if he has esophageal spasms or if his lower esophageal sphincter is unable to relax, which occurs with achalasia.[5]

Case Follow-Up

Obtaining a detailed history is essential to establish and prioritize a workable differential diagnosis. Critical diagnoses related to ACS are time dependent since "time is muscle." If a patient presents with atypical chest pain that is due to a myocardial infarction, taking steps to revascularize the myocardium with either stents or thrombolytics is vital. Differentials related to the respiratory system also need to be quickly identified in order to prevent a life-threatening situation such as hypoxia or respiratory failure. Once the life-threatening diagnoses are eliminated, the list of diagnoses can be sorted system by system to avoid overlooking a potential cause. My goal as I approached this patient with "chest pain" was to avoid "satisfaction of search." Satisfaction of search occurs when a provider stops considering other possible differentials, after identifying a single most likely cause. With this patient, I might have been tempted to diagnose GERD without carefully considering the possibility of cardiac disease, or I might have rushed the patient to a cardiac catheterization without considering the gastrointestinal disorders that can cause these symptoms. In this case GERD is very likely the final diagnosis, but one needs to also be aware that this patient may be having esophageal spasms, which could put the patient at risk for aspiration, or Barrett esophagus, which is associated with a risk of esophageal cancer.

What are the next steps for this patient? Cardiac disease has not been completely eliminated. This patient does have risk factors, but his stress echocardiogram is negative, so he is stable for discharge the following morning. Prior to discharge the patient is instructed to avoid foods that trigger reflux and to keep a food diary, as well as begin taking omeprazole 40 mg daily. He is also encouraged to document any further episodes of chest pain and any associated activities or other symptoms that accompany chest discomfort. While this patient had a negative stool guaiac, the possibility of a peptic ulcer has not been fully ruled out, hence I do not begin this patient on a prophylactic aspirin regimen related to his cardiovascular history until the upper endoscopy confirms the absence of an ulcer. If the upper endoscopy is normal and this patient remains symptomatic, the next test to consider would be an esophageal manometry.[5] This test will document esophageal motility and possible issues related to the lower esophageal sphincter (LES) such as an inability for the LES to relax or an increase in LES tone. The last differential diagnosis to consider for this patient is cancer. This patient denies any weight loss, his symptoms appear to be positional, and while they are increasing in severity this is the first time he has sought medical treatment. If I thought that gastric or esophageal cancer was a high probability I would order an abdominal ultrasound in the ED, and a CT scan following the stress test. However, given his symptoms, his negative stool guaiac, a normal abdominal examination, and no weight loss, I would first treat this patient with a proton-pump inhibitor and then reevaluate him in 2 weeks to determine if the symptoms have resolved.

References

1. O'Gara PT, Hushner FG, Ascheim DD, et al. 2013 ACF/AHA guideline for the management of ST-elevation myocardial infarction. *J Am Coll Cardiol*. 2013;61(4). http://content.onlinejacc.org.
2. Godara H, Hirbe A, Nassif M, Otepka H, Rosenstock A, eds. Ischemic heart disease. *The Washington Manual of Medical Therapeutics*. Philadelphia, PA: Lippincott Williams & Wilkins; 2014:112-170.

3. McPhee SJ, Papadakis MA, eds. Liver, biliary tract and pancreatic disorders. *Current Medical Diagnosis & Treatment*. New York, NY: McGraw-Hill; 2012:475-519.

4. McPhee SJ, Papadakis MA, eds. Gastrointestinal disorders. *Current Medical Diagnosis & Treatment*. New York, NY: McGraw-Hill; 2012;546-643.

5. Hiltz SW, Black E, Modlin IM, et al. American Gastroenterological Association Medical Position Statement on the management of gastroesophageal reflux disease. *Gastroenterology*. 2008;135: 1383-1391.

CASE 30

Charles Fisher

Charles Fisher works as an ACNP in the Medical ICU at the University of Virginia and previously was an ACNP in the MICU step-down unit caring for long-term critically ill patients. His background spans many years as a critical care nurse in a thoracic-cardiovascular ICU.

CASE INFORMATION
Chief Complaint

A 69-year-old male with a history of alcoholic cirrhosis presented in the emergency department (ED) with recent bloody bowel movements and worsening abdominal, scrotal, and leg swelling. He is anemic with hemoglobin of 8.9 g/dL (male normal = 13.5–16.5) on ED admission, but his hemoglobin is now 6.4 g/dL. I am called for a medical intensive care unit (MICU) consultation and for possible transfer to the MICU service.

❓ What are the potential causes of this patient's symptoms?

The patient's history and drop in blood count are concerning for a gastrointestinal bleed (GIB), in either the upper or lower gastrointestinal tract. The best way for me to ensure that I arrive at an appropriate diagnosis is to begin with a comprehensive differential for both upper and lower GIB. But prior to doing so I must determine if he is in imminent life-threatening danger from bleeding. If he is, emergent intervention is necessary. I must evaluate his current status quickly. To do so I take a general survey of the patient.

CASE INFORMATION
Initial Survey

I first see the patient in the ED. The ED service obtained a stat complete blood count, type and screen, and the patient's consent for blood transfusions. He is currently being transfused with his first of 2 units of packed red blood cells. He has two large bore peripheral lines in place. The patient is alert and interactive, able to answer questions, and denies pain or shortness of breath. His vital signs are blood pressure 109/55 mm Hg lying at 45° head elevation with a mean arterial pressure (MAP) of 73 mm Hg, heart rate 95 beats per minute, respiratory rate 26/min.

Case Analysis: His admission hemoglobin was extremely low and he clearly requires transfusions. At this point his condition is somewhat stable but he will require close monitoring of his vital signs, frequent checks of his blood counts, a thorough history, and physical to determine the source of the bleed, and rapid treatment to prevent further bleeding. I quickly consider potential causes of GI bleeding and separate them into upper and lower causes.

Comprehensive Differential Diagnoses for Patient With Upper GIB[1]

- Peptic ulcer disease (commonly due to infection with *Helicobacter pylori*)
- Gastritis: nonsteroidal anti-inflammatory drugs (NSAIDs), steroids, alcohol, burns, and trauma.
- Esophageal varices: liver disease, alcoholic liver cirrhosis, portal vein thrombosis
- Mallory-Weiss tear: forceful vomiting or retching, coughing, lifting, straining, childbirth, or even laughing
- Cancer: early sign of esophageal or stomach cancers
- Inflammation: NSAIDs, aspirin, alcohol, and cigarette smoking promote gastric ulcer formation

Comprehensive Differential Diagnoses for Patient With Lower GIB[2]

- Diverticulosis: One of the most common causes of GI bleed, occurs when outpockets (diverticula) form in the wall of the colon and with constipation and strain during a bowel movement, begins to bleed.
- Angiodysplasia: Another common cause of lower GI bleeding with malformation of blood vessels in the GI tract. Seen in the elderly and patients with chronic kidney failure.
- Colitis: Infectious, ischemic colitis and inflammatory bowel disease (IBD) can all present initially with hematochezia.
- Infectious colitis: The most common of the causes of infectious colitis are *Salmonella*, *Campylobacter*, and *Shigella*, identified by stool culture.
- Inflammatory bowel disease: Inflammatory bowel disease refers to both Crohn disease and ulcerative colitis. Hematochezia is a more common initial presentation with ulcerative colitis.
- Cancers: An early sign of colon or rectal cancers will be bloody stools. Cancer bleeding tends to be low-grade and recurrent. Bright red blood suggests left-sided lesions as opposed to right-sided lesions with maroon blood or melena.
- Polyps: Noncancerous tumors of the GI tract mostly in people older than 40 years of age, and these may transform into cancer.
- Hemorrhoids, anal fissures, and miscellaneous disorders: Hemorrhoids are swollen veins proximal to the anus with bleeding that is intermittent

and bright red. Anal fissures, or tears in the anal wall, may also cause bright red blood and occur with forceful straining and constipation or hard stools. Other disorders associated with bleeding include solitary rectal ulcers, rectal varices, and Dieulafoy lesions.

- Radiation telangiectasia or proctitis: Radiation therapy of abdominal and pelvic cancers can lead to lower gastrointestinal bleeding as either an early or late complication of radiation damage. Ulceration or cancer recurrence can also be seen as late complications following radiation therapy. These entities must be excluded in patients with rectal bleeding.

- Following biopsy or polypectomy: Bleeding following endoscopic biopsy or polypectomy is usually self-limited, although active arterial bleeding can occur acutely.

- Pharmacology induced: Bleeding occurs secondary to anticoagulant or antiplatelet medications, such as aspirin and clopidogrel. Warfarin interactions with aspirin, NSAIDs, antiplatelet agents (eg, clopidogrel), antibiotics, amiodarone, statins, fibrates also increases the risk of GI bleeding.

While this patient's drop in hemoglobin could have other causes, gastrointestinal bleeding is the most likely to cause this degree of change and the patient reports blood in his stools. The patient's cirrhosis contributes to his risk of GIB in two important ways. First, portal hypertension causes pressure in the vessels of the gastrointestinal track creating varices, which are friable and bleed easily. In addition, compromised intrinsic liver function causes a deficit of clotting factors, which leads to elevated clotting times, so that any bleeding that occurs may result in a large volume loss. An additional consideration is that the excessive alcohol consumption that led to this patient's cirrhosis is also a risk factor for GI cancers including esophageal, colorectal, and liver carcinomas.[3] After reviewing all the possible causes of GI bleeding, I begin collecting more data from the patient. Although I know from my initial survey that he is hemodynamically stable, I consult the GI service as I am fairly confident that he will require endoscopic evaluation to determine the source of his bleeding. I also initiate transfer to the MICU for further stabilization and management. I write admission orders and start twice daily intravenous pantoprazole 40 mg (a proton-pump inhibitor) as its use has demonstrated improved clinical outcomes by stabilizing blood clots and reducing gastric pH levels.[4]

CASE INFORMATION

History of Present Illness

The patient states that he saw his primary care provider 2 weeks ago and had routine blood work done. After the appointment, his doctor called and told him that his potassium level was 5.9 (Normal = 3.5–5.2 mEq/L) and his creatinine was 1.6 (Normal = 0.7–1.4 mg/dL) (above his baseline of 1.2). The PCP advised discontinuing Lasix, spironolactone, and potassium supplementation. In the subsequent 2 weeks, the patient developed increasing swelling in his legs, abdomen, and scrotum, and most recently, bloody bowel movements. These symptoms prompted his visit to the emergency department (ED) today. He denies dizziness, hematemesis, and recent NSAID or aspirin use. ED laboratory values of note included a sodium of 124 (Normal = 135–147 mEq/L), potassium of 5.0 mmol/L, blood urea nitrogen (BUN) 36 mg/dL (Normal = 7–20 mg/dL), and a creatinine of 1.8 mg/dL (Normal = .5–1.4 mg/dL). His initial ED complete blood count (CBC) showed a hemoglobin of 8.9 g/dL and hematocrit 24.1% (male normal = 41%–50%) but a second CBC drawn 2 hours later showed a hemoglobin of 6.4 g/dL, a hematocrit of 19.5%, and a platelet count of 107 × 10³/µL. He was transfused with 2 units of blood and transferred to the MICU for management of his GI bleed.

Past Medical History

Past medical history includes hepatic encephalopathy, esophageal varices, portal hypertensive gastropathy, ascites, peptic ulcer disease, and history of alcohol abuse since a teenager. He was diagnosed with alcoholic cirrhosis over 7 years ago. Three months prior to this admission he was admitted with an upper GI bleed. At that time, he underwent esophagogastroduodenoscopy (EGD) showing a 1.3-cm duodenal ulcer with a visible oozing vessel, which was injected with epinephrine, clipped and cauterized during the EGD. He also had a prophylactic embolization of his gastroduodenal artery by interventional radiology. He was discharged home to the care of his primary care provider on day 4, and has had no further bleeding since. The hospital record also shows that he had an EGD done 4 years ago, which showed two columns of low-grade varices but none were in evidence during his last admission.

Social History

- Nonsmoker.
- Quit alcohol 7 years ago when diagnosed with cirrhosis.
- Family: He has no close immediate family, but a designated health care power of attorney is in the chart.
- Allergies: No known allergies

Home Medications

- Lactulose 30 g four times a day
- Spironolactone 25 mg daily (on hold)
- Furosemide 40 mg daily (on hold)
- Potassium 10 mEq daily (on hold)
- Esomeprazole 40 mg capsule, two times daily

- Folic acid 1 mg daily
- Magnesium oxide 400 mg tablet, two tablets daily
- Thiamine 100 mg tablet, one tablet daily
- Multivitamin one tablet once a day

? What are the pertinent positives from the information given so far?

- Acute drop in hemoglobin and hematocrit.
- Recent history of hematochezia.
- Three months ago, he had a GI bleed and there were varices seen on an endoscopy 4 years ago.
- He is fully oriented and cooperative showing no signs of hepatic encephalopathy.
- The patient was taken off home diuretics 2 weeks ago.
- The patient has swelling in his abdomen, legs, and scrotum.
- The patient's labs show mild acute kidney injury, slightly worse than baseline despite discontinuing diuretics.

? What are the significant negatives from the information given so far?

- The patient is not hypotensive or tachycardic.
- No current hematochezia or hematemesis.
- He has no other significant chronic conditions at this time, is fully capable of self-care, and adheres to his medical therapy and primary care provider management strategies.

? Given the information so far what is your problem representation? How does this information affect the list of possible causes?

The problem representation in this case might be: This 69-year-old man with known alcoholic cirrhosis and GIB in the past is now admitted with an acute GIB of undetermined location requiring transfusion and probable acute kidney injury (AKI) and electrolyte disturbances due to chronic diuretic use.

Case Analysis: This patient presents with what is likely to be an upper GI bleed secondary to his cirrhosis such as from varices. But he has also had ulcers in the past so they cannot be ruled out as the cause. And lower GI causes must also be considered. Gastroenterology examination with an EGD and possible colonoscopy to visual the lower GI tract is the gold standard for diagnosing the source of a GI bleed. Based on his history, I can rule out medication-related bleeding (he is not on warfarin, NSAIDs, or any other blood thinners) and this is not bleeding that results from radiation exposure, trauma, or recent procedures as he has none of these in his history. I will need to do a complete history and physical to further consider the diagnoses on my differential. In addition to closely following his blood counts and knowing that anemia can be multifactorial, I will order labs to evaluate for iron deficiency anemia including serum iron, ferritin, and vitamin B_{12}.

When caring for patients with acute blood loss, consideration also needs to be given to the consequences of blood loss on the patient's other systems. For this reason, I order an ECG and cardiac enzymes to evaluate for myocardial infarction or stress on the myocardium due to loss of oxygen-carrying capacity due to his low hemoglobin. I also order oxygen at 2 liters per minute per nasal cannula to protect him from hypoxemia. Patients with GI bleeding can lose a lot of blood quickly so he will need continuous monitoring in the ICU. My admission orders include CBC to be drawn every 4 hours, along with serial chemistries, coagulation studies, and ionized calcium every 8 hours; a type and screen to be repeated every 3 days, normal saline IV boluses as needed to keep MAP over 65 mm Hg, and nothing by mouth pending evaluation by gastroenterology.

I am also concerned about his renal function, given the rising creatinine and BUN noted initially by his primary care provider. One explanation is that the patient had some blood loss prior to the lab work done by the primary care provider and the accumulation of blood in his stomach caused his BUN and creatinine to rise. Other considerations are pre-renal kidney injury due to hypovolemia, intrinsic kidney disease due to damage to the kidney tissue itself, or an obstructive process such as prostatic hypertrophy that blocks the flow of urine out of the bladder. This patient's most likely cause of AKI is pre-renal since he has lost fluid with bleeding. If this is the case, then his kidney function should stabilize with appropriate fluid resuscitation. I need to also consider the possibility that his liver disease has progressed and is transitioning to hepatorenal failure, which is the result of changes in intestinal circulation that alter blood flow and blood vessel tone in the kidneys. If he is now in hepatorenal failure he may require additional treatment, including the possible use of continuous renal replacement therapy. For this reason, I will consider consulting the Nephrology Service.

CASE INFORMATION

Review of Systems

- Constitutional: Negative for fevers, chills or weight loss, nausea or vomiting.
- Head/eyes/ears/nose/throat: Negative for sore throat, rhinorrhea, tinnitus, or hearing loss. Negative for blurred vision and double vision. Wears glasses for reading.
- Cardiovascular: Negative for chest pain or palpitations, positive for bilateral leg swelling.

- Pulmonary: Negative for shortness of breath or wheezing.
- Gastrointestinal: Negative for nausea, vomiting, abdominal pain, diarrhea, constipation. Positive for blood on toilet paper after wiping prior to admission. He has been having three to six dark bowel movements/day and is taking lactulose three times a day.
- Genitourinary: Negative for dysuria, urgency, and frequency. Positive for scrotal edema. Reports decrease in urine output since stopping diuretics with slightly darker urine.
- Integumentary: Skin intact. Negative for itching and rashes. Positive for jaundice, unknown duration.
- Musculoskeletal: Negative for myalgias, back pain, and joint pain.
- Neurological: Negative for dizziness, sensory changes, speech changes, or focal weakness. He denies episodes of confusion but has had day-night reversal for the last week. Denies falls.
- Endocrine: Denies diabetes, or thyroid disorder.

Physical Examination

- Vital signs: Blood pressure 101/56 mm Hg sitting, 105/60 mm Hg lying, pulse 89 beats per minute, temp 35.6°C (96.1°F) oral, respirations 19/min, 96% saturation on room air. Mildly anxious adult male, no acute distress, and well nourished, weight 12 lb higher than at the primary care provider visit 2 weeks ago.
- Head/eyes/ears/nose/throat: Oropharynx is clear with moist mucous membranes, scleral icterus, neck supple, and no lymphadenopathy.
- Cardiovascular: Regular rate and rhythm, no rubs or gallops, 2/6 systolic murmur lower sternal boarder (LSB).
- Pulmonary: Respirations even and unlabored. Crackles at bilateral bases.
- Gastrointestinal: Distended, normoactive bowel sounds, soft, nontender, no flank dullness, negative for fluid wave. Rectum: Dark brown stool with minimal streaks of old dark blood, no hemorrhoids noted with direct rectal examination, guaiac positive.
- Genitourinary: Scrotal edema otherwise normal.
- Integumentary: Warm and dry, no rashes, jaundice, erythema, bruising.
- Musculoskeletal: No clubbing or cyanosis, 3+ edema to hips and on abdomen, 2+ ankle edema, 2+ pulses bilaterally.
- Neurological: Alert and oriented to person, place, and time, no asterixis, no clonus.
- Lymphatic: No lymphadenopathy.
- Psychiatric: Normal mood and affect.

CASE INFORMATION

Diagnostic Testing

- After 2 units of blood, hemoglobin = 8.2 g/dL and hematocrit = 25.4%. Platelets stable at 121 × 103/μL.
- INR = 2.2
- BUN = 45 mg/dL Creatinine = 2.2 (N = 0.7–1.4 mg/dL)
- Albumin = 1.8 g/dL (N = 3.5–5 g/dL)
- Ammonia level 12 mg/dL (N = 15–45 μg/dL)
- Troponins: negative
- ECG: normal sinus rhythm, no ischemic changes

Case Analysis: Given the information collected so far, I suspect an upper GIB is the likely source as he has cirrhosis, a history of varices, and a prior EGD that found a duodenal ulcer. His cirrhosis is well controlled at this time, but he may need lactulose enemas if he shows signs of encephalopathy, and his acute bleed increases the risk of encephalopathy. He will remain nothing by mouth (NPO) for the EGD, and if the EGD is negative he will be prepped for a colonoscopy in the morning. My main concern is maintaining a stable hemoglobin and hematocrit until the EGD is done. I will follow all the labs, give fluids to promote urine output, and provide transfusions to keep his hemoglobin >8 and hematocrit >25. Though I cannot rule out a lower GI bleed without further testing, I am less concerned that this is a lower GI bleed.

He has generalized anasarca and this is likely due to his hypoalbuminemia because his liver is not producing adequate albumin stores. This in combination with his elevated BUN and creatinine suggest acute kidney injury (AKI), which I suspect is due to pre-renal causes including bleeding (hypovolemia) and third spacing which refers to the movement of intravascular fluid into the tissues or extravascular space. Fluid and blood infusions will improve his pre-renal volume depletion and his renal function will be monitored carefully. My task now is to determine the cause of his GI bleed while I support him hemodynamically.

❓ What diagnostic tests would be helpful at this point and in what order?

The decision related to what diagnostic test should be done emergently for an acute brisk bleed is made in consultation with the GI service and the interventional radiology (IR) team. A key consideration is the availability of the specialists and the speed with which a procedure can be performed. If the GI team is ready to perform an endoscopy, then that is the usual route taken, particularly in case like this, where upper GI bleed is likely based on the patient's history. In addition, EGD offers the opportunity to both diagnose and treat the bleed, with direct cauterization, banding of varices, hemoclips, or the injection of epineph-rine.[4-6] The choice of therapy is based on the findings of the EGD.

An alternative to EGD, particularly if the patient does not respond to transfusion and appears to be continuing to bleed at a brisk pace, is transfer to the IR department.[4] In IR, the site of the bleeding can be identified via angi-ography with a femoral sheath in place, allowing insertion of coils for emboli-zation, once again permitting simultaneous diagnosis and treatment. A third option is to send the patient for a computerized tomography vascular scan to identify arterial or venous bleeding. This is usually done when patients have recurrent drops in hemoglobin over several days, indicating a persistent slow bleed.[5] The downside of starting with a CT scan is that this procedure requires contrast, and further IV contrast will need to be provided if the patient is then taken to IR for embolization. Doubling the exposure to contrast is far from ideal given that I already have concerns about this patient's kidney function. A final diagnostic study to consider at this point is a tagged red blood cell study, which will identify the source of a bleed, if the bleeding is occurring at a rapid pace.[5] The downside of tagged red blood cell studies is that if the bleeding is not brisk, the results are inconclusive. The discussion of planned procedures should always take into account the likely source, success in finding a bleed, and the amount of radiopaque dye load required.

Colonoscopy is the gold standard for evaluating for lower GI bleed, including diverticulosis, angiodysplasia, colitis, cancers, polyps, and the rarer disorders such as rectal ulcers, rectal varices, and Dieulafoy lesions.[6] This patient does not have hemorrhoids, nor has he had diarrhea or radiation therapy or a recent procedure and his medication history does not suggest a causal agent. For these reasons lower GI bleed is less likely to be the source of this patient's acute anemia. Colonoscopy also requires bowel preparation for complete visualization of the lower GI tract. The patient does not have a history of cancer but his age and his history of alcohol use are significant risks for new malignancy. If no source of bleeding is identified with EGD or colonoscopy, a full CT of the abdomen and pelvis will be needed to further evaluate for tumor sites.

Management: GI Bleed

In consultation with the GI service, we proceed with EGD as the diagnostic and therapeutic modality of choice. Prior to undergoing this procedure, I consider the need to intubate the patient for airway protection. Airway is often a concern in patients with upper GI bleed, particularly if they are vomiting blood, and requiring sedation for procedures. This patient was known to tolerate EGD without intuba-tion in the past, and he is not vomiting or reporting any nausea. The GI service proceeds with EGD using conscious sedation and identifies a bleeding gastric ulcer. This is treated with epinephrine injection, and the patient tolerates the procedure without any complication. He is placed on a pantoprazole infusion following the procedure and there is no evidence of further bleeding.[4]

A key consideration in the management of this patient with large volume GI bleed is the frequency of monitoring. Prior to the EGD, I continue to draw labs at 4-hour intervals to assess for bleeding, and every 8 hours to check chemistry and ionized calcium. The reason for checking ionized calcium is to replace the calcium should the ionized level fall as banked blood has citrate phosphorus dextrose adenine added as an anticoagulant preservative. This chemical quickly reduces the blood level of ionized calcium as it binds with the calcium in blood transfusions. The drop in ionized calcium can lead to further hypotension during acute bleeding and must be monitored and replaced as needed. Once the hemoglobin/hematocrit has stabilized, the frequency of lab draws is reduced to every 6 hours postprocedure, then to every 12 hours if completely stable 24 hours after the procedure.

My management of this patient's GIB included the infusion of IV fluid boluses as well as transfusions. So I need to evaluate his fluid status carefully. I order a complete abdomen ultrasound to determine the volume of ascites present, and to evaluate the kidneys, liver, and liver portal vein flow to rule out obstructive kidney disease and evaluate for worsening cirrhosis. I also obtain a chest film to evaluate for pulmonary edema, especially given the presence of bilateral crackles on examination. These results are reassuring. There is an insufficient volume of fluid in his abdomen to require paracentesis and his chest x-ray shows only mild pleural effusions. In addition, with fluid resuscitation, his BUN and creatinine fall, suggesting that his acute kidney injury was pre-renal due to volume depletion and making further work up unnecessary.

The patient's cirrhosis and recent bleed create a risk of hepatic encephalopathy so ongoing monitoring of his neurological status is warranted. Once the procedure is over and he is able to take medications by mouth, I resume his home dose of lactulose and add an as needed dose so that the nurses can titrate to ensure he has at least two to three loose to soft bowel movements per day. The patient's cirrhosis and mild ascites create a risk of spontaneous bacterial peritonitis (SBP), a frequent cause of morbidity in this patient population. Per guidelines, I start him on IV ceftriaxone for SBP prophylaxis.[7]

Case Follow-Up

Over the course of his remaining hospital stay, the patient's hemoglobin/hematocrit remains stable and he is transferred to the floor and followed by the GI service. Orders for labs to be drawn every 12 hours (as described earlier) are written upon transfer. His diuretics are resumed on his third day in the hospital and his edema is negligible prior to discharge. The GI service elects to schedule a colonoscopy at a later date for routine screening based on his age. He is scheduled for a follow-up appointment in 1 week with his primary care provider and in 4 weeks with the GI service with weekly labs to follow his hemoglobin/hematocrit and chemistries. His BUN and creatinine continue to fall during the hospital course and return to his prior levels. These will be followed for the next few weeks with resumption of his diuretics.

References

1. Rockey DC, Feldman M, Travis A. Major causes of upper gastrointestinal bleeding in adults. UpToDate Web site. http://www.uptodate.com/contents/major-causes-of-upper-gastrointestinal-bleeding-in-adults. Updated August 14, 2013. Accessed August 29, 2014.

2. Strate L. Etiology of lower gastrointestinal bleeding in adults. UpToDate Web site. http://www.uptodate.com/contents/etiology-of-lower-gastrointestinal-bleeding-in-adults. Updated November 15, 2013. Accessed November 4, 2014.

3. Alcohol and cancer risk. National Cancer Institute Web site: http://www.cancer.gov/cancertopics/factsheet/Risk/alcohol. Reviewed June 24, 2013. Accessed Nov 26, 2014.

4. Saltzman JR, Feldman M, Travis AC. Overview of the treatment of bleeding peptic ulcers. UpToDate Web site. http://www-uptodate-com.proxy.its.virginia.edu/contents/overview-of-the-treatment-of-bleeding-peptic-ulcers. Updated November 21, 2014. Accessed November 26, 2014.

5. Saltzman JR, Feldman M, Travis AC. Approach to acute upper gastrointestinal bleeding in adults. UpToDate Web site. http://www.uptodate.com/contents/approach-to-acute-upper-gastrointestinal-bleeding-in-adults. Updated May 16, 2014. Accessed August 29, 2014.

6. ASGE Standards of Practice Committee, Early DS, Ben-Menachem T, et al. Appropriate use of GI endoscopy. *Gastrointest Endosc.* 2012;75(6):1127.

7. Alaniz C, Regal RE. Spontaneous bacterial peritonitis: a review of treatment options. National Center for Biotechnology Information Web site. http://www.ncbi.nlm.nih.gov/pmc/articles/PM2697093/. Accessed November 27, 2014.

CASE 31

Cynthia Wolfe

Cynthia Wolfe works as an ACNP in a step-down cardiac surgery unit at the University of Virginia. Cynthia's main focus is the care of postsurgical patients.

CASE INFORMATION

Chief Complaint

Day 8, post-op from bioprosthetic aortic valve replacement, the patient tearfully states, "I thought this surgery would make me feel better but it hasn't. I still have trouble breathing."

❓ What are the potential causes?

Shortness of breath following open heart surgery with a complicated post-operative course has a long list of potential causes. My highest priority is to determine if the patient has a life-threatening condition requiring urgent intervention.

> **Comprehensive Differential Diagnoses for Patient With Dyspnea[1]**
> • Neurologic: acute stroke, neuromuscular disease
> • Cardiovascular: myocardial infarction, aortic dissection, valve failure, pericardial tamponade, acute on chronic systolic heart failure, cardiac arrhythmias, failing aortic valve, fluid overload, atrial fibrillation
> • Pulmonary: pulmonary embolism, pulmonary hypertension, hypoxia, pleural effusion, pneumothorax, ventilator-associated pneumonia, chronic obstructive pulmonary disease, asthma
> • Gastrointestinal: ascites, gastroesophageal reflux disease
> • Renal: acute kidney injury
> • Hematologic: anemia due to blood loss or chronic disease
> • Psychological: anxiety, panic attacks
> • Physiologic: deconditioning, obesity

CASE INFORMATION

History of Present Illness

This is a 55-year-old woman with a past medical history of morbid obesity, diabetes mellitus type 2, sleep apnea (uses bilevel positive airway pressure, BiPAP, at night), heart failure, and aortic stenosis who successfully received a bioprosthetic aortic valve replacement 8 days ago. She is being transferred from the ICU to the cardiovascular intermediate care unit for further postoperative management and care. This is the patient's second hospital admission for aortic valve stenosis. One month ago, she was admitted with progressive dyspnea on exertion and was found to have severe aortic stenosis with a valve area of $0.80 \, cm^2$ (normal: $3.0-4.0 \, cm^2$). At that time, she declined surgery and was discharged home. On this admission, the patient presented with reports of weight gain, progressive shortness of breath, and increased BiPAP requirements. She was admitted to the coronary care unit and evaluated by the cardiac surgery team. Preoperatively, she underwent cardiac catheterization, which showed normal coronary arteries, severe pulmonary hypertension, and confirmed severe aortic stenosis. Her pulmonary function tests prior to surgery showed restrictive lung disease, and computed tomography (CT) scan of the chest showed mild bronchial thickening, air trapping, and small bilateral pleural effusions. She was deemed a surgical candidate and this time the patient agreed to surgical management. The intraoperative course was without complications; however, postoperatively, she developed atrial fibrillation and was started on carvedilol (Coreg) and amiodarone (Pacerone). She also had hypotension, heart failure, and acute kidney injury (AKI). Her hypotension was treated with albumin and her heart failure symptoms were treated with intravenous bumetanide (Bumex). Nephrology was consulted to help manage her AKI. The Bumex doses were decreased to minimal doses and nephrotoxic medications were held.

Her problem list on admission to the step-down unit is as follows:
1. Aortic stenosis
2. Heart failure
3. Atrial fibrillation
4. Hypotension
5. Acute kidney injury
6. Diabetes mellitus type 2
7. Asthma

Case Analysis: As I review the HPI information available to me, I am aware that this patient's clinical course has been complicated and that I will need additional information to manage her many existing problems and evaluate her for any new, recurrent, or persistent conditions that may negatively affect her recovery. A complete review of her history is necessary to identify existing conditions and how they were treated during her postoperative course in the ICU. And, a current review of systems and complete physical examination are essential to evaluate her status now. Because her complaint of shortness of breath may indicate an emergent situation, I start with an immediate general survey of the patient.

CASE INFORMATION

General Survey

The patient is a well-developed and well-groomed obese 55-year-old female. She does not appear to be in any respiratory distress and is able to carry on a conversation and maintain her oxygen saturation of 97% on 3 L/min via nasal cannula. I ask her how her night was. She breaks into tears and states, "I'm tired and I did not sleep well. I thought this surgery would make me feel better but it hasn't. I'm still having trouble breathing." I also notice that she has significant bilateral lower extremity edema. I ask the patient how far she is able to walk. She states, "I can walk to the nurses' station, but I get short of breath." She denies any chest pain or palpitations. I palpate her legs and ask if she has any pain or tenderness and she says "no."

❓ What are the pertinent positives and significant negatives from the information given so far?

Pertinent Positives

- Dyspnea that is worse with exertion
- Fatigue and unable to sleep
- Leg swelling
- Past medical history of CHF, sleep apnea, and asthma
- Recent acute kidney injury
- New onset atrial fibrillation while post-op in ICU
- Requires 3 L of oxygen to maintain normal oxygen saturation

Significant Negatives

- The patient does not appear to be in acute respiratory distress
- The patient is not having chest pain or palpitations
- The patient denies leg tenderness

❓ What might the problem representation be at this point?

At this point, the problem representation is: a 55-year-old female, day 8 following a bioprosthetic aortic valve replacement, with complaints of continued shortness of breath with activity and lower extremity edema.

Case Analysis: While I am concerned that the patient is still experiencing shortness of breath with activity, I am relieved to see that she is not in respiratory distress, has a normal oxygen saturation, and has no chest pain. Based on her appearance, I am less inclined to think that she has a pulmonary embolism (PE), a pneumothorax, cardiac tamponade, or valve failure. She just is not that uncomfortable. Her statement that she expected her "breathing to improve and it has not," suggests to me that her current dyspnea is similar to the symptoms she experienced prior to admission. I need to gather more information before I can rule out items on my differential list, but at the moment I tend to favor an exacerbation of one of her chronic health problems, such as heart failure or maybe chronic obstructive pulmonary disease (COPD). The association of leg swelling certainly suggests that she may have fluid overload impacting her breathing. Additional data I can collect in relation to her heart failure include her weight, her recorded intake and output, and her echocardiogram results. In addition, I will need to proceed with a full history and physical examination, particularly a lung examination to determine if she has abnormal breath sounds suggestive of heart failure or COPD.

CASE INFORMATION

Past Medical History

Diabetes mellitus, type 2, obesity, asthma, sleep apnea (wears BiPAP at home), gastric polyp, colon polyp, heel fracture, and pseudotumor cerebri.

Past Surgical History

Hernia repair, cholecystectomy, cesarean section, and pseudotumor cerebri with burr hole and insertion intracranial pressure monitoring.

Medications, Prior to Admission

- Albuterol 4 mg twice a day
- Aspirin 81 mg tablet daily
- Diazepam 10 mg twice daily as needed
- Docusate sodium 100 mg twice daily
- Fluticasone 110 µg/act inhaler: inhale one puff twice daily
- Furosemide 40 mg tablet twice daily
- Gabapentin 300 mg capsule four times daily
- Glargine 100 unit/mL injection: inject 75 units twice daily
- Ipratropium 0.5 mg: albuterol 2.5 mg—inhale 3 mL every 4 hours as needed

- Metformin 1000 mg twice daily with meals
- Omeprazole 20 mg capsule twice daily before meals
- Oxycodone-acetaminophen 10 mg/ 325 mg one tablet every 8 hours as needed
- Polyethylene glycol packet twice daily
- Potassium chloride 40 mEq twice daily
- Simethicone 80 mg tablet four times daily as needed
- Simvastatin 80 mg tablet once a day at bedtime

Inpatient Medications

- Amiodarone 400 mg every 8 hours
- Aspirin 325 mg daily
- Bumex 3 mg IV every 6 hours × 2 doses
- Coreg 6.25 mg twice daily
- Fluticasone one puff inhalation twice a day
- Gabapentin 300 mg four times daily
- Heparin 5000 units subcutaneous every 8 hours
- Insulin glargine 38 units subcutaneous every morning
- Lispro 5 units subcutaneous before meals, three times a day
- Lispro sliding scale, three times a day as needed according to blood glucose
- Ipratropium (0.5 mg)—albuterol (2.5 mg) 3 mL inhalation every 6 hours
- Lidocaine transdermal patch daily, on 12 hours, off 12 hours
- Pantoprazole 40 mg daily before breakfast
- Potassium chloride 20 mEq twice a day × 2 doses
- Senna 2 tablet nightly
- Simvastatin 20 mg oral nightly
- As-needed medications include bisacodyl, dextrose, glucagon HCl, labetalol, magnesium hydroxide concentrate, naloxone, ondansetron, and oxycodone

Allergies: Reactions

- Strawberries: anaphylaxis
- Theophyllines: short of breath and swelling
- IV contrast: severe convulsions
- All artificial sweeteners: rash

Family History

- Heart attack: brother age 30 at onset
- Heart attack: maternal uncle age 50 at onset
- Diabetes: mother
- Colon cancer: father

Social History
- Marital status: divorced
- Children 1: disabled
- Smoking: former smoker 1 pack/day for 16 years. Quit 9 years ago

Review of Systems
- Constitutional: The patient reports fatigue. No fever or chills.
- Head/eyes/ears/nose/throat: Negative.
- Cardiovascular: Denies chest pain or palpitations. Positive for lower extremity swelling.
- Pulmonary: The patient reports shortness of breath on exertion but denies shortness of breath at rest. Denies cough. History of asthma and sleep apnea.
- Gastrointestinal: No nausea or vomiting. History of cholecystectomy.
- Genitourinary: Negative.
- Musculoskeletal: Negative.
- Integumentary: Negative.
- Psychiatric: No history of anxiety or depression.
- Neurologic: Negative.
- Endocrine: Reports diabetes.
- Hematological: Negative.

Physical Examination
- Vital signs: temperature 36.6°C oral, heart rate 96 beats per minute, respirations 18 to 22 breaths/min, blood pressure 92/64 mm Hg, oxygen saturation 97% on 3 L via NC
- Height 1.6 m (5'3"), weight 148.5 kg (327 lb 6.1 oz), BMI 57.8
- Intake/output: 550/6800 over the past 24 hours, net 33,981 since admission (although the I and Os do not correlate with her documented 10 lb weight gain since CCU admission and transfer to step-down unit)
- General appearance: interactive, well developed, out of bed to chair, morbidly obese, no acute distress, 10 lb weight gain between CCU admit and admit to step-down unit
- Head/eyes/ears/nose/throat: normocephalic, atraumatic, extraocular movements intact, oral mucosa membranes are pink and dry, no scleral icterus
- Neck: supple, no tracheal deviation, normal range of motion, jugular venous distension at 45° 5 cm, no bruits
- Pulmonary: respiratory pattern eupneic, percussion difficult due to body habitus, bibasilar crackles, no wheezing or rhonchi
- Cardiovascular: S1,S2, irregular rhythm, II/VI systolic ejection murmur heard best at the right upper sternal border, no rubs or gallops

- Gastrointestinal: normoactive bowel sounds, soft nontender, no hepatosplenomegaly
- Genitourinary: Foley catheter, no hematuria, straw color urine
- Neurological: alert and oriented, no focal deficits, strength 5/5
- Integumentary: mid-sternal incision well-approximated without redness, swelling, or drainage
- Extremities: 3+ edema bilaterally in lower extremities to mid-calf, warm, 2+ pedal pulses, (−) Homans sign
- Musculoskeletal: full range of motion
- Psychiatric: tearful at times

Labs

- Complete blood count normal with the exception of an anemia (Hct 28%) and coagulation studies normal (because she had a bioprosthetic [tissue] valve she does not require Coumadin or other anticoagulants).
- Basic metabolic panel shows normal electrolytes with exception of blood urea nitrogen (BUN) elevated at 45 mg/dL (normal 10–20 mg/dL) and creatinine elevated at 1.4 mg/dL (normal 0.8–1.2 mg/dL).

Imaging

- Echocardiogram prior to surgery showed ejection fraction of 30% to 35%.
- Cardiac catheterization prior to surgery showed a pulmonary artery pressure of 77/38 mm Hg with a mean of 54.
- ECG done this morning: atrial fibrillation at 93 beats per minute.
- Postoperative transthoracic echocardiogram: "Left ventricle: Normal cavity size. There is mild concentric hypertrophy present. Ejection fraction is 20% to 25%. Left ventricular systolic global function is severely decreased. Severe diastolic dysfunction. Elevated left atrial pressure. Aortic valve: Aortic valve not well visualized. The peak aortic velocity was measured in the apical view. There is a 21-mm St Jude Trifecta pericardial bioprosthetic valve present. The prosthetic valve is normal. Since the prior study there is no significant change in left ventricular (LV) function now s/p aortic valve replacement."
- CT chest: atelectasis of the right lower lobe and a moderate-sized right pleural effusion.

❓ What are the pertinent positives and significant negatives from the review of systems and physical examination?

Pertinent Positives

- The patient's ambulation is limited by shortness of breath and fatigue. She can only walk short distances without stopping.

- The patient has significant lower extremity edema.
- Systolic murmur on cardiac examination.
- The patient has bibasilar crackles on lung examination and CT shows atelectasis of the right lower lobe and a moderate-sized right pleural effusion.
- She had post-op atrial fibrillation and continues to be in atrial fibrillation.
- She has an EF of 20% to 25% and severely impaired LV function.
- She is a diabetic type 2 on insulin.
- She has severe pulmonary hypertension with pulmonary artery pressure 77/38 mm Hg on cardiac catheterization prior to her surgery.
- She is morbidly obese.

Significant Negatives
- She has no fever and her white blood cell count is normal.
- She is sitting in the chair and able to carry on a conversation.
- She denies chest pain or palpitations.
- She has no slurred speech and no facial droop.
- She has no history of DVT or PE.
- She has no surgical fractures.

? Given the information you have so far, what are the potential causes of these symptoms?

It is important that I consider both cardiac and noncardiac reasons for this patient's symptoms. At this point, I can easily rule out a stroke or a neuromuscular disorder as she has symmetric strength, full range of motion in all extremities, and no neurological deficits. Her lab work also shows that her kidney function is actually improving so I cannot attribute her shortness of breath solely to acute kidney injury. She is anemic, but looking back through her records, her blood count has been stable in the week since her surgery so this probably does not account for her new sensation of shortness of breath. Her examination shows no evidence of ascites and her description of her symptoms is not consistent with gastroesophageal reflux so I can rule out gastrointestinal causes of her symptoms.

The patient's ECG, chest CT, and echocardiogram results assist in ruling out, or putting much lower, several of the pulmonary and cardiac diagnoses on my list. Based on these results, the patient does not have a new arrhythmia, a pneumothorax, cardiac tamponade, or valve failure. The pneumothorax would be visible on the chest CT, and the echocardiogram would show cardiac tamponade or valve failure. However, it does show that she has a right pleural effusion and some atelectasis. These are not uncommon findings s/p valve surgery and may be contributing to her dyspnea but I do not think they are the sole reason. While many patients experience shortness of breath with atrial fibrillation, this patient has been in this rhythm since early in the postoperative course and the shortness of breath just started today. Pulmonary embolism is unlikely in the setting of adequate DVT prophylaxis and/or the absence of a surgical fracture but she is obese and her activity is limited, so while I think it is an unlikely cause, I put it lower on my differential. Asthma exacerbation is also a consideration in this patient with a known history of asthma but given the absence of wheezing and the association of her dyspnea with activity and not at rest, I rule out this diagnosis. I can also rule out pneumonia based on her normal temperature and white blood cell count, and the absence of infiltrates on her chest CT.

At this point the diagnosis that is most likely to be causing her symptoms is congestive heart failure. This is based on the presence of lower extremity edema, bilateral effusions on chest CT, the 10 lb weight gain, and the fact that the shortness of breath is qualitatively the same as what she experienced pre-operatively. Her recorded intake and output suggest that she is already net negative but I am not confident that her intake has been accurately captured. In addition, her acute kidney injury and hypotension in the ICU were managed by cutting back on her diuresis which may have caused the fluid accumulation she is experiencing now.

❓ Given the information so far what is your new problem presentation?

The problem representation in this case is "a 55-year-old female with morbid obesity, diabetes mellitus type 2, sleep apnea (uses BiPAP), heart failure, aortic stenosis who underwent an aortic valve replacement now experiencing acute on chronic systolic heart failure."

Management of Acute on Chronic Systolic Heart Failure

At this point, I obtain a consultation from the heart failure team. The team recommends a furosemide infusion and basic metabolic profiles every 12 hours. Carvedilol (Coreg) is switched to metoprolol (Lopressor) to decrease the hypotensive effect associated with Coreg.[2] Spironolactone, a potassium sparing diuretic, is added to decrease potassium loss and provide diuresis. I continue amiodarone for atrial fibrillation and start apixaban (Eliquis) for anticoagulation. This medication is used in patients who have atrial fibrillation to decrease the risk of blood clots and strokes. She responds well to the furosemide infusion, with increased urine output. An angiotensin-converting enzyme inhibitor (ACE-I) such as lisinopril can be added to her regimen for vasodilation, neurohormonal modification, and to improve left ventricular ejection fraction.[3] The patient's heart failure symptoms gradually improve. At discharge, she is enrolled in the "Hospital to Home" (H2H) nurse practitioner clinic program, which provides transitional care to patients with congestive heart failure, because that diagnosis is associated with a high rate of hospital readmission. Patients enrolled in the H2H clinic are seen within 7 days of discharge and receive extra support during the month after their hospital stay. This patient successfully transitions back home and is not readmitted in the subsequent three months. I believe if I had not consulted the heart failure team, the patient would have been readmitted to the hospital within 30 days.

In the heart failure population, symptom management is imperative to maintaining quality of life. Strategies to control heart failure include educating patients on the importance of medication adherence, monitoring daily weights (if the patient gains 5 lb in 1 week or 2 lb in 1 day to call the physician), restricting fluid and sodium (2 L of fluids in a 24-hour period), and maintaining an appropriate activity level. Patients are educated in the hospital, on admission, and throughout their hospitalization. Some patients may benefit from cardiac resynchronization therapy if they meet the criteria such as a prolonged QRS.[4] This patient did not have a prolonged QRS so she did not qualify for a biventricular implantable cardiac defibrillator (ICD). A BNP (B-type natriuretic peptide) is a blood test to determine the severity of acute on chronic heart failure.[5] While useful in differentiating heart failure from other causes of shortness of breath, such as COPD, the BNP is less helpful in patients who are in decompensated heart failure.[5] This patient is in decompensated heart failure so the heart failure team does not check a BNP.

Every day during the remainder of her hospital stay, I educate the patient on the regimen advised by the heart failure team. We discuss medication management, daily weights, fluid and sodium restriction, and activity level. Noting the distress she was in when I first met her, I encourage her to take a proactive approach to the management of congestive heart failure. The surgery will help but her own vigilant attention to her health is essential in preventing further episodes of volume overload.

References

1. Kuzniar T, Lim K, Kasibowska-Kuzniar K. Evaluation of dyspnea. Epocrates essentials. Epocrates, Inc; Ver 14.10. https://online.epocrates.com/noFrame/showPage?method=diseases&MonographId=862&ActiveSectionId=11 Accessed October 18, 2014.
2. Sanderson J, Chan KW, Yip G, et al. Beta-blockade in heart failure: a comparison of carvedilol with metoprolol. *J Am Coll Cardiol*. 1999;34(5):1522-1528. doi:10.1016/S0735-1097(99)00367-8.
3. Dumitru I, Baker MM, Windle ML, Ooi HH. Heart failure treatment & management. Medscape. http://emedicine.medscape.com/article/163062-treatment#aw2aab6b6b3. Updated June 9, 2014. Accessed December 4, 2014.
4. Saxon L, DeMarco T. Cardiac resynchronization therapy indications. UpToDate. http://www.uptodate.com/contents/cardiac-resynchronization-therapy-in-heart-failure-indications. Updated September 19, 2014. Accessed September 10, 2014.
5. Writing Committee Members, Yancy CW, Jessup M, et al. 2013 ACCF/AHA guideline for the management of heart failure: a report of the American College of Cardiology Foundation/American Heart Association Task Force on practice guidelines. *Circulation*. 2013;128; e240-e327. doi: 10.1161/CIR.0b013e31829e8776.

CASE 32

Denise Buonocore

Denise Buonocore works in a community teaching hospital in Bridgeport, CT, as a Heart Failure Service NP. Denise previously taught ACNP students in the Acute and Specialty Care Program at Yale University.

CASE INFORMATION

Chief Complaint

A 75-year-old male presents to the emergency room with complaint of pain and swelling of both legs.

❓ What is the potential cause?

When a patient presents with pain and swelling of the lower extremities both local and systemic disease processes should be considered. Important first steps are to inquire about the location, duration, intensity, associated symptoms such as fever, and any aggravating and alleviating factors, such as leg position or ambulation. If all the symptoms are local and the presentation is acute, consider deep vein thrombosis (DVT) first. Edema of the lower extremities can also occur in systemic disease such as heart, liver, kidney, or vascular lung disease so questions about chronic systemic disease are also very important.

Edema is the swelling that is produced by the expansion of the interstitial fluid volume. Edema does not become apparent until interstitial volume has increased by 2.5 to 3 liters.[1] Factors that affect interstitial volume include capillary hydrostatic and oncotic pressures, capillary permeability, serum albumin levels, and the lymph and vascular systems. As with any presenting symptom, consideration must be given to medication side effect and related retention of sodium and water by the kidneys. The most common causes of generalized edema are heart failure, cirrhosis, nephrotic syndrome, premenstrual edema, and pregnancy.[1] The first three can be life threatening. My approach is to rule out the life-threatening conditions first. Often, edema is not the only issue, particularly in patients who have multiple comorbidities, so it may be necessary to rule out several causes simultaneously.

> ### Comprehensive Differential Diagnoses for Edema of Lower Extremities[1]
>
> **Increased capillary hydrostatic pressure**
> - Increased plasma volume due to renal failure or sodium retention
> - Heart failure including cor pulmonale

- Medications: NSAIDs, glucocorticoids, fludrocortisones, thiazolidinediones, insulin, estrogen, progestins, androgens, testosterone, tamoxifen, vasodilators (hydralazine, minoxidil, diazoxide), calcium channel blockers
- Refeeding edema
- Early hepatic cirrhosis
- Pregnancy and premenstrual edema
- Idiopathic edema, when diuretic induced
- Sodium or fluid overload: parenteral antibiotics or other medications with large amounts of sodium, sodium bicarbonate, or excessive or overly rapid fluid replacement

Venous obstruction

- Cirrhosis or hepatic venous obstruction
- Acute pulmonary edema
- Local venous obstruction, such as a deep vein thrombosis

Arteriolar vasodilatation

- Medications: vasodilators, calcium channel blockers, α_1-blockers, sympatholytics, nondihydropyridine calcium channel blockers
- Idiopathic edema

Hypoalbuminemia

- Protein loss
- Nephrotic syndrome
- Protein-losing enteropathy
- Reduced albumin synthesis
- Liver disease
- Malnutrition

Increased capillary permeability

- Idiopathic edema
- Burns
- Trauma
- Inflammation or sepsis
- Allergic reactions including certain forms of angioedema
- Adult respiratory distress syndrome
- Diabetes mellitus
- Interlukin-2 therapy
- Malignant ascites

Lymphatic obstruction or increased interstitial oncotic pressure

- Lymph node dissection
- Nodal enlargement due to malignancy
- Hypothyroidism
- Malignant ascites
- Primary lymphedema

Other medications

- Anticonvulsant: gabapentin, pregabalin
- Antineoplastic: docetaxel, cisplatin
- Antiparkinson: pramipexole, ropinirole

CASE INFORMATION

History of Present Illness (HPI)

A 77-year-old African American male with atrial fibrillation and sleep apnea arrives in the emergency room with leg swelling and leg pain. He reports this is a recurrent problem; he has had occasional leg swelling and leg ulcers in the past, mostly in the summer when it is very hot and humid. This particular episode started about 2 months ago. He went to the walk-in clinic 1 month ago and was placed on an antibiotic (he does not know the name) for 10 days. This did not help the pain or the swelling; in fact, the swelling has gotten worse over the last several days. The swelling is in both legs but slightly worse in the left leg. The pain is localized to the left leg where there is an open wound, induration, and erythema. The pain is described as an ache or throbbing type pain and he rates it as a 4 or 5 on a 10-point scale. He has taken ibuprofen once a day on most days and this does help the discomfort but never completely alleviates it. The pain and the swelling are worse toward the end of the day; he notes he still has the swelling in the morning but it is considerably diminished. He denies fever or chills, denies new onset of numbness or tingling in his legs and color changes in his feet or legs. He has had no recent injuries or surgery.

Past Medical History (Reported by Patient and Found in the Electronic Medical Record)

- Allergies: none
- Morbid obesity

- Paroxysmal atrial fibrillation (PAF)
- Obstructive sleep apnea (OSA) not on continuous positive airway pressure (CPAP)
- Hypertension (HTN)
- Chronic kidney disease (CKD) stage 2
- Diabetes mellitus (DM) type 2
- Gout
- Hyperlipidemia

Social History

- Former smoker
- Currently drinks a 12 pack of beer most days of the week
- Former drug use including marijuana and cocaine but no current use

Case Analysis: Clearly, this is not premenstrual edema or pregnancy-related edema but I need more information to consider the other items on my differential list. My general approach is to let the patient tell the story in their own words with little prompting as I do a general survey of the patient from head to toe while they are speaking. This gives me an overview of other issues that may be present and a chance to determine the degree of the patient's distress. He appears slightly disheveled, and diaphoretic. He moves slowly and is somewhat short of breath when speaking although appears comfortable at rest. Considering the list of possible differentials, there are several red flags in the history of this illness. One is his obesity, and history of OSA not on CPAP; his edema may be the result of untreated pulmonary hypertension. He also has a history of PAF so I wonder about anticoagulation, and the possibility of a clot, although the gradual onset of symptoms and the presentation with bilateral edema make arterial embolism less likely. Deep vein thrombosis (DVT) is a consideration in that he is not very mobile and his pain is localized to one leg. Cellulitis is also high on my list due to the presence of a wound, with pain and erythema. At this point, my leading theory is that heart failure is causing his symptoms; he has multiple risk factors for heart disease including diabetes, hypertension, chronic kidney disease, hyperlipidemia, and smoking history. The swelling is in both legs and worsens through the day, which suggests a systemic process rather than a local one. Another systemic disease to consider is acute on chronic kidney disease especially given his report of recent ibuprofen use, which can worsen kidney disease but can also independently cause swelling. I wonder also about liver disease as he drinks quite a bit and has a large belly that, on my general survey, I think may be ascites.

CASE INFORMATION

Medication List

I ask about medications and he initially hesitates to answer. I inquire about a medication list and he then supplies one. Of note, I also ask about over-the-counter medications and herbal preparations because many patients only list their prescribed medications.

• Allopurinol 100 mg PO daily

• Amlodipine 5 mg PO daily

• Atorvastatin 20 mg PO daily

• Carvedilol 12.5 mg PO twice daily

• Colchicine 0.6 mg daily as needed

• Losartan 50 mg PO daily

• Flomax 0.4 mg PO daily

• Saxagliptin 2.5 mg PO daily

• Warfarin 5 mg alternating with 2.5 mg every other day

• Ibuprofen 400 mg once or twice a day as needed

Because of his hesitation, I question if he has run out of any of his medications. In addition to finding out what medications a patient takes, an accurate history must include an assessment of adherence to the medication regimen. Often I will ask, "With so many medications, patients sometimes miss doses or forget to fill their prescriptions. How many times a week do you think you have missed doses? Are you having any problems refilling your prescriptions?" Using this nonjudgmental approach helps patients open up and be honest about their adherence. In this case, the patient replies that he ran out a few weeks ago and tried to get refills but was unable. I realize that when I develop this patient's transitional plan I will need to involve social services and pharmacy to ensure he gets his prescriptions.

Review of Electronic Health Record

A review of the electronic health record (EHR) shows that he has been seen three times in the last 2 years in our emergency room. Twice he complained of dizziness and was found to have high blood sugar; he was treated and then he was released. He has had one observation stay for PAF that converted to sinus rhythm on its own with oral meds. On that admission he was also hypertensive and medications were added to his regimen. He was discharged with a recommendation to follow up with a cardiologist for an echocardiogram and stress test. He states that he did have this testing done and it all was "good." I make a note to obtain copies of the results of these tests. The EHR also shows that he went to a local walk-in clinic several times for gout flairs and for this leg swelling; however, records for those visits are not available. His primary care provider is at a local community clinic. He gets his INR checked about once a month, but states he has not had one done since before the swelling issue started. Follow-up monitoring for his anticoagulation therapy will also need to be addressed in his transitional plan of care.

What are the pertinent positives and significant negatives found in the information obtained so far?

Pertinent Positives

- Acute on chronic bilateral leg swelling, left greater than right.
- Leg swelling occurring on and off over the last 2 months and worsening recently.
- Pain and erythema localized to the left leg, with an open wound.
- Multiple chronic medical problems including PAF, CKD, DM, OSA, and obesity that could be contributing to his swelling.
- His OSA is currently not being treated.
- He has two ER visits with hyperglycemia.
- Medication regimen includes an angiotensin receptor blocker and a β-blocker, which suggests a history of heart failure.
- He is on multiple medications that could also be contributing to his swelling, including amlodipine and ibuprofen.
- He has a recent history of nonadherence to prescribed medications.

Significant Negatives

- Treatment with antibiotics did not improve pain or swelling.
- His pain is not acute, and he is still able to walk.
- He is uncomfortable but not in acute distress.
- He has no fever, no chills, no color changes, and no numbness or tingling in his legs.
- He has had no recent accident, injury, or surgery that may lead to this problem.
- He has no history of pelvic or abdominal malignancy.
- He reports a normal echocardiogram and stress test completed recently.

❓ Can the information gathered so far be restated in a single sentence highlighting the pieces that narrow down the cause?

Putting the information obtained so far in a single statement—a problem representation—sets the stage for gathering more information and determining the cause.

In this case, the problem statement would be: A 77-year-old male with a history of DM, CKD, HTN, HL, and PAF on anticoagulation, OSA not currently treated presenting with a 2-month history of worsening bilateral leg swelling, and localized pain in one leg with an open wound, and observed to be short of breath with exertion.

Case Analysis: Based on the information so far, I do not believe the patient's edema is due to malignancy, trauma, or nutritional issues because his history so far does not suggest problems in these areas. While the medications on his list can cause edema, he describes issues with adherence so medication side effect is less likely to be the cause of his symptoms. At this point I am thinking that the wound probably is not causing the swelling, but that the wound, in the absence of any trauma, is a result of chronic swelling. With only mild to moderate pain, and no paresthesias or pallor, an arterial embolism is unlikely. Because the swelling is chronic over the last 2 months and worsening recently, I am leaning more toward a systemic issue as the cause, with possibly a superimposed local cellulitis causing the pain.

❓ What diagnostics are important to obtain and in what order?

The patient's history of DM (based on his ER visits) is not controlled and his nonadherence to his current medical regimen for hypertension and hyperlipidemia make me concerned about a cardiac process, specifically heart failure, myocardial infarction (MI), or other acute coronary syndrome (ACS). I will order a chest x-ray, an ECG, a comprehensive metabolic panel including calcium and magnesium, which will show his kidney function and a liver function panel with albumin level, a troponin because he has multiple cardiac risk factors, and a brain-natriuretic peptide (BNP) or NT-proBNP to help me determine if he has heart failure. I will also order a PT/INR because of his warfarin therapy and a complete blood count (CBC) and blood cultures because I cannot yet rule out sepsis. Given the chronic nature of this swelling, I am less inclined to think he is septic, but it is a life-threatening diagnosis and so it is crucial to rule this out definitively. I will also obtain a TSH to rule out hypothyroidism as a cause and a HgbA1c to assess his DM control. While I await those results, I will proceed with a full history and physical, keeping in mind that I am still concerned about the possibility of liver disease, kidney disease, or vascular disease, though these are lower on my list than a cardiac process.

CASE INFORMATION

Review of Systems

- Constitutional: Denies fever, chills, and change in appetite. He has had some problems sleeping at night, waking several times per night. Does have daytime sleepiness and takes a short nap in the afternoon. Has always been a big man but has gained more than 50 lb in the last year.

- Head/eyes/ears/nose/throat: No vision or hearing problems, no throat or neck pain or tenderness, no swallowing problems.

- Cardiovascular: Denies any chest pain, pressure, tenderness. Does have leg swelling as outlined in HPI, improves overnight, worse in the evening. He does not feel short of breath but on further questioning notes that for the last 6 months he stops to rest after climbing the five stairs into his house. He sleeps on two pillows, but he sleeps well during daytime nap in his recliner chair, which is actually more comfortable than lying in bed at night. Denies any history of circulatory problems, DVT, blood clots. Able to walk around the house without leg cramps but states when he goes grocery shopping he has to rest because his legs get tired.

- Pulmonary: Shortness of breath as described above. Also occasionally awakens from sleep "startled" and takes a few minutes to catch his breath. He did get tested for sleep apnea approximately 5 years ago but did not like the mask so he returned the machine.

- Gastrointestinal: Denies nausea, vomiting, and abdominal pain but complains of early satiety. Bowel movements are daily and normal without bleeding but he admits to often feeling bloated.

- Genitourinary: Denies blood or foul smelling urine, does not feel that he makes as much urine as he used to but thinks it is because he does not drink enough water. States he knows he has a kidney problem but so far they are doing ok.

- Musculoskeletal: Occasional pain in his big toes that he attributes to gout, but improved when he started on the allopurinol. Also improved with discontinuing a water pill, he thinks it was hydrochlorothiazide (HCTZ). Pain as in HPI, localized to left lower extremity open area. Pain is partially relieved with elevation of the limb and taking ibuprofen.

- Neurological: Denies headache, falls, seizure, stroke, and transient ischemic attacks. Reports numbness on the soles of both feet which has been present for years, and which he attributes to diabetes. No extremity weakness.

- Integumentary: Only issue has been the wound on his left leg that brought him to the ER. He had a similar problem a few years ago.

- Lymphatic: Denies any nodes.

- Endocrine: Rarely tests his blood sugar. His glucose monitor is not currently functioning. He does not know his last A1C. Denies excessive thirst, excessive hunger, or excessive urination.
- Functional Status: The patient describes himself as being fairly active up until 6 to 8 months ago when he put on more weight after his spouse died. He relates it to being too much of a bother to go out, and when he does go out it "just wipes me out." He cooks his own meals or orders out from a local restaurant. He has a son and a neighbor, and one of them helps him with the grocery shopping.

Physical Examination

- Vital signs: Blood pressure 109/57, pulse 78 regular, respirations 24, O_2 sat 99% on room air, temperature is normal, height 172 cm, weight 128 kg, BMI 43.3.
- Constitutional: Appears his stated age, obese, slightly anxious, and diaphoretic. He also appears slightly short of breath when answering questions.
- Head/eyes/ears/nose/throat: Unremarkable, no thyromegaly, short thick neck noted.
- Pulmonary: Lungs clear but decreased sounds at bases.
- Cardiovascular: Slight heave is noted left sternal border at four intercostal space. Point of maximal impulse is slightly laterally displaced. Normal S1 and S2. No S3 or S4; there is a 2/6 holosystolic murmur noted at left sternal border. This murmur does not radiate. He is not aware of any history of a murmur. It is difficult to appreciate jugular venous distention due to his neck size and body habitus, but on applying pressure to his abdomen a positive hepatojugular sign is elicited. Bilateral swelling of both legs but left leg is somewhat greater than right, 4+ pitting edema noted up to mid-thighs bilateral. There is no toe or foot edema noted.
- Peripheral vascular: Pulses intact on radial, brachial, femoral, pedal pulses both dorsal pedis and posterior tibial 2+. Auscultation of carotid and femoral pulses reveal no bruits. Extremities are warm to touch and color is normal for race.
- Gastrointestinal: Abdomen is large, distended, and somewhat firm. + bowel sounds, + fluid wave, cannot appreciate liver borders. Rectal examination is negative.
- Genitourinary: Unremarkable except some degree of scrotal edema noted.
- Integumentary: Intact except for area of induration and erythema on left lower extremity, with a 3 cm open wound that is draining serous clear fluid. Skin on bilateral legs below the knee is hyperpigmented, dry, and scaling. Left lower leg is warm to touch below the knee.
- Musculoskeletal: Walks slowly, hesitant, but able to move all extremities to resistance, equal strength bilaterally.

- Neurological: No focal neurologic deficits except decreased sensation of both feet in stocking pattern. Reflexes are normal.
- Lymphatic: Difficult to ascertain due to body habitus.

Results of Preliminary Diagnostic Testing

ECG: normal sinus rhythm, rate 75, left ventricular hypertrophy, and right atrial enlargement

Chest x-ray: difficult to assess heart size due to body habitus, slight blunting of the costophrenic angles bilaterally

---

❓ What elements of the review of systems and the physical examination should be added to the list of pertinent positives? Which items should be added to the list of significant negatives?

Pertinent Positives

- Dyspnea on exertion (DOE)
- Orthopnea and paroxysmal nocturnal dyspnea (PND)
- 50 lb weight gain
- New heart murmur
- 4+ Pitting edema up to his upper thighs
- + Hepatic jugular reflux
- + Fluid wave and abdominal distention
- Warmth, redness, and induration of open area on left lower extremity

Significant Negatives

- No chest pain and no ECG changes or symptoms to suggest an MI or ACS (although he could have silent ischemia since he has diabetes).
- Afebrile.
- He is not hypoxic and his lungs sound clear.
- Chest x-ray shows no active disease.

❓ How does this information affect the list of possible causes?

The patient's review of systems and physical examination show that his fluid accumulation is not limited to lower leg swelling; in fact his swelling extends to his thigh and he has ascites and signs of total body anasarca. This suggests a systemic process such as heart failure, cirrhosis, CKD, or nephrotic syndrome. The patient has risk factors for all of these conditions; his atrial fibrillation and hypertension create a risk for heart failure, and his medication regimen suggests that another provider may have made this diagnosis; his alcohol use creates a risk for liver disease, and his poorly controlled DM has likely worsened his renal function.

Regarding the possibility of heart failure, I consider both right- and left-sided heart failure and pay particular attention to his respiratory status. While he does have significant respiratory symptoms of DOE and PND, he has no signs of acute pulmonary edema as he is not hypoxic and his chest x-ray does not show pulmonary vascular congestion. The absence of crackles on lung examination is also significant but does not rule out pulmonary edema in a person with heart failure. Patients with chronic HF may have increased venous capacitance and enhanced lymphatic drainage of fluid from the lungs; crackles are often absent in right-sided heart failure. His cardiac examination also increases my concern for right heart failure; the presence of a parasternal lift suggests right ventricular hypertrophy. While he does have lateral displacement of his PMI suggesting left ventricular hypertrophy, the absence of an S3 or S4 makes volume overload from left-sided heart failure less likely. The presence of a hepatojugular reflux is a key finding. This is not commonly present in cirrhosis, which is a concern in this patient due to his history of alcohol use, but is present in both right heart failure and renal disease.

While this patient's anasarca suggests a systemic process, my examination of his left lower extremity is concerning for a concurrent acute local process. He is at risk for a clot based on his inconsistency with anticoagulation therapy. My examination confirms that there is no evidence of arterial embolism but the disproportionate swelling and tenderness in his left extremity make me concerned for a DVT. Additionally, while he does not appear acutely septic since he has a normal blood pressure, heart rate, and temperature, I will keep cellulitis in the differential based on the appearance of his left leg. I also note that his blood pressure is relatively low for someone who has not taken his medications, and has a history of hypertension.

At this point a restatement of his problem representation is: A 77-year-old male nonadherent to medical regimen with history of uncontrolled DM, HTN, hyperlipidemia, PAF on anticoagulation but no recent INR testing, alcohol abuse, and untreated OSA presenting with anasarca, and left greater than right leg swelling for the last 2 months

❓ What diagnostic tests should be done and in what order?

I have already ordered basic lab tests including electrolytes, blood urea nitrogen (BUN), creatinine, liver function tests (LFTs)—which are all part of a comprehensive metabolic panel, a complete blood count (CBC), troponins (to rule out MI), BNP, and blood cultures. Because of my concern about his left leg, I order a D-dimer and an ultrasound to rule out a DVT. Additional information can be obtained with a bedside echocardiogram (ECHO). This noninvasive study can assess for signs of volume overload including chamber dilation, lung fluid, and vena cava dilatation to confirm a diagnosis of heart failure. A formal ECHO will give additional information on heart function, including ejection fraction (EF), as well as the condition of the valves and any signs of endocarditis.

CASE INFORMATION

Diagnostic Testing Results

- Stress test: Completed 1 month ago obtained electronically showed no sign of ischemia and gated EF estimate of 45%.
- CMP: Normal electrolyte panel, mild renal function impairment with a BUN of 10 (Normal = 7–20 mg/dL) and creatinine of 1.4 mg/dL (Normal = 0.7–1.4 mg/dL), an estimated GFR of 57 (Normal = >60 mL/min),
- LFT: elevation of both AST and ALT but less than two times above the normal level.
- Serum bilirubin: Mild elevation.
- Alka phosphatase: Normal.
- Serum albumin: Normal.
- TSH: Normal.
- Troponin: Negative.
- BNP: 246 pg/mL (Normal < 100 pg/mL).
- HgbA1c: 8.2 mmol/L (Normal = ≤5.4).
- D-dimer: Normal.
- Ultrasound with Doppler of lower extremities: No DVT.
- Echocardiogram: EF of 45%, no wall motion abnormalities, evidence of diastolic dysfunction, biatrial enlargement, both RV and LV dilatation, moderate tricuspid regurgitation, and moderate pulmonary hypertension with a pulmonary systolic pressure of 50 mm Hg.

Case Analysis: With the addition of the results of the tests I can further hone my diagnoses. A negative troponin together with his normal ECG, recent negative stress test, and normal wall motion on ECHO confirms that he does not have an acute MI or acute coronary syndrome. Mild renal dysfunction may indicate renal disease as he has both DM and HTN, but typically mild renal dysfunction does not lead to this degree of total volume overload.

The mild elevation in liver function tests including elevated serum bilirubin level, but normal albumin and alkaline phosphatase, helps differentiate liver congestion versus biliary obstruction. This pattern of liver dysfunction is most likely due to passive congestive hepatopathy from right-sided heart failure and is not consistent with liver damage causing the ascites. The normal albumin level rules out two other diagnoses, nephrotic syndrome and malnutrition, where swelling occurs because of hypoalbuminemia and third spacing. A normal TSH and no signs of lymphedema on physical examination such as marked toe and foot edema or lumpy rough thick skin make lymphatic obstruction less likely. His BNP while not extremely elevated in comparison to his degree of anasarca may be relevant as lower levels of BNP than anticipated are often found in obese patients with heart failure. In patients with A-fib, values greater than 200 are consistent with heart failure. The patient's chest x-ray indicated small bilateral pleural effusions, which may be due to heart failure although there was no evidence of central pulmonary congestion. D-dimer is normal, making pulmonary embolism less likely. The ultrasound of the lower extremities with Doppler ruled out a DVT.

At this point with the current test results I am ready to state that my patient has acute heart failure, with more right-sided heart failure than left sided. The cause of the right heart failure at this point is unknown. The most common cause of right heart failure is left heart failure and he does have evidence on the recent gated stress test of overall abnormality with mildly reduced EF, which is also confirmed with his ECHO results. By definition the patient has heart failure with preserved EF (HFpEF). Pulmonary embolism can cause signs of right heart failure, but his ECG and echo do not support that diagnosis nor is he hypoxic. There is no evidence of a DVT source and he has a normal D-dimer, all making pulmonary embolism less likely.

Diagnosis and Treatment: Acute Right Heart Failure

The diagnosis of acute right heart failure (RHF) in this patient could represent an exacerbation of chronic HF, but at this point we are unclear of any previous diagnosis. Other causes of RHF need to be considered including constrictive pericarditis, mitral stenosis, tricuspid regurgitation (which can lead to hepatic congestion because of transmission of elevated right ventricular pressure to the hepatic veins), cor pulmonale, and cardiomyopathy. Echocardiogram results help with differentiating the cause of his heart failure. The patient's echocardiogram results showed an EF of 45%, evidence of diastolic dysfunction, biatrial enlargement, indicating elevated filling pressures and volume overload, both right ventricular and left ventricular dilatation, moderate tricuspid regurgitation, and moderate pulmonary hypertension with a pulmonary systolic pressure of 50. There was no evidence of intraventricular septum shift to the left, which would suggest a diagnosis of cor pulmonale. The untreated OSA could cause cor pulmonale but usually that only occurs with coexisting daytime hypoxemia, and this patient's oxygen saturation on this examination is normal. To definitely determine the cause of this patient's RHF, I would need to order a right heart catheterization but based on the echo results, I suspect that his elevated pulmonary artery pressures and right heart disease are due to left-sided dysfunction.

According to the American Heart Association/American College of Cardiology guidelines, the treatment of HFpEF focuses on treating the symptoms of edema and shortness of breath as well as controlling and treating existing comorbidities and contributing factors.[2] Edema and shortness of breath can be managed initially with either intravenous or oral diuretics. Diuresis requires close monitoring in patients with right HF since they may be preload dependent. Overdiuresis can cause decreased right ventricular filling and reduced cardiac output. Diuresis can also lead to electrolyte abnormalities especially potassium and magnesium, so close monitoring of serum electrolytes is important. Long-term treatment of HFpEF includes managing hypertension, treating coronary artery disease, if present, and controlling atrial fibrillation. According to the guidelines, blood pressure control in HFpEF is the most important management strategy. Angiotensin converting enzyme (ACE) inhibitors or angiotensin receptor blockers are first-line drugs for controlling blood pressure in HFpEF. But HFpEF often requires treatment with several medications in order to adequately control blood pressure. Beta-blockers may be used in addition to ACE inhibitors or angiotensin receptor blockers. Treatment of OSA may also be helpful in controlling BP. Current guidelines for treatment of A-fib in HFpEF do not recommend a rate control versus rhythm control strategy as there have been no long-term trials to confirm one strategy over the other. It is recommended that tachycardia be controlled as a rapid rate may shorten diastolic filling time and contribute to worsening HF.

Case Follow-Up

This patient was given IV furosemide twice a day for 3 days with close monitoring of intake and output, daily weights and electrolytes, BUN and creatinine levels and his blood pressure, all of which remained stable. He exhibited an effective diuresis with a 10 lb weight loss. BUN and creatinine levels stabilized and on day 4 he was transitioned to an oral diuretic regimen and continued to diurese. His blood pressure was controlled using a combination of carvedilol and losartan, as previously prescribed. His A-fib remained rate controlled and his INR remained therapeutic on warfarin. His fasting lipid panel was obtained and recorded for use in follow-up management. Preparations for discharge that began on day of admission included social work and pharmacy intervention for identifying barriers to home medication adherence and anticoagulation monitoring. The local infection of his left leg was treated with a 7-day course of cephalexin and dramatically improved once the edema improved. Plans for close monitoring of his INR were put in place since antibiotics can alter the metabolism of warfarin, resulting in INR elevations. The patient and family received education regarding heart failure signs and symptoms, medications, importance of daily weights, sodium and fluid restrictions, activity, who to call for worsening symptoms, and the importance of close follow-up. He was given a glucometer and DM management instructions. Follow-up appointments were made with the Heart Failure Clinic nurse practitioner for 2 days postdischarge and within a week with his primary care provider. Referral was made to sleep study center for testing and fitting of proper device, mask, or nasal prongs for use with nighttime CPAP. Patient and family comprehension of instructions were validated by teach back method and demonstrated a good understanding. On the day of discharge, he no longer had a positive hepatojugular reflex, his edema was much improved and he was no longer short of breath with exertion or when lying flat.

References

1. Sterns, R. Pathophysiology and etiology of edema in adults. 2014. www.uptodate.com.
2. Yancy CW, Jessup M, Bozkurt B, et al. ACCF/AHA guideline for the management of heart failure: a report of the American College of Cardiology Foundation/American Heart Association Task Force on Practice Guidelines. *J Am Coll Cardiol*. 2013;62(16):1495-1539.

CASE 33

Jie Chen

Jie works for the abdominal solid organ transplant service at University of Virginia Medical Center. She has been working with the abdominal organ transplant patient population since 2006, first as a bedside nurse and then as an NP.

CASE INFORMATION

Chief Complaint

A 57-year-old female with nonalcoholic steatohepatitis (NASH) cirrhosis presents with increased abdominal fullness and decreased urine output as a direct admit from the transplant clinic.

❓ What is the potential cause?

Ascites is one of the signs of decompensated cirrhosis, which is caused by portal hypertension. An increase in ascites as noted in this patient, in combination with decreased urine output, is a sign of potential acute kidney injury (AKI) and is a very serious and urgent condition. Patients with decompensated cirrhosis are inclined to develop AKI as a result of a number of conditions including dehydration due to diuretics use with or without vomiting or diarrhea, gastrointestinal bleeding due to esophageal varices, spontaneous bacterial peritonitis, or hepatorenal syndrome (HRS).[1] While I am already thinking that this is the cause of the oliguria, I still must rule out other reasons. First and foremost, I need to assess how she is tolerating the abdominal fullness and evaluate the severity of her oliguria.

Oliguria in adults is defined as a urine output that is less than 400 mL in 24 hours. It is a sign of renal failure and has been used as a criterion for diagnosing and staging AKI. According to Acute Kidney Injury Network (AKIN), AKI is defined as any of the following: increase in serum creatinine by ≥0.3 mg/dL within 48 hours, or increase in serum Cr to ≥1.5 times baseline, which is known or presumed to have occurred within the prior 7 days, or urine output <0.5 mL/kg/h for 6 hours.[2] At onset, oliguria is frequently acute in all patients regardless of etiology. However, it is often reversible and does not progress to chronic renal failure, provided the reversible causes are identified and treated early.[3] I need to quickly determine if my patient meets the criteria for AKI and identify the underlying causes so that I may treat them and prevent worsening renal function. Because of the urgency of this patient's condition I start by generating a complete list of differential diagnoses for AKI and categorize them into three causal groups: pre-renal, intrinsic renal, and postrenal.

Differential Diagnoses for Patient With Acute Onset Oliguria

Pre-renal: these causes include severe volume depletion and hypotension in a patient with otherwise intact nephrons.

- Volume depletion: overdiuresis, vomiting, diarrhea, GI bleeding,
- Decreased cardiac output: heart failure, pulmonary embolus, acute myocardial infarction, severe valve disease, abdominal compartment syndrome
- Systemic vasodilatation: sepsis, drug overdose
- Afferent arteriolar vasoconstriction: hypocalcemia, drug use such as NSAIDs, and hepatorenal syndrome (HRS)

Intrinsic: this category refers to the kidney's response to cytoxic, ischemic, or inflammatory insults and results in structural and functional damage to the nephrons.

Postrenal: caused by obstruction of the urinary tract, such as stones, strictures, or tumors

CASE INFORMATION

General Survey and History of Present Illness

Having a list of differential diagnoses in mind prepares me to consider specific questions to ask when interviewing the patient. When I walk in the room, the patient is in a half sitting position in bed holding her abdomen with both hands. Her facial expression tells me that she is uncomfortable. I start by asking her the reason she came to the hospital. She says, "My belly started feeling really tight 3 days ago and I have not been making much urine. I take medications that would normally make me go, but they don't seem to work anymore. I have gained 8 pounds in 3 days, and my hands and ankles are swelling." I ask her if she has trouble lying down. She says, "I can't lie down because my belly is too big for me to lie down comfortably; it hurts when I try to lie flat". She admits that she has some shortness of breath but denies chest pain. I ask her if she has had fever or chills. She says, "I have had chills and some night sweats but have not had my temperature checked". She denies nausea or vomiting, but she does have loose stools because she takes lactulose. When asked if she has had a paracentesis in the past, and how often, she replies that she has had paracentesis since she got sick and was diagnosed with NASH cirrhosis a year ago, but it has not been done regularly. The last time she had it done was 2 weeks ago, In addition, I ask about her urine output. She says that she only urinated two to three times yesterday, and only a small amount at each time. Her urine is dark but she denies dysuria, hematuria, urgency, or frequency.

Past Medical History

She denies known heart disease or kidney disease, but does have type 2 diabetes which was well controlled until her liver function started to decline. She is in the process of being evaluated for a liver transplant. I review the hospital's electronic medical records and learn that as she stated, she underwent a paracentesis 2 weeks ago and had 10 L of ascites fluid removed. She received 50 g of 25% albumin postprocedure. At that time, her serum creatinine (Cr) was 0.9 mg/dL.

Family/Social History

She states that she has a family history of diabetes (both her mother and father have type 2 diabetes). Her mother also had NASH cirrhosis and had a liver transplant but is now deceased. Her sister who is younger was diagnosed with fatty liver but is fairly healthy. The patient denies any alcohol use currently or in the past. She used to work as a lab technician. She is married and her husband brought her to the hospital.

Current Medications

The patient denies any known medication allergies. She is prescribed the following medications and reports she does not miss any doses:
• Furosemide 40 mg once a day
• Spironolactone 50 mg twice a day
• Propranolol 10 mg three times a day
• Lactulose 30 g two to four times a day as needed to produce two to three loose stools a day
• Glucophage 1000 mg twice a day

❓ What are the pertinent positives from the information given so far?

• The patient has abdominal pain
• Tightness in her abdomen while on dual diuretic therapy
• Decreased urine output and concentrated urine
• Weight gain of 8 lb in 3 days
• Swelling in hands and ankles
• Chills and night sweats
• Having trouble lying flat due to distended abdomen

- Shortness of breath
- Loose stools
- Recent paracentesis with albumin replacement postprocedure
- History of diabetes and on metformin

❓ What are the significant negatives from the information given so far?

- No nausea or vomiting
- No chest pain
- No dysuria, urinary urgency or frequency
- No history of heart disease or kidney disease
- Patient's serum Cr was within normal range 2 weeks ago

❓ Can the information gathered so far be restated in a single sentence, a problem representation, highlighting the pieces that narrow down the cause?

The problem representation in this case might be: "a 57-year-old female with decompensated NASH cirrhosis and history of diabetes who presents with worsening ascites, weight gain, and new onset of decreased urine output."

Case Analysis: According to the information I have so far, the patient's acute oliguria is less likely caused by cardiac or pulmonary diseases but I will need to gather more information, including a complete review of systems and physical examination before I can definitively rule out these potential etiologies. After reviewing the patient's medications and talking to her I can eliminate drug overdose and nonsteroidal anti-inflammatory use as causes of intrinsic kidney injury.

At this point a pre-renal cause is most likely. Her shortness breath, orthopnea, weight gain, and swelling in all extremities are likely to be caused by her liver failure and worsening ascites. She has not had diarrhea or vomiting but does have large sequestration and third spacing of fluid into her abdomen and tissues. In severe liver failure, albumin is not produced adequately and intravascular oncotic pressures are decreased, resulting in the movement of fluid out of the vascular space. The result is a decrease in intravascular fluid volume and a subsequent decrease in flow to the kidneys, thus potentiating the development of AKI.

Hepatorenal syndrome (HRS) is a possibility and very concerning. HRS represents the end stage of a progressive reduction in renal perfusion as liver function increasingly declines. Portal hypertension triggers arterial vasodilation in the splanchnic circulation presumably caused by increased production or activity of vasodilators, such as nitric oxide. Thus, the vasodilators cause a reduction in total vascular resistance, which activates the renin-angiotensin and sympathetic nervous systems. As a result, renal arteries constrict.[4] HRS can be classified as type 1 and type 2 based on the rapidity of the acute kidney injury and the degree of renal impairment. Type 1 is more severe, which is defined as at least a twofold increase in serum Cr to >2.5 mg/dL during a period of less than 2 weeks. Without therapy, most patients with HRS die within weeks of the onset of the renal impairment.[1,4,5] However, it is often overdiagnosed due to a misunderstanding of the disease processes. HRS is a diagnosis of exclusion. The next step is to do a thorough review of systems and physical examination so that I have a full picture of contributing factors for my patient's acute oliguria, and can make an accurate diagnosis and initiate appropriate and timely treatment.

CASE INFORMATION

Review of System

- Constitutional: Denies known fever, recent illness, or sick contacts. Endorses chills, night sweats, fatigue, and malaise.
- Cardiovascular: Denies chest pain or palpitations. Endorses leg swelling and difficulty breathing while lying down.
- Pulmonary: Denies cough or wheezing. Endorses shortness breath on exertion.
- Gastrointestinal: Denies heartburn, nausea, vomiting, constipation, or blood in stools. Endorses abdomen pain (tightness/fullness), and loose stools because of taking lactulose. She also endorses that she has not been eating or drinking fluids much because her stomach feels full all the time.
- Genitourinary: Denies burning while urinating, urgency, frequency, or blood in her urine, endorses decreased amount of urine and notes that it is tea colored. She is not able to state exactly how much she voids in a 24-hour period.
- Musculoskeletal: Noncontributory.
- Neurological: Denies headache, weakness, or tremors.
- Endocrine: Endorses that her sugar has been in the 110 to 120s in the last 3 days, denies polydipsia and polyphagia.

Physical Examination

- Vital signs: Pulse 78 beats per minute, blood pressure 124/75 mm Hg, respirations 19/minute, and temperature 99°F oral, oxygen saturation by pulse oximeter is 98% on room air, and finger-stick blood glucose is 112 mg/dL.
- Well developed, not in distress but does appear to be uncomfortable with both hands holding her abdomen, appears tired.
- Head/eyes/ears/nose/throat: Normocephalic and atraumatic, pupils equal, round, reactive to light, sclera icterus, buccal mucosa and oropharynx moist.

- Cardiovascular: Regular heart rate and rhythm, no murmur, gallops, or rubs, cardiac apex 4/5 intercostal space, mid-clavicular line, 1+ nonpitting edema to bilateral upper extremities, 2+ nonpitting edema to bilateral lower extremities, pulses equal and intact throughout.
- Pulmonary: Respiratory rate and rhythm are normal, no use of accessory muscles, lungs diminished at bases to auscultation, no crackles or wheezing.
- Gastrointestinal: Abdomen firm and distended, normoactive bowel sounds, positive for shifting dullness and fluid wave, mild diffuse tenderness, no guarding or rebound.
- Skin: Intact, no lesions, warm and dry.
- Neurological: No focal neurologic deficits, face symmetric, alert, oriented to person, time, and place, answers questions and follows commands appropriately, moves all extremities. No asterixis.

❓ What elements of the review of systems and the physical examination should be added to the list of pertinent positives? Which items should be added to the list of significant negatives?

- **Pertinent positives:** fatigue and malaise, decreased oral intake of food and fluids, abdominal distension that is mildly firm, shifting dullness, fluid waves, mild tenderness throughout abdomen
- **Significant negatives:** normal vital signs and oxygen saturation, respiratory effort normal, no crackles or wheezing, no cough, no melena, no abdominal guarding or rebound, no hematuria, normal neurological examination

❓ How does this information affect the list of possible causes?

Given that she has normal vital signs, oxygen saturation and pulmonary and cardiac examination findings, pulmonary embolism, acute myocardial infarction, abdominal compartment syndrome, and sepsis are unlikely. Volume depletion due to gastrointestinal bleeding is less likely as well since the patient denies any hematemesis or bloody or dark stools. The description of her abdominal pain and her denial of hematuria makes urinary obstruction less likely. Heart failure could cause orthopnea, ascites, and edema, but she has no history of heart failure and her pulmonary and cardiac examinations do not support it. For now a cardiac cause is lower on my differential. I am still thinking that pre-renal causes may have contributed to the oliguria and am suspicious that HRS is a likely diagnosis. I need to obtain additional diagnostic data.

? What diagnostic testing should be done and in what order?

I order a complete blood count (CBC) with differential, comprehensive metabolic panel (CMP), protime with international normalized ratio (PT/INR), blood culture, urine analysis (UA), urine electrolytes, urine creatinine, urine urea, and urine culture. I also order an abdominal ultrasound focusing on the kidneys to rule out a hydronephrosis, which would suggest a postrenal cause of oliguria. In addition I order strict recording of the patient's intake and output so that the exact amount of urine the patient is producing can be accurately calculated.

CASE INFORMATION
Results

CBC With Differential		
Test	Patient Value	Lab Reference Range (Normal)
WBC	8.38	4.0–11.0K/μL
Band percent	0.6	0%–7%
Band absolute	0.08	
RBC	2.74	4.20–5.20M/μL
Hb	8.6	12.0–16.0g/dL
Hct	25	35.0%–47.0%
PLT	91	150–450k/μL
Comprehensive Metabolic Panel		
Na	128	136–145mmol/L
K	4.7	3.4–4.8mmol/L
Cl	106	98–107mmol/L
CO_2	18	22–29mmol/L
BUN	55	9.8–20.1mg/dL
Cr	1.7	0.6–1.1mg/dL
Glucose	114	74–99mg/dL
GFR	33	
Total bilirubin	4.9	0.3–1.2mg/dL
Alkaline phosphatase	96	40–150U/L
AST	36	<35U/L
ALT	16	<55U/L
Protime	34.5	9.8–12.6s
Protime INR	3.1	0.9–1.2

Urinalysis		
Color	Dark yellow	Yellow
Specific gravity	1.010	1.005–1.030
PH	6.0	5–8
Protein	Negative	Negative
Glucose	Negative	Negative
Ketone	Negative	Negative
Bilirubin	Negative	Negative
Nitrite	Negative	Negative
Leukocyte esterase	Negative	Negative
RBC	Rare	<3/HPF
WBC	7	<2/HPF
Cast	Negative	<1/LPF
Bacteria	Negative	Negative
Urine sodium	<10 mmol/L	
Urine urea	560 mg/dL	
Urine creatinine	109.2 mg/dL	

❓ What does the information provided from the diagnostics tell you about the patient's status?

CBC and differential: The patient's WBC is within normal limits and there are no bands to suggest infection. Her hemoglobin is low and is likely due to her chronic condition but at the current level of 8.6 she does not meet the criteria for blood transfusion. Comparing this to past labs, this value is stable for this patient.

Blood culture: The blood cultures are pending. Regardless I have not found evidence of infection yet but cannot rule out spontaneous bacterial peritonitis (SBP). A sample of peritoneal fluid from either a palliative or diagnostic paracentesis will be necessary to rule this in or out.

Metabolic panel: The patient's panel has a number of abnormalities. The sodium is low and blood urea nitrogen (BUN) and creatinine are elevated. While hyperkalemia and/or high BUN may require dialysis, the patient's values are not high enough to warrant this intervention. Creatinine level alone is not a sufficient indicator of kidney function in patients with liver failure but a progressive rise in serum Cr level is one of the diagnostic criteria for HRS. This patient's serum Cr was 0.9 mg/dL 2 weeks ago and now it is up to 1.7 mg/dL, which meets the criteria for AKI.[2] The serum bicarbonate (CO_2) is decreased, demonstrating a metabolic acidosis, and is likely due to AKI. Last the patient's glucose is elevated but not excessively so. I will monitor subsequent glucose levels but do not need to do anything at this point.

Hepatic panel: Generally these labs do not completely correlate with liver function but rather inflammation. It is useful to trend changes in liver status. The patient's AST is only slightly elevated and the ALT is normal.

Urine analysis and culture: It is possible for patients to have a normal urine analysis (no white blood cells) but still have a positive urine culture. Thus it is helpful to get both at the same time to ensure that if infected, the patient is treated appropriately with antibiotics. The UA can also give information about existing proteinuria, hematuria, or sediment. With HRS the UA may be without sedimentation and have minimal or no proteinuria.[4] This patient's UA is negative for protein, bacteria, and sediment, and has only rare red blood cells. Her urine culture is pending. Since the patient has been on diuretics, a fractional excretion of sodium (FENa) to assess for pre-renal or postrenal levels of sodium will be inaccurate. Thus a fractional excretion of urea (FEUrea) should be calculated instead.[6] Her FEUrea is 15.9% which indicates a pre-renal etiology. Low urine sodium is another diagnostic criterion for HRS. The patient's urine sodium is less than 10 mEq/L. I hold her diuretics to prevent further loss of sodium and volume. Metformin should also be held as well to prevent further metabolic acidosis and rhabdomyolysis.

Now that I have my patient's labs I can calculate her Model of End-Stage Liver Disease (MELD) score. The MELD score is used to stratify the severity of chronic liver disease and ranges from 6 to 40. The greater the number, the higher is the probability of death. It is used by the United Network for Organ Sharing (UNOS) to determine prognosis and prioritization for receipt of a liver transplant.[7] If my patient has HRS, I know that she has advanced liver failure and she may need a liver transplant. To calculate the score I need a bilirubin, Cr, and INR level. Using the results of her labs I calculate her MELD score, which is 30. During her hospitalization I will calculate this daily to continue to monitor her progression.

Abdominal ultrasound: The patient's ultrasound is normal with the exception of a very large amount of ascites. The ultrasound is a useful noninvasive test to help exclude hydronephrosis and intrinsic renal disease. For this patient, the test helps me assess the volume of ascites and can be used to mark the site for a paracentesis. A paracentesis is essential for my patient for both therapeutic and diagnostic reasons. Ascites fluid is sent for cell count profile and culture to diagnose spontaneous bacterial peritonitis (SBP). SBP is often complicated by AKI associated with acute tubular necrosis, but it can also be a precipitant of HRS.[4] The American Association for the Study of Liver Disease guidelines recommends that ascites fluid drained during a paracentesis should be replaced with 25% albumin. Any amount greater than 4 L is replaced with 6 to 8 g/L 25% albumin immediately postprocedure to prevent acute kidney injury, or worsening kidney function.

CASE INFORMATION

The patient undergoes paracentesis and 13 L serous fluid is removed. The ascetic fluid white blood cell count is 92 cells/mm³ and the Gram stain is negative for bacteria. In addition to 100 g of 25% albumin, she receives 5% albumin and normal saline for repletion. No free water was used to avoid third spacing.

The following day, the patient is more comfortable, due to the paracentesis and her vital signs remain stable. Her cultures are negative, ruling out infection. Her labs are stable except for a rise in creatinine to 1.9 mg/dL. Her urine output was less than 400 in the past 24 hours despite volume repletion with albumin and saline.

Hepatorenal Syndrome: Diagnosis and Treatment

The diagnosis of HRS as opposed to other etiologies of AKI is associated independently with a high mortality but 3-month mortality rates of HRS differ significantly. Establishing the etiology of AKI in patients with cirrhosis is critical for guiding therapy.[1] For this patient, a diagnosis of HRS can be made based on[4]:

- Advanced liver failure and portal hypertension

- A progressively rising Cr and low GFR

- Oliguria

- Urine sodium <10 mEq/L

- Absence of proteinuria and normal urine sediment

- Absence of: shock, ongoing bacterial infection, fluid losses, and current treatment with nephrotoxic medications

- Absence of obstructive uropathy or intrinsic parenchymal disease on ultrasound

- No improvement in renal function after diuretic withdrawal and a trial of fluid repletion

Albumin, midodrine (a selective α_1 adrenergic), and octreotide (a somatostatin analog) therapy is initiated to improve renal and systemic hemodynamics. The goal of this therapy is to provide adequate volume and reverse the vasoconstriction that contributes to HRS. The patient undergoes expedited evaluation for a liver transplant and is placed on the waiting list. Daily CBC, BMP, magnesium, phosphate, hepatic panel, and PT/INR are trended for changes. Octreotide therapy is discontinued after 24 days of treatment if the patient does not improve.[4,5]

Case Follow-up

Unfortunately, this patient's kidney function did not improve with medical therapy; this is often the case with HRS. Research is ongoing to determine if additional medical interventions can stabilize kidney function in patients with HRS and provide a bridge to transplant. Fortunately, this patient underwent a deceased donor liver transplant during this admission because of her high MELD score. Posttransplant, continuous renal replacement therapy (CRRT) was used in the ICU, and then she was transitioned to intermittent hemodialysis. She was discharged to a transitional care hospital after 2 weeks. In a few weeks following her transplant, she was able to come off dialysis.

References

1. Belcher JM, Parikh CR, Garcia-Tsao G. Acute kidney injury in patients with cirrhosis: perils and promise. *Cilin Gastroenterol Hepatol.* 2013;11:1550-1558.
2. KDIGO. Clinical practice guidelines for acute kidney injury. *Kidney Int Suppl.* 2012;2:19-36. doi:10.1038/kisup.2011.32.
3. Devarajan P. Oliguria. Medscape. http://emedicine.medscape.com/article/983156-overview. Updated June 10, 2014.
4. Runyon BA. Hepatorenal syndrome. UpToDate. 2014. http://www.uptodate.com/contents/hepatorenal-syndrome.
5. Davenport A, Ahmad J, Al-Khafaji A, Kellum JA, Genyk YS, Nadim MK. Medical management of hepatorenal syndrome. *Nephrol Dial Transplant.* 2012;27:34-41.
6. Carvounis CP, Nisar S, Guro-Razuman S. Significance of the fractional excretion of urea in the differential diagnosis of acute renal failure. *Kidney Int.* 2002;62:2223-2229; doi:10.1046/j.1523-1755.2002.00683.x.
7. Bambha K, Kamath PS. Model for end-stage liver disease (MELD). UpToDate. 2014. http://www.uptodate.com/contents/model-for-end-stage-liver-disease-meld.

CASE 34

Michelle A. Weber

Michelle A. Weber works in General Surgery, providing perioperative care for patients undergoing complex abdominal wall reconstructions, foregut operations, and bariatric procedures.

CASE INFORMATION

Chief Complaint

A 38-year-old male complains of a painful bulge in right groin after lifting an 80-lb box at work.

Upon first meeting a patient, it is important to consider a broad list of differential diagnoses, guided by the patient's chief complaint(s).

> **Comprehensive Differential Diagnoses for Patient With Acute Onset Unilateral Groin Pain[1]**
> - Inguinal hernia, including those that are incarcerated or strangulated
> - Femoral hernia, including those that are incarcerated or strangulated
> - Muscle strain/musculoskeletal pain
> - Inguinal lymphadenopathy
> - Epididymitis
> - Testicular torsion
> - Groin abscess/soft tissue infection
> - Sexually transmitted infection
> - Lipoma
> - Hydrocele/varicocele

This list of differential diagnoses will serve as a guide while interviewing and assessing the patient. It will be modified as additional subjective and objective data are obtained.

CASE INFORMATION

History of Present Illness and Survey

Mr D is a 38-year-old male, who presents to the emergency department with complaints of a 4-hour history of a new nonreducible right groin bulge. He initially noted severe groin pain, rated "9" out of 10 at its worst, while lifting an 80-lb box at work. He notes that his job requires repetitive, frequent heavy lifting. While lifting, he felt a pulling sensation in his right groin, followed by a "pop," and then a sharp pain. He now describes the pain as a constant "strong ache" that is aggravated by any activity, including standing, walking, and sitting. Pain has not worsened since initial event. Pain has minimally improved since he took 600 mg ibuprofen about 1 hour ago and applied an ice pack to his right groin. After this event, he noted a tender, nonreducible bulge in his right groin. Denies difficulty or pain with urinating, blood in urine, other abdominal pain, nausea, vomiting, fever, chills, and history of previously diagnosed hernias, hernia repairs, or groin operations. He is tolerating oral intake without difficulty, is passing flatus, and his last bowel movement was this morning. Upon meeting Mr D, he appears slightly uncomfortable and is hunched forward, but is not in any acute distress.

Case Analysis: The heavy lifting that preceded the onset of his acute groin pain and new groin bulge raises clinical suspicion that his symptoms may be related to an inguinal hernia. An inguinal hernia occurs when a piece of intraperitoneal fat or intestine pushes through a weakened area at the inguinal ring, which is the opening to the inguinal canal. The contents of a hernia are typically surrounded by a sac-like structure, commonly referred to as the hernia sac, which is made up of the membrane that naturally lines the body cavity through which the hernia is protruding.[2] Inguinal hernias may occur at any time in life from infancy to late adulthood and are more common among males than females, with a male-to-female ratio greater than 10:1.[1,3] The lifetime prevalence is approximately 25% for males and approximately 2% for females.[1]

There are two different types of inguinal hernias—indirect and direct. Indirect hernias are the most common type, accounting for approximately two-thirds of all inguinal hernias,[1] and are considered congenital as they are often related to a weakness that remains in the abdominal wall if the inguinal ring does not close as it should after birth. Indirect hernias pass through the internal ring, following the spermatic cord in males and the round ligament in females.[1] Direct hernias, on the other hand, result from tissue degeneration and weakening of the posterior wall of the inguinal canal. They are typically associated with repeated stress on the muscle, such as repetitive heavy lifting, frequent coughing, or straining.[2,3] It is often difficult, if not impossible, to determine whether a hernia is direct or indirect based solely on a physical examination.[1] A third type of groin hernia is the femoral hernia that tracks below the inguinal ligament through the femoral canal. Femoral hernias constitute approximately 2% to 4% of all groin hernias with 70% occurring in women.[1,2,4,5]

Additional questions for Mr D should also focus on other potential causes of groin pain in males of this age category to aid in further narrowing of the differential diagnoses.

CASE INFORMATION

History of Present Illness (continued)

The patient reports that he has been in a monogamous relationship for the past 11 years. Has two total lifetime partners. Denies history of sexually transmitted infections, penile or urethral discharge, scrotal or testicular swelling or pain, or blood in semen. Prior to today, has never noted any lumps or bumps, skin changes or discoloration, or infections in groin.

History

- Past medical history: asthma, seasonal allergies
- Past surgical history: tonsillectomy (4 years old); laparoscopic appendectomy (15 years old); left rotator cuff repair (24 years old)
- Social history: married; two young children; works in a factory; nonsmoker; drinks two to four beers weekly; no recreational drug use currently or in the past
- Family history: father and eldest brother have had groin hernia repairs in the past
- Medications: Zyrtec, albuterol as needed
- Allergies: no known drug allergies

Review of Systems

- Noncontributory, except as noted in history of present illness

Physical Examination

- Vital signs: blood pressure 130/75 mm Hg, heart rate 78 beats per minute, respiratory rate 14/min, T 98.4°F oral, O_2 saturation 98% on room air.
- Constitutional: Alert, no acute distress.
- Head/eyes/ears/nose/throat: Normal.
- Cardiovascular: Regular rate and rhythm, S1/S2.
- Extremities: Warm, well perfused, no peripheral edema.
- Pulmonary: Unlabored respiratory effort; clear to auscultation bilaterally.
- Gastrointestinal: Abdomen is soft, nontender, nondistended. Laparoscopic port sites from the previous surgery are well healed and without evidence of incisional hernia. + tender, palpable, nonreducible right inguinal hernia. No skin changes, erythema, or warmth noted over area of hernia. No evidence of inguinal or femoral hernia on the left side.
- Genitourinary: Testes descended and nontender, without edema or palpable abnormalities. Urethral meatus without discharge.
- Integumentary: Warm and dry. No rashes or discoloration noted.
- Neurological: Alert, oriented.
- Psych: Pleasant, appropriately interactive.

? **Given the information provided so far, what are the pertinent positives and significant negatives?**

Pertinent Positives

- Acute onset of pain that occurred during strenuous activity
- Bulge noted soon after heavy lifting
- Bulge is nonreducible
- Job requires significant and repetitive heavy lifting

Significant Negatives

- Denies GU complaints, nausea, and vomiting
- Scrotal and testicular examination unremarkable
- No skin changes noted over hernia site
- Afebrile
- No evidence of tachycardia

? **How does the information gathered so far affect the list of possible causes?**

Given the information obtained thus far—the patient's report of a precipitating event, and subjective and objective data—suspicion remains high that the cause of his pain is likely related to an incarcerated right inguinal hernia. While assessing a patient with a hernia of any type, I look for signs and symptoms of both incarcerated and strangulated hernias. A hernia is said to be reducible if the contents of the visible bulge are able to be massaged back into the abdomen when gentle external pressure is applied. An incarcerated hernia is one that is not able to be reduced,[3,4] but does not show signs of bowel ischemia. An incarcerated hernia may become strangulated if bowel is present in the hernia and its blood supply becomes compromised. Common assessment findings when strangulation is present include extreme tenderness over the herniated area with pain out of proportion to examination, redness of the skin over the bulge, acute onset of pain that worsens in a short duration of time, fever, and tachycardia related to bowel ischemia or gangrene.[1,4] If a strangulated hernia is not properly identified and treated, nausea, vomiting, death of the bowel, and life-threatening infection may result.[3]

Considering the pertinent pieces of information listed above, at this point in time, the following diagnoses are less likely: epididymitis, testicular torsion, sexually transmitted infection, groin abscess/soft tissue infection, lipoma, hydrocele, and varicocele. In addition, given the available information, the patient does not demonstrate signs or symptoms that his inguinal hernia is strangulated.

❓ Can the information gathered so far be restated in a single sentence highlighting the pieces that narrow down the cause?

Given the information acquired so far the problem presentation is: "a 38-year-old male who presents with acute onset unilateral groin pain and a new nonreducible, right-sided groin bulge consistent with an incarcerated inguinal hernia."

❓ What diagnostic testing should be done for this patient and in what order?

If a patient presents with signs or symptoms of either hernia incarceration or strangulation, the following laboratory studies are considered[2]:

- Complete blood count: Leukocytosis with a left shift may be present if strangulation has occurred.
- Basic chemistry: Important to assess a patient's hydration and electrolyte status if he/she has presented with GI complaints such as nausea and vomiting.
- Urinalysis: May be useful to look for other possible causes of groin pain regardless of whether or not a hernia is present.
- Lactate level: Useful especially if strangulation is suspected. A normal lactate level does not rule out strangulation, but elevated levels should raise the suspicion for hypoperfusion.

In addition, if during a comprehensive physical examination, the main technique used to evaluate for and diagnose an inguinal hernia cannot be completed due to pain or a patient's body habitus, or if examination findings are inconclusive, a CT scan or ultrasound may be useful to aid in diagnosis of a hernia.[1,2] One of the primary differences between these two studies is that an ultrasound is a more dynamic study, meaning that the technician may have the patient cough, change positions, or Valsalva during the study, similar to what might be done during a physical examination. A CT scan, on the other hand, is a static or nondynamic study in which the patient will be lying still while the imaging is obtained. Before deciding whether to order an ultrasound or CT, I would also consider that performing an ultrasound and subsequently ruling in or out a hernia is somewhat operator dependent and therefore may not be readily available at all times. Advantages of an ultrasound include that it is less expensive than other forms of imaging such as CT or MRI and it does not expose the patient to radiation. If there is clinical suspicion for concurrent abdominal processes, such as bowel obstruction, a CT scan may be the better study as it provides additional diagnostic findings.

Although Mr D does not currently exhibit signs or symptoms of bowel ischemia such as fever, tachycardia, systemic toxicity, or skin changes over the new bulge[2] or signs and symptoms of a bowel obstruction such as nausea and vomiting, a CBC is ordered as leukocytosis will raise my concern for a strangulated hernia.

CASE INFORMATION

Laboratory Results

Complete Blood Count	Normal Range	Today
White blood cell count (WBC)	4,000–11,000 cells/μL	6,400
Red blood cell count (RBC)	3.9–5.2 10_6 cells/μL	5.0
Hemoglobin	11.2–15.7 g/dL	14.5
Hematocrit	34%–45%	43
Mean corpuscular volume	80–100 fL	90
Mean corpuscular Hgb	25.6–32.2 pg	28.4
Mean corpuscular Hgb concentration	32–36 g/dL	34
Red cell distribution width	11.6%–14.4%	13.6
Platelet count	163–369 10e3/μL	202

Case Analysis: Definitive treatment for both direct and indirect inguinal hernias is surgical repair, which generally has minimal short-term morbidity, meaning most patients return to their presurgery baseline fairly rapidly. For uncomplicated hernias, the timing and technique (open versus laparoscopic approach) remain controversial.[5] However, with time, hernias tend to get larger and subsequently, more difficult to repair. Each year, more than 20 million inguinal and femoral hernia repairs are performed worldwide, 700,000 of these occurring in the United States. Almost 90% of these are performed on males.[2,5]

CASE INFORMATION

Given the presence of a hernia, acute onset of symptoms, and that Mr D's hernia was not reducible on initial examination, a surgical consultation is obtained. While awaiting this consultation, efforts were made to attempt spontaneous reduction of hernia contents. To do so, the patient was administered a combination of sedation and analgesia,[6] placed in Trendelenburg position,[1] and cold packs were applied to the hernia for 20 to 30 minutes. Unfortunately, spontaneous reduction was unsuccessful, so the general surgeon therefore attempted manual reduction, implementing the three techniques discussed above in addition to the following: placing the patient in a supine position with a pillow under knees to relax the abdominal wall musculature and externally rotating and flexing the opposite leg. Once the patient was positioned, firm, steady pressure was applied to the herniated contents close to the defect itself.[2] This resulted in hernia reduction and Mr D reported significant improvement in his groin pain. If pain had not improved after the hernia was reduced, the suspicion for strangulation remains high.

When an incarcerated hernia is reduced nonsurgically, the patient needs to be observed closely for the development of peritonitis caused by perforation or ischemic changes of a loop of strangulated bowel. Mr D remained afebrile, had a normal WBC, and noted continued pain relief following manual reduction of the hernia. He also tolerated oral intake, and his abdominal examination remained benign. As a result, the decision is made to discharge home. Discharge instructions for a patient following reduction of an inguinal hernia include specific signs and symptoms that should lead the patient to seek additional care. In this particular case, Mr D is instructed to return to the emergency department if he experiences any of the following: increased groin pain associated with a recurrent nonreducible bulge, nausea, vomiting, inability to tolerate oral intake, or fever. He is to follow-up in the General Surgery Clinic in the next 1 to 2 days for further evaluation and surgical planning/preparation.

Management of Groin Hernia

In general, elective repair of uncomplicated groin hernias should be done when possible as there is significantly higher morbidity and mortality associated with incarceration and strangulation.[1,4] Compared to elective repair, emergent surgical intervention for an incarcerated or strangulated hernia is accompanied by higher morbidity and mortality,[6] often related to the viability of the bowel entrapped within the hernia.[4] Further, there are relatively few contraindications to inguinal hernia repair and typically, the main contraindication relates to the anesthesia required for the surgery itself. For patients with significant comorbidities, such as a significant cardiac or pulmonary history, surgery may be performed with a combination of monitored anesthesia care and local anesthetic,[5] using an open approach to repair. Potential complications following inguinal hernia repair include, but are not limited to, the following: bleeding, hematoma formation, infection, damage to adjacent structures (for instance, blood supply to the testicle), blood clots, chronic pain/nerve injury, hernia recurrence, complications from anesthesia, heart attack, stroke, and even death. Another contraindication to hernia repair is active infection or systemic sepsis if the hernia repair will involve implantation of a prosthetic mesh, which is commonly used so that the end result is a tension-free repair, decreasing the risk of hernia recurrence. Preoperative antimicrobial prophylaxis is indicated if mesh will be implanted.[5]

Urgent or emergent hernia repairs are indicated when there are signs and symptoms of strangulation. To prevent loss of bowel due to strangulation, surgery is often needed within 4 to 6 hours of symptom onset.[5] If a patient exhibits signs and symptoms of strangulation and emergency surgery occurs, he/she should also be treated based on the nature of hernia complication. For example, if bowel perforation is suspected, broad spectrum antibiotic therapy should be initiated and narrowed when possible as intraoperative culture results become available.[1,2,5] Nasogastric decompression as well as correction of fluid status and electrolyte abnormalities may be necessary if bowel obstruction is present.[1]

References

1. Melman L, Matthews BD. Hernia. In: Klingensmith ME Aziz A, Bharat A, Fox AC, Porembka MR, eds. *Washington Manual of Surgery*. 6th ed. Philadelphia, PA: Lippincott Williams & Wilkins; 2012.
2. Nicks BA. Hernias. Medscape. April 10, 2014. http://misc.medscape.com/pi/iphone/medscapeapp/html/A775630-business.html. Accessed June 13, 2014.
3. Inguinal hernia. National Digestive Diseases Information Clearinghouse (NDDIC) Web site. http://digestive.niddk.nih.gov/ddiseases/pubs/inguinalhernia/inguinalhernia.pdf. Published December 2008. Accessed June 13, 2014.
4. Alvarez JA, Baldonedo RF, Bear IG, Solis JAS, Alvarez P, Jorge JI. Incarcerated groin hernias in adults: presentation and outcome. *Hernia*. 2004;8:121-126. doi: 10.1007/s10029-003-0186-1.
5. Brooks DC. Overview of treatment for inguinal and femoral hernias in adults. UpToDate. October 31, 2013. http://www.uptodate.com/contents/overview-of-treatment-for-inguinal-and-femoral-hernia-in-adults. Accessed June 13, 2014.
6. Harissis HV, Douitsis E, Fatouros M. Incarcerated hernia: to reduce or not to reduce? *Hernia*. 2009;13:263-266. doi: 10.1007/s10029-008-0467-9.

CASE 35

Mary M. Brennan

Mary M. Brennan is the Coordinator of the Adult ACNP Program at New York University. Dr Brennan practices in a cardiology service where patients are managed by NPs in collaboration with cardiologists.

CASE INFORMATION

Chief Complaint

A 67-year-old African American male is transported via ambulance from a primary care clinic to the nearest emergency room (ER) with a severely elevated blood pressure of 228/120 accompanied by confusion.

The emergency medical responders report that the patient has a long-standing history of uncontrolled hypertension (HTN), type 2 diabetes mellitus (DM), and hypercholesterolemia. He was seen by his primary care nurse practitioner (NP) who noted the patient had an elevated blood pressure of 230/120 associated with acute confusion. An ambulance was called to transport the patient to the nearest ER.

When evaluating a patient who presents with acute confusion, assessing hemodynamic stability is the first priority. I initially evaluate the patient's airway, breathing, circulation and vital signs including the blood pressure, pulse rate, respiratory rate, and oxygen level. Assessment of vital signs is not only a prudent first step in the assessment of the patient, but also the first step in determining the cause of the confusion. Hypotension, hypertension, tachycardia, bradycardia, tachypnea, apnea, and hypoxia may all contribute to the development of acute confusion. If the patient is hemodynamically unstable, immediate measures to correct any of the aforementioned derangements are warranted. For example, if the patient's blood pressure is decreased, intravenous fluids and vasopressors may be needed to restore the blood pressure to a normal range even before a diagnosis is established.

❓ What is the potential cause?

When patients present to the ER with acute confusion accompanied by a severely elevated blood pressure a broad spectrum of diagnoses are considered. Life-threatening causes of acute confusion such as a hemorrhagic stroke, embolic stroke, or transient ischemic attack (TIA) will need to be ruled out first. Hypertensive emergency, the presence of target organ damage in conjunction with a severely elevated blood pressure, will need to be differentiated from hypertensive urgency, severely elevated blood pressure in the absence of target organ damage. Target organ damage may manifest as confusion related to encephalopathy, blurred vision associated with papilledema, chest pain associated with acute coronary syndrome, a "tearing" pain consistent with a ruptured thoracic aorta, and renal failure. In this case, the presentation of acute confusion in the setting of severe hypertension strongly suggests a neurovascular cause, such as acute stroke, or encephalopathy as a result of the hypertensive emergency. Alternatively, common causes of confusion such as acute drug/alcohol toxicities, hyperglycemia, hypoglycemia, or hypoxia should also be considered. Differentiating among these possibilities is imperative since treatment of each is variable and complicated, and may or may not require reduction of the blood pressure.

List of Differential Diagnoses for Acute Confusion[1]

A comprehensive list of all possible diagnostic differentials is listed below.

- Neurologic: Neurologic possibilities top the differential list at this point. Stroke, transient ischemic attack (TIA), hypertensive encephalopathy, and traumatic head injury are priority diagnoses and will need to be considered and ruled out. Other considerations are migraine headache, dementia, brain tumor, postictal state, and Wernicke encephalopathy.
- Cardiovascular: Myocardial infarction, cardiac tamponade, thoracic aortic dissection, heart failure, valvular disorders, coarctation of the aorta.
- Pulmonary: Acute respiratory failure, hypoxemia, hypercarbia.
- Gastrointestinal: Abdominal aortic aneurysm.
- Genitourinary: Acute renal failure, obstructive renal disease, pyelonephritis, urinary tract infection.
- Metabolic: Hypoglycemia, hyperglycemia, illicit drugs, alcoholic or diabetic ketoacidosis, hepatic encephalopathy, renal failure, hypernatremia, hyponatremia, hypercalcemia.
- Endocrine: Adrenal crisis, thyrotoxicosis, myxedema coma, Cushing disease, adrenal crisis, hyperaldosteronism, pheochromocytoma.
- Musculoskeletal: Trauma.
- Infectious: Acute systemic infection, meningitis, encephalitis, brain abscess, neurosyphilis.
- Exogenous: Acute intoxication, withdrawal of antihypertensive agents; illicit drug use including cocaine, amphetamines, sympathomimetic drugs
- Other: Dehydration, constipation.

In this case, a search for the cause will be pursued at the same time that treatment measures are being considered to reduce the blood pressure. Asking questions as to when the patient was last seen without confusion provides a timeline of events and helps pinpoint when the symptoms first began. I will also need to ask his wife about any associated symptoms such as weakness or difficulty speaking to narrow the list of potential causes.

CASE INFORMATION

General Survey

The patient's vital signs, on admission to the ER are: blood pressure 228/116 mm Hg, heart rate of 78 beats per minute (bpm), normal sinus rhythm on the monitor, a respiratory rate of 18/min, and a room air oxygen saturation of 96%. He is lethargic but easily arousable, disoriented to time and place and therefore unable to give a reliable history. I will need to gather data from his wife and the electronic health record (EMR).

History of Present Illness

The patient's wife denies that the patient experienced weakness, paresis, or paralysis of extremities, dysarthria, aphasia or other signs that may indicate a stroke, but notes that the patient started acting "strangely" at approximately 8 PM the night before admission. This morning, he was confused about the day and year, and forgot many of the details about his daughter's recent wedding. She was concerned so took him by taxi to the primary care office, where the NP called 911. She reports there is no recent history of falls or trauma, or substance use. She endorses that the patient has hypertension and diabetes, as reported by the primary NP, and denies any history of cancer or heart disease. She also reports that he stopped taking his blood pressure medications approximately 6 months ago because they caused excessive fatigue. She is unsure if he is taking his other prescribed medications.

Past Medical History

• Hypertension, diabetes, high cholesterol

Past Surgical History

• Per wife and EHR the patient has never had surgery

Social History

• Patient's wife reports he has never smoked, does not drink, does not use drugs

Medications

• No allergies to any medications
• Lipitor 10 mg by mouth daily
• Metformin 500 mg by mouth twice daily
• Per EHR: he is prescribed amlodipine, a calcium channel blocker, 10 mg by mouth daily and Toprol, a selective β-blocker, 50 mg by mouth daily, but has not filled his prescriptions for the last 6 months

Given the information obtained so far, what are the pertinent positives and significant negatives?

Pertinent Positives

- The patient is 67 years of age.
- The patient is presenting with progressively worsening confusion of 12 to 16 hours duration.
- The patient's blood pressure is severely elevated to 228/116 mm Hg.
- The patient stopped taking his blood pressure medications about 6 months ago. The EHR reveals he has not filled his prescriptions for the last 6 months.
- The patient's risk factors for cardiovascular and neurovascular disease include male gender, African American ethnicity, older age, diabetes, and hypertension.

Significant Negatives

- The patient's wife denies knowledge of recent trauma or falls.
- The patient's past medical history is negative for cancer or heart disease.
- There is no history of substance use or abuse.

 How does this information affect the list of possible causes?

Summarizing the salient points from the case information allows the nurse practitioner to focus on the important aspects of the case.

I rephrase my problem representation as: "This is a 67-year-old male with a past medical history significant for hypertension, type 2 diabetes, and medication nonadherence who presents with progressively worsening confusion in association with a severely elevated blood pressure of questionable etiology."

The patient's long-standing history of hypertension increases his risk for the development of hypertensive emergency. Essential hypertension can cause hypertensive emergency in Caucasians; however, the risk is increased in African Americans and males.[2] The physical examination will provide additional information as to the potential etiology of the confusion and hypertension. Conducting a rapid survey from head-to-toe will help me identify signs of trauma, such as bruising, erythema, or swelling of the extremities, signs that may signal a recent fall with a head injury. Assessment of the cranial nerves may help identify possible neurovascular or stroke symptoms. Evaluation of the cardiovascular system including listening for carotid bruits may reveal a clinically significant carotid stenosis. Assessment of the jugular veins, and auscultation of heart sounds, S1 and S2, may indicate the presence of valvular disorders such as aortic stenosis or mitral regurgitation, and may lead me to consider a diagnosis of heart failure. Muffled heart sounds may provide evidence of cardiac tamponade with a resultant decrease in cardiac output contributing to consequent confusion. Examining the abdomen may identify the presence of abdominal bruits, an indication of disease of the aorta, renal arteries, or iliac arteries. Diminished or absent pulses including radial, brachial, femoral, popliteal, dorsal pedis may help identify a dissection of the aorta, or an obstructive mass, such as a tumor, or thrombus.

CASE INFORMATION

Review of Systems

The patient is not able to answer all of the questions; some of the information is obtained from the patient's wife.

- Constitutional: Denies fever, chills.
- Cardiovascular: Denies chest pain, chest pressure, shortness of breath, palpitations.
- Pulmonary: Denies shortness of breath.
- Gastrointestinal: Denies abdominal discomfort; unable to determine last bowel movement.
- Genitourinary: Denies burning with urination.
- Musculoskeletal: Denies pain of extremities.
- Neurological: The patient is not able to provide a timeline as to the onset of confusion; per wife, the patient started acting strangely after dinner— "quiet, noncommunicative, not answering questions—said he didn't feel well, but would not elaborate." This morning, his wife was concerned when he appeared dazed and confused. He was disoriented to day and time. Wife reports acute change in short- and long-term memory.
- Endocrine: Denies thirst, excessive urination, or excessive hunger, does not check blood glucose at home.

Physical Examination

- Vital signs: Repeat blood pressure is 200/120 mm Hg in both the right and left arms; heart rate is 78 beats per minute; respiratory rate is 16 breaths per minute; oxygen saturation on room air is 95%.
- Weight: 90 kg; height 5'10", body mass index (BMI) is 28.1.
- Fingerstick glucose is 92.
- Constitutional: Obese male, appears stated age, lethargic, disoriented to time and place, oriented to person, arouses easily, able to answer simple questions with a "yes" or "no."
- Head/eyes/ears/nose/throat: Normocephalic, anicteric, funduscopic examination reveals exudates and cotton wool spots consistent with grade III retinopathy, no carotid bruits, no thyromegaly or thyroid nodules.
- Cardiovascular: S1, S2, no murmurs, no gallops, no rubs, + displaced PMI. Pulses present bilaterally +2/+2 femoral pulses, +2/+2 right and left dorsalis pedis and posterior tibial pulses.

- Pulmonary: Respirations even and unlabored, breath sounds are clear, equal throughout.
- Gastrointestinal: Normoactive bowel sounds, abdomen is soft, nontender, no hepatosplenomegaly, + left epigastric abdominal bruit—systolic-diastolic bruit.
- Musculoskeletal: Nontender spine; + systolic-diastolic bruit—located at the mid to lower left of the spine.
- Neurological: Limited neurologic examination due to the patient's inability to follow commands. Cranial nerves II-XII intact, however, unable to examine extraocular movements due to the patient being unable to follow commands; otherwise grossly nonfocal, able to move both arms and legs; no facial asymmetry, no dysarthria.

? What additional information from the review of systems and clinical examination should be added to the list of pertinent positives and significant negatives?

- **Pertinent positives:** On examination, the patient has a number of physical characteristics that indicate a long-standing history of hypertension such as a displaced point of maximal impulse (PMI), and grade III retinopathy. The finding of a left-sided abdominal bruit in the presence of severe hypertension supports the diagnosis of renal artery stenosis as the etiology of the hypertensive emergency.
- **Significant negatives:** Equal blood pressures on both right and left arms, palpable pulses in all extremities, absence of focal neurological deficits, normal cardiac and pulmonary examinations, normal blood glucose.

? How does the above information help to narrow the list of possible etiologies?

The presence of significant comorbidities, such as hypertension and type 2 diabetes, in association with a severely elevated blood pressure, raises the suspicion for serious neurological and cardiovascular causes. Acute coronary syndrome, stroke, and hypertensive encephalopathy are top diagnostic possibilities that must be considered and excluded immediately.

? What diagnostic testing should be done and in what order?

While there is no evidence of focal neurological deficits, a noncontrast-enhanced computed tomography (CT) scan of the head is needed to definitively rule out a stroke.

The American Heart Association/American Stroke Association recommends that a CT be performed within 25 minutes of the patient's presentation.[3] CT is reliably able to visualize areas of parenchymal hemorrhage, thus ruling in a hemorrhagic infarct and excluding eligible patients from receiving fibrinolytic therapy. If the CT is negative for a hemorrhage and reveals findings associated with an embolic stroke, this patient would still not be eligible for fibrinolytic therapy due to the duration of his symptoms, exceeding the usual window of 3 hours, and in some cases 4.5 hours, from symptom onset. CT may provide evidence of an early infarct, such as loss of gray-white differentiation; however, these infarct signs are apparent in fewer than two-thirds of patients.[3] Changes associated with hypertensive encephalopathy may be apparent, including alterations in white matter. While other diagnostic examinations such as an MRI of the brain have superior sensitivity and specificity for detecting an acute infarct, the ease of performing an CT, in combination with widespread availability of this technology and the relative low risk in comparison to other diagnostic technologies, makes CT the preferred initial diagnostic test.

The next priority, after the CT, is a 12-lead electrocardiogram (ECG) and continuous telemetry monitoring to rule out acute coronary syndrome and possible atrial or ventricular arrhythmias. A series of cardiac troponin levels is ordered to determine if myocardial damage has occurred. A chest radiograph is ordered to address the possibility of a ruptured or dissecting thoracic aortic aneurysm. Abnormal chest x-ray findings of the aorta and mediastinum such as a widened mediastinum are associated with a 90% sensitivity for the presence of a thoracic aortic aneurysm.[4] Since an infectious etiology is also a concern, a dipstick urinalysis is done and a urine culture is sent. While the patient's wife denies a history of alcohol or substance use or abuse, a toxicology screen will be sent along with a complete blood count (CBC) and a basic metabolic panel (BMP) to corroborate the history and determine if renal failure or electrolyte derangement is contributing to this patient's confusion. His history of diabetes mellitus suggests that both hyperglycemia and hypoglycemia are considerations but his fingerstick on admission is normal at 92, effectively ruling out these causes.

The presence of an abdominal bruit strongly supports the diagnosis of renal artery stenosis as the precipitating cause of the severely elevated blood pressure. A renal ultrasound is the preferred noninvasive test and a Class I, Level of Evidence (LOE) C recommendation in the diagnostic workup for renal artery stenosis, particularly in patients who may have renal disease.[5] Diagnostic studies have determined that the presence of an abdominal bruit is moderately sensitive for the diagnosis of renal artery stenosis, with sensitivities ranging from 39% to 63% and specificities of 90% to 99%.[6] Other diagnostic considerations given the presence of an abdominal bruit include an abdominal aortic aneurysm, splenic arteriovenous fistula, and pancreatic carcinoma.[6] If renal artery stenosis is excluded, another consideration is pheochromocytoma, a tumor of the adrenal gland that synthesizes, stores, and then secretes catecholamines erratically throughout the day and can thus cause severely elevated blood pressure. Cushing disease, an increase in glucocorticoids, and hyperaldosteronism, both of which may cause or worsen hypertension, are additional possibilities.

CASE INFORMATION

Preliminary Diagnostic Results

12-lead ECG reveals NSR of 78 beats per minute; PR interval 0.14, QRS interval 0.06; QT interval 0.40 with left ventricular hypertrophy; CXR demonstrates borderline cardiac enlargement; negative for a widened mediastinum.

NECT: Negative for bleeding; diffuse white matter changes consistent with cerebral encephalopathy.

Laboratory

Today	One Year Ago
Troponin 0.01 ng/mL	
Na 140 mEq/L	Na 136 mEq/L
K 4.4 mEq/L	K 4.2 mEq/L
Cl 105 mEq/L	Cl 107 mEq/L
CO_2 24 mEq/L	CO_2 21 mEq/L
Total cholesterol 200 mg/dL	Total cholesterol 261 mg/dL
LDL 139 mg/dL	LDL 156 mg/dL
HDL 32 mg/dL	HDL 25 mg/dL
Triglycerides 300 mg/dL	Triglycerides 402 mg/dL
BUN 40 mg/dL	BUN 23 mg/dL
Creatinine 2.5 mg/dL	Creatinine 1.0 mg/dL
WBC 6,900 cells/μL	WBC 7,600 cells/μL
Hgb 12.7 g/dL	Hgb 13.8 g/dL
Hct 35.5%	Hct 38.5%
Glucose 92 mg/dL	Glucose 105 mg/dL
HgbA1c 8.5	HgbA1c 7.0
Glomerular filtration rate (GFR)= 36 cc/min	Glomerular filtration rate (GFR) = 87 cc/min

Today: urinalysis: specific gravity 1.020, pH 5.0, color clear, protein 100 mg/dL, leukocyte esterase negative, nitrite negative, ketones negative, red blood cells negative.
Toxicology screen: negative.

Case Analysis and Diagnosis

A review of the patient's clinical, laboratory, and diagnostic test data allows me to cross off several items on my differential diagnosis list. First, the CT is negative for hemorrhage, ruling out hemorrhagic stroke. The CT does show white matter changes, suggesting hypertensive encephalopathy as the cause of his persistent confusion. The lack of focal neurological deficits in conjunction with the CT report diminishes the likelihood of an embolic stroke. The absence of chest pain, pulse deficits, and a widened pulse pressure, in conjunction with a normal chest radiograph, makes ruptured aortic aneurysm very unlikely. Myocardial infarction is similarly ruled out based on the normal troponin level and absence of ischemic changes on ECG. On examination, there is no evidence of heart failure, respiratory failure, or acute infection; the patient's white blood cell count is normal. The patient's lab values also rule out electrolyte imbalance as the cause of his confusion.

The laboratory results show an increased creatinine of 2.5, which is 2.5 times the baseline serum creatinine, consistent with acute kidney injury (AKI). The glomerular filtration rate (GFR) is 36 cc/min, a significant reduction from last year's GFR of 87 cc/mL; however, in the setting of AKI, a calculated GFR is less reliable. I suspect that the elevated creatinine is due to hypertensive emergency, but I must consider the possibility of urinary obstruction as well. I order an ultrasound to evaluate for kidney stones, an enlarged prostate, or a mass, all of which may obstruct the flow of urine in the urinary tract and contribute to AKI. Additional causes of AKI include dehydration, hypotension, infections, glomerular diseases, medications, rhabdomyolysis, and vasculitis—all of these are less likely in this patient than hypertensive emergency. An absence of hematuria, red blood cells, and red blood cell casts helps exclude glomerular causes. A negative urine leukocyte-esterase and lack of white blood cells rule out a urinary tract infection.

A severely elevated blood pressure with the associated findings of confusion and an increase in the serum creatinine and blood urea nitrogen (BUN) lead me to conclude that the patient has hypertensive emergency, which is hypertension causing target organ damage. This damage is the result of a critical rise in systemic blood pressure causing injury to the vascular endothelium, with a subsequent reduction in circulating vasodilators, such as nitric oxide, and an increase in systemic vasoconstrictors, including the renin-angiotensin-aldosterone system. The damage to the endothelium also activates the coagulation system with increases in clotting factors such as thrombin, fibrin, and platelets, all of which lodge in the damaged endothelium and obstruct vessels. Widespread vascular damage also contributes to an increase in the release of cytokines and proinflammatory factors, such as IL-6, causing further damage, vascular permeability, and a serious reduction in the perfusion to critical organs, such as the brain, the kidney, and the heart.

The brain is particularly sensitive to abrupt changes in blood pressure. Cerebral perfusion pressure is maintained in hypertensive patients by vasoconstriction and by shifting the mean pressure needed to maintain perfusion from 60 to 120 mm Hg to 110 to 180 mm Hg. Changes above this pressure contribute to vasodilation, hyperperfusion, and cerebral edema, the changes associated with hypertensive emergency.

Management of Hypertensive Emergency with Encephalopathy and Nephropathy

Reducing the blood pressure is of paramount importance; however, in most cases of severely elevated blood pressure, it is important not to reduce the blood pressure too quickly, as this may contribute to a significant decline in the cerebral perfusion pressure. Although there are no evidence-based guidelines for blood pressure control in hypertensive emergency, reducing the mean arterial blood pressure (MAP) by 20% or less within the first hour is considered safe.[7] The exception to this rule is the treatment of aortic dissection when rapid reduction of the blood pressure to a goal systolic pressure of less than 120 mm Hg and a reduction in the heart rate of less than 65 bpm are indicated.

For this patient, presenting with encephalopathy and kidney injury, immediate treatment is instituted to reduce the diastolic pressure to between 100 and 110 mm Hg within the first hour. Reducing the blood pressure in hypertensive emergency is very effective in relieving the associated symptoms of encephalopathy including confusion, headache, and blurred vision and decreases the risk of irreversible neurologic deficits. Over the next 24 hours, the goal is to reach the patient's target systolic blood pressure of 140 mm Hg or less, and a diastolic pressure of 90 mm Hg or less. These goals are consistent with the latest Eighth Joint National Committee (JNC VIII) guidelines for treating hypertensive patients with diabetes.[8]

There are a number of intravenous antihypertensive infusions that may be used to treat hypertensive encephalopathy with associated renal involvement. Fenoldopam, a dopamine (DA) receptor agonist, is a rapid acting vasodilator and acts on both DA1 and DA2 receptor sites. DA1 stimulation causes significant vasodilation of both the systemic circulation and the renal circulation, lowering blood pressure within a few minutes. Favorable vasodilator effects on both the afferent and efferent arterioles make Fenoldopam an effective option for this patient who has acute kidney injury. Since Fenoldopam is excreted by the kidneys, caution must be exercised in the prolonged use of this medication due to concerns over accumulation of the agent. Increases in intraocular pressure, hypokalemia, tachycardia, and hypotension may occur. Nicardipine, an intravenous dihydropyridine calcium channel antagonist, is also an option. Other intravenous agents that may be considered are labetalol, an α-adrenergic and β-adrenergic antagonist, indicated for the treatment of aortic dissection and Enalaprilat, an angiotensin-converting enzyme inhibitor (ACE-I), which may be particularly suited for the treatment of acute heart failure. In this case, ACE-Is are contraindicated due to acute kidney injury. Nitroprusside, an arteriolar and venous vasodilator, is effective in reducing blood pressure, however, should be used with caution in patients with possible renal disease.

? What is the etiology of the hypertensive encephalopathy?

The question remains as to the etiology of the hypertensive emergency. The patient's history of hypertension and clinical examination reveal manifestations of long-standing, and poorly controlled HTN as evidenced by a displaced PMI, grade III retinopathy, and a left abdominal systolic-diastolic bruit suggestive of renal artery stenosis with mild proteinuria. Prolonged, uncontrolled hypertension, obesity, age, gender, and African American ethnicity constitute risk factors for the development of cardiovascular disease, including renal artery stenosis and increases the patient's risk for hypertensive emergency.

Once the blood pressure is stabilized, a duplex ultrasonography of the abdomen is ordered to evaluate for the presence of renal artery stenosis, a Class I, Level of Evidence (LOE) B indication for individuals who experience hypertensive emergency and/or the sudden onset of severe hypertension.[5] Doppler ultrasonography has excellent sensitivity and moderate to high specificity for accurately diagnosing renal artery stenosis.[9] An ultrasound of the abdomen with Doppler ultrasonography reveals a shrunken left kidney, a peak systolic velocity (PSV) in the left renal artery of 220 cm/s without a detectable Doppler signal, consistent with a significant stenosis of the left renal artery. In addition, the ultrasound excludes an obstruction of the urinary tract as the cause of his AKI.

Renal Artery Stenosis

Patients with multiple risk factors for the development of cardiovascular disease, such as obesity, diabetes, older age, and hypertension are at increased risk of developing atherosclerotic renal artery stenosis, which is the most common form of the disease. Fibromuscular dysplasia (FMD), a disease that weakens the media component of the renal artery, is the second most common cause of renal artery stenosis, usually affecting younger individuals, particularly females. The cause is unknown. FMD accounts for up to 10% of all cases of renal artery stenosis, and is often not associated with cardiovascular risk factors.[10]

In this case, the patient most likely has atherosclerotic renal artery stenosis, severe enough to interrupt the blood flow to the left kidney as evidenced by atrophy of the affected kidney. A consult to a nephrologist and/or interventional radiologist is warranted to determine if the patient is a candidate for revascularization, through either angioplasty or stenting. To date, large randomized controlled trials have not shown endovascular interventions to be superior to traditional risk factor reduction and medical therapy, perhaps owing to the inherent bias of many of the trials.[10] Therefore, strict risk factor reduction and medical therapy are central to the treatment of all patients with atherosclerotic renal artery stenosis. In this patient's case, once the acute hypertensive emergency is addressed, improved compliance with both nonpharmacologic and pharmacologic therapies is needed to reduce and prevent further cardiovascular and neurovascular atherosclerotic complications.

References

1. Pisani MA, Murphy TE, Araujo KL, Van Ness PH. Factors associated with persistent delirium after intensive care unit admission in an older medical patient population. *J Crit Care*. 2010 Sep;25(3):540. e1-7. doi: 10.1016/j.jcrc.2010.02.009. Epub 2010 Apr 22.
2. Varon J, Marik PE. Clinical review: the management of hypertensive crises. *Crit Care*. 2003;7(5): 374-384.
3. Jauch EC, Saver JL, Adams HP, et al. Guidelines for the early management of patients with acute ischemic stroke: a guideline for healthcare professionals from the American Heart Association/ American Stroke Association. *Stroke*. 2013;44:870-947.
4. Klampas MJ. Does this patient have an acute aortic dissection? *JAMA*. 2002;287(17):2262-2272.
5. Anderson JL, Halperin JL, Albert NM, et al. Management of patients with peripheral artery disease (compilation of 2005 and 2011 ACCF/AHA Guideline Recommendations). *J Am Coll Cardiol*. 2013;61(14):1555-1570.

6. Rosner MH. Renovascular hypertension: can we identify a population at high risk? *South Med J.* 2001;94(11):1058-1064.

7. Johnson W, Nguyen ML, Patel R. Hypertension crisis in the emergency department. *Card Clin.* 2012;30(4):533-543.

8. James PA, Oparil S, Carter BL, et al. 2014 Evidence-based guideline for the management of high blood pressure in adults report. Report from the panel members appointed to the Eighth Joint National Committee (JNC 8). *JAMA.* 2014;311(5):507-520. doi:10.100/jama.2013.284427.

9. Chain S, Luciardi H, Feldman G, et al. Diagnostic role of new Doppler index in assessment of renal artery stenosis. *Cardiovasc Ultrasound.* 2006;(4)4: doi:10.1186/1476-7120-4-4.

10. Shetty R, Biondi-Zoccai GGL, Abbate A, et al. Percutaneous renal artery intervention versus medical therapy in patients with renal artery stenosis: a meta-analysis. *EuroIntervention.* 2011;7:844-851.

CASE 36

Donna W. Markey

Donna W. Markey is an ACNP caring for adult hematology and oncology patients in a university-based community cancer center. She has a vast background in critical care, digestive health, surgical and medical oncology, is a preceptor of NP students, and coordinates survivorship care in her practice.

CASE INFORMATION

Chief Complaint

A 50-year-old female was seen by her primary care physician (PCP) earlier in the week with the complaint of frequent bruising over the past 3 months. A complete blood count (CBC) revealed platelets of 11,000/μL (normal = 100,000–450,000/μL). An urgent hematology consultation is requested and I see the patient in my office.

❓ What is the potential cause of bruising?

Bruising and bleeding are nonspecific signs with a variety of medical and non-medical etiologies. A comprehensive differential list of possible etiologies will guide me in gathering relevant information from the patient and her family during history taking.

Differential Diagnoses for Frequent Bruising

Quantitative or functional platelet disorders, hemophilia, malignancy, clotting factor disorders, liver dysfunction, recent infection, vaccine exposure, adverse drug reactions, tissue trauma from potential physical abuse, and vitamin C deficiency.

Differential Diagnoses for Thrombocytopenia

For this patient, I also know that she is thrombocytopenic; in other words, her platelet count is low. Thrombocytopenia is a condition that is generally classified as being the result of (1) impaired or decreased production of platelets, (2) increased platelet destruction, or (3) disorders related to distribution or dilution of platelets. These categories may be further expanded as follows:

1. Impaired or decreased platelet production is associated with numerous congenital disorders, neonates, viral exposure, drug-induced or acquired factors.

2. Increased platelet destruction is associated with acute and chronic immune thrombocytopenia purpura (ITP), drug-induced immunologic thrombocytopenia, heparin-induced thrombocytopenia (HIT), posttransfusion isoimmune thrombocytopenia, secondary autoimmune thrombocytopenia. Nonimmune causes can include preeclampsia and thrombocytopenia in pregnancy, human immunodeficiency virus (HIV) infection, thrombotic thrombocytopenia purpura (TTP), disseminated intravascular coagulation, hemolytic uremic syndrome, and drugs causing nonimmune mechanisms of platelet destruction.

3. Disorders related to distribution or dilution include splenic sequestration, hypothermia, and loss of platelets due to massive blood transfusions or extracorporeal circulation.[1]

Establishing the most likely cause of the patient's bruising will inform my diagnostic decision making and the development of my treatment plan.

CASE INFORMATION

General Survey and History of Present Illness

With a mental list of the potential causes for thrombocytopenia, I begin to gather data, from the patient and her family. Experience allows me to focus and prioritize the assessment, so that it is organized efficiently and effectively. Before I see the patient I review the CBC performed at her PCP's office that reveals normal red blood cell indices with normal mean corpuscular volume (MCV) and red blood cell distribution width (RDW). There is an isolated thrombocytopenia and no other abnormal findings.

I begin with a general survey of the patient upon entering the examination room. She is seated comfortably with another woman whom she introduces as her close friend. Her husband is out of town. The patient explains that her family doctor told her that her platelet count is low and that she should see a hematologist. She states she never had bruising like this before and even when she had gallbladder surgery 3 years ago, she had no problem with bleeding. However, recently she had a steroid injection into her hip for pain relief and while the steroid did help the pain, she bruised heavily. She denies any recent illnesses or taking any medications other than occasional ibuprofen for "stiff joints" which she presumes is arthritis. On the Internet she learned that low platelets can be associated with bleeding and cancer and she is very nervous about this. I explain to her that we need to consider all the possible causes of low platelets and bruising and that we will move through her evaluation quickly to find the answers and help her with this problem. The potential causes for low platelets serves to guide me in formulating my questions as I begin a comprehensive history and physical.

Past Medical History

She has never had a blood transfusion, and denies any medical problems including heart disease, liver disease, diabetes, or cancer. She is up to date with health screening and vaccinations, has had her annual mammogram, gynecologic follow-up, and first screening colonoscopy within the prior 6 months.

- Past surgical history: Laparoscopic gallbladder surgery 3 years ago, no increased bruising or bleeding.
- Social history: Lives with husband, monogamous relationship. She does not drink alcohol now or in the past and does not smoke or use recreational/illicit drugs. She denies HIV and hepatitis risk factors.
- Family history: Adopted—does not know family history, two adult children alive and well (vaginal deliveries without complications).
- Allergies: None known.
- Medications: Ibuprofen as needed, no medications taken on a regular basis.

Review of Systems

The patient is an excellent historian.

- Constitutional: Denies fevers, chills, drenching sweats, does endorse hot flashes consistent with menopause. Appetite is generally good, states anxiety presently suppressing appetite; weight is stable. Tires more easily but able to meet work and personal obligations; has not missed time from work in the past 3 months. Sleeps well at night and denies any pain. No recent travel or recent illnesses.
- Head/eyes/ears/nose/throat: Wears glasses for reading, denies nosebleeds or gingival bleeding.
- Cardiovascular: Denies chest pain or palpitations, no history of heart problems or hypertension.
- Pulmonary: Denies cough, shortness of breath.
- Gastrointestinal: Occasional nausea, no vomiting, reflux associated with dietary indiscretion, commonly avoids spicy foods, denies bright red blood or melena with bowel movements, bowel movements three to four times per week baseline, drinks limited fluids during work day.
- Genitourinary: Denies blood in urine, frequency or urgency, no incontinence. Endorses perimenopause, no menses in 4 months.
- Integumentary: No skin rashes, but endorses bruising and small splattered red spots on arms and legs, reports increased bruising over last 3 months, which appear without provocation. Denies falls, trauma, or physical abuse.
- Musculoskeletal: Occasional stiff joints, particularly fingers and knees. Recent left hip pain, received steroid injection with relief but noted heavy bruising.

- Neurological: Denies history of stroke, occasional headaches, described as "tension" relieved with ibuprofen, two to three times per week. No vision changes, altered thought processes, no falls or seizures. Reports occasional dizziness with quick movement from bending to standing or seated to standing. No weakness, numbness, or tingling.
- Lymphatic: Denies swelling or "enlarged glands."
- Endocrine: Denies diabetes, increased hunger, thirst or urination, reports stable weight.

Physical Examination

- Vital signs: blood pressure 98/60, heart rate 88 beats per minute, temperature 98.8 oral, respiratory rate 20 breaths per minute, height 5ft 3 inches, weight 109 lb (49.5 kg)
- Constitutional: well appearing, well groomed, developed, petite statured, appears stated age, makes eye contact, and engaged in discussion
- Head/eyes/ears/nose/throat: normocephalic, atraumatic, pupils equal, round, and reactive to light and accommodation, oral mucosa moist, no lesions or thrush, dentition in good repair, petechia on dorsum of tongue
- Cardiovascular: S1, S2, normal, no murmurs, rubs, or gallops, rate and rhythm regular
- Pulmonary: respirations even and unlabored, clear breath sounds bilaterally
- Gastrointestinal: normoactive bowel sounds, no rebound or guarding, mild tenderness left upper quadrant, splenic tip palpable 1 cm below costal margin
- Genitourinary: normal
- Integumentary: skin warm and dry, ecchymosis of differing ages noted, left arm at elbow 3 × 4 cm bruise; left hip 5 × 4 cm bruise associated with recent injection. Scattered petechiae on bilateral lower extremities. 2 × 2 cm bruise right knee
- Musculoskeletal: no edema or tenderness, full range of motion in all joints
- Neurological: alert, oriented to person, place, and time, no focal deficits, speech clear and fluent, upper and lower extremity strength 5/5 throughout; cranial nerves 2–12 intact
- Lymphatics: no palpable lymphadenopathy
- Psychiatric: normal mood and affect

❓ What are the pertinent positives and the significant negatives in the information we have obtained so far?

Pertinent Positives

- New and progressive scattered bruising
- Decreased platelet count
- Fatigue increased above baseline over the preceding 3 months
- History of headaches of longer duration than bruising, relationship unknown
- Occasional nausea, indigestion
- Mild left upper quadrant tenderness, with prominent/palpable spleen

Significant Negatives

- The patient is not in any acute distress
- No active bleeding
- No known history of bleeding or bruising prior to this incident
- No weight loss, fevers, drenching sweats
- No history of alcohol use, liver disease, HIV, hepatitis, or infection
- No recent medication use or changes
- No abdominal pain to suggest splenomegaly
- With exception of abdominal findings and bruising the examination is normal

❓ Can the information presented thus far be restated in a single sentence highlighting the pieces that narrow down the cause?

A single problem representation statement sets the stage for gathering more information and determining the cause. The problem representation statement in this case might be: A 50-year-old woman in generally good health presents with a recent 3-month history of increased fatigue, easy bruising, and thrombocytopenia.

Case Analysis: Now I have lots of data with which to compare the potential different causes of my patient's thrombocytopenia and begin to do so by evaluating them based on the categories described earlier.

Impaired or decreased platelet production: The patient's prior good health, stable weight, and absence of fevers or night sweats make malignancy a less likely explanation for her low platelet count. Likewise she has not had any viral illnesses in the preceding 6 months and has no history of HIV or hepatitis infections, making these unlikely explanations for her low platelets. This does not mean testing for these is unnecessary as either could cause low platelets. If present, treating them may result in correction of the problem.[2] Given her history, alcohol and liver disease are also not likely explanations for her thrombocytopenia. Because she takes no regular prescription medications or illicit drugs, a medication side effect is not likely. But she does take ibuprofen for headaches periodically, which can interfere with platelet function and she will need to stop this medication. Regardless it is unlikely this is the cause of her thrombocytopenia. And at the age of 50 it is highly unlikely that a congenital disorder would emerge now.

Disorders related to distribution or dilution: Hypothermia and loss of platelets due to massive blood transfusions or extracorporeal circulation are not supported by her history and I eliminate them from my list. Splenic sequestration generally presents with a much larger spleen than I found on my physical examination and upper abdominal complaints of discomfort are more common.

Increased platelet destruction: As her story unfolds, I recognize that the potential cause for her thrombocytopenia is most consistent with a platelet destruction process. An immune-mediated cause is high on my differential as this is the leading cause of platelet destruction problems. Over the last 3 months that she has noticed bruising, it is possible that her spleen has been sequestering platelets as they are destroyed, thus resulting in the very mild splenomegaly I detected. But there are other nonimmune causes of platelet destruction as well. At this point in my diagnostic evaluation, I need additional data to determine the cause of her platelet destruction.

❓ What diagnostic testing should be done?

A complete blood cell count with differential is a requisite for anyone with a bleeding or bruising disorder and it may detect anemia and potential infection. A peripheral smear provides details about the number and types of cells, the shape of the cells, and whether there are cell fragments that suggest cell lysis. These data provide further clues to the diagnosis and nature of platelet dysfunction. A normal platelet count is 150,000 to 300,000/μL. Bleeding can occur if platelets are below 50,000. Pancytopenia (low red blood cell count, low white blood cell count, and platelet counts) indicates bone marrow failure. If this is the case, a vitamin B_{12} level should also be checked, as B_{12} deficiency can lead to anemia and platelet depletion.

Depending on the results of the CBC with differential and smear, I will consider a platelet function analysis, which screens for von Willebrand deficiency. The von Willebrand factor (vWF) is the superglue of platelets, allowing platelets to adhere to injured blood vessel walls and activate the migration of platelets to an injured area. vWF is also the plasma carrier of clotting factor VIII. A decrease in vWF causes decreased circulating factor VIII.[2]

I draw a prothrombin time (PT) and activated partial thromboplastin (aPTT) and international normalized ratio (INR) to help identify alterations in the extrinsic and intrinsic clotting pathways. PT and aPTT are basic measures of coagulation to evaluate increased bruising or bleeding. A PT of 11 to 16 seconds indicates normal extrinsic pathway coagulation. Factors I, II, V, VII, and X can be assessed using the INR, where 1 is normal, and 2 to 3 is therapeutic on warfarin therapy. An aPTT of 33 to 45 seconds indicates a normal functioning intrinsic pathway. This measures factors XII, XI, X, IX, VIII, and V. The aPTT is also used to monitor heparin therapy.

A complete chemistry profile is one of the most comprehensive tests as it includes electrolyte, liver, and kidney function values. A total bilirubin is the combination of the indirect bilirubin (preliver) and the direct bilirubin (liver). In cell lysis, the indirect bilirubin is often elevated as is LDH. The direct bilirubin is elevated in liver disease. ALT, AST, and alkaline phosphatase are also elevated in cases of liver inflammation and cell lysis. BUN and creatinine may be elevated in renal disease and with dehydration. A haptoglobin is an additional test for hemolysis, I need not draw that yet. A low haptoglobin indicates red blood cell destruction due to hemolysis.

A urine analysis (UA) may be helpful to look for protein which may be two times higher than normal in patients with renal failure. Hemolysis or liver disease can result in the presence of urinary bilirubin and hemoglobinuria. Hematuria suggests bleeding from the kidney, ureter, or bladder.

According to the American Society of Hematology HIV and HCV should also be tested in any patient with a bleeding disorder[1] regardless of risk factors.

CASE INFORMATION

Results and Analysis

The patient's CBC reveals a normal white blood cell and red blood cell profiles, but the patient's platelets are 10,000/μL. Her CMP reveals normal BUN, creatinine, total bilirubin, and liver enzymes. The PT, INR, and aPTT are all normal. B_{12} is 410 pg/mL (normal). With these findings I can rule out liver or renal dysfunction as well as a clotting factor defect. Because of these results I defer the UA and any further platelet dysfunction testing. At this point I am ready to list immune (idiopathic) thrombocytopenia purpura (ITP) as the diagnosis. ITP is usually diagnosed by excluding other possible causes of bleeding and a low platelet count, such as an underlying illness or medications. I have ruled out bone marrow causes as well as clotting disorders.

Idiopathic Thrombocytopenia Purpura: Management

I explain these results to the patient and also tell her that in the absence of active bleeding we do not recommend transfusions or an inpatient admission. Treatment recommendations are influenced by appraisal of the patient's ability to comply with treatment and frequent monitoring of the CBC. Conservative first-line treatment includes observation, corticosteroids, and IVIG (intravenous immunoglobulin). She will start prednisone 75 mg daily and she will return in 48 hours to obtain a repeat CBC.

I teach her about the side effects of prednisone and the importance of immediately seeking medical care if she begins to experience active bleeding. She is advised not to work for now; I write a directive to that effect for her employer. In addition I caution her about activities that may result in injury. If there is no improvement in her platelet count in 48 hours we will consider initiating IVIG infusions. This will help accelerate a rise in platelets. Additional treatments for refractory ITP unresponsive to steroids or IVIG include rituximab (Rituxan), new thrombopoietin stimulating agents, and potentially splenectomy.

Case Follow-Up

The patient's platelets initially responded with a rise to 60,000/µL, then fell once again below 20,000/µL at which time we proceeded with IVIG. This did not result in a durable response and she was treated with rituximab, weekly for 4 weeks. She did not respond to rituximab and is presently on eltrombopag, an oral thrombopoietic agent. Her platelets have been stable for the past 4 weeks at 55,000/µL. She has had no further bleeding or bruising. We will maintain her on this agent as long as she tolerates it and it maintains her counts. If this becomes ineffective we will consider alternate agents or splenectomy.

References

1. Karnath B. Easy bruising and bleeding in the adult patient: a sign of underlying disease. *Hosp Physician*. January 2005;41(1):35-39.
2. American Society of Hematology. 2011 Quick reference: clinical practice guideline on the evaluation and management of immune thrombocytopenia. www.hematology.org/practiceguidelines.

CASE 37

Elizabeth S. Gochenour

Elizabeth Gochenour is an ACNP on the Wound Ostomy Care team at the University of Virginia Medical Center in Charlottesville, VA.

CASE INFORMATION

Chief Complaint

Ms S presents to the emergency department (ED), with the chief complaint of "I don't feel good" and "my ostomy bag leaks all of the time." I am called to see the patient by the ED physician.

History of Present Illness

The patient is a 38-year-old female with a past medical history of hypertension, hyperlipidemia, diabetes mellitus type 2, and factor V Leiden disorder who was discharged 6 days ago following an exploratory-laparotomy and small bowel resection for a small bowel infarction secondary to superior vein thrombosis mesenteric ischemia. She returned to the OR on day 3 for a reexploration, end ileostomy, and fascial closure. Her hospitalization was complicated by the development of bilateral lower extremity deep vein thrombosis (DVT). She is on enoxaparin sodium injections bridging to oral warfarin (Coumadin).

? What is the potential cause of the patient's symptoms?

The patient's complaints of "not feeling well" and a leaking ostomy appliance may be related. Because Ms S is recently status post an exploratory laparotomy I must quickly determine if there is a surgical complication such as bleeding, pulmonary embolus, or sepsis that may be causing her to "not feel good." Once I rule these out, I will look at other less urgent potential causes.

Initial Differential Diagnoses

- Pulmonary embolus
- Cardiac conditions: arrhythmias, heart failure, MI
- Infection and sepsis
- Mesenteric thrombosis
- Electrolyte disturbances
- Anemia

- Dehydration
- Hemorrhage
- Hypovolemia
- Hyper/hypoglycemia
- Acute renal failure
- Perforated bowel
- Small bowel obstruction

CASE INFORMATION

General Survey

With all of these possible causes in mind, I will begin to narrow down my list of possible causes by gathering data and eliminating some of these diagnoses.

In this case I begin with a general survey of the patient. She is an obese female, appearing to be well nourished and well developed. She does not appear to be in any distress. She is independently mobile and able to answer questions, and is smiling and conversant with me. Her mother is with her and they express concern that they cannot get the patient's ostomy bags to stay on for more than a few hours. Ms S denies fever, chills, or night sweats. She denies palpitations as well. She states she has felt generally tired and weak ever since she returned home. She also says she has lost her appetite and has only been able to drink about three to four glasses of fluid per day and feels nauseated and dizzy most of the time. She has felt particularly bad since last night at bedtime. Nothing makes her feel better or worse. When questioned about her ileostomy output she and her mom state that more than 2 L per day is being produced. She describes her urine output as "ok."

I continue to gather information for the history of present illness but I suspect at least part of her problem is that she is not taking enough fluids to stay adequately hydrated given her ileostomy output. At this point I am thinking that the "not feeling well" is directly related to her state of hydration. However, given her complicated surgical history, I must rule in, or out, other causes.

❓ What are the pertinent positives from the information gathered up to this point?

- Ms S is dizzy, tired, and weak
- Ms S has a poor appetite
- Ostomy output >2000 mL/day for the last 4 days

- Nausea and poor oral intake
- Urinary output fair per patient report

? What are the significant negatives?

- No apparent distress
- Well nourished, well developed
- No cardiac history
- Denies palpitations

? Can the information gathered so far be restated in a single sentence highlighting the pieces that narrow down the cause?

By putting the information in a concise statement—a problem presentation—the stage is set for gathering more data and determining the cause. The problem representation in this case might be: "A 38 year-old female s/p recent ileostomy presents to the ED with high ileostomy output, nausea, dizziness, and weakness."

? How does this information affect our differential diagnosis?

Because Ms S is in no apparent distress I am thinking that the symptoms are urgent but not life threatening at this point. Regardless, I must quickly collect additional information to better hone my differential. Since she has a history of DVT and factor V Leiden disorder, I must consider the potential for a pulmonary embolism (PE). While I doubt that this is the cause given her stable state, and the fact that she is on enoxaparin and warfarin, it stays on my differential for now until I gather more information. Perforated bowel, mesenteric thrombosis, and sepsis are also life-threatening conditions but I would expect the patient to look much sicker with any of these disease processes, so they are low on my differential at this point. A cardiac cause also cannot be ruled out but is less likely given her age and stable state. An obvious potential cause of her symptoms is the high ileostomy output, which can cause both fluid and electrolyte imbalance. I will explore this further because I am especially concerned about her fluid status and electrolytes, specifically her potassium. I need more information so will proceed to a comprehensive history and physical.

CASE INFORMATION

History and Physical Examination

Past medical history: As noted in HPI plus irritable bowel syndrome and endometrial cancer. She lives with her sister who is supportive, but is expressing significant challenges caring for the patient postoperatively.

Past surgical history: Uterine fibroid surgery followed by hysterectomy in 2010.

Family history: Type 2 diabetes in maternal grandmother, mother, sister, and brother. Hypothyroid disease and clotting disorders in her father.

Social history: Denies alcohol or tobacco use; occupation: works as a cashier at a department store but has not returned to work since her surgery.

Review of Systems (ROS)

- Constitutional: has had chills, denies fever
- Cardiovascular: denies chest pain, palpitations, diaphoresis, neck pain
- Pulmonary: denies shortness of breath, cough, or recent pulmonary infections
- Gastrointestinal: endorses nausea and liquid stool; denies abdominal pain, blood in stool, or emesis
- Genitourinary: denies dysuria, urinary frequency, blood in urine
- Neurological: endorses dizziness and light-headedness, denies confusion, memory loss, motor/sensory deficit, loss of consciousness, gait changes, or seizure activity
- Integumentary: notes that she has a rash around her stoma and the ileostomy bags will not stay on

Medications

- Acetaminophen 650 mg by mouth every 4 hours as needed for pain
- Amlodipine 5 mg by mouth daily
- Aspirin 81 mg by mouth daily
- Atorvastatin 40 mg tablet daily by mouth
- Enoxaparin 100 mg/mL injection 1.1 mL subcutaneously every 12 hours
- Insulin aspart (NovoLog FlexPen) 100 unit/mL : 8 units before meals unless blood sugar is over 200 then take 13 units; insulin glargine 100 units/mL injection: take 50 units subcutaneously at bedtime
- Warfarin 2.5 mg one tablet by mouth daily
- Imodium 2 mg two tablets before each meal and at bedtime

Allergies

Vancomycin: decreased kidney function (elevated BUN and creatinine)

Physical Examination (PE)

- Vital signs: Blood pressure 100/56 mm Hg, pulse 110 beats per minute, temperature 36.4°C (97.5°F), respiration 16 breaths per minute, weight 226 lb BMI 37, SpO_2 98% on room air.
- Constitutional: Obese female, appears stated age, in no apparent distress.
- Head/eyes/ears/nose/throat: Normocephalic, atraumatic, extraocular movements normal, pupils equal, round, reactive to light, no injection

or scleral icterus. Dry mucous membranes. No oral erythema, lesions, or exudate.

- Neck: Supple, full range of motion.
- Cardiovascular: Regular rate, tachycardic at 110, no murmurs, rubs, or gallops.
- Pulmonary: No accessory muscle use, clear to auscultation in all lung fields.
- Gastrointestinal: Abdomen obese nondistended, positive bowel sounds, stoma in right upper quadrant, pink moist, with liquid fecal effluent. Abdomen soft, to palpation and nontender to moderate pressure, no rebound or guarding,
- Musculoskeletal: Moves all extremities freely. Strength is 4/5 throughout.
- Integumentary: No edema, no rashes, warm and dry, denudement noted on peristomal skin. Abdominal incision well healed and pink, without exudate.
- Neurological: Awake, alert, and oriented. Appears calm and comfortable, easily engaged, answering questions and smiling occasionally. Thought process coherent. She does indicate she is tired as well as frustrated with the frequent bag changes and the irritation around her stoma. Cranial nerves II-XII intact. No pronator drift noted. Gait not assessed.
- Psychiatric: Normal mood and affect.

❓ What elements of the review of systems and physical examination should be added to the list of pertinent positives? Which items should be added to the list of significant negatives?

- **Pertinent positives:** positive for dizziness and light-headedness, positive for chills, poor oral intake, nausea, dry mucous membranes and liquid stool, denuded skin around stoma, tachycardia with heart rate of 110, blood pressure 100/60 mm Hg is low given history of hypertension
- **Significant negatives:** afebrile, abdomen examination benign, no respiratory distress, heart sounds normal, no neurological deficits noted

---

❓ How does this information affect our potential causes?

The patient's examination is essentially normal with the exception of her ileostomy output and irritation around her stoma. I rule out bowel ischemia or perforation at this point. Bowel obstruction is eliminated as well since her ostomy output is high (even while taking maximum doses of Imodium). She is not in any respiratory distress and has no signs of a potential deep vein thrombosis such as leg swelling or redness, so I am comfortable moving pulmonary embolism lower on my differential. Sepsis seems less likely given the absence of fever, and there is no clear source of infection but I will need additional diagnostics to rule this out or in. Anemia could cause some of her symptoms though there is no sign of obvious bleeding. Regardless, she is on warfarin so I cannot eliminate this yet. Laboratory studies will help me rule this in, or out. Dehydration is high on my list given her dry mucous membranes, high ostomy output, and tachycardia. I also am concerned about her electrolytes. I order a peripheral intravenous access to be placed and a 500 mL infusion of 0.9% NS over an hour followed by intravenous fluids of 0.9% NS at 100 mL per hour. I ask the nurse to place her on a bedside monitor which shows sinus tachycardia, no arrhythmias, but high peaked T waves are present. At this point I must obtain some diagnostics to further evaluate the patient.

❓ What diagnostics are needed at this time and in what order?

- ECG: I am very concerned about the peaked T waves so a stat ECG is essential. I will compare this to her preoperative ECG.

- Chest x-ray: Her respiratory examination is normal but a baseline is important because I have initiated fluid repletion and suspect she will require more fluids. I want to watch for changes in volume that may cause pulmonary edema.

- Laboratory tests: I order a comprehensive metabolic profile (CMP) to evaluate her electrolytes, glucose and renal function, and a lactic acid to evaluate for acidosis that may be associated with an ischemic bowel. A complete blood count (CBC) with a differential is necessary to look for anemia and leukocytosis consistent with an infection. Because she is on anticoagulation with warfarin, I need a baseline should she have an occult bleed and need to be reversed with blood products. I will obtain a urinalysis to evaluate for a urinary tract infection. I also draw an arterial blood gas (ABG) to determine her acid-base status, specifically her pH.

CASE INFORMATION

Results of Diagnostics

ECG: sinus tachycardia and peaked Ts, no signs of ischemia
Chest x-ray: no acute cardiopulmonary disease, heart size normal, lungs clear

Laboratory Findings

- CBC with differential (abnormal values noted)
- RBC 3.3 (normal = 4–4.9 × 10⁶/mL), Hgb 9.3 (normal = 12–15 g/dL), Hct 28 (normal = 36–44)
- WBC 14,000 (normal = 4,000–11,000 cells/μL), neutrophils 70% (normal = 54%–62%), bands 4% (normal = 3%–5%)

- Comprehensive metabolic panel:
  - glucose 180 (normal = 70–110 mg/dL)
  - potassium 6.6 (normal = 3.5–4.8 mEq/L)
  - CO_2 18 (normal = 22–29 mEq/L)
  - Na 131 (normal = 135–147 mEq/L)
  - Cl 105 (normal = 98–107 mEq/L)
  - blood urea nitrogen (BUN) 70 (normal = 7–18.7 mg/dL)
  - creatinine 3.1 (normal = 0.6–1.1 mg/dL)
- Anion gap 14.6 (N: 5–15)
- Albumin 3 (normal = 3.2–5 g/dL)
- Coagulation: PT 20.7 (normal = 9.8–12.6), INR 1.8 (normal = 0.9–1.2)
- Lactic acid 2.4 (0.5–2.2 mEq/L)
- ABG: pH 7.30, $PaCO_2$ 32, bicarbonate 15 mEq/L, PaO_2 92 (room air)
- Urinalysis: color yellow, appearance turbid (normal = clear), specific gravity 1.028 (normal = 1.002–1.030), pH 5, protein trace (normal = negative), blood trace (normal = negative), glucose negative, ketones negative, bilirubin negative, RBC 4 (normal <3), WBC 17 (normal <2), casts 8 (normal <1), bacteria negative, epithelial cells 24 (normal <9)

Case Analysis: The patient's CBC confirms that Ms S is anemic. However, her postoperative hemoglobin and hematocrit were 8.7 and 27.2 respectively. Her current blood count is higher but it is likely due to hemoconcentration from her dehydration. I suspect her count will drop with rehydration so I will need to monitor this. None of her examination suggests an active bleeding site. Her WBCs are elevated and her neutrophils are elevated which could also be related to hemoconcentration. Stress from her recent surgery as well as smoking and steroid use can also cause elevated neutrophils; however, Ms S is not a smoker and not taking steroids presently. Her bands are normal but I cannot rule out infection at this time. She may potentially have an infection at the peristomal skin breakdown site, or another source. I keep infection on my list and also consider sepsis as a potential cause of her symptoms.

Her glucose and potassium are elevated most likely from hemoconcentration and should improve with fluid resuscitation. She is showing signs of acute kidney injury (AKI) as her BUN and creatinine are both elevated likely due to extreme dehydration, a common cause of pre-renal AKI. She also has an elevated potassium level, low sodium and bicarbonate levels, slightly elevated lactic acid but no anion gap acidosis at this time. In addition her pH demonstrates a partially compensated metabolic acidosis. I suspect this is due to dehydration but will need a renal consult as I continue to monitor and rehydrate the patient.

At this point I am confident that the diagnosis is significant dehydration due to inadequate fluid intake and excessive ileostomy output. This combination can account for her elevated potassium, lactic acidosis, and AKI.

I confer with the primary team attending physician and he agrees that admission is necessary to continue to work up and manage the patient.

❓ What interventions are necessary at this time?

While waiting for transfer to the medical intensive care unit, I know I must treat her potassium of 6.6 (moderate hyperkalemia). She has ECG signs (peaked Ts) that are ominous and which can transition to cardiac arrest. I follow ED management guidelines and treat her with 20 mL of 10% calcium gluconate intravenously over 5 to 10 minutes, 10 units of insulin, and 40 g of glucose intravenously as a bolus. I do not give sodium bicarbonate as it does not lower potassium in the first hour and is only used for severe acidosis (pH <7.20).[1] While hemodialysis is a preferred method to lower critical potassium levels, her potassium will decrease with rehydration should her kidneys continue to respond. If not, hemodialysis will be initiated. Ms S also requires more intravenous fluids; she reports subjective improvement with the NS bolus so I order two more liters. Because of her ECG changes, I keep her in a monitored bed in the ED until transfer.

Diagnosis and Treatment: Dehydration due to Excessive Ileostomy Output

Dehydration is the most common cause of readmissions in the postoperative ileostomy patient.[2] For severe dehydration it is initially essential to obtain peripheral IV access and provide 20 mL/kg of an isotonic crystalloid.[3] Because hyperkalemia due to acute kidney injury and electrolyte imbalance from ileostomy output can be a prelude to heart block and asystole, patients with hyperkalemia must be continuously monitored until the potassium is normal. Myocardial manifestations of hyperkalemia are (1) myocardial depression resulting in contractility and conduction disturbances, (2) arrhythmias including heart block and bradycardia, (3) hypotension, and (4) asystole.[4] Serial labs are followed to monitor changes in potassium and other electrolytes with rehydration.

Because the patient has acute kidney injury, a renal consult is warranted. Hypovolemia and hypotension have led to her pre-renal condition but should improve with rehydration. During the rehydration period, laboratory tests that are essential to monitor include urinary sodium (should be <10 mEq/L), specific gravity (should be less than 1.020), serum BUN to creatinine ratio (between 10:1 and 20:1). If there is no improvement in urine output then a renal ultrasound is warranted to rule out an obstruction.[5] But in this case it is likely that once the patient is normotensive and her cardiac output is optimized, her urine output will increase and her AKI will resolve.[5]

My patient's glucose is high but this will likely also decrease with hydration. I initiate an insulin infusion per our hospital protocol to maintain her glucose between 120 and 150. For now her home insulin regimen is on hold. I also order ondansetron (Zofran) for nausea and to increase oral rehydration, and strict intake and output including careful monitoring of the ileostomy output. Additional medical management for the high output from her ileostomy includes diphenoxylate/atropine (Lomotil) 5 mg four times daily (total of 20 mg a day) and loperamide (Imodium) 10 mg with each meal and at bedtime. Once the goal of fecal consistency of mush or oatmeal is met, the dosage may be decreased. Fecal output should be evaluated daily and the Lomotil titrated. The effects of Lomotil should be apparent after 48 hours.[6]

It is essential to accurately measure the ileostomy output and per the patient she is changing her appliance several times per day. An ostomy appliance should last 3 to 5 days. If it does not, then assessment for a different appliance is required. Now that I have addressed her more urgent problems, I can evaluate her ostomy and determine how we will manage it.

Care of an Ileostomy

As noted in Figure 37-1, Ms S's stoma is flush with the peristomal skin. When the stoma is not protruding or budded then the stool seeps under the ileostomy wafer and compromises the seal. The objective of the stoma is for fecal effluent to come up and out and into the appliance. In Ms S's case she is in need of convexity. Convex appliances have a "bump" or firm ring protruding circumferentially around the hole that is cut to fit the stoma (Figure 37-2). There is also a great deal of denudement around her stoma and typically these areas weep a moderate amount of serosanguineous drainage, which can also compromise the seal of the ostomy appliance. The use of ostomy powder to dust over the area assists in providing a dry top layer to achieve a seal.

Case Follow-Up

The patient's potassium decreased to normal and her urinary output increased rapidly in the MICU. The renal team followed her case and hemodialysis was not required. On day 3 of admission she was transferred to a medical floor for continued management. Her intravenous fluids were discontinued shortly thereafter because she was able to take adequate oral fluids. Her BUN and creatinine returned to baseline by day 5 and her sodium and potassium normalized by day 6.

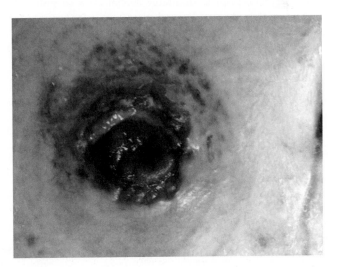

Figure 37-1 Denuded ileostomy site. Note the tissue damage related to exposure of fecal effluent.

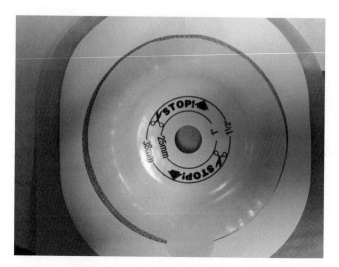

Figure 37-2 The convex wafer. In contrast to a standard flat appliance, the purpose of convexity is to apply pressure circumferentially around a stoma. This causes the stoma to stand at attention and improves how the stoma protrudes into the pouch. The goal is to have the effluent go up and into the bag and not allow it to seep under the wafer and cause premature leakage.

The application of the convex pouching system (described above) allowed Ms S to wear the appliance for 2 days without leaking and within 4 days her peristomal skin was much improved. Her ileostomy output decreased to 750 mL/day with the Imodium and Lomotil regimen. She was provided further education about the importance of drinking 8 to 10 glasses of fluids daily and was transitioned to her home insulin regimen prior to discharge. Social work consulted secondary to Ms S's sister's concern that she could not adequately care for her at home. The social worker arranged for Ms S to be cared for in a skilled nursing facility following discharge. She was scheduled for a follow-up visit to her colorectal team 7 days after discharge. She has since had her ileostomy reversed and is doing well.

References

1. Ahee P, Crowe AV. The management of hyperkalaemia in the emergency department. *J Accid Emerg Med.* 2000;17:188-191. doi:10.1136/emj.17.3.188. http://emj.bmj.com/content/17/3/188.full. Accessed April 3, 2015.
2. Messaris E, Sehgal R, Deiling S, et al. Dehydration is the most common indication for readmission after diverting ileostomy creation. *Dis Colon Rectum.* 2012;55(2):175-180. doi: 10.1097/DCR.0b013e31823d0ec5.
3. Phillips E. Volume resuscitation. Medscape. December 8, 2014. http://emedicine.medscape.com/article/2049105-overview#aw2aab6b2b4. Accessed March 31, 2015.
4. Burns S, ed. *AACN Essentials of Critical Care Nursing.* 3rd ed. New York, NY: McGraw-Hill Publishers; 2014:389, chap 15.
5. Nazar CMJ, Bashir F, Izhar S, Anderson J. Overview of management of acute renal failure and its evaluation; a case analysis. *J Nephropharmacol.* 2015;4(1):17-22.
6. Epocrates Online. https://online.epocrates.com/noFrame/showPage?method=drugs&MonographId=1813&ActiveSectionId=8.

CASE 38

Michelle Beard

Michelle Beard is an ACNP who works in the University of Virginia's Cancer Care clinics in Charlottesville and Farmville. She manages hematology/oncology patients suffering from a variety of illnesses.

CASE INFORMATION

Chief Complaint

A 46-year-old woman presents to her primary care physician (PCP) with a several month history of fatigue. A complete blood count reveals pancytopenia. I am the acute care nurse practitioner working collaboratively with the attending in the hematology/oncology outpatient consult service. I ask the PCP to send the patient to the clinic for evaluation.

? What are the potential causes of fatigue?

Fatigue is a nonspecific symptom and the list of potential etiologies is quite broad. In this particular patient she is also presenting with pancytopenia that is likely contributing to her symptom of fatigue. However, to be sure we are not missing something I want to keep in mind that some patients will present with separate issues occurring simultaneously. So, I will consider both problems separately before fully deciding that they are correlative. Fatigue in and of itself does not require emergent consult. However, with the discovery of pancytopenia this should prompt an urgent workup to determine the underlying etiology of low counts as this person is at heightened risk for life-threatening complications.

Fatigue is in the top 10 most commonly seen complaints at PCP visits. Fatigue associated with a long, full day or physical and mental strain is common and a normal physiologic response. Prolonged fatigue is abnormal and should lead to further investigation. Some principal underlying disorders to consider when working up fatigue are infections, anemia, sleep disorders, endocrinopathies like diabetes, hypothyroidism, and adrenal insufficiency, side effects from medication, and malignancy. Hormonal changes from menopause in women or low testosterone in men can lead to fatigue.

Fatigue associated with an underlying organic etiology is often constant and only improved with decreasing activity level and rest. Fatigue from anxiety and depressive disorders will most often improve with activity/exercise but is not typically relieved with rest.[1]

❓ What are the potential causes of pancytopenia?

The differential for pancytopenia includes aplastic anemia, viral infections such as parvovirus B19, HIV, hepatitis, Epstein-Barr, cytomegalovirus, dengue fever, medication side effect, autoimmune diseases, alcoholism, hypersplenism, vitamin deficiency, bone marrow infiltrating neoplasms, bone marrow fibrosis.[2,3]

Now that I have considered my differential diagnosis for both fatigue and pancytopenia, I will want to proceed with a thorough discussion and review of systems with the patient. This will help me rule out possible causes, and make other diagnosis more likely.

CASE INFORMATION

History of Present Illness

The patient tells me that over the past 2 to 3 months she has noticed a diminished energy level that has progressively worsened over the past 2 weeks. She finds it hard to do any activity without stopping to rest. She denies any difficulty with sleeping and in fact she feels that she can sleep any time during the day if she could. She has noted an intermittent sore throat over the past week. She denies chemical exposures, prior chemotherapy, radiation therapy, and recent foreign travel. No other ill family members. She denies HIV risk factors. She brings with her a copy of the labs done by her PCP today, which show the following: white blood cell count (WBC) 1.57K/μL, red blood cell count (RBC) 2.13M/μL, hemoglobin 7.9 g/dL, hematocrit 23.1%, mean corpuscular volume 86 fL, platelet count 28K/μL. A white blood cell differential was not done and no other blood work was obtained.

Past Medical and Surgical History

She denies medical problems in the past. I review the notes from her PCP. She is not seen there routinely. Two years ago she went in for a well-visit examination. Blood work done at that time including CBC, comprehensive metabolic panel (CMP), thyroid-stimulating hormone, and lipid profile were normal. She had a mammogram after that visit which was normal but she has not had one this year. Her pap smear was normal at that time. She has not had any other health care visits except twice annual dental cleanings in the past 2 years. She reports she has not had laboratory studies done at outside locations. Her only surgical history is an appendectomy at age 12.

Family and Social History

She is a nonsmoker and drinks a glass of red wine about five nights out of the week. She has never been a heavy drinker. She is married and has no children. She has three siblings in good health. Her parents are both living and reported to be in good health with the exception of hypertension and glaucoma in her father. She works full time as an administrative assistant. Family history is negative for malignancy or hematologic disorders.

Medications

She has no allergies to any medications that she knows of, and she is not currently taking any prescription medications. She takes a multivitamin and calcium with vitamin D.

Review of Systems

- Constitutional: She ambulates independently into the clinic accompanied by her husband. I notice that she is pale and appears tired. She is nervous but alert and pleasant.
- Cardiovascular: No chest pain, cough, orthopnea, heart palpitations. Denies swelling.
- Pulmonary: She has some mild dyspnea with walking short distances or a flight of steps but no shortness of breath at rest.
- Gastrointestinal: She denies abdominal pain. She notes a slight decrease in her appetite over the past 1 to 2 weeks but no weight loss. Food does not taste as good. No excessive thirst. No change in bowel pattern. No rectal bleeding or melena.
- Genitourinary: No change in bladder pattern. No urinary frequency or dysuria. No hematuria. Her menstrual bleeding was heavy this month but no current vaginal bleeding.
- Musculoskeletal: She has some discomfort "in my thigh bones." No other sites of pain. She describes the pain as constant, dull, and aching. She rates the pain at 4/10. She has tried Tylenol on occasion and that does help somewhat. It is not interfering with sleep.
- Neurological: She denies headaches, visual changes, unsteady gait, unilateral weakness, or speech changes.
- Endocrine: She denies any fevers or drenching sweats. No cold or heat sensitivity. No polydipsia, polyuria, or polyphagia.
- Skin: She reports easy bruising and some gum bleeding with brushing her teeth. No tick or insect bites, skin rashes, or new lumps or bumps.

❓ What are the pertinent positives from the information given so far?

- Abnormal CBC: pancytopenia
- Worsening fatigue
- General weakness
- Dyspnea with exertion

- Gum bleeding, easy bruising, heavy menses
- Intermittent sore throat
- Decreased appetite and taste changes
- Thigh pain
- One glass of wine, five nights a week

❓ What are the significant negatives from the information obtained?

- No known exposures
- No weight loss, fevers, sweats (no B symptoms except fatigue)
- No chest pain
- No neurologic symptoms
- No apparent active bleeding
- Normal blood work 2 years prior
- No family history of malignancy
- Nonsmoker

❓ Can the information gathered so far be restated in a single sentence highlighting the pieces that could narrow down the cause?

A problem representation sets the stage for determining the cause and revealing additional information that may need to be gathered.

The problem representation in this case might be: "An otherwise healthy 46-year-old woman presents with new onset pancytopenia and progressive fatigue."

❓ How does the information affect our list of differential diagnoses?

The patient has no past medical history to suggest the etiology of her current problem. This appears to be an acute or new onset diagnosis. Since I did a thorough review of systems I can now move through the list of differential diagnosis fairly quickly and develop an efficient diagnostic workup. The two things common to both differential diagnosis lists are infection and malignancy. My leading hypothesis is that the fatigue is directly related to the low blood counts and most of my focus will be on getting to the bottom of her pancytopenia since the underlying cause can be life threatening. Also, treating the underlying cause of her low counts will most likely help the secondary fatigue.

She takes no medications associated with myelosuppression or fatigue. As such, I am able to quickly rule out medication toxicity. I confirmed that she takes no herbal supplements. She has no history of sleep disorders and nothing in her review of systems to suggest diabetes, thyroid, or other hormone-related issues. Vitamin deficiency is unlikely since her MCV is normal. She has no symptoms of neuropathy, sore tongue, pica, or restless legs. I would expect to see microcytosis in iron deficiency and macrocytosis in folate and/or B_{12} deficiency. However, if she has both deficiencies this can mask a change in the MCV. She has no history of gastrointestinal surgery or disorder to suggest a malabsorption state and given the rapidity of her symptoms this would seem unlikely especially with this level of myelosuppression and the absence of expected associated symptoms. Nonetheless, I will not rule this out yet, and testing is straightforward.

Alcohol consumption can lead to vitamin deficiencies, and direct bone marrow suppression. The toxic effects on the bone marrow from alcohol are dose dependent. She is considered a moderate drinker by the American dietary guidelines on alcohol use.[4] As such, I do not believe alcohol is playing a major role in her bone marrow suppression or fatigue and am comfortable ruling out alcohol as the culprit.

Since she does not live in an area associated with mosquitos carrying dengue fever, nor has she traveled to an affected area, I can rule this out. The other infections on my differential can be insidious and difficult to detect so I cannot rule them out at this time. She does report intermittent sore throats, so I will need to include inspection of her pharynx and palpation of her cervical lymph nodes in my physical examination. For now, infection remains on my differential. Autoimmune disorders and malignancies will stay on my differential as well. I will proceed with my physical examination with these pathologies in mind.

CASE INFORMATION

Physical Examination

- Vital signs: Blood pressure is 104/68, pulse is 88, respiratory rate is 20, and temperature is 98.9°F tympanic, oxygen saturation by pulse oximeter is 96% on room air.
- Constitutional: She is well developed, but appears fatigued. She is nervous but otherwise in no apparent distress.
- Head/eyes/ears/nose/throat: Pupils are equal, round, and reactive to light. Extraocular movements are intact. Funduscopic examination reveals no hemorrhages or white plaques. The conjunctivae are pale. Sclera are anicteric. Oropharynx is moist without significant erythema and no lesions. She does have oral candidiasis on her tongue. No gingival hypertrophy. Teeth are in good repair. Mucous membranes are pale.
- Neck: Supple without rigidity. No swelling. No parotid, occipital, submental, submandibular, cervical, or supraclavicular adenopathy. No thyromegaly.

- Cardiovascular: Heart rate and rhythm are regular. No murmurs, rubs, or gallops. No jugular venous distension. No carotid bruits. No edema, cyanosis, or clubbing.
- Pulmonary: Clear to auscultation and percussion. No wheezing, crackles, or rhonchi. No use of accessory muscles.
- Breasts: No skin or nipple changes. No discharge. No masses, thickening, or pain. No axillary adenopathy.
- Gastrointestinal: Normoactive bowel sounds. Tympanic on percussion. Soft and nontender without masses or hepatosplenomegaly. No inguinal adenopathy.
- Integumentary: General pallor. Warm and dry. Nail beds are pale. No rashes or erythema. Multiple small bruises on her forearms and lower legs. No petechiae.
- Musculoskeletal: No joint tenderness or swelling. Normal range of motion. Strength 5/5 × 4. No spinous process tenderness. No reproducible pain in her thighs or obvious abnormalities.
- Neurological: No focal deficits. Cranial nerves II-XII are intact.
- Psychiatry: Normal mood and affect. Interactive and maintains eye contact.

? Are there elements of the physical examination that should be added to the list of pertinent positives or significant negatives?

- **Pertinent positives:** oral candidiasis and pallor.
- **Significant negatives:** afebrile, normal vital signs, no masses, adenopathy, organomegaly, joint redness or swelling. No findings to explain thigh pain.

? Does this information from her physical examination affect the differential diagnosis list?

The oral candidiasis is suggestive of alteration of the immune system. Therefore, this finding does not alter my remaining list of possible causes since viral infections, autoimmune diseases, and malignancy can affect immune function. The finding of pallor is expected in someone with a significant anemia and does not change the possible causes at this time. The lack of masses or adenopathy is not unexpected given my remaining list of causes. I would expect a patient with a solid tumor that has spread to the bone or bone marrow to present with additional symptomatology. For example, a patient with advanced lung cancer that has metastasized to the bone or bone marrow would likely be experiencing weight loss, cough, and possible hemoptysis. However, the majority of viral illness, bone marrow disorders, autoimmune diseases, and vitamin deficiencies will not present with palpable masses or adenopathy.

There was no enlargement of her liver or spleen on physical examination. Enlargement of the spleen is a cardinal finding in hypersplenism. Sequestration of cells from an overactive spleen leads to engorgement of the spleen and secondary cytopenias. Splenomegaly can be seen in infections such as mononucleosis, tuberculosis, HIV, and hepatitis to name a few. Splenomegaly also occurs in portal hypertension from underlying liver disease, and in splenic infiltration with cancer cells from leukemia and lymphomas. Hypersplenism has now become a much less likely cause of her presentation.

There are no findings on clinical examination to suggest an autoimmune disease. However, there are more than 80 different types of autoimmune diseases. In considering several of the most common ones I recognize that none fit my patient's clinical presentation. They include lupus, rheumatoid arthritis, Graves disease, type 1 diabetes, psoriasis, inflammatory bowel disease, Hashimoto disease, and pernicious anemia. I am fairly confident that the cause of her symptoms is not from an underlying autoimmune disease.

Myelofibrosis is one of the chronic myeloproliferative neoplasms of the bone marrow in which an abnormal clone of stem cells does not mature properly, leading to thickening or scarring of the reticulin fibers of the bone marrow. This leads to a steady decline in hematopoietic function. To compensate, the liver and spleen begin to make blood cells, leading to enlargement of both organs. Early in the disease process the laboratory findings may reveal leukocytosis, anemia, and thrombocytosis. The majority of patients present with severe fatigue, marked splenomegaly, fevers, bone pain, weight loss, night sweats, and sometimes pruritus. Later in the disease process thrombocytopenia becomes more common. Both the World Health Organization and the Italian Society of Hematology consider the presence of splenomegaly to be criteria for diagnosis.[5,6] As for our patient, she has some of the presenting symptoms but is without splenomegaly. For now, we will move this to the bottom of the differential.

The term aplastic anemia is a misnomer. It is a disease reflecting deficiency of the production of stem cells in the bone marrow leading to peripheral pancytopenia, not just anemia, and to bone marrow hypoplasia. This can be a congenital or acquired bone marrow failure. The majority of cases are acquired following exposure to drugs, chemicals, ionizing radiation, or certain viruses. Presenting symptoms are typical for someone with pancytopenia: fatigue, dyspnea on exertion, recurrent infections (usually bacterial), and bleeding. Physical findings on examination are limited to pallor and bruising or petechiae. The liver, spleen, and lymph nodes are not involved.

? How does the information gathered and analyzed so far change the problem representation?

I now reexamine my problem representation. The new problem representation reads: "A 46-year-old female presenting with new onset pancytopenia resulting in progressive fatigue." At this point, I have narrowed the list of differential diagnosis to aplastic anemia, infiltrating bone marrow neoplasms, and less likely, infections and fibrosis of the bone marrow. As mentioned before viral illness can be insidious, and therefore, this will be left on the list of differential diagnosis. This list requires diligent and timely pursuit of the underlying disorder to ensure best possible outcome for the patient.

❓ What diagnostic testing should be done and in what order?

My first priority is to repeat the CBC and include the differential. This can be done easily in the office and results will be available within minutes. At the time the CBC is done I will prepare a smear for microscopy. Leukemias and myelofibrosis have distinct cellular characteristics that can be identified by simple microscopy. Aplastic anemia has no morphological abnormal cells and evaluation of the peripheral smear does not help to support the diagnosis. However, all patients presenting with pancytopenia should have a peripheral blood smear examined. Findings on the peripheral smear can help determine additional diagnostic workup. Most patients with this presentation will require bone marrow aspirate and biopsy. I can prepare for this as well.

CASE INFORMATION

Results of Diagnostic Tests

A repeat CBC reveals very similar results to those done earlier at her PCP's office. The differential reveals neutropenia with an absolute neutrophil count (ANC) of 340. Examination of her peripheral smear reveals multiple myeloblasts with Auer rods. Myeloblasts are large cells with high nuclear-to-cytoplasmic ratio and nucleoli. Auer rods are elongated structures seen in malignant cells of the neutrophil lineage and are really just linear groupings of primary granules. This finding is highly suggestive of acute myeloid leukemia. I recognize that without therapy my patient's condition is fatal. I discuss my findings and plan of action with the patient and her husband.

Diagnosis and Treatment: Acute Myeloid Leukemia (AML)

My patient has a typical presentation of symptoms related to the complication of pancytopenia from an underlying leukemic process. Her progressive fatigue, pallor, gingival bleeding, bruising, and oral thrush are all related to her low blood counts. Thigh pain or pain in the long bones, ribs, and sternum are a result of the increasing pressure from the proliferation of the leukemic cells within the bone marrow. A finding of peripheral myeloblasts with Auer rods is highly suggestive of AML and I would consider this AML unless proven otherwise. A bone marrow aspirate and biopsy will be required to confirm the diagnosis and to obtain additional information including morphologic, cytogenetic, immunophenotypic, and molecular studies for classification using the World Health Organization (WHO) classification system. Prognosis and selection of treatment options is also determined based on these different classifications. A diagnosis of AML is confirmed when the marrow demonstrates 20% or greater infiltration with blasts and the blasts are myeloid in origin.

Without therapy, AML is fatal since normal hematopoietic function becomes severely impaired as the bone marrow becomes progressively infiltrated or "packed" with leukemic cells. Patients have a high likelihood of succumbing to infections or bleeding. Patients with acute myeloid leukemia require admission in a tertiary hospital that has experience and appropriate resources to manage the complexity of this disease. Careful physical examination is important to determine involvement of leukemia in other body systems like eyes, skin, gums, organs, and central nervous system. Additional laboratory studies will be required since AML can cause metabolic and electrolyte abnormalities such as tumor lysis syndrome which is an oncologic emergency. Disseminated intravascular coagulation (DIC) is another complication of leukemia placing the already compromised patient at high risk for both bleeding and clotting.

In addition to a bone marrow analysis on my patient, the following admission labs will be obtained: renal and liver function, LDH, electrolytes including phosphorus and calcium levels, uric acid and lactic acid levels, and coagulation studies to detect the presence of DIC. The clotting studies are important to obtain in order to prepare for central venous catheter placement in anticipation of treatment with systemic chemotherapy. I will also check serology for herpes simplex virus, cytomegalovirus, hepatitis profile, and HIV infection. Human leukocyte antigen (HLA) typing will also be performed in anticipation of possible bone marrow transplantation.

Once the diagnosis and classification of AML is made, the patient is prepared for induction chemotherapy with the goal of achieving remission. The standard "7 + 3" induction regimen is a combination of cytarabine and daunorubicin. The patient remains hospitalized during and after therapy to monitor and manage side effects, toxicity, and complications of the treatment. The patient requires intensive support during this time.

The majority of patients will achieve complete remission following induction chemotherapy. However, without additional consolidative therapy virtually all patients will experience a rapid relapse. Additional therapy is provided to eliminate any additional leukemic cells that may have survived induction but are not detectable by current surveillance studies. Three options for post-remission therapy are consolidative chemotherapy, autologous stem cell transplant, or allogeneic transplant.

Following completion of post-remission therapy the patient will be monitored closely at routine intervals especially during the first 2 years when the disease has the highest incidence of relapse. Long-term prognosis is variable and dependent on risk stratification obtained during our initial workup of karyotype and cytogenetic analysis.

References

1. Fatigue. UpToDate. http://www.uptodate.com/contents/approach-to-the-adult-patient-with-fatigue?source=search_result&search=fatigue&selectedTitle=1%7E150. Updated October 29, 2014.

2. Pancytopenia. UpToDate. http://www.uptodate.com/contents/search?search=pancytopenia&sp=0&searchType=PLAIN_TEXT&source=USER_INPUT&searchControl=TOP_PULLDOWN&searchOffset=. Updated October 21, 2014.

3. Weinzierl EP, Arber DA. The differential diagnosis and bone marrow Evaluation of new-onset pancytopenia. *Am J Clin Pathol*. 2013;139:9-29. doi: 10.1309/AJCP50AEEYGREWUZ.

4. Alcohol-related morbidity and mortality. National Institute on Alcohol and Alcohol Abuse. http://pubs.niaaa.nih.gov/publications/arh27-1/39-51.htm. Published December 2003.

5. Chronic myeloproliferative neoplasms treatment (PDQ). National Cancer Institute. http://www.cancer.gov/cancertopics/pdq/treatment/myeloproliferative/HealthProfessional/page4. Updated December 3, 2014.

6. Myelofibrosis. UpToDate. http://wwwuptodate.com/contents/myelofibrosis. Updated January 13, 2014.

CASE 39

Charles Fisher

Charles Fisher works as an ACNP in the Medical ICU at the University of Virginia and previously was the ACNP in the MICU step-down unit caring for long-term critically ill patients. His background spans many years as a critical care nurse in a thoracic-cardiovascular ICU.

CASE INFORMATION

Chief Complaint

A 26-year-old African American female is brought to the emergency department (ED) with a chief complaint of a 1-month history of intermittent joint pain without swelling.

? What is the possible cause?

The causes range from fairly benign, such as pain from overexercising, to life threatening such as malignancy. I will first think through all the possible causes and then gather more information from the patient to help me rule out, or rule in, the potential causes on my list.

> ### Differential Diagnoses for Joint Pain
>
> - Trauma or overuse injury
> - Infectious conditions such as Lyme disease, septic arthritis, HIV, cytomegalovirus, mononucleosis
> - Autoimmune disorders such as systemic lupus erythematosus, rheumatoid arthritis, antiphospholipid syndrome, mixed connective tissue disease
> - Malignancy with bone metastasis or leukemia, lymphoma
> - Underlying organ dysfunction such as glomerulonephritis or chronic liver disease
> - Fibromyalgia or chronic fatigue syndrome
> - Depression

CASE INFORMATION

History of Present Illness

The patient reports pain in her knees, hips, shoulders, and elbows. This has occurred off and on for the past month, and seems to be getting worse.

The patient denies any change in activity level or recent injury. The pain is not specifically associated with movement, nor with time of day and has not limited her activities of daily living, though some days all she wants to do is lie down. She has not noted any redness or swelling at the sites of pain, but she has had swelling in her ankles. She reports that massage, heat, cold, and over-the-counter analgesics including Tylenol and Advil do not alleviate the pain at all. Her associated symptoms include fatigue, low-grade fevers, urinary frequency and urgency, ankle swelling, and a rash on her face, which she thought was due to spending time in the sun but it has persisted for a full week. She denies any new soap, make up, or other facial products.

Her vital signs in the emergency room, heart rate of 105 beats per minute, systolic blood pressure 99 mm Hg, and temperature 38.1°C orally, trigger the best practice "sepsis alert." Blood drawn in the emergency room shows a hemoglobin level of 8.2 g/dL (12.0–15.0 g/dL) and white blood cell count of 4,200 cells/μL (4,500–10,000 cells/μL); platelet count 79×10^3/μL (100–450×10^3/μL), creatinine level is 1.9 mg/dL (0.5–1.4 mg/dL), and blood urea nitrogen (BUN) level is 52 mg/dL (7–20 mg/dL). Urinalysis reveals 3+ blood, 3+ protein, + nitrites, numerous bacteria, 15 dysmorphic red blood cells per high-power field (RBCs/HPF), and 22 RBC casts. She is started on ceftriaxone, 1 g intravenously every 24 hours[1] and admitted to the medical ICU for possible sepsis of urinary origin due to her fever, leukopenia, and acute kidney injury.

General Survey

Prior to doing a full history and physical, I survey the patient to determine her level of distress, particularly given the concern for sepsis that her initial presentation generated. She is alert, oriented, in no distress, receiving normal saline intravenously. Her most recent blood pressure is now 122/70 mm Hg and her heart rate is down to 90 beats per minute. Her face is discolored with patches of redness on each cheek that extend to the bridge of her nose.

Previous Medical History

The patient reports she has generally been in very good health, sees her primary care provider regularly, and had a routine physical 2 months ago. She was found to be anemic at that time and started on iron.

She has a history of two miscarriages over the last 3 years, while attempting to become pregnant. Evaluation by a fertility specialist is underway but she has not initiated any treatment.

Social History

She is married, no children, and lifetime nonsmoker, no alcohol use.

Family History

Her mother and father are living. Mother has diabetes, father has hypertension, and neither smokes. Two siblings are alive and well.

Medications

The patient has no known allergies and is not taking any prescription medications. She takes over-the-counter multivitamins with an iron supplement on irregular basis due to forgetting to take them. She also takes acetaminophen (Tylenol) and ibuprofen (Advil) on an as-needed basis.

? What are the pertinent positives from the information so far?

- Bilateral joint pain at multiple sites.
- Urinalysis shows urinary tract infection.
- The patient has mild ankle edema, no swelling in any other joint.
- Fatigue for the past month.
- Bilateral facial redness on both cheeks and bridge of nose.
- Pancytopenia.
- Acute kidney injury (elevated BUN and creatinine).
- Recurrent miscarriages.

? What are the significant negatives from the information given so far?

- The patient is afebrile.
- No signs of shock after fluid bolus.
- No other symptoms or organ systems involved at this time.

? Given the information so far what is your problem representation?

The problem representation in this case might be: "a 26-year-old female presents with possible sepsis of urinary origin, mild renal failure of an uncertain etiology based on the BUN and creatinine levels, and systemic symptoms of joint pain, facial rash, and fatigue."

Case Analysis: While initial results from the ER workup confirm the presence of a urinary tract infection (UTI), I also need to consider that this diagnosis does not explain the patient's presenting complaint of joint pain with profound fatigue for the past month. I review the care of patients with a urinary tract infection and find that ceftriaxone is appropriate for patients with sepsis of urinary origin and for pyelonephritis, both of which are more likely to cause the systemic symptoms this patient has.[1,2] The usual symptoms of urinary tract infection are dysuria, frequency, urgency, suprapubic pain, and/or hematuria; however, a patient with pyelonephritis may also experience fever, chills, flank pain, costovertebral angle tenderness, and nausea and vomiting. I will evaluate this further on full history and physical examination. The course of pyelonephritis can be insidious with nonspecific symptoms occurring over several weeks without progression to sepsis, organ failure, or shock.[1] At the moment, pyelonephritis seems the most likely diagnosis. My plan is to await the urine culture and switch the patient to an appropriate oral antibiotic. Assuming she improves on the ceftriaxone and her blood urea nitrogen and creatinine decrease with intravenous fluids I will likely transfer her from the intensive care unit to the general medical floor.

Reviewing my list of differential diagnoses, I am confident I can cross off injury, trauma, and depression. The patient denies any history of trauma or change in activity level and her lab results and vital signs demonstrate the presence of a physical disease process so I do not think depression is the primary issue. Based on the information gathered so far, an infectious process or an autoimmune process seems most likely. Certainly her fatigue and ankle swelling could be the result of her kidney injury, demonstrated by her elevated BUN and creatinine and her low hemoglobin. But this is a young otherwise healthy woman and a new onset of renal dysfunction is an unusual finding.

❓ What diagnostic testing should be ordered?

The patient's vital signs triggered a sepsis alert, although the alterations were mild and not indicative of a septic state. Her systolic blood pressure is above 90 mm Hg and her fever, while significant, is not over the standard 38.3°C threshold.[3] In addition, her heart rate came down to the low 90s on subsequent vital sign checks. It appears she is experiencing a systemic inflammatory response and it may be to the UTI, but I need to do a thorough history and physical to determine if another process is causing this alteration. I will follow up on urine and blood cultures, and do a chest x-ray to rule out a pulmonary source of infection. A renal ultrasound will also be helpful, to look for an obstruction that might cause her acute kidney injury and contribute to pyelonephritis. Plain films of her joints to determine a source of her pain may also be helpful, although the bilateral diffuse nature of the pain makes injury or dislocation unlikely. Given her history, a pregnancy test is needed; this would explain only some of her symptoms but could profoundly affect her care.

Her pancytopenia and low hemoglobin could be anemia due to her menses and possible iron deficiency anemia. I will obtain laboratory values from the primary care provider for comparison. Another consideration is that she has sepsis due to the urinary tract infection or another source and this has caused elevated BUN/creatinine levels, thrombocytopenia, and low WBC levels.[3] Some viral infections lead to low white blood cell count, and this may explain her facial rash as well.

CASE INFORMATION

Review of Systems

- Constitutional: Denies fevers, chills, or weight loss. Reports stable appetite, fatigue for the last month, where she wants to lay down even in the middle of the day but still does not feel rested. No recent change in activity, no falls, no trauma.
- Head/eyes/ears/nose/throat: Denies sore throat, rhinorrhea, tinnitus, or hearing loss. Denies changes in vision, blurriness, or double vision, does not wear glasses.
- Pulmonary: Denies shortness of breath, cough, or wheezing.
- Cardiovascular: Denies chest pain or palpitations. Endorses bilateral leg swelling.
- Gastrointestinal: Denies nausea, vomiting, abdominal pain, diarrhea, constipation, and melena.
- Genitourinary: Denies dysuria, but endorses urgency and urinary frequency. Also notes a decrease in urine output. Last menses 2 weeks ago.
- Musculoskeletal: As noted in HPI, she endorses bilateral joint pain at multiple sites that is unrelieved by rest or over-the-counter medications.
- Integumentary: Denies wounds, itching, or lesions. Endorses red facial rash, most recently started a week ago, not related to use of sunscreen, new cosmetics, soaps, or lotions. She has not had this rash before and does note that she has sunburned more easily in the past few months, and her primary care provider advised using high level of sunscreen on her face when she is outdoors.
- Neurological: Negative for dizziness, sensory change, speech change, and focal weakness.

Physical Examination

- Vital signs: Blood pressure 129/82 mm Hg, pulse 96 beats per minute, temperature 38.1°C (100.6°F), respirations 21/min, 98% saturation on room air; estimated body mass index is 20.8 kg/m^2 as calculated from the following: height 1.73 m (5' 7"); weight 60.0 kg (133 lb).
- Constitutional: No apparent distress, well developed, well groomed, well nourished, calm, cooperative African American female, with weight up 6 lb since her last check outpatient appointment visit.
- Head/eyes/ears/nose/throat: Normocephalic and atraumatic. Pupils are equal, round, and reactive to light. Extraocular muscles intact. Sclera is nonicteric. Oropharynx is clear. Moist mucus membranes, no oral lesions or dental problems.
- Neck: Neck supple. No lymphadenopathy.

- Cardiovascular: Regular rate and rhythm with no murmurs, rubs, or gallops. 2+ radial pulses, mild nonpitting edema of both ankles, equal bilaterally.
- Pulmonary: Eupneic respiratory rate and pattern, lungs are clear to auscultation bilaterally.
- Gastrointestinal: Bowel sounds present, normoactive, abdomen soft, nondistended, nontender. No rebound/guarding, shifting dullness, and +fluid wave.
- Musculoskeletal: Strength 5+ in all extremities, normal range of motion.
- Neurological: Alert and oriented to person, place, and time. No focal neurological deficits, sensation intact, cranial nerves intact.
- Skin: Warm, dry, and intact. Rash on her face on both cheeks and the nose sparing the nasolabial folds, erythematous, nonblanching, flat red patches, cool, nontender, and not on other areas of face, torso, or limbs. There is no facial edema or pruritus or other facial abnormalities.

Diagnostic Testing

Laboratory results on admission to the intensive care unit: hemoglobin level of 7.9 g/dL (12–15 g/dL) and white blood cell count of 3.2×10^3 cells/μL (4.5–10×10^3 cells/μL); platelet count is 71×10^3/μL (100–450), creatinine level is 1.9 mg/dL (0.5–1.4 mg/dL), and blood urea nitrogen level is 45 mg/dL (7–20 mg/dL). Urine culture initial Gram stain returns as gram-negative bacilli. The spot urine protein to creatinine ratio is 1.6.

Blood cultures drawn on admission show no growth to date.

Serum human chorionic gonadotropin test is negative.

Imaging

A renal ultrasound shows normal appearing kidneys. Plain radiologic films of her joints reveal no erosions as in rheumatoid arthritis, and her distal joints are not affected. A plain chest radiograph indicates clear lungs without cardiomegaly, effusions, or interstitial lung disease.

❓ What are the pertinent positives from the review of systems and physical examination?

- Rash and increased sensitivity to sunlight
- Bilateral ankle edema
- Pancytopenia and worsening renal function despite intravenous fluids
- Six pound weight gain
- Fever of 100.6 F

❓ **What are the significant negatives?**

- Negative pregnancy test.
- No history of abdominal, flank pain, nausea, or vomiting to suggest pyelonephritis.
- No prior renal disease.
- Renal ultrasound rules out hydronephrosis and obstruction.
- Chest radiography is normal.
- Blood culture shows no growth to date.
- Review of systems and examination do not suggest any other source for infection.

With the information collected so far, I believe she has a urinary tract infection, most likely due to *Escherichia coli,* resulting in a systemic inflammatory response with possible bacteremia sepsis. The sepsis has resolved with antibiotic and fluids, but the other symptoms, fatigue and joint pain, so are not explained by this diagnosis, and are nonspecific so may have a different cause. In addition, her acute renal failure did not improve with intravenous hydration, suggesting she may have intrinsic kidney injury, not just pre-renal failure due to infection. Her normal renal ultrasound rules out an obstructive uropathy. Her facial rash is an interesting finding and suggests a possible autoimmune process. The "butterfly rash" of systemic lupus erythematosus (SLE) can be transient or persistent, and is present in up to one-half of cases.[4] Other potential causes of the rash include rosacea, seborrhea, atopic, and contact dermatitis, but her history makes contact dermatitis unlikely as she denies any new medications or topical agents.[5] Other acute cutaneous lesions include generalized facial erythema with various lesions or pustules that she does not have.

I am thinking that this patient has renal failure of an uncertain etiology but that her pertinent positives including the facial rash, edema, fatigue, and joint pain in combination with her significant negatives of no history of prior renal disease, absence of hydronephrosis, and the nonspecific "sepsis" signs suggest an autoimmune disorder, especially with the specific "butterfly rash" facial finding.[6] However, when considering diagnostics necessary to hone my differential, I need to also consider other autoimmune causes of her symptoms in addition to SLE. These include rheumatoid arthritis, rhupus, mixed or undifferentiated connective tissue disease, systemic sclerosis, and other disease states.[6,7] A renal biopsy may be indicated to confirm the diagnosis.

SLE is a diagnosis of exclusion; other autoimmune disorders and infection must be ruled out. However, the patient fits the profile for a diagnosis of SLE as it is most prevalent among African American females of childbearing age. The constellation of nonspecific symptoms makes diagnosis difficult and I know I will need to exclude all other causes, infection, and other autoimmune disorders with thorough laboratory testing. I can start by ordering an antinuclear antibody (ANA) test, a sensitive test but not a specific test for SLE. Then I consult a rheumatologist to assist with this diagnosis and also to provide the ongoing long-term follow-up and care that is needed for SLE.[7]

CASE INFORMATION

The rheumatologist notes that the patient's recent miscarriages, pancyto-penia, and elevated creatinine are all potential signs of SLE. The ANA test is positive and further testing is done, in accordance with the 2012 Systemic Lupus International Collaborating Clinics.[7] Per the recommendation of the rheumatologist I call nephrology to consider a renal biopsy. Among the bat-tery of lab work that was done, the patient's anti-double stranded DNA and anti-smooth muscle antibody are both positive. These tests are highly spe-cific for SLE, and present in 70% and 30% of patients with SLE, respectively.[7]

Additional tests are done to rule out other causes of the patient's symp-toms. Per the recommendation of the rheumatologist, I order a rheumatoid factor and anti-cyclic citrullinated peptide (CCP) antibodies to exclude rheu-matoid arthritis. I also order testing for human parvovirus B19, hepatitis B virus, hepatitis C virus, Lyme disease, and Epstein-Barr virus, which rules out an infectious cause of the patient's symptoms. Creatinine kinase is within normal limits, ruling out myositis. Based on these results as well as the positive ANA, positive anti-dsDNA, and positive anti-SM tests, the patient is diagnosed with SLE. A renal biopsy was deferred at this time due to her recent infection.

Management of SLE

SLE, or lupus, is a chronic disease that can progress to life-threatening with mul-tiorgan system involvement. Lupus is more common in younger women and non-Caucasians. Women are nine times more likely than men to develop lupus. The disease typically begins during the childbearing years, between the ages of 15 and 45. Lupus occurs three times more often in African American women than in Caucasians. It is also more common in Hispanics, Asians, and Native Americans.[8] The patient with SLE may present as in this case with a mild set of symptoms, a new infection, and not have major organ failure. SLE patients will require a lifetime of clinical monitoring by a specialist in rheumatology, and other disciplines for spe-cific organ involvement.

The management of SLE is based on the severity of symptoms. Current thera-pies for any severity of disease activity include hydroxychloroquine or chloroquine to help relieve constitutional, musculoskeletal, and mucocutaneous manifesta-tions. In addition, for mild SLE symptoms, nonsteroidal anti-inflammatory med-ications or short-term glucocorticoids of less than 7.5 mg prednisone equivalent per day may be helpful.[9] Patients with moderate lupus symptoms are treated with higher doses of steroids or azathioprine or methotrexate for additional suppres-sion of the autoimmune process. Moderate lupus symptoms include significant but non-organ-threatening disease of constitutional, cutaneous, musculoskeletal, or hematologic systems. The therapy is usually hydroxychloroquine or chloroquine plus short-term therapy with doses of 5 to 15 mg of prednisone equivalents daily. Prednisone taper begins once hydroxychloroquine or chloroquine has taken effect, and a steroid-sparing immunosuppressive agent such as azathioprine or methotrexate is often used for symptom control.

Manifestations that are severe or life threatening, including renal and central nervous system involvement, are managed with high-dose steroids along with immunosuppressants and added biologic agents such as mycophenolate, cyclophosphamide, or rituximab. The aim of these therapies is to reduce the autoimmune process, but careful monitoring is required because side effects of immunosuppression, including increased risk of infection, is a significant cause of morbidity in SLE patients.[9] Treatment is usually with a short duration of high-dose systemic glucocorticoids at 1 to 2 mg/kg/day of prednisone or equivalent or intermittent intravenous methylprednisolone alone or in combination with other immunosuppressive agents to limit organ damage. The advantage of high-dose glucocorticoid therapy is it quickly reduces inflammation, leading to rapid disease control. If needed, immunosuppressive agents such as mycophenolate, cyclophosphamide, or rituximab are added. Once this initial high-dose therapy is completed it is followed by a longer period of less intensive maintenance therapy to reduce SLE flares and achieve remission. Throughout ongoing maintenance therapies reduced prednisone equivalent doses are used and there is close monitoring of clinical symptoms and laboratory values for SLE activity. The complexity of therapies requires ongoing care by a rheumatologist and other specialists as needed depending on which organs are affected.

Pregnancy is a key consideration in this patient as this alters the medications used for SLE. The medication regimen must be adjusted to avoid teratogenic agents. Patients with SLE are often advised to avoid attempts to get pregnant during an acute flare and for up to 6 months after a flare.[9] Additional lifestyle considerations include smoking cessation, and avoiding medications that can cause an SLE flare-up. Coordination of care is a key consideration in SLE. For this patient, since she is attempting to get pregnant she will need her fertility specialist, primary care physician, and any other specialists to communicate with her rheumatologist regarding the management of her SLE during pregnancy.

Treatment for SLE, including immunosuppression, is used to prevent flare-ups, limit organ damage, and provide improved quality of life for this lifelong disease; there is no cure for SLE. However, with early diagnosis and current available therapy, SLE has a survival rate that is greater than 90% for the first 5 years.[9] Patients with renal involvement have a poorer prognosis, so close monitoring of renal function and early referral to nephrology are key elements of care. Despite improvements in care, SLE patients face an overall two to five times higher mortality than the general population, so ongoing lifelong care by a specialist in the management of SLE is essential.[9]

References

1. Hooton TM. Acute uncomplicated cystitis and pyelonephritis in women. UpToDate Web site. http://www.uptodate.com/contents/acute-uncomplicated-cystitis-and-pyelonephritis-in-women. Updated and literature review current as of October 2014. Accessed December 2, 2014.

2. Ceftriaxone: drug information Lexicomp®. UpToDate Web site. http://www.uptodate.com/contents/ceftriaxone-drug-information?source=search_result&search=ceftriaxone+drug+information&selectedTitle=1%7E150. Accessed December 2, 2014.

3. Neviere R. Sepsis and the systemic inflammatory response syndrome: definitions, epidemiology, and prognosis. UpToDate Web site. http://www.uptodate.com/contents/sepsis-and-the-systemic-inflammatory-response-syndrome-definitions-epidemiology-and-prognosis?source=search_result&search=sepsis+and+the+inflammatory+res&selectedTitle=4%7E150. Updated and literature review current as of October 2014. Accessed December 2, 2014.

4. Schur P, Moschella SL, Callen J, Ramirez MP, Ofori AO. Mucocutaneous manifestations of systemic lupus erythematosus. UpToDate Web site. http://www.uptodate.com/contents/mucocutaneous-manifestations-of-systemic-lupus-erythematosus?source=search_result&search=Mucocutaneous+manifestations+of+systemic+lupus+erythematosus. Literature review current July 2014. Updated April 16, 2014. Accessed December 7, 2014.

5. Dahl MV. Approach to the patient with facial erythema. UpToDate Web site. http://www.uptodate.com/contents/approach-to-the-patient-with-facial-erythema?source=search_result&search=approach+to+the+patient+with+facial&selectedTitle=1%7E150. Updated and literature review current as of November 2014. Accessed December 7, 2014.

6. Schur PH, Gladman DD, Pisetsky DS, Ramirez MP. Overview of the clinical manifestations of systemic lupus erythematosus in adults. UpToDate Web site. http://www.uptodate.com/contents/overview-of-the-clinical-manifestations-of-systemic-lupus-erythematosus-in-adults?source=search_result&search=Overview+of+the+clinical+manifestations+of+systemic+lupus+erythematosus+in+adults. Literature review current July 2014. Updated January 23, 2013. Accessed date December 7, 2014.

7. Schur P, Wallace DJ, Pisetsky DS, et al. Diagnosis and differential diagnosis of systemic lupus erythematosus in adults. UpToDate Web site. http://www.uptodate.com/contents/diagnosis-and-differential-diagnosis-of-systemic-lupus-erythematosus-in-adults. Updated and literature review current as of July 01, 2014. Accessed December 7, 2014.

8. Yesterday, today, tomorrow: NIH research timelines. NIH Web site. http://report.nih.gov/nihfactsheets/ViewFactSheet.aspx?csid=47. Accessed December 13, 2014.

9. Schur PH, Wallace DJ. Overview of the management and prognosis of systemic lupus erythematosus in adults. UpToDate Web site. http://www.uptodate.com/contents/overview-of-the-management-and-prognosis-of-systemic-lupus-erythematosus-in-adults?source=search_result&search=lupus&selectedTitle=2%7E150. Updated and literature review current as of November 1, 2014. Accessed December 13, 2014.

CASE 40

Lynn A. Kelso

Lynn A. Kelso is an Assistant Professor of Nursing at the University of Kentucky College of Nursing in Lexington. She started the ACNP Program at UK and served as its coordinator for a number of years before focusing on undergraduate education. She holds a clinical appointment with the Department of Pulmonary, Critical Care and Sleep Medicine, practicing in the Medical ICU at the University of Kentucky Chandler Medical Center.

CASE INFORMATION

Chief Complaint

A 24-year-old female is admitted to the intensive care unit (ICU) from the emergency department (ED) with a generalized seizure, now in status epilepticus. She is sedated and intubated in the ED prior to transfer to the ICU.

❓ What are my initial thoughts?

The first concern is making sure the patient has a protected airway and is breathing adequately. Intubation is not typically needed for an isolated seizure, but once someone has a second seizure or develops status epilepticus, intubation is needed to ensure a protected airway.

Beyond this, I begin to consider what could have caused these seizures. I first consider two possibilities, either this patient has a known history of seizures or this is new. If she has a history of seizures, I question if there has been a recent change in medical management (new regimen, change in dosing, weaning or discontinuation of medications) or patient nonadherence. If there is no history of seizure activity, because of her age, I initially think of illicit drug use, drug withdrawal, infection, trauma, a new space-occupying lesion such as a tumor, or a cerebral vascular event.

Because this patient in status epilepticus is sedated, intubated, and on mechanical ventilation, I am hoping that there are family members present. Trying to uncover the cause of a new onset seizure can be daunting, but needs to be done quickly. Being able to talk with the family and obtain information related to the patient will help focus my examination.

Differential Diagnoses for an Adult Patient With New Onset Seizures[1-3]

In patients with no known history of epilepsy, the cause of a new seizure is likely to be an acute medical condition, including drug intoxication or withdrawal, sepsis, kidney or liver failure, and electrolyte abnormalities, or an acute neurological event, including traumatic brain injury, meningitis, or anoxic encephalopathy. A tumor or cerebral vascular accident (hemorrhagic or ischemic) may also be considered. Considerations for status epilepticus include:

- Antiepileptic drug withdrawal or nonadherence (with history of seizures)
- Alcohol or drug withdrawal, including barbiturates and benzodiazepines
- Central nervous system structural abnormality, acute or chronic
- Metabolic derangement including hypo- or hyperglycemia, uremia, hepatic encephalopathy, hyponatremia, and vitamin B_6 (pyridoxine) deficiency
- Drug overdose including drugs of abuse such as cocaine and tricyclic antidepressants

CASE INFORMATION

History of Present Illness

With initial evaluation of the patient, I can begin to refine my thought process. This begins with determining what information has already been gathered.

The patient was at a party when the first seizure occurred and emergency medical services (EMS) was called. EMS gave her 4 mg of lorazepam, which initially stopped the seizure, and transported her to the ED. Upon arrival to the ED, she had another generalized seizure, which necessitated an additional 2 mg of lorazepam intravenously and intubation for airway protection. Her initial ED management included placing intravenous access, administrating a dose of 50% dextrose, and a dose of thiamine, and initiating a propofol infusion, which was titrated to 40 µg/kg/min in order to control her seizure activity. She also received a loading dose of fosphenytoin of 20 mg/kg. Initial labs were sent, including a urine and serum drug screen, pregnancy test, and blood cultures.

The ED team then ordered a computed tomography (CT) scan of her head to rule out acute head injury, intracranial mass, or cerebral vascular accident. However, prior to transporting her to CT scan, her systolic blood pressure dropped to 80 mm Hg. Her hypotension improved with decreasing the propofol dose and giving an infusion of a normal saline (NS) fluid bolus. Because propofol can cause hypotension, especially at higher doses, she was switched to a midazolam infusion at 5 mg/h. Her blood pressure stabilized and she was safely transferred to the CT scan. Unfortunately, by the time she returned to the ED, she had resumed generalized seizure activity. Despite an increase in the midazolam to 10 mg/h, the seizure activity continued. In anticipation that she might require propofol again to control the seizures, a central venous catheter was placed so that vasopressors could be safely infused if necessary.

The initial presentation of frequent seizure activity, without return to her neurological baseline, progressed to continuous seizure activity, lasting longer than 5 minutes. Both of these criteria meet the definition of status epilepticus.[1]

The head CT showed no acute process or structural abnormality. Her initial bloodwork, which included a chemistry panel, and liver function studies is all within normal limits. Her blood alcohol level is negative as is her pregnancy test. Her complete blood count shows an elevated white blood cell count (WBC) count of 20,000 cells/µL with 78% neutrophils and 17% lymphocytes.

❓ What are the pertinent positives and significant negatives obtained from the information so far?

Pertinent Positives

- Frequent seizures without return to baseline neurological status progressing to continuous seizure activity lasting longer than 5 minutes
- Continued seizure activity despite propofol and midazolam infusions and a fosphenytoin loading dose
- Elevated WBC count with increased neutrophils

Significant Negatives

- Negative head CT
- Normal chemistry panel and liver function
- Negative pregnancy test

❓ Given this information what is the problem representation?

The patient is a 24-year-old female with new onset generalized seizures, now in status epilepticus, despite propofol, midazolam, and fosphenytoin.

Case Analysis: The CT results rule out an acute or chronic structural abnormality and the chemistry and liver function studies are normal, ruling out metabolic derangements. The toxicology screen is pending and is important given her age and the setting in which her symptoms started. For now I cannot rule out drug intoxication or withdrawal as a cause. The WBC count and neutrophil percentage are increased, which makes me consider the possibility of an infectious process. A lumbar puncture (LP) is now higher on my list of diagnostics to evaluate for a central nervous system (CNS) infection such as meningitis or encephalitis.

The longer seizures continue, the more likely the patient is to experience permanent brain damage. I need to control the seizure activity and develop a plan for treating the most likely underlying cause or causes. Because of the continued seizure activity, a lumbar puncture cannot safely be performed at this time but based on her WBC, it is essential that I initiate empiric antimicrobial coverage for possible bacterial meningitis.

Initial Antimicrobial Therapy for Suspected Bacterial Meningitis[4]

Empiric antibiotic treatment is started based on the most likely bacteria given a person's age and health status, and the suspected site of infection. The most common organisms causing bacterial meningitis include *Staphylococcus pneumoniae*, *Neisseria meningitides*, group B *Streptococcus*, *Haemophilus influenza*, and *Listeria monocytogenes*, which is typically more common in persons >80 years; however, it has been increasing in incidence.[5]

Initial therapy for this patient includes ceftriaxone (Rocephin) to cover *Streptococcus (pneumococcal) pneumoniae* and *Neisseria meningitidis* and vancomycin to cover *Staphylococcus aureus*, including methicillin-resistant *Staphylococcus aureus* (MRSA), and *Staphylococcus epidermidis*. These are the most common organisms responsible for bacterial meningitis. The recommended drug for covering suspected *Listeria* infection is ampicillin although alternate drugs include gentamycin, imipenem, or meropenem. Carbapenems, which have a broad spectrum of antimicrobial activity, can lower seizure threshold and so are avoided in this patient. For suspicion of viral meningitis, empiric acyclovir may be given until herpes simplex virus (HSV) results are received.

Antimicrobial coverage is not held in order to perform an LP in a patient suspected of having bacterial meningitis as this infection is life threatening and delay in treatment will lead to increased morbidity and mortality. My initial antimicrobial orders include ceftriaxone, vancomycin, and acyclovir, to cover possible herpetic meningitis/encephalitis. I continue to think through possible causes for her continued seizure activity.

CASE INFORMATION

When her family arrives I am able to obtain pertinent information about her history. They inform me that she was doing well until the previous day when she was just a bit more tired than normal. She complained about her neck and back hurting her, which she attributed to lying in an uncomfortable position and sleeping longer than usual.

Past Medical History

- Bike accident 15 years ago, leading to a splenectomy
- Emergency department visit a month before this admission for dehydration after vomiting for 36 hours, treated with fluids and ondansetron (Zofran)
- Recent urinary tract infection (UTI) treated with a 5-day course of an unknown antibiotic
- Related to her splenectomy, her most recent Pneumovax vaccine was 3 years prior and she sees her primary care provider annually and as needed.

Allergies

Amoxicillin (hives), Bactrim (rash)

Social History

- Occasional smoker, less than half of a pack per day
- No alcohol or drug use that the family is aware of
- Volunteers at the local animal shelter and has been hiking with friends throughout the summer

Review of Systems

Questions are addressed to the patient's family and are negative except for the neck and back pain, increased fatigue within the last 24 hours, and recent UTI and probable gastritis.

Medications

She takes no medications; recently completed an antibiotic prescription for her UTI.

❓ What are the pertinent positives and significant negatives obtained from the new information?

Pertinent Positives

- Recent increase in fatigue followed by neck and back pain
- Recent infection with antibiotic use
- Food poisoning 1 month ago, possible gastroenteritis
- Volunteers at animal shelter
- Recent hiking

- Allergies to amoxicillin and Bactrim
- Splenectomy; has had recent Pneumovax vaccine

Significant Negatives

- No history of drug or alcohol abuse
- No history of seizure disorder or other significant medical history

---

❓ How does this information affect the list of possible causes?

The information provided by the family describing new onset fatigue, neck and back pain, supports the suspected diagnosis of meningitis, and the need to complete the LP. Her history of splenectomy increases her risk of pneumococcal meningitis (*S pneumonia*); however, this is most frequently seen in patients who are not adequately vaccinated.[6,7]

In patients who have undergone a splenectomy, there is an increased risk of infection from encapsulated organisms. Encapsulated organisms include *Streptococcus (pneumococcal) pneumoniae, Neisseria meningitidis, Klebsiella pneumonia, Haemophilus influenzae* type b, Group B *Streptococcus*, and *Salmonella typhi*.[6] The spleen processes these organisms so that phagocytic WBCs engulf and remove them. The greatest risk of severe infection is from *Streptococcus pneumonia*, and, to a lesser extent, *H influenza* and *N meningitidis*, which is why it is recommended that asplenic patients be vaccinated for these organisms.[6,7]

She was vaccinated against *Streptococcus (pneumococcal) pneumoniae* within the last 3 years and had a flu shot the previous fall. She has not been vaccinated against meningococcus. Because of her work in the animal shelter and recent hiking history, I need to consider broadening my antimicrobial coverage to include *Listeria*, Lyme disease, Rocky Mountain spotted fever (RMSF), and other atypical organisms. I add doxycycline, for coverage of Lyme disease and RMSF, and meropenem, to cover *Listeria* and also increase coverage for atypical organisms such as *Pseudomonas*.[4] I choose meropenem over imipenem because while it still is associated with lowering seizure threshold in some cases, it is less likely to do so than imipenem.[8] However, I still need to be very cautious and make sure that I avoid medications that may contribute to her seizure activity, if at all possible.

CASE INFORMATION

Physical Examination

- Vital signs: Pulse 106 beats per minute, blood pressure 126/86 mm Hg, respiratory rate 16 breaths per minute, oral temperature 97.4°F.
- Bedside monitoring: Pulse oximetry 100% on pressure-regulated, volume-controlled (PRVC) ventilation: rate 12, tidal volume 400 mL, PEEP 5, FiO$_2$ 0.5, telemetry—sinus tachycardia without ectopy or ST elevation.

- Constitutional: Well-developed adult female who appears her stated age.
- Head/eyes/ears/nose/throat: Normocephalic and atraumatic; sclera white, ears, oropharynx, and nasopharynx all unremarkable; good dentition; mucous membranes pink.
- Neck: Stiff, no jugular venous distension noted.
- Pulmonary: Orally intubated, symmetrical expansion, bilateral breath sounds clear.
- Cardiovascular: Normal S_1, S_2; no murmur, rubs, gallops; telemetry shows sinus tachycardia, trace amount of pedal edema.
- Gastrointestinal: Abdomen soft, nondistended without organomegaly on palpation, normoactive bowel sounds in all four quadrants.
- Genitourinary: Urinary catheter in place and draining clear, pale yellow urine.
- Integumentary: Skin is pink, warm, and dry, normal hair distribution, there are no bites or scratch marks found on the skin surface, there are no ticks found.
- Neurological: Continues generalized tonic-clonic seizure activity; pupils equal, round, and reactive to light at 2 mm, although sluggish, no blink or lash reflex, weak cough with suctioning; no focal neurological deficits noted.
- Lymphatics: No lymph node enlargement noted.
- Toxicology screen: Positive only for benzodiazepines. This result can be attributed to the lorazepam she was initially given to control the seizure activity, and the midazolam she is currently receiving.

Because of the continued seizure activity, a second antiepileptic drug is added to the regimen; a 2 g loading dose of levetiracetam is given.

❓ Given the information to this point, what elements of the physical examination should be added to the lists of pertinent positives and significant negatives?

- **Pertinent positives:** tachycardia, continuous generalized seizures, pupils reactive, breath sounds clear
- **Significant negatives:** afebrile, stable blood pressure, normal skin examination without bite or scratch marks, no ticks noted, examination normal other than neurologic system, toxicology screen is negative

The patient's pupils remain equal and reactive and there are no focal neurologic deficits. Her breath sounds are clear, which suggests she did not aspirate with her seizure activity or subsequent intubation. A thorough examination of her skin finds no markings to suggest a bite or scratch by an animal in her volunteer work caused her current illness. Because of her recent hiking, I carefully check for ticks or tick bites which can transmit rickettsial and other diseases. However, I am not going to decrease my antimicrobial coverage based solely on the physical examination. I still need more diagnostic confirmation to ensure I am treating the patient correctly.

❓ What diagnostic testing should be done and in what order?

The two most important diagnostic tests that still need to be completed at this time are continuous electroencephalograph (cEEG) monitoring and an LP. The cEEG needs to be initiated as soon as possible to evaluate the effect of levetiracetam. If the tonic/clonic activity is controlled, I must also assess whether the EEG shows that the seizures are under control. Subclinical seizures occur when there is no longer any muscle movement or visible signs of seizure yet increased abnormal electrical activity in the brain continues.

The LP is the second diagnostic test that needs to be completed, to confirm the diagnosis of meningitis and identify the causative organism so that my empiric antibiotic choices can be narrowed. Because the patient continues to have seizure activity, I choose to give her a short-acting neuromuscular blocking agent so that I can safely complete the LP. I select rocuronium, a nondepolarizing agent. Seizure activity stops with a 50 mg dose and I am able to perform an LP without difficulty. This is the only dose of a paralytic agent that I use, as it is essential that I am able to continuously monitor both her motor seizure activity and electrical brain activity.

Diagnostic Results and Treatment

The cEEG continues to show epileptic activity in the brain. Valproic acid is started as a third antiepileptic agent. An initial bolus is given followed by a continuous infusion. Close collaboration with neurology is essential in the care of this patient. They provide expert recommendations for antiepileptic therapy and are invaluable partners in determining optimal interventions to stop the seizure activity.

The patient's LP results support the diagnosis of bacterial meningitis (Table 40-1). However not all of the results will be back within the first 24 hours. Thus I continue broad-spectrum empiric antimicrobial coverage until I receive the final results. Also, because of the severity of her status, and the difficulty in controlling the seizure activity, I consult an infectious disease specialist to make sure I am covering all possible organisms, which may be causing her meningitis. The Gram stain is consistent with strep. Because the seizures are refractory to the current regimen, the infectious disease specialist recommends changing vancomycin to linezolid (an oxazolidinone) to provide better coverage for vancomycin-resistant *Enterococci*.

Over the next 48 hours, the patient's seizure activity is brought under control with the three initially prescribed antiepileptic medications: fosphenytoin, levetiracetam, and valproic acid. She is slowly weaned from the propofol and midazolam

Table 40-1   LP Values Consistent With Bacterial Meningitis[9]

LP Normal Values	Reference Values for Bacterial Meningitis	Patient's Values
WBC	1000–5000/μL	1045/μL
0–5 cells/μL	Majority neutrophils	92% neutrophils
Glucose	<40 mg/dL	8 mg/dL
40–70 mg/dL		
CSF/serum ratio 0.6		
Protein	>500 mg/dL	97 mg/dL
15–45 mg/dL		

infusions while the cEEG remains in place to monitor the brain's electrical activity for subclinical seizure activity. Unfortunately there is an increase in abnormal electrical brain activity each time sedation is decreased, so the weaning process takes a total of 6 days before the propofol and midazolam infusions can be safely discontinued. The cEEG monitoring continues for an additional 24 hours after the infusions are stopped to ensure an absence of further seizure activity.

Additional LP results are available within 48 hours. Viral cultures including herpes simplex, cytomegalovirus, and Epstein-Barr are all negative so the acyclovir is discontinued. Later that same day, the culture from the LP shows *Enterococcus faecium*, which is a rare cause of meningitis in otherwise healthy adults with no CNS trauma or devices. The minimum inhibitory concentration (MIC) on the sensitivity shows that the organism is sensitive to vancomycin. However, because the seizure activity continued when the patient was treated with vancomycin, and improved when linezolid was started, the infectious disease specialist recommends keeping the linezolid and adding gentamycin for a synergistic effect. The infectious disease specialist also recommends discontinuing the meropenem, doxycycline, and ceftriaxone. Although the CT scan of the head did not show any acute or chronic process, which could have led to her seizure activity, enterococcal meningitis is rare in an otherwise healthy adult. So once the cEEG is stopped, I obtain an MRI of the brain to rule out potential disorders which the initial CT did not show such as tumor or ischemic stroke. The MRI shows no acute or chronic abnormalities in the brain.

Case Follow-Up

Once the seizure activity is controlled, physical therapy (PT) and occupational therapy (OT) are consulted to address the patient's functional status by maintaining flexibility and muscle activity. As soon as the patient began to recover from the sedative medications, more aggressive PT and OT was done to increase her strength and stamina. Throughout her illness, enteral nutrition is given to maintain her nutritional status. Following extubation, the patient is seen by speech therapy to evaluate her ability to take nutrition by mouth.

Throughout the patient's illness, keeping the family informed of potential outcomes, both good and bad, is a key aspect of her care. For example, we discussed the fact that prolonged seizure activity may result in significant neurological deficits and necessitate the placement of a tracheostomy should she be unable to be weaned from the ventilator. We also discussed the possible need to place a percutaneous gastrostomy tube for continuous feeding if she had dysphagia.

Fourteen days after admission, she is discharged to an acute rehabilitation center. A peripherally inserted central catheter (PICC) line is placed to complete the course of linezolid and gentamycin. Prior to discharge, the patient reported memory lapses and difficulty in concentrating and remained weak but was able to ambulate with assistance. She continued on antiepileptic medications and was scheduled for follow-up appointments with neurology and infectious disease.

References

1. Ortega-Gutierrez S, Desai N, Claassen J. Status epilepticus. In: Lee K, ed. *The Neuro ICU Book*. New York, NY: McGraw-Hill; 2012:52-76.

2. Drislane FW. Convulsive status epilepticus in adults: classifications, clinical features, and diagnosis. UpToDate. 2015. http://www.uptodate.com/contents/convulsive-status-epilepticus-in-adults-classification-clinical-features-and-diagnosis?source=search_result&search=status+epilepticus&selectedTitle=2%7E150.

3. Schachter SC. Evaluation of the first seizure in adults. UpToDate. 2015. http://www.uptodate.com/contents/evaluation-of-the-first-seizure-in-adults?source=search_result&search=seizures+adult&selectedTitle=1%7E150.

4. Tunkel AR. Initial therapy and prognosis of bacterial meningitis in adults. UpToDate. 2015. http://www.uptodate.com/contents/initial-therapy-and-prognosis-of-bacterial-meningitis-in-adults?source=search_result&search=bacterial+meningitis+adult&selectedTitle=3%7E150.

5. Dzupova O, Rozsypal H, Smiskova D, Benes J. Listeria monocytogenes meningitis in adults: the Czech Republic experience. *BioMed Res*. 2013;2013:1-4. doi: 10.1155/2013/846186.

6. Pasternack MS. Clinical features and management of sepsis in the asplenic patient. UpToDate. 2014. http://www.uptodate.com/contents/clinical-features-and-management-of-sepsis-in-the-asplenic-patient?source=search_result&search=asplenic+sepsis&selectedTitle=1%7E150.

7. Adriani KS, Matthijs CB, van der Ende A, van de Beek D. Bacterial meningitis in adults after splenectomy and hyposplenic states. *Mayo Clin Proc*. June 2013;88(6):571-578. doi:10.1016/j.mayocp.2013.02.009.

8. Smith BT. Pharmacology of antimicrobial drugs. In: Smith BT, ed. *Pharmacology for Nurses*. Burlington, MA: Jones & Bartlett Learning; 2016:411-456.

9. Zomorodi M. Acute intracranial problems. In: Lewis SL, Dirksen SR, Heitkemper MM, Bucher L, eds. *Medical-Surgical Nursing: Assessment and Management of Clinical Problems*. St Louis, MO: Elsevier; 2014:1356-1387.

CASE 41

Kelly Wozneak

Kelly Wozneak has been an RN since 1985. She works in the MICU at the University of Virginia as part of an ACNP team.

CASE INFORMATION

Chief Complaint

A 70-year-old female presents to the emergency room via emergency medical service (EMS) with confusion and abdominal pain, progressing to somnolent state.

❓ What is the potential cause?

The reasons for confusion are many and may be associated with abdominal pain. My approach initially will be to address potential causes by developing a differential for altered mental status.

> **Differential Diagnoses for Altered Mental Status[1]**
>
> - Drugs: intoxication or withdrawal from opioids, alcohol, sedatives, or antipsychotics
> - Metabolic: hypoxia, hypoglycemia, hyperglycemia, hypercalcemia, hypernatremia, hyponatremia, uremia, hepatic encephalopathy, hypothyroidism, hyperthyroidism, vitamin B_{12} or thiamine deficiency, carbon monoxide poisoning, Wilson disease
> - Infectious: meningitis, encephalitis, bacteremia, urinary tract infection, pneumonia, neurosyphilis
> - Structural: space-occupying lesion, eg, brain tumor, subdural hematoma, hydrocephalus
> - Vascular: stroke, subarachnoid hemorrhage, coronary ischemia, hypertensive encephalopathy, CNS vasculitis, thrombotic thrombocytopenic purpura, disseminated intravascular coagulation, hyperviscosity
> - Psychiatric: schizophrenia, depression
> - Other: seizure, hypothermia, heat stroke, ICU psychosis, "sundowning"

I am immediately concerned about her acute somnolence. I order a stat head CT without contrast while the nurse is obtaining her vital signs and then call her daughter to obtain more information.

CASE INFORMATION

History of Present Illness

Per her daughter, the patient's illness began 4 days ago with complaints of lower abdominal and lower back pain and increased urinary frequency. Yesterday her mother's mentation started to change with the daughter describing her as "talking out of her head." Her daughter took her to her primary care provider (PCP) yesterday morning where she was found to have a urinary tract infection (UTI) and was discharged home with a 7-day course of trimethoprim/sulfamethoxazole (Bactrim). After returning home from the PCP office, the patient's abdominal pain grew more severe to the point where she could no longer stand up, she reported epigastric pain that radiated to her chest and she had an episode of vomiting. The daughter called EMS.

The daughter lives with her mother and saw her frequently during the 4-day illness. She denies that her mom had any period of slurred speech, weakness on one side, or change in facial expressions. She has not known her mother to experience blood in stool, diarrhea or constipation, seizure-like activity, loss of consciousness, recent falls or trauma, or changes in breathing. She does not have a thermometer but said her mom might have felt a little feverish to touch last night and this morning. The daughter states that to her knowledge there is no history of heart attack or arrhythmias, stroke, depression, dementia, psychiatric illnesses, diabetes, liver or kidney disease. She does have a history of hypertension, breast cancer treated with lumpectomy and radiation over 20 years ago, and uterine cancer treated with total abdominal hysterectomy 16 years ago, with no known recurrence of either. She has smoked for 50 years and is a current 1 pack per day smoker; she also drinks heavily on the weekends (seven cans of beer/week), but has not had any alcohol for the last 3 days.

Toward the end of our conversation, the daughter mentions that 3 weeks ago she brought her mother to the emergency room with generalized abdominal pain. The patient was found to have a UTI and given a prescription for 7 days of trimethoprim/sulfamethoxazole (Bactrim) and the pain resolved. When I check the record, I see that the patient underwent abdominal computed tomography (CT) imaging, revealing some thickening in her colon. At the appointment yesterday, the PCP saw the CT scan result and completed a referral to see a gastroenterologist for an esophagogastroduodenoscopy (EGD) and colonoscopy.

General Survey of the Patient

She is a well-nourished well-developed appropriately groomed female in moderate distress, her face is symmetric, and she is able to move all extremities. She is somnolent and groaning occasionally with her hand on her abdomen and does not make eye contact when spoken to. She does not respond to questions.

Review of Hospital's Electronic Medical Record

Notes from the patient's prior visit to the emergency room confirm the past medical history given by the patient's daughter. The daughter reports that her mother has not sought care at any other facility. The medical record from the primary care provider's office is in the eletronic medical record and I quickly review her last visit.

Current Medications

• Bactrim DS one tablet twice a day—prescribed but not yet started
• Ranitidine 150 mg twice a day
• Omeprazole 20 mg daily for 6 weeks
• Hydrochlorothiazide 25 mg once a day

Allergies

There are no documented food or medication allergies or adverse reactions in her records and the daughter denies any known allergies also.

❓ What are the pertinent positives from the information given so far?

- The patient was treated 3 weeks prior for a UTI with abdominal pain and appeared to respond to the antibiotic as evidenced by resolution of her symptoms.
- She has a 4-day history of urinary frequency with lower abdominal and lower back pain resulting in her PCP visit yesterday morning and was again prescribed an antibiotic, which she has not begun taking.
- Yesterday evening she became acutely confused/altered with worsening abdominal pain to the point of being unable to stand and had one episode of vomiting.
- Prior to becoming somnolent, she reported epigastric pain radiating to her chest.
- She had an abdominal CT scan 3 weeks ago showing thickening of the transverse and proximal colon.
- She is presently somnolent and does not respond to questions.
- She appears to be in pain at presentation.
- She has a remote cancer history.
- She regularly drinks seven beers a week, mostly on the weekends

---

❓ What are the significant negatives from the information given so far?

- The patient has no known history of dementia, psychiatric illnesses, seizures, heart disease, or stroke.
- No facial droop, no slurred speech. No noted seizure activity.
- According to her PCP records her hypertension was controlled with medications.
- No known recent falls, trauma, or exposure to chemicals or gases.
- No history of diarrhea, constipation.
- Prior to the past 3 weeks she was in good health and able to care for her own basic needs, living with her daughter who provides her transportation.

❓ Given the information obtained so far, what might the problem representation be?

At this point, the problem representation in this case might be: "a 70-year-old female with a history of hypertension, remote history of breast cancer and uterine cancer who presents with altered mental status and abdominal pain."

Case Analysis: Altered mental state, especially in an older adult, is a non-specific symptom and the list of possible causes is long. The causes that are life threatening and/or require immediate intervention are the ones to rule out first. Her history and general survey findings make me less concerned for stroke; however, this must be confirmed first, since prompt treatment of stroke has a huge impact on survival and recovery. The head CT, which will help rule out intracranial bleed and embolic stroke, is the top priority. Similarly, myocardial ischemia/infarction (MI) must be diagnosed quickly to initiate appropriate treatment. MI can cause altered mental state if there is associated decrease in perfusion to the brain. Her cardiac risk factors include her age, her history of hypertension, her smoking history, and her report of epigastric pain prior to becoming somnolent. An ECG and troponin levels will help rule out this cause and this will be done immediately after head CT.

Her abdominal pain is also significant and the etiology of that symptom could be a factor in her altered mental status. Sepsis with an abdominal origin is high on my list at this point. In addition, meningitis from any cause needs to be considered; a lumbar puncture is the best test to rule this out, and I will need the head CT result before proceeding to this step. Sepsis of urinary origin is also a possibility, given her recent history of UTI. Her worsening abdominal pain with known colonic thickening is concerning for ischemic bowel, though this is an unusual diagnosis. Her history of cancer raises concern for metastatic disease, such as a slow-growing tumor from her prior malignancy. The head CT can assist in ruling out a brain tumor though I may need to order an MRI to exclude this diagnosis completely. The head CT can also determine if she has a traumatic brain injury which could cause a progressive alteration in mental status change, and though the daughter is not aware of any trauma, there may have been a fall or an injury that was not witnessed. Uncontrolled hypertension presenting as hypertensive emergency can cause posterior reversible encephalopathy syndrome (PRES) or hypertensive encephalopathy and result in altered mental status and this requires urgent treatment, but this can be ruled out quickly with blood pressure monitoring.

There could be a metabolic cause of her confusion such as electrolyte disarray from dehydration due to her vomiting and urinary tract infection, especially as she takes a diuretic to manage her blood pressure. She may have new onset thyroid disorder, diabetes, kidney or liver disease causing an encephalopathy. A comprehensive metabolic panel will determine if this is the cause of symptoms. Hepatic encephalopathy also presents as progressive altered mental state and somnolence, and though she has no history of liver disease, this may be her first presentation with this diagnosis. I will need to order an ammonia level and liver studies to rule this out. Medication side effect is also possible, but less likely based on the history obtained from the daughter. At this point I also doubt drug intoxication or withdrawal based on the fact that her daughter witnessed the progression of her confusion and did not see any misuse of medication. According to our records, the patient was not prescribed any narcotics, anxiolytics, or psychiatric medications. Thus far, pyelonephritis or sepsis of urinary origin seem most likely, but I need to gather more information, particularly a neurological examination to determine if there are focal deficits, and an ECG since cardiac ischemia needs urgent intervention. The head CT result should be back any minute.

CASE INFORMATION

Review of Systems

History per daughter due to patient's altered mental status.

- Constitutional: Endorses probable fever, her appetite is normally good but has not eaten since breakfast yesterday except for a bite of food last night. No recent falls, no trauma.
- Cardiovascular: Earlier today, the patient endorsed epigastric pain radiating to her chest. Denies leg swelling, or difficulty breathing when lying down.
- Pulmonary: Denies shortness of breath or cough.
- Gastrointestinal: Endorses nausea/vomiting beginning last night, last bowel movement yesterday morning, denies blood in stools. Endorses frequent indigestion for which she takes medicine.
- Genitourinary: Denies blood in her urine, change in urine smell or amount. Endorses increased urinary frequency and had episode of incontinence this morning with foul-smelling urine.
- Musculoskeletal: Daughter states, "She has the usual old folks ache and pains and occasionally takes Tylenol for that." Today was the first time she was unable to stand up, normally she walks without assistance.

- Neurological: Denies headache but did complain of neck stiffness, no falls, no history of seizure disorder or stroke, the daughter is not aware of any numbness, tingling or extremity weakness, or change in speech. Daughter has not noted any facial changes.
- Endocrine: Denies increased hunger, thirst. Endorses increased urinary frequency—but not amount of urine produced.

Physical Examination

- Vital signs: Pulse is 110, blood pressure is 111/79 (both arms with similar readings), respiratory rate is 26, and temperature is 39.6°C (103.3°F) axillary, oxygen saturation by pulse oximeter is 95% on room air, and a fingerstick blood glucose is 108. Her weight is 55 kg (approximately 121 lb), height 1.524 m (5 ft).
- Constitutional: Somnolent, unable to follow commands. Appears uncomfortable, groaning occasionally with hand on abdomen.
- Head/eyes/ears/nose/throat: Normocephalic/atraumatic, pupils are equal, round, reactive to light, buccal mucosa moist, oropharynx is moist and posterior pharynx rises symmetrically, poor dentition noted with some missing teeth. Strong cough and gag reflex, able to protect airway at this time.
- Neck: No nuchal rigidity, no carotid bruits.
- Cardiovascular: Tachycardic, rhythm regular, no murmurs, no gallops, no jugular venous distension, no lower extremity edema.
- Pulmonary: Mildly tachypneic, respirations even and regular, no use of accessory muscles, lungs clear to auscultation and resonant to percussion bilaterally.
- Gastrointestinal: Normoactive bowel sounds, tympanic on percussion, abdomen soft with moderate tenderness worse in right upper quadrant on deep palpation, with guarding. No masses, negative Murphy sign.
- Extremities: Pulses strong throughout, brisk capillary refill.
- Integumentary: Very warm and dry, intact, no rashes, lesions or sores, normal skin turgor.
- Neurological: (Limited by mentation) unable to answer questions or follow commands, moves all extremities, no focal deficits assessed.

Results of Diagnostics

The ECG shows sinus tachycardia with mild ST depression in V4 and V5 (comparing to old ECG, the ST depression is new).

Head CT result: no evidence of acute intracranial abnormality, unable to obtain further details except verbal confirmation from the radiologist that there are only normal atrophic changes associated with aging.

❓ What are the pertinent positives and significant negatives from the review of systems and physical examination?

- **Pertinent positives:** Acutely confused and weakened and now somnolent, temperature of 103, heart rate of 110, respiratory rate of 25. Appears to be uncomfortable. ECG concerning for ischemia, but not infarction.

- **Significant negatives:** The review of systems and the limited physical examination are both negative for focal neurological deficits. There is no nuchal rigidity or recent headache. There is no loss of consciousness or seizure activity. Negative Murphy sign, abdomen soft and nondistended. Normal oxygen saturation, normal blood glucose.

❓ How does this information affect the list of possible causes?

Reviewing the pertinent positives, the patient meets criteria for systemic inflammatory response syndrome (SIRS) and it is likely that infection is the cause of her current state. To diagnose SIRS, a patient must meet two or more of the following criteria: increased respiratory rate, tachycardia, hypo- or hyperthermia, altered mental state, elevated white blood cell count, and elevated blood glucose.[2] I do not have her blood count yet, but based on her assessment, she meets four of the criteria for SIRS: she is tachypneic, tachycardiac, has a fever and an altered mental state. Rapid identification of the infection causing SIRS and potentially sepsis is essential. She will need blood cultures, urine culture, and a chest x-ray to look for pneumonia. Because the patient's primary complaint is progressive confusion in the setting of SIRS, a lumbar puncture to look for central nervous system infection is indicated. The patient did also complain of abdominal pain, according to the history from her daughter, so I also need to consider gastrointestinal sources of infection. I think this is less likely, however, based on the fact that her abdominal examination is unremarkable and a recent CT scan showed only colon thickening. If she has diarrhea, I will order stool studies, including *Clostridium difficile*. The cultures I order will take time to grow and treatment of this patient's altered state needs to begin as soon as possible so I will empirically initiate broad-spectrum antibiotics and plan to tailor the antibiotic therapy once I have identified a specific source of infection. The patient's oxygen level is normal and she appears to be breathing comfortably and able to protect her airway so I will hold on intubation for now.

Based on the information I have gathered, I can rule out some of the diagnoses on my list. The head CT confirms that the patient did not have a stroke or intracranial bleed that is the cause of her symptoms. There is no evidence of mass on the CT, making primary or metastatic brain tumor less likely. I would need to do further imaging to definitively rule out a malignancy, but that is a lower priority since the CT is normal. In addition, the patient's altered mental state is not due to hypoxia or hypoglycemia, or hypertensive encephalopathy as her oxygen saturation, blood glucose, and blood pressure are all normal. There is evidence of possible ischemia on her ECG, but no evidence of acute ST-elevation myocardial infarction (STEMI). I will need to gather more information, additional ECGs, and troponin levels, to rule out NSTEMI. I also need to obtain further lab work before I can rule out other metabolic causes of altered mental state such as thyroid dysfunction, renal failure, or hepatic encephalopathy.

Because she is febrile, had an episode of vomiting and takes a diuretic to manage her blood pressure, electrolyte abnormalities such as hypernatremia or hyponatremia could be contributing to her somnolent state. The history from the patient's daughter does indicate significant alcohol intake and this too could be contributing to her altered state. I need to monitor her closely for withdrawal from alcohol over the course of this hospital stay. Fortunately, our institution has a protocol for monitoring for alcohol withdrawal that includes a scoring tool and as-needed orders for benzodiazepines if the patient begins to show evidence of withdrawal. I institute this protocol so the nurses will begin routine monitoring.

Sepsis of urinary origin is still at the top of my list, as she is elderly and presents with confusion, fever, abdominal pain, and increasing frequency of urination, which are all symptoms[3] of sepsis of urinary origin.

Reexamining the Problem Presentation

This is a 70-year-old female with a part medical history of breast cancer (s/p lumpectomy and radiation more than 30 years ago), uterine cancer presenting with abdominal pain, fever, probable UTI, and acutely altered and worsening mental status.

❓ What other diagnostic testing should be done and in what order? What treatment will I initiate now?

At this point, the patient requires continuous cardiac monitoring and continuous pulse oximeter, with oxygen titrated to keep her saturation greater than 94%. She also needs immediate intravenous access, which is now established by the nurses. I authorize a Foley catheter to monitor urine output and obtain urinalysis and urine culture. I order blood cultures, complete blood count with differential, comprehensive metabolic panel, coagulation studies, alcohol level, lactic acid, troponin, amylase, liver enzymes, lipase and arterial blood gas, and ammonia level. I also order stat abdominal and chest x-rays and ask the emergency room staff to begin preparing for a lumbar puncture (LP). Once the cultures are drawn, the patient will be given IV ceftriaxone, to cover *S pneumoniae*, *N meningitides*, and *H influenzae*, which are the most common pathogens causing adult meningitis.[1] Per our hospital antibiogram, ceftriaxone is also appropriate empiric treatment for complicated UTI.[4] Depending on LP results, I will add vancomycin and ampicillin, and possibly acyclovir if there is concern for viral meningitis. As adjunctive therapy, I will also order dexamethasone, 0.15 mg/kg q6h for 2 to 4 days with the first dose to be administered 10 to

20 minutes before, or at least concomitant with, the first dose of antimicrobial therapy. Dexamethasone is used to minimize the inflammatory response within the brain, which can be particularly damaging after the antibiotic activity begins.[5]

CASE INFORMATION

Results of Diagnostic Testing

- Her abdominal and chest x-rays are normal.
- Troponin drawn in conjunction with the ECG is elevated at 0.14 ng/mL.
- The comprehensive metabolic panel shows normal blood urea nitrogen, normal creatinine, normal blood glucose, and normal electrolytes, with the exception of low magnesium at 1.4 mEq/L (Normal = 1.6–2.4) and phosphorus at 1.9 mg/dL (Normal = 2.5–4.5).
- Her bilirubin, liver function tests, albumin, and ammonia level are normal.
- Her complete blood count shows an elevated white blood cell count of 16,000 cells/μL (Normal = 4500–10,000) but her hemoglobin, hematocrit, and platelet count are all normal.
- Urinalysis shows positive leukocyte esterase, positive nitrates, greater than 10 white blood cells per mL, and many bacteria.
- Her lactic acid level is elevated at 2.9 mEq/L (Normal = 0.7–2.1).
- The LP shows clear cerebrospinal fluid (CSF) and without elevated opening pressure at 60 mm H_2O (normal adult value 70–180 mm H_2O).
- CSF glucose is low at 13 mg/mL (normal 50–80 mg/100 mL, or greater than two-thirds of blood glucose level).
- CSF protein is elevated at 98 mg/dL (normal 15–60 mg/dL).
- CSF white blood count is 1520 in bottle 1, and 2020 in bottle 2 with a predominance of neutrophils at 89% (Normal = 0–5 cells/mm³).
- The Gram stain shows 3+ white blood cells and no bacteria.
- No red blood cells seen in CSF fluid.
- Herpes simplex virus polymerase chain reaction (PCR) and cryptococcal antigen are sent.

Case Analysis: The results of the LP confirm a diagnosis of meningitis as evidenced by elevated protein, elevated white blood count with a predominance of neutrophils (89%), and decreased glucose in the patient's cerebrospinal fluid. With these results, the most likely diagnosis is bacterial meningitis and less likely fungal or viral; however, due to her altered mental status, unless the offending organism is isolated, empiric coverage is necessary.[6] Additional lab results confirm that the patient does not have a significant electrolyte imbalance, renal impairment, or hepatic encephalopathy contributing to her altered mental state.

Treatment of Meningitis

Per the Infectious Disease Society of America, the most common pathogens for causing meningitis in patients over 50 years old are *S pneumoniae*, *N meningitides*, *L monocytogenes*, and aerobic gram-negative rods. The recommended empiric antibiotic therapy is vancomycin, starting at 15 mg/kg every 8 hours, with a target trough level of 15 to 20 µg/mL, in addition to ampicillin 2 g every 4 hours, and a third-generation cephalosporin such as ceftriaxone 2 g every 12 hours or cefotaxime 2 g every 4 or 6 hours.[7]

For this patient, we also add acyclovir to treat possible viral meningitis due to herpes simplex virus (HSV). This is a less common cause of meningitis but it carries a very high morbidity and mortality in all age groups. The risks of giving acyclovir to a patient who does not have HSV meningitis are far less than the risk of failing to treat this infection early on. So we will give acyclovir until the PCR test confirms or rules out HSV.

Fluid resuscitation is also a key component in the management of SIRS and sepsis. Per current clinical practice guidelines, initial fluid resuscitation for a patient with SIRS is 30 mL/kg infused over 1 hour[2] to treat hypotension and address a lactate level of greater than 4 mEq/L. The average amount of fluid given initially is approximately 1 L of normal saline over 15 minutes, with repeat boluses given the same way every 15 minutes for mean arterial pressure of less than 60 mm Hg or systolic blood pressure <90 mm Hg, for a maximum of 3 L total in the first hour. The lactic acid is reassessed after the first hour to aid in deciding if more fluids are needed. Central venous pressure (CVP) measurement with goal >8 mm Hg is also mentioned in the guidelines but this parameter can be unreliable. An alternative way to determine the impact of fluid resuscitation is ultrasound measurement of the inferior vena cava.[2]

Case Follow-Up

The patient is transferred from the ER to the intensive care unit for further care. Her troponin level peaks at 1.54 confirming an NSTEMI and she is started on aspirin 81 mg a day, atorvastatin, and a heparin drip. Her abdominal CT shows resolution of bowel wall thickening but is positive for distended bladder, bilateral hydroureter, and mild hydronephrosis, confirming probable UTI.[8] I suspect this is the cause of her pain, and I leave the Foley catheter in place to prevent further urinary retention. She continues on intravenous fluids and antibiotics to manage SIRS, sepsis, and meningitis and shows gradual improvement. Occasional agitation is managed with as-needed lorazepam (Ativan), and the nurses monitor her for alcohol withdrawal according to our institution protocol. Her magnesium and phosphorous are repleted with her IV hydration and the patient is also given thiamine and folate with her intravenous fluids as these vitamin deficiencies are common with alcohol use. After 4 days, the acyclovir is discontinued because her PCR comes back negative.

Due to her altered mental state, the patient is initially given nothing by mouth. Her first swallow study shows high risk for aspiration so I place a nasogastric tube and begin feedings. Initially she develops mild refeeding syndrome, so I adjust the rate and volume of the feeding. As her mental status improves, a repeat swallow study shows she is safe to take medications and nutrition by mouth, the tube is removed and I change her thiamine, folate, and PRN lorazepam to oral doses. She works with physical therapy and demonstrates the ability to safely ambulate. A PICC line is placed in anticipation for discharge home to complete her intravenous antibiotics with a home health nurse.

While the patient's cerebrospinal fluid culture and urine culture showed only normal flora, her course of intravenous antibiotics for meningitis is continued because of the substantial improvement the patient showed once this treatment was initiated. At discharge the patient is advised to keep appointments with her primary care physician, scheduled for 2 weeks after discharge, and with cardiology scheduled for 4 weeks after discharge. Her alcohol use is discussed with her and her daughter and I advise them that this probably contributed to this illness and will increasingly affect her overall health. Resources for behavioral health treatment are provided.

This patient fooled me at first, as I was sure she had urosepsis causing her confusion and somnolence. This case is a good example of how diligently pursuing the proper differential diagnoses is crucial to ensuring proper care and treatment.

References

1. Zeiger RF. McGraw-Hill's Diagnosaurus 4.0. http://accessmedicine.mhmedical.com.proxy.its.virginia.edu/diagnosaurus.aspx. Accessed August 3, 2014.

2. Surviving sepsis campaign. International guidelines for management of severe sepsis and septic shock. http://www.sccm.org/Documents/SSC-Guidelines.pdf. Published 2012. Updated 2012. Accessed August 7, 2014.

3. Cetti R, Venn S. The management of adult urinary tract infection. In: Dawson C, Nethercliffe J, eds. *ABC of Urology*. 3rd ed. London: John Wiley & Sons, 2012.

4. University of Virginia Health System. 2012. Antimicrobial susceptibility profiles of selected aerobic isolates all sources ICUs (NNICU, CCU, TCVPO, SICU, MICU, MSICU, STICU, 3N, 4N, 5N). http://www.healthsystem.virginia.edu/pub/medlabs/lab-handbook-test-directory/2010-antimicrobial-susceptibility-profiles/ICUs%202010.doc/view?searchterm=antibiogram. Accessed September 5, 2014.

5. Jaffe J, Ratcliff T. Chapter 42. Infectious disease emergencies. In: Stone CHR, ed. 7th ed. New York, NY: McGraw-Hill; 2011. http://accessmedicine.mhmedical.com/content.aspx?bookid=385&Sectionid=40357258. Accessed August 3, 2014.

6. Web link for analysis of CSF from The Royal College of Pathologists of Australasia. http://www.med.uottawa.ca/procedures/lp/e_interpretation.htm. Accessed October 10, 2014.

7. Tunkel AR, Hartman BJ, Kaplan SL, et al. ISDA guidelines. Practice guidelines for the management of bacterial meningitis. http://www.idsociety.org/uploadedFiles/IDSA/Guidelines-Patient_Care/PDF_Library/Bacterial Meningitis(1).pdf.

8. Coats J, Rae N, Nathwani D. What is the evidence for the duration of antibiotic therapy in gram-negative bacteraemia caused by urinary tract infection? A systematic review of the literature. *J Glob Antimicrob Resist*. 2013;1(1):39-42.

CASE 42

Allison Walton

Allison works at the University of Virginia Health System in the Department of Neurosurgery Skull Based Cerebrovascular Division where she cares for a variety of patients suffering from brain aneurysm rupture, hemorrhagic stroke, and other cerebrovascular problems.

CASE INFORMATION

Chief Complaint

A 54-year-old African American female presents to the emergency department complaining of a severe headache (9/10 on 0–10 pain scale) with left arm weakness, nausea, and vomiting.

? What is the potential cause?

Headache is an extremely broad, sometimes vague complaint with a seemingly endless list of potential causes. The highest priority is to eliminate the lethal causes of the symptom, which would require a noncontrast head computed tomography (CT) scan to evaluate for bleeding or cerebral edema. Once I eliminate these causes I must continue to comprehensively and quickly evaluate other causes starting with those that are most serious. I use a system-by-system approach to develop a differential diagnosis for severe headaches.

Comprehensive Differential Diagnoses for Severe Headache[1]

- Neurologic: subdural hematoma, epidural hematoma, giant cell arteritis, ischemic stroke, hemorrhagic stroke, venous sinus thrombus, arterial dissection (carotid or vertebral arteries), malignant hypertension, trigeminal neuralgia, occipital neuralgia, meningitis, Chiari malformation, idiopathic intracranial hypertension (increased intracranial pressure), intracranial hypotension, moyamoya, cerebrospinal fluid leak, vasculitis, brain tumor, concussion/trauma, acute hydrocephalus, migraine, cluster headache, tension-type headache
- Cardiovascular: acute coronary syndrome, preeclampsia/eclampsia
- Pulmonary: obstructive sleep apnea
- Infectious: brain abscess, fungal infection in the brain, neurocysticercosis, sinusitis, otitis media, dental caries, and wisdom tooth impaction

- Musculoskeletal: cervical spine disorder, temporomandibular joint syndrome, and cervical paraspinal muscle tenderness/muscle spasms
- Endocrine: pituitary apoplexy, menstrual headache
- Metabolic: thyroid disorder, carbon monoxide poisoning, and dehydration
- Miscellaneous: medication related (side effects), medication overuse, and acute angle-closure glaucoma

In this case of a middle-aged African American female complaining of a severe headache (9 out of 10 on pain scale) with left arm weakness associated with nausea and vomiting, I am concerned because her age, race, and presentation make me think stroke is a possible cause. Hemorrhagic stroke or intracranial hemorrhage (ICH), subarachnoid hemorrhage (SAH), and ischemic stroke are all possibilities. If any of these are the cause of her pain, emergent interventions will be necessary. To that end, I order a stat CT scan of her head without contrast and continue my evaluation of the patient. There are many essential questions that will help me focus on the cause of her headache and I will try to obtain answers as I proceed through my history and physical, as the patient's condition allows (see Table 42-1).

Table 42-1 Questions to Help Focus on Severe Headache Causes with Symptoms of Nausea and Vomiting

When did it start?

What were you doing when the pain began?

Were there any visual, auditory, or other unusual changes that you noticed before you had the headache? (This question is to determine if a prodrome or aura was present.)

What does the pain feel like?

How long has the headache continued?

What were you doing before you got the headache?

Anything make the pain better or worse (foods, alcohol, activities, sleep medications)?

Have you had this pain before?

Has the pain limited your activity?

Are you on birth control and if so what method?

If you are having periods what are they like (regular, irregular, amenorrhea)?

Any new physical environment changes such as carpets, construction, etc?

Any recent changes in vision with or without the headache?

Any recent trauma?

Any recent changes in weight, diet, exercise, or sleep patterns?

Any changes in work or lifestyle?

Any new stressors in your life?

CASE INFORMATION

History of Present Illness

I go to the patient's bedside and she appears uncomfortable, has her eyes closed, and has the lights off. I am particularly interested in learning that her pain started a few days ago, and is not like her normal sinus headache pain which she says occurs during the spring and fall. She reports her headaches do not occur typically more than once or twice a week and acetaminophen or ibuprofen manages the pain. Her current pain is primarily on the right side, throbbing in nature, and over the last few hours has gotten increasingly intense. She has tried nonsteroidal anti-inflammatory agents, acetaminophen, and acetaminophen with aspirin and caffeine (Excedrin). The Excedrin gave her relief that lasted for a half day. She denies any history of migraines. She reports her arm has been weak since the headache began, 3 days ago. When I ask her why she came to the ED today she reports the pain is getting the best of her, in addition to "feeling crummy" because of the nausea and vomiting. She then says that talking makes her nauseated so she asks her husband to talk to me.

Her husband reports her headaches have never been this severe or lasted this long. Typically he says her headaches resolve in about 2 to 3 hours after taking acetaminophen or ibuprofen and only occur once or twice a week in the spring and fall. He thinks they are related to allergies. On rare occasions she tries over-the-counter sinus medications such as Advil "cold and sinus" if the pain does not subside after 2 hours. He cannot remember her having nausea and vomiting with prior headaches and states she has never had weakness associated with her headaches. He reports she has not gone to work in 2 days because of the pain, and has spent that time lying in bed with the lights off. He finally convinced her to come to the hospital to get evaluated and treated.

Her stat CT scan of the head is negative for bleeding or edema. Now I can focus on obtaining much more information to help work through my differential. I continue with my evaluation.

❓ What are the pertinent positives elicited so far?

- Headache pain is severe and unlike her usual sinus headaches.
- Headache is associated with nausea, vomiting, and photophobia.
- Left arm weakness noted for the full duration of her headache.
- Headache pain present for 36 hours, but increasing in intensity over the past several hours.

? What are the pertinent negatives from the information gathered so far?

- No blood or edema on head CT
- Gradual onset of headache—not sudden onset, not the worst headache of her life
- No head trauma
- No changes to lifestyle, job, routine, medications

? Can the information gathered so far be restated in a single sentence highlighting the pieces that narrow down the cause or diagnosis?

Putting the information obtained so far in a single sentence—a problem-focused presentation—sets the stage for gathering more information and determining the cause/diagnosis. The problem presentation might be: "This is a 54-year-old African American female presenting with a headache of 36 hours duration, increasing in intensity over the past several hours, and associated with nausea, vomiting, photophobia, and left arm weakness."

The gradual onset of her pain and the negative head CT scan rule out a hemorrhagic stroke. But, I must fully evaluate her to determine the cause of her headache. I need to complete my history and physical keeping my differential in mind.

CASE INFORMATION

Past Medical and Surgical History

Osteopenia, hypertension, sinus headaches, and hysterectomy 5 years ago.

Allergies

None known.

Medications

Lisinopril/hydrochlorothiazide 20/12.5 mg, one tablet daily, calcium 600 mg twice a day, multivitamin one tablet daily, glucosamine, vitamin D 2000 IU, one tablet daily, Naprosyn as needed, Tylenol as needed.

Social History

No tobacco products, two glasses of wine on weekends, no other drug use. Married, three adult children, works as a bank teller. Heats house with electric heat pump, no fireplace, natural gas, or wood in the house.

Family History

Hypertension diabetes mellitus, myocardial infarction. Denies family history of stroke, cancer, or migraines.

Review of Systems

- The patient is an adequate historian but becomes nauseated when speaking so her husband reports much of the review of systems.
- Constitutional: Denies fever, chills, recent falls, trauma. Endorses poor appetite and poor oral intake since start of headache. Denies change in sleep patterns.
- Head/eyes/ears/nose/throat: Denies recent colds or sinus infections, no nasal drainage or postnasal drip, no pain when bending over, no ear pain. Reports regular dental visits, without any recent dental work other than routine cleaning. Denies any jaw pain, ear pain, clicking while eating, clenching or grinding of teeth. Denies any fluid dripping from nose or salty taste in her mouth.
- Cardiovascular: Denies chest pain, leg swelling, and shortness of breath when lying down.
- Pulmonary: The patient does not smoke, denies cough, shortness of breath, wheezing, or sputum production.
- Gastrointestinal: Reports nausea/vomiting since headache began, denies blood in stool, blood in emesis, reports regular bowel movements.
- Genitourinary: Denies blood in urine, pain with urination, discoloration of urine, foul smelling urine, and incontinence.
- Musculoskeletal: Reports occasional knee and hip pain, states it is likely arthritis due to sports and running when younger, nonsteroidal anti-inflammatory agents do alleviate the pain; no changes in gait pattern, or ability to ambulate.
- Endocrine: Denies excessive thirst, unexpected weight loss/weight gain, increased urination, denies temperature intolerance.
- Neurologic: Reports headaches without aura, denies seizures, vision changes, tingling, numbness, facial droop, speech difficulties.
- Miscellaneous: Denies exposure to infectious diseases, denies travel outside of the United Sates, denies eating raw fish or undercooked meat, particularly pork.

Physical Examination

- Vital signs: Height 5'8", weight 210 lb, BMI 31.9, pulse 78 beats per minute, respirations 18 breaths per minute, blood pressure 146/69, temperature 37.2°C orally, oxygen saturation via pulse oximeter 98% on room air, blood glucose via finger stick is 90 mg/dL.
- Constitutional: Ill appearing, appears stated age, interactive, and assisted by husband despite feeling poorly, lying on a stretcher in a dimly lit room, minimal eye contact due to photophobia.
- Head/eyes/ears/nose/throat: Pupils equal, round, reactive to light and accommodation, 3 mm with brisk response, buccal and oral mucosa dry

appearing, no thyromegaly, and no carotid bruits auscultated. Sinuses clear with bedside transillumination, no tenderness upon palpation, and throat without erythema, discharge, swelling, or exudate. Ears: external canal is clear, small amount of cerumen, tympanic membranes translucent pearly gray, no fluid behind tympanic membrane. Oropharynx: without any missing, broken, rotten teeth. No clicking audible while talking, no clicking felt upon jaw movement.

- Cardiovascular: Heart rate and rhythm regular, no murmur, gallop, or rub. No edema, pulses palpable throughout extremities. Nail beds pink, fingers cool to touch with brisk capillary refill.
- Pulmonary: Respiratory rate regular, no use of accessory muscles, lungs resonant on percussion, clear to auscultation throughout.
- Gastrointestinal: Normally active bowel sounds, tympanic on percussion, abdomen soft, and no tenderness with palpation.
- Integumentary: No rashes, lesions, or sores noted. Decreased skin turgor, mild tenting noted.
- Lymphatics: No lymphadenopathy.
- Neurologic: Cranial nerves 2 to 12 intact, no focal neurologic deficits except left arm, strength 4/5 throughout. Alert and oriented to person, place, time, and situation. No nuchal rigidity. Kernig and Brudzinski signs negative. Finger to nose examination within normal limits. Tandem gait within normal limits, negative Hoffman sign, upper and lower reflexes 2+ throughout, no clonus, down going toes bilaterally. No spine tenderness upon palpation. Unable to do Romberg due to discomfort.

❓ What elements of the review of systems and the physical examination should be added to the list of pertinent positives?

- The patient appears uncomfortable, lights are off, left arm weakness, cool fingertips, decreased skin turgor, headache, nausea, vomiting, history of seasonal allergies.

❓ Which items should be added to the list of significant negatives?

- Nonsmoker, has not traveled outside the United States, no vision changes, no consumption of raw meat or fish, no recent traumas, no new life stressors. No recent surgeries or illnesses. Teeth and dental work in good condition. No use of wood heating, uses electric heat pump.
- No nuchal rigidity. Kernig and Brudzinski signs negative. Hoffman negative. No clonus, reflexes 2+ throughout, downgoing toes.

❓ How does this information affect the list of possible causes?

I have done a CT scan to rule out immediate life-threatening causes of her headache such as a subdural hemorrhage, epidural hemorrhage, or intracerebral bleed but there are still many potential neurologic causes that I cannot eliminate yet such as intracranial hypertension or hypotension, temporal arteritis, Chiari malformation, infection, or vasculitis.

Another cause of headache on my differential, hydrocephalus, is very unlikely as this usually presents with lethargy, confusion, urinary incontinence, and gait disturbances. The patient is nauseated and uncomfortable and thus I was unable to perform the Romberg test during my physical examination. However, the patient and her husband deny any gait problems and she has not exhibited incontinence or confusion so I rule this out. A tumor is possible but is lower on the differential given her history of a headache beginning over the past 36 hours. If other information does not identify the cause of her symptoms, I will obtain an MRI with and without contrast to evaluate for a tumor as well as venous sinus thrombus, arterial dissection, intracranial hypotension due to cerebral spinal leak or intracranial hypertension caused by intracranial venous stenosis, or congenital Chiari malformation.

Infection, specifically meningitis is potentially life-threatening but her symptoms do not make me think she has meningitis as she has not been febrile, has no rashes, no nuchal rigidity and has negative Kernig and Brudzinski signs (both of which demonstrate meningeal irritation). Brain abscess or neurocysticercosis is very low on the differential since there is no evidence of sinus infection, dental disease, no third world country travel, and she denies consuming raw or undercooked meat. I have not ruled out metabolic causes yet such as hyper- or hypothyroidism so these are still on my differential but are low for now.

I do not find any evidence of medication overuse or side effects from a medicine, as she denies any use of illicit drugs, significant nonsteroidal anti-inflammatory use, or recent narcotic use. She is not diabetic and only takes lisinopril-hydrochlorothiazide for hypertension. She does not smoke or have sleep apnea. She denies any recent illness or surgeries and no known allergies with the exception of possible seasonal allergies. All of these are eliminated from my differential. The findings from the physical examination reveal no cardiac abnormality, no murmur or arrhythmia, thus eliminating a cardiac source for headache pain. Her physical examination is unremarkable for any spine abnormalities with no clonus, normal reflexes, negative Hoffman sign, no clicking with jaw movement. She also denies any recent falls, trauma, or spine tenderness. I remove musculoskeletal causes from my differential.

The patient's history is also notable for the absence of chronic daily headache, tension-type headaches, or cluster headaches. Other types of headaches, however, are possible. The patient's symptoms do not fit the usual description of cluster headaches as these usually start on one side around the eye or temple; the pain comes on quickly, over a few minutes. The pain is generally described as excruciating and gets to its peak in minutes. It is also described as deep, continuous, and explosive. The patient is typically able to continue doing whatever they were doing prior to the headache. The pain can last 30 minutes to several hours. Typically patients have eye redness or tearing in the same side as the pain. The nose can run, or get stuffy, the pupils can dilate, but patients do not usually have any focal neurologic deficits associated with the pain. Cluster headache is exclusively a clinical diagnosis but her picture is not consistent with this type of headache.

Tension-type headache is also low on the differential because this pain is typically bilateral, described as tightness or pressure that comes and goes. There is no pattern to the duration of pain. Tension-type headaches do not cause neurologic deficits, such as arm weakness so I will rule out that diagnosis. Sinus headache typically is reported as a deep and constant pressure around the eyes, nose, and face. The pain is worsened with bending over, straining, coughing, or sudden head movement, and is typically associated with fever, facial swelling, nasal discharge, and feelings of fullness in the ears. While my patient has a history of sinus headaches, her physical examination and description of the pain do not fit this diagnosis. Carbon monoxide poisoning is eliminated as there is no propane, natural gas, or wood stove in the house. The house is heated with an electric heat pump. If there were a significant concern for this a carboxyhemoglobin would be drawn.

Migraine-type headaches cause an intense throbbing or pulsation in the head commonly associated with nausea and vomiting in addition to severe light and sound sensitivity. Some migraine headaches are preceded by an aura; these can be flashing lights tingling sensations in an arm or leg, or blind spots. The pain can last hours or days. Patients who suffer from migraines typically seek out dark quiet rooms to lie down.

The patient is exhibiting a headache lasting 36 hours associated with light sensitivity, nausea, and vomiting in addition to left-sided weakness. While she does not describe an aura, these symptoms are leading me to consider migraine very high in my differential. However, migraine is typically a diagnosis of exclusion and I am still concerned about her left-sided arm weakness. Thus, I must obtain additional diagnostic tests to rule in or out remaining diagnoses in my differential.

❓ What diagnostic testing should be performed and in what order?

As stated earlier, a STAT head CT is performed as soon as possible. Hemorrhagic stroke and malignant cerebral edema are life-threatening conditions that need to be addressed immediately. That done, additional studies are necessary and I order the following:

Labs: Chemistry panel with hepatic panel, complete blood count with differential, coagulation times, B_{12} level, B_1 (thiamine) level, troponins, sedimentation rate, C-reactive protein (not high sensitivity), thyroid-stimulating hormone, free T4, urinalysis with reflex culture, ECG, and chest x-ray.

CASE INFORMATION

Diagnostics and Results

Sedimentation rate and C-reactive protein are normal, which rules out an inflammatory process such as an infectious cause, or vasculitis, or temporal arteritis. The complete blood count with differential is normal. The thyroid-stimulating hormone and free T4 reveal appropriate thyroid function. Troponin is less than 0.02, suggesting no injury to the heart. I can rule out a metabolic cause as the patient's hepatic, coagulation, and chemistry studies are normal with the exception of an elevated BUN at 34 mg/dL (normal 10–20 mg/dL) indicating dehydration. Her B_{12} is normal and the B_1 and thiamine tests (low thiamine can contribute to headache pain) take a week or so to return.

The chest x-ray is clear without any obvious consolidation, effusion, or pulmonary edema, which makes a pulmonary disorder less likely. While the patient has no history of sleep apnea, she is obese and may have undiagnosed sleep apnea. While sleep-related pulmonary disorders cannot be seen on an x-ray, patients with sleep apnea often develop right-sided heart failure and pulmonary edema, which would show up on chest x-ray. In addition, this patient's headache lasts all day and is not worse in the morning, whereas the headache associated with sleep apnea typically occurs upon waking and improves as the day progresses. I can rule out sleep apnea and other pulmonary causes for headache.

Case Analysis: The information gathered in the history and physical, and the diagnostic test results make me confident that I have excluded all life-threatening and serious conditions from my differential. At this point my findings are most consistent with the diagnosis of migraine headache as the cause of her symptoms. The patient's left arm weakness places the migraine in the hemiplegic migraine category or complex migraine category. Patients can have weakness associated with migraines headaches. However, an MRI with and without contrast still needs to be performed to rule out any other underlying cause of the weakness and migraine pain and finalize my diagnosis. I obtain an MRI following evaluation of the diagnostics and it is also negative. My diagnosis is migraine with hemiplegia.

Migraine Headache: Diagnosis and Treatment

The diagnosis of migraine, as demonstrated by my patient, is often a diagnosis of exclusion. All life-threatening potential causes are eliminated first. A key to reaching the correct headache diagnosis is the history, review of systems, and physical examination.

As in the case of my patient, however, the arm weakness, escalating headache pain and duration, of necessity, increased my concern that other serious conditions may have been the cause. Once the diagnosis is determined, then treatment can be addressed. Commonly migraines are diagnosed in the emergency department setting and in specialty or primary care clinics. Treatment options vary and are described below.

Treatment of Migraine Headache: Emergency Department

There are many abortive treatments for migraine headache. Patients come to the emergency department and are given many different "cocktails" of intravenous or intramuscular medications. These cocktails may include a narcotic with an antiemetic such as prochlorperazine 10 mg or promethazine 12.5 or 25 mg. Diphenhydramine 25 or 50 mg may also be used. Dexamethasone 4 mg and/or lorazepam 2 mg may also be included, and ketorolac 15 mg IV or IM is also a common drug of choice. Typically the combination of drugs used is at the discretion of the treating provider.[2,3]

UpToDate[2] guidelines for the treatment of acute migraine are separated into two main categories. For mild to moderate attacks simple analgesics such as nonsteroidal anti-inflammatory drugs (NSAIDS) or combination analgesics (aspirin with acetaminophen and/or NSAID, and/or caffeine) are used initially. Many of the medications can be given via a non-oral route in the patient who is suffering with nausea and vomiting or gastric stasis due to the migraine pain. For moderate to severe attacks the recommendations include the use of triptans or combination triptans/nonsteroidal anti-inflammatory agents. In the emergency room setting, the recommendations are to initially begin with the less expensive NSAID or combination medications, if they can tolerate the medications. Antiemetics are more easily administered in combination with these medications as an adjunctive treatment in the emergency setting. Ergotamines are also effective when used orally; non-oral routes demonstrate poor absorption and bioavailability. Dexamethasone does not show any significant benefit to immediate abortive therapies; however, use of the drug is associated with a decrease in early recurrence of migraine pain in the following 24 to 72 hours. Opioids and barbiturates should be used as a last resort medication in all circumstances. For a patient who is in status migrainosus (migraine pain lasting >72 hours)—DHE (dihydroergotamine 45) can be administered via daily infusions for 5 days. DHE is an ergotamine that has weaker arterial vasoconstriction and more potent venoconstriction that oral ergotamine, in addition to fewer side effects.

Management: Specialty and Primary Care Clinics

For patients diagnosed with migraine headaches by a primary care provider or neurologist in the outpatient setting, the triptans can be effective abortive medications if taken at the onset of an aura or immediately at the onset of migraine symptom. If these are not effective, β-blockers may be used for preventative maintenance. However, β-blockers may be contraindicated in patients with very low heart rate or blood pressure. To date medications specifically developed for migraine headaches have not been developed, however anti-seizure medications are often effectively used. Currently the mainstay of outpatient treatment consists of medications such as topiramate (Topamax), carbamazepine (Tegretol), lamotrigine (Lamictal), and divalproex (Depakote). Unfortunately there are many associated side effects, which limit the escalation of the doses of these medications.

Narcotics are not used for chronic migraine headache pain because they are not effective. Occasionally naproxen (Naprosyn) 500 mg twice a day for 5 to 7 days may be given to abort a headache. Some also use a Medrol dose-pack to stop the headache cycle.

For tension-type headaches, nonsteroidal anti-inflammatory agents or combination over-the-counter preparations such as Excedrin, BC powders or Goody's powders can be effective to stop the pain. These combinations contain aspirin, acetaminophen, and caffeine. For the patient that has frequent tension-type headaches, preventative measures can be utilized such as tricyclic antidepressants and stress management techniques, with other forms of behavioral therapy.[2]

Cluster headaches fall into the general category of trigeminal autonomic cephalalgias. Sumatriptan subcutaneous injections and oxygen therapy are the mainstay first-line abortive treatment. Ergots, lidocaine, and octreotide have revealed some effectiveness in the treatment if cluster headache. Verapamil is the agent of choice for prevention of cluster headaches. Glucocorticoids, lithium, topiramate (Topamax), and methysergide (Sansert) show limited effectiveness as preventative medications.[2]

In patients with chronic daily headache (daily headache for 15 or more days a month for at least 3 months) the challenge is to identify the underlying cause of the headache pain and determine the diagnosis. "Chronic daily headache" is not a specific type of headache pain. The treatment depends on the root cause of the headache pain.

Headaches come in many forms and have numerous causes. The discussion above focuses on some of the more serious types. Other causes can be reviewed at http://www.headaches.org/press/NHF_Press_Kits/Press_Kits_-_The_Complete_Headache_Chart.

Case Follow-Up

During her stay in the emergency room, a neurologist and I both evaluate the patient. We prescribe diphenhydramine (Benadryl) 25 mg intravenously, prochlorperazine (Compazine) 10 mg intravenously, and intravenous fluids at 125 mL/h times 2 L.[2,3] After hydration and medication, the pain decreases to 2/10, and the nausea, vomiting and left arm weakness resolve. She was discharged the following morning from the ED with prescriptions for diphenhydramine (Benadryl) 25 mg by mouth every 6 hours and prochlorperazine (Compazine) 10 mg by mouth every 6 hours, both to be taken together for migraine pain. She is to follow up with her PCP in the next 2 days, with a follow-up appointment with the neurologist in 2 weeks' time.

References

1. Epocrates Rx Online [database on the Internet]. Epocrates, Inc, San Mateo, CA. 2003. www .epocrates.com. Web-based; continuous content updates. Accessed September 12, 2014.
2. Bajwa ZH, Sabahat A. Acute treatment of migraine in adults. In: Swanson JW, ed. UpTo Date. Waltham, MA. http://www.uptodate.com/contents/acute-treatment-of-migraine-in-adults. Accessed October 24, 2014.
3. Kostic MA, Gutierrez FJ, Rieg TS, Moore TS, Gendron RT. A prospective, randomized trial of intravenous prochlorperazine versus subcutaneous sumatriptan in acute migraine therapy in the emergency department. *Ann Emerg Med.* 2010 Jul;56(1):1–6. doi: 10.1016/j.annemergmed. 2009.11.020. Epub January 4, 2010.

CASE 43

Michelle Beard

Michelle Beard is an ACNP who works in the University of Virginia's Cancer Care clinics in Charlottesville and Farmville. She manages hematology/oncology patients suffering from a variety of illnesses.

CASE INFORMATION

Chief Complaint

HC is a 60-year-old Caucasian male presenting to urgent care with back pain. He was seen by his primary care doctor 2 weeks prior for the same complaint and was treated for back strain with heat, nonsteroidal anti-inflammatory drugs (NSAIDs), and exercises.

❓ What is the potential cause?

Back pain is a very common complaint that spans the continuum of all practice settings. The potential etiology of back pain is extensive and a challenge for the clinician to determine cause. In addition, management varies depending on whether it is a benign condition that might be treated conservatively or a potential life-altering condition that may require an aggressive workup and treatment.

Back pain is the leading cause of disability in Americans under 45 years old. More than 26 million Americans between the ages of 20 and 64 experiences frequent back pain.[1] In 2008, nearly 7.3 million ED visits and over 2.3 million hospital inpatient stays were related to back problems.[2] The importance of the nurse practitioner's knowledge base related to this common complaint of back pain is essential and is demonstrated in this case.

For this patient it is imperative that I determine whether he has an underlying condition causing his back pain that may require immediate intervention to ensure an optimal outcome. This is his second visit with the same complaint, indicating that conservative measures did not yield adequate results and increasing my level of concern about his need for urgent evaluation.

Comprehensive Differential Diagnoses for a Patient With Back Pain

Back pain can be categorized into mechanical, nonmechanical, and visceral disease.
• Mechanical causes of back pain include degenerative spine disease, herniated disk, spinal stenosis, kyphosis, osteoporosis, spondylolysis/spondylolisthesis, lumbar strain, fractures.

- Nonmechanical causes of back pain include infections such as osteo-myelitis, paraspinous abscess, epidural abscess, bacterial endocarditis. Inflammatory arthritis, osteochondrosis, Paget disease, and cancers such as lymphoma, leukemia, metastatic carcinoma, multiple myeloma, and retroperitoneal cancers can also cause back pain.
- Visceral diseases such as abdominal aortic aneurysm, nephrolithiasis, pancreatitis, penetrating/perforated ulcer, prostatitis, pelvic inflamma-tory disease can secondarily lead to back pain.[3]

Considering all the possible etiologies for persistent back pain I now need to proceed with a careful history and physical examination. I begin with the history of this symptom but move quickly into an extensive review of systems and thorough examination to rule in or out some of the possible causes of my patient's back pain. The information I gather will also guide what additional diagnostic studies are warranted.

CASE INFORMATION

History of Present Illness

The patient reports a 2- to 3-month history of intermittent dull aching of his lower back. Over the past couple of weeks the pain has intensified and become constant. He denies initiating new physical activities, and denies any recent injury, trauma, or falls. He rates his back pain as 7 on a 10-point scale. There is minimal relief with ibuprofen 600 mg three times a day. Resting or lying down does not help alleviate the symptoms and even light activity like walking exacerbates his pain. As the pain has intensified he also notes pain radiating down his left buttocks, outer thigh, and sometimes to the top of his foot. The radiating pain is described as shooting/burning pain with tingling and decreased sensation of his thigh. He feels that his legs are weak and at times may not hold his weight. He is not able to work as a maintenance supervisor with the local school system because of his pain. His wife reports a dramatic decline in his overall activity level over the past 2 weeks. He is requiring help to get dressed and other activities of daily living. She reports that prior to the onset of this pain, he was very active at home even after a full day at work.

Medical and Surgical History

The patient has no prior back problems. He does have hypertension but denies diabetes, heart disease, or history of cancer. He has had no recent procedures or surgeries. His only past surgical history is a tonsillectomy at age 8. He is up to date on prostate and colon cancer screening. He reports his last annual physical examination was 9 months ago and everything was normal.

A review of his electronic medical records confirms that 9 months ago he had a normal complete blood count with differential, comprehensive metabolic profile and lipid panel, prostate specific antigen, and ECG. No laboratory studies or radiology studies have been done in the interval.

Family and Social History

No one in his family suffers from back issues. He has never been a smoker and drinks alcohol in small amounts once or twice a month. He denies any illicit drug use.

Medication List

- The patient has no known drug allergies.
- Amlodipine 5 mg once a day—last dose was this morning.
- Aspirin 81 mg once a day—last dose was yesterday.
- Ibuprofen 600 mg three times a day for his back pain—last dose was 2 hours before his arrival.

CASE INFORMATION

Review of Systems

- Constitutional: No fevers, recent infections, or medical procedures. He complains of trouble sleeping due to pain. He has fatigue and a sense of general weakness, which he attributes to his lack of sleep. He denies weight loss but has had early satiety and "disinterest" in food over the past 3 to 4 weeks. He denies night sweats.
- Cardiovascular: No chest pain, cough, shortness of breath, or orthopnea. He does note swelling equal in both legs over the past 2 to 3 weeks.
- Pulmonary: No cough or resting shortness of breath. Admits to mild dyspnea on exertion but believes this is related to his fatigue.
- Gastrointestinal: He notes mild nausea but no vomiting, melena, or bright red rectal bleeding. He does note early satiety, a sense of bloating, and recent constipation. Last bowel movement was 2 days ago. Previously he had a daily bowel movement.
- Genitourinary: Denies hematuria, frequency, dysuria, incontinence, or retention.

- Musculoskeletal: Back pain as described in the history of present illness; the patient initially denies any other sites of bone pain. His wife reminds him that he has mentioned having some pain in his right lateral rib cage. He reports that this is mild and the "least of my worries." He denies pain with deep breathing but does note some increase in the rib pain with coughing or sneezing.
- Integumentary: No spontaneous bruising, pruritus, ulcers, change in moles.
- Neurologic: Denies headaches or visual changes. He does endorse "foggy thinking" but attributes this to his lack of sleep. As above, he has paresthesia of the left buttocks and leg with weakness of his legs and loss of sensation of his left outer thigh. No history of stroke or change in speech. His wife notes that his memory is not as good since his pain has increased. She reports having to repeat things to him on multiple occasions and reports that at times he seems confused.
- Endocrine: No cold or heat intolerance. He does report polydipsia, but no polyuria or polyphagia.
- Lymphatic/hematologic: Denies excessive bleeding, history of anemia, enlarged or tender lymph nodes. His wife notes that he has appeared pale to her over the last month.

Physical Examination

- Vitals: BP is 174/88, heart rate 90, respiratory rate is 18, and temperature is 98.7 F tympanic, oxygen saturation by pulse oximeter is 98% on room air.
- General: Appears weak and tired and in moderate distress from pain. He repositions frequently and has facial grimacing. He is conversant.
- Head/eyes/ears/nose/throat: Pupils equal, round, reactive to light and accommodation, sclera anicteric, oropharynx with dry mucous membranes, no ulcerations, good dentition, normal soft and hard palate.
- Neck: Trachea mid-line. Normal range of motion, no thyromegaly. No cervical lymphadenopathy.
- Pulmonary: Clear to auscultation and percussion. Symmetric lung expansion and no intercostal muscle retraction.
- Cardiovascular: S1, S2 with regular rate and rhythm and without murmurs, gallops, or rubs. Peripheral pulses intact. Trace bilateral ankle edema.
- Gastrointestinal: Hypoactive bowel sounds, tympanic, mild distention with no fluid wave, no tenderness, and no hepatosplenomegaly. No pulsatile masses. No bruits. No inguinal adenopathy.
- Musculoskeletal: No joint deformity, erythema, swelling. Spinous process tenderness of the L4 region. No reproducible rib cage pain. Decreased strength of the left leg.
- Integumentary: General pallor. Warm. Pale nail beds with brisk capillary refill. No rashes or ulcerations. Poor skin turgor.

• Neurologic: Oriented to person, place, and time. His speech is slow but clear. Cranial nerves II-XII intact, muscle strength and tone of the upper extremities 5/5, right leg 4/5 and left leg 3/5 with slight muscle atrophy of the left thigh. Weakness with left hip abduction, left knee flexion, and left foot dorsiflexion. Hyporeflexia of the left patellar and left Achilles reflexes noted 1/4. All other reflexes are normal; 2/4. Decreased light touch sensation of the left lateral thigh, left calf, and dorsum of the left foot. Negative Babinski. Cerebellar testing intact: finger to nose, rapid alternating movements.

? What are the pertinent positives from the history and physical examination?

• Progressive back pain with motor and sensory changes
• Pain not improved with rest/lying down or NSAIDs
• Tenderness over his lumbar spine at L4 region
• Fatigue/weakness
• Pallor
• Poor skin turgor
• Mild anorexia with abdominal distention and constipation
• Changes in memory and possible intermittent confusion
• Hypertensive
• Rib pain with cough/sneezing

? What are the significant negatives from the history and physical examination?

• No prior back problems
• No recent injury or new activities to explain back pain
• Absence of chronic health problems such as heart disease, cancer, pulmonary disease
• Had been in good health
• No weight loss
• No lymphadenopathy
• No confusion on current presentation
• No central nervous system abnormalities on examination
• Normal laboratory studies and ECG 9 months ago

❓ Can the information gathered so far be restated in a single sentence—problem presentation—highlighting the pieces that narrow down the cause?

The problem presentation in this case might be: "a 60-year-old male with worsening back pain presenting with motor and sensory changes leading to declining performance status and debility."

❓ How does the information affect the list of possible causes?

The patient's presentation of pain crisis and peripheral neurologic changes requires immediate intervention, not only for patient comfort but to prevent a further decline in his motor and sensory function. He has limited medical history and his hypertension does not seem to be a key factor in his current health situation. Although he is clearly hypertensive, he is not having a hypertensive crisis and has no symptoms or clinical findings to suggest that this is playing any role in his chief complaint. He does not have any specific central nervous system findings. On the other hand, his pain and current circumstances are the more likely etiology of his blood pressure elevation. For now I will simply treat his pain, monitor his blood pressure, and continue to consider potential diagnoses to explain his symptoms.

At this time, the priority is pain control to lessen the patient's suffering and maximize his ability to undergo diagnostic imaging studies. Nonsteroidal anti-inflammatory medications have not been helpful and I am not certain of his current renal function. Since he is in a controlled environment with proper monitoring, I decide to move forward with intravenous narcotic administration until the patient is more comfortable. It is also essential that I order selected laboratory studies since he has been on NSAIDs, it has been 8 months since last lab assessment, and he has some clinical findings of concern, such as pallor, dry mucous membranes, vague abdominal findings, and complaints of anorexia in addition to his back pain.

In considering the current information obtained so far, his symptoms do not appear to be related to mechanical or visceral causes. Typically, mechanical causes of back pain improve with rest or lying down. A herniated disk can lead to nerve root impingement causing motor and sensory deficits but here again symptoms are typically improved with rest. There is no indication of fracture since there have been no falls or trauma and he is not at heightened risk of osteoporotic fracture given his medical history and medication list. Lumbar strain does not typically involve nerve involvement. He has no specific symptoms to suggest a visceral etiology. He does have some abdominal symptoms but none of which are clearly indicative of causality. A perforated ulcer, pancreatitis, abdominal aneurysm, or kidney stones each have specific clinical findings or symptoms that are not currently present, and tenderness over his lumbar spine does not fit with a visceral etiology, making these diagnoses unlikely. This helps me narrow my workup. I now am considering a nonmechanical spine disease such as neoplasia, infections like paraspinous, epidural abscess, or septic discitis more likely in my differential. Inflammatory arthritis cannot be ruled out yet but is lower on differential because he has no other findings on his musculoskeletal examination. I know that cancers that have a propensity to spread to bone emanate from the lung, prostate, breast, and kidney. Cancers that may originate in the bone are multiple myeloma and sarcomas. His normal prostate specific antigen, lack of pulmonary symptoms, and no breast complaints argue against prostate, lung, and breast cancer. Kidney cancer will need to stay on the differential since direct invasion to the spine is possible. He does not report gross hematuria. Given the current considerations, I will add an erythrocyte sedimentation rate to his laboratory workup. This is a nonspecific and inexpensive test for inflammation, malignancy, infection, and autoimmune diseases. I will also check a urinalysis for microscopic blood or infection.

? What diagnostic testing should be done and in what order?

The laboratory studies are easy to obtain during initiation of intravenous access. IV access is necessary since he appears dehydrated and requires pain medication. While pain control is being obtained, blood work can be processed. I order a complete blood count with differential, comprehensive metabolic profile that will include electrolytes, renal and liver function, albumin, and total protein. Erythrocyte sedimentation rate and urinalysis will be done as well. The peripheral neurologic deficits warrant rapid assessment by imaging. I would consider magnetic resonance imaging (MRI) over computed tomography (CT) or plain x-rays in this circumstance. MRI is the preferred modality for evaluating the lumbar spine (L-spine) because it more clearly demonstrates the bones, muscles, nerves, discs, and other connective tissues of the spine, as well as the spinal cord and the alignment of these structures. Since there is evidence of peripheral neurologic deficit on physical examination, a plain x-ray or CT scan would not be the most efficacious radiographic studies to use at this time. The other consideration when ordering a test is my level of concern in finding pathology and the need for involvement of other specialists. In this case, given his clinical presentation, I already suspect he will need an urgent neurosurgery consult and they will require MRI in considering treatment modalities. By ordering the correct test to start with, I can ultimately save time and money and increase patient comfort. On the other hand, if my index of suspicion is low for identifying potentially significant findings in the setting of a normal clinical examination, it would be reasonable to start my workup with plain radiographs of his spine.

CASE INFORMATION

Since patient comfort is a priority I want to administer pain medication. Oral administration is not a reasonable option given his pain score and vague GI symptoms. I will keep him off oral medications for now and provide parenteral pain medications. Since we are awaiting laboratory studies including renal function and I suspect dehydration I want to consider options of pain control that will not be toxic if renal impairment is an issue. Therefore, I opt to provide the patient with hydromorphone 2 mg intravenous push every 15 minutes until he reports an acceptable pain score and providing his vital signs remain stable. Typically, in a narcotic naïve patient, the requirement is small. This patient requires only two doses or 4 mg total and his pain score comes down to 2. His vital signs are good; blood pressure is 134/72, and respiratory and heart rates are stable. His oxygen saturation remains greater than 95%. He appears much more comfortable. He is now able to tolerate diagnostic studies.

Results of Diagnostic Tests

CBC With Differential and Sedimentation Rate		
Test	Reference Range	Patient Value
Erythrocyte sedimentation rate	0–22 mm/h	124 mm/h
RBC	4.00–6.00 M/µL	2.92 (L)
Hemoglobin	11.0–18.0 g/dL	8.4 (L)
Hematocrit	35.0%–50.0%	24.6 (L)
MCV	80.0–99.9 fL	82.8
MCH	27.0–31.0 pg	31
MCHC	33.0–37.0 g/dL	33
RDW	11.6%–13.7%	13.6
Platelets	150–450 K/µL	325
WBC	4,500–10,500 cells/µL	6,800 cells/µL
Neutrophils percent	54%–62%	60.1
Lymphocytes percent	24%–44%	31.1
Monocytes percent	3%–6%	8.8
Neutrophils absolute count	1.4–6.5 K/µL	3.20
Lymphocytes absolute count	1.2–3.4 K/µL	1.60
Monocytes absolute count	0.1–0.6 K/µL	0.50

Electrolytes-Basic Metabolic		
Test	Reference Range	Patient Value
Glucose	74–99 mg/dL	102 (H)
Sodium	136–145 mmol/L	139
Potassium	3.4–4.8 mmol/L	4.2
Chloride	98–107 mmol/L	106
CO_2	23–31 mmol/L	19 (L)
BUN	8.4–25.7 mg/dL	26 (H)
Creatinine	0.7–1.3 mg/dL	2.0 (H)
Calcium	8.5–10.5 mg/dL	13.5 (H)
Total protein	5.8–8.1 g/dL	12.5 (H)
Albumin	3.2–5.2 g/dL	2.9 (L)
Total bilirubin	0.3–1.2 mg/dL	1.1

Liver Enzymes		
Test	Reference Range	Patient Value
Alkaline phosphatase	40–150 U/L	253 (H)
ALT	<55 U/L	18
AST	<35 U/L	25

Urinalysis		
Test	Reference Range	Patient Value
Color, UA	Yellow	Yellow
Clarity, UA	Clear	Cloudy
pH, UA	5.0–8.0	5.5
Spec grav, UA	1.001–1.030	≥1.030
Protein, UA	Negative	120 (H)
Glucose, UA	Negative	Negative
Ketones, UA	Negative	Negative
Bilirubin, UA	Negative	Negative
Nitrite, UA	Negative	Negative
Leukocytes, UA	Negative	Negative
Blood, UA	Negative	Moderate
Urobilinogen, UA	0.1–1.0 EU	0.2

MRI: results are pending.

Case Analysis: At this point in his workup I have a high level of suspicion for an underlying malignancy with spine involvement. An ESR above 100 is suggestive of malignancy. Multiple myeloma is my leading diagnosis at this point since he has some characteristic laboratory findings of myeloma such as anemia, renal insufficiency, hypercalcemia, and elevated total protein. His low albumin will need to be taken into account as this will alter his true serum calcium level. I do the calculation to correct his calcium and his calcium is actually 14.38 mg/dL. [Corrected calcium = serum calcium + 0.8 (4 − serum albumin)]. There is a mnemonic that may help in remembering symptoms associated with multiple myeloma: CRAB (C = elevated calcium, R = renal insufficiency, A = anemia, B = bone lesions).

He has an oncologic emergency of hypercalcemia, which requires immediate intervention. I order an ECG to ensure that the high calcium is not affecting his heart. The key to management at this point is prioritizing his care since I suspect he has another oncologic emergency: impending spinal cord compression. I begin with hydration using normal saline at 200 cc/h, recognizing this to be the first-line therapy in management of hypercalcemia. Hydration repletes volume and promotes sodium diuresis, which leads to calciuresis. I keep in mind that the rapidity of the elevated calcium levels plays a role in deciding the urgency of treatment. His calcium levels were likely rising over weeks to months versus days. Nonetheless, without treatment this is a life-threatening abnormality and will need additional therapy urgently.

CASE INFORMATION

Diagnostic Test Results

The ECG reveals no abnormality such as shortening of the QT interval, flattening of the T wave, the presence of Osborn waves (J waves) or ventricular ectopy. This result confirms that clinically, the patient is stable from his high calcium levels with no ECG changes, seizures, psychosis. So, I hold off on further treatment with bisphosphonates for now until after his MRI.

The MRI of his lumbar spine reveals widespread lytic lesions in his lumbar spine consistent with metastatic cancer or myeloma. There is near complete replacement of L4 vertebrae from tumor with invasion into the epidural space and impingement of the nerve root. Impending cord compression from invasion of the epidural space from adjacent vertebral metastasis is an oncologic emergency. The findings from the MRI further support my suspicion of underlying malignancy with multiple myeloma.

Multiple Myeloma Diagnosis and Treatment

Multiple myeloma is a complex malignancy of the plasma cells. A *plasma cell* is a mature B lymphocyte that is specialized for antibody (immunoglobulin) production.

In multiple myeloma a single abnormal plasma cell clone replicates within the bone marrow. By infiltrating the bone marrow these renegade plasma cells impede normal marrow functioning, leading to myelosuppression. The infiltrated bone marrow also leads to a cascade of events that activate osteoclasts that in turn lead to bone resorption (breakdown), causing osteopenia and lytic bone lesions. This breakdown of bone leads to release of calcium, causing hypercalcemia and its associated symptoms. Proteins secreted by the malignant cells can cause abnormal elevation of serum protein. As these proteins are filtered through the tubules of the kidneys they can join with another protein normally found in the urine. The combination of proteins is large and can block the tubules, resulting in an inflammatory process that in turn leads to renal damage or cast nephropathy. Hypercalcemia causes nephrocalcinosis, which also contributes to renal dysfunction. The total immunoglobulin level is typically elevated in myeloma but the majority is ineffective in antibody production, leading to increased risk of opportunistic infections.

The diagnosis of myeloma is made by laboratory studies including serum protein electrophoresis, serum-free light chain assay, quantitative immunoglobulins, β_2-microglobulin, CBC with differential, calcium, albumin, LDH, renal function, electrolytes, 24-hour urine for protein, urine protein electrophoresis. Additional diagnostic tests include skeletal survey, bone marrow aspirate, and biopsy. MRI and PET/CT are used as clinically indicated.[4,5]

The incidence of myeloma remains steady at about 5 cases per 100,000 and accounts for approximately 10% of all hematologic malignancies. African Americans are twice as likely to develop myeloma as Caucasians and men have a slightly greater incidence than women. The median age at diagnosis is 66 years.[4]

Multiple myeloma is a heterogeneous disease and distinguishing stage, risk, and prognosis at the onset is helpful in determining median survival as well as determining immediate need to initiate therapy versus an active surveillance strategy. Not all patients presenting with myeloma require therapy at the onset. For the sake of this case, I will focus on active or symptomatic myeloma that requires therapy.

HC is in immediate danger of spinal cord compression from the tumor replacing the L4 vertebral body, which can lead to collapse of the spine. He also has direct invasion of his epidural space. Initial therapy includes administration of corticosteroids intravenously in a loading dose. Typically, dexamethasone is the steroid of choice. The loading dose is followed by oral therapy every 6 hours and tapered during the course of definitive therapy for the underlying malignancy. The steroid administration will have some added benefit in treating the hypercalcemia since myeloma is a malignancy that is responsive to steroid therapy. However, this is typically a temporary benefit and more definitive therapy is required. While hydration continues, I will also provide a dose of pamidronate or zoledronic acid to help bring down his calcium levels. Bisphosphonate dosing requires adjustment for his creatinine clearance. The bisphosphonate therapy administration has proven benefit in helping reduce bony pain and decrease skeletal related complications from cancer over time. Once stabilized, HC will remain on bisphosphonate therapy monthly to counteract the excess bone resorption activity from his myeloma.

HC requires several urgent consults including radiation oncology, neurosurgery, and medical oncology. He will also need to be seen by nephrology as well.

Typically, these patients are best served by urgent radiation therapy to shrink the tumor that is invading the epidural space. However, it is helpful to have the neurosurgeon's input to ensure the patient does not require spinal stabilization and to follow the patient's neurologic status once treatment is underway. The radiation will palliate symptoms of pain and help minimize further neurologic decline as the tumor shrinks. Medical oncology will perform a bone marrow aspirate and biopsy as well as review and interpret his laboratory workup. In our case, HC's serum protein electrophoresis confirms a monoclonal protein production of 4 g/dL. As well as the other abnormal labs seen by initial CBC, CMP, ESR, his β_2-microglobulin is elevated at 5.5. His bone marrow analysis confirms 30% infiltration of the marrow with plasma cells consistent with multiple myeloma. A skeletal survey indicates some additional lytic lesions to several of his right ribs and a right humeral lesion. No impending fracture apparent to the right humeral lesion.

HC's hospital course of 4 days is remarkable for good control of his pain with successful conversion to oral narcotic therapy, correction of his hypercalcemia resulting in resolution of his constipation, some of his fatigue, and generalized weakness, and clearing of his mild confusion and memory deficit. His renal function improves but he continues with stage III renal insufficiency, making treatment with erythrocyte-stimulating agents a good option to treat his underlying anemia. His appetite improves. He experiences no further neurologic deficit and begins having less motor and sensory nerve dysfunction by day #4 of radiation therapy. He will continue his palliative radiation therapy as an outpatient; follow up with medical oncology to begin definitive therapy for his myeloma per National Comprehensive Cancer Network guidelines.[5] Part of his plan will likely include a consult with the bone marrow transplant team since he is under age 70 and otherwise in good health. He will follow up with nephrology and neurosurgery as needed.

Additional interventions for HC include physical and occupational therapy consults, social work, chaplaincy, advanced practice nursing for disease and treatment education, palliative medicine consult for symptom management. Treating malignancy often includes a multidisciplinary approach especially in a complex malignancy like multiple myeloma, where the expected goal of therapy is not typically curative.

The acute care NP in oncology plays a vital role with the patient and family monitoring and managing disease-related complications and treatment-related side effects as well as helping the patient with treatment decisions throughout the course of his disease.

References

1. Chartbook on trends in the health of Americans, special feature: pain. National Center for Health Statistics, Centers for Disease Control and Prevention Web site. http://www.cdc.gov/nchs/data/hus/hus06.pdf. Published November 2006.
2. Statistical Brief #105. Healthcare cost and Utilization Project Web site. http://www.hcup-us.ahrq.gov/reports/statbriefs/sb105.pdf. Published February 2011.
3. Multiple myeloma: key statistics. American Cancer Society Web site. http://www.cancer.org/cancer/multiplemyeloma/detailedguide/multiple-myeloma-key-statistics. Revised January 23, 2015.
4. Multiple myeloma: Uptodate. http://www.uptodate.com/contents/clinical-features-laboratory-manifestations-and-diagnosis-of-multiple-myeloma?source=search_result&search=multiple+myeloma&selectedTitle=1~150. Accessed Oct 2015.
5. NCCN—evidence based cancer guidelines. Version 3. 2015. National Comprehensive Cancer Network. http://www.nccn.org/professionals/physician_gls/pdf/myeloma.pdf. February 11, 2015.

CASE 44

Janet H. Johnson

Janet H. Johnson practices in a Cardiology Telemetry Service that admits over 9000 patients a year and manages patients with acute coronary syndrome, congestive heart failure, and cardiac arrhythmias. She is also preceptor for ACNP students.

CASE INFORMATION

Chief Complaint

A 66-year-old man with a significant history of coronary artery disease (CAD) presents to the emergency department (ED) with a complaint of intermittent chest pain that radiates to jaw and down left arm. With the chest pain episodes, he experiences shortness of breath and back discomfort.

❓ What is the potential cause?

Chest pain can have many etiologies from benign indigestion to a life-threatening acute condition. Prompt recognition of acute coronary syndrome (ACS) is essential because treatment is most beneficial when initiated soon after presentation. Any patient who presents to the ED with complaints of chest pain or severe epigastric pain that is not due to trauma needs to be evaluated immediately for potential ACS. Chest pain symptoms that may indicate ACS include substernal pressure, crushing chest pain, tightness, heaviness, cramping or aching sensation; unexplained indigestion, belching, epigastric pain; pain that radiates to neck, jaw, shoulder, or one or both arms; associated dyspnea or associated diaphoresis. If the patient presents with any of these symptoms, an electrocardiogram (ECG) and a focused assessment of the patient's risk for cardiac disease are immediate priorities. The patient should be questioned about past medical history of coronary artery bypass graft; percutaneous coronary intervention (PCI); CAD; angina on effort; myocardial infarction (MI); cardiac risk factors including smoking, hyperlipidemia (HLD), hypertension (HTN), diabetes mellitus (DM), family history of CAD; cocaine and methamphetamine use; use of nitroglycerin to relieve chest pain; and regular and recent medication use. If the patient is a female, diabetic, or elderly, symptoms of ACS may be atypical. ACS protocol should be initiated if appropriate.

Comprehensive Differential Diagnoses for Patient With Chest Pain[1,2]

- Acute coronary syndrome (ACS): ST-segment elevated myocardial infarction (STEMI), non-ST-segment elevated myocardial infarction (NSTEMI), unstable angina (UA)—definite, probable, or possible

- Non-ACS cardiovascular condition: pericarditis, myocarditis, acute aortic syndrome, cardiac amyloid, mediastinitis, sternal wound post-CABG, sternal wound infection
- Noncardiac condition with another specific disease: chest pain secondary to hyperadrenergic states, stress-induced cardiomyopathy, cocaine intoxication, methamphetamine intoxication, pheochromocytoma
- Gastrointestinal: gastroesophageal reflux disease; esophageal hypersensitivity; abnormal motility patterns and achalasia; esophageal rupture, perforation, and foreign bodies; esophagitis
- Pulmonary: pulmonary vasculature disease related to acute pulmonary embolism, pulmonary hypertension, cor pulmonale; lung parenchyma related to pneumonia, cancer, sarcoidosis; asthma and chronic obstructive pulmonary disease, pleural and pleural space related to pneumothorax, pleuritis, pleural effusion
- Noncardiac condition that is undefined: chest wall pain, musculoskeletal pain related to isolated musculoskeletal pain syndrome, rheumatic disease, nonrheumatic disease; skin and sensory nerves
- Psychogenic/psychosomatic: panic disorder, anxiety

Since my patient presented with chest pain, a focused history and ECG will be done immediately.

CASE INFORMATION

The patient reports he had an MI 3 years ago, and a subsequent cardiac catheterization showed two-vessel CAD. A review of his past medical records revealed that a percutaneous coronary intervention (PCI) was performed and two drug eluting stents were placed in proximal and mid-right coronary artery (RCA). The patient reports additional past medical history of hypertension, hyperlipidemia, diabetes, and chronic systolic heart failure but denies chronic obstructive pulmonary disease, asthma, esophageal reflux, or substance use. Regarding the current illness the patient reports intermittent substernal chest pain occurring over the last 2 to 3 months, worse in the morning and on exertion. The episodes last for a few minutes to 10 to 20 minutes and are usually relieved by taking one sublingual nitroglycerin tablet. The patient reports recent travel from Honduras where he resides. While on the plane, he experienced an episode of severe chest "burning," which was more intense than his prior episodes, and felt similar to the pain he had when he had his MI. He also noted discomfort in his left arm and up to his jaw. His back was achy, but he thought that was due to the plane seats. He took a sublingual nitroglycerin with only minimal relief.

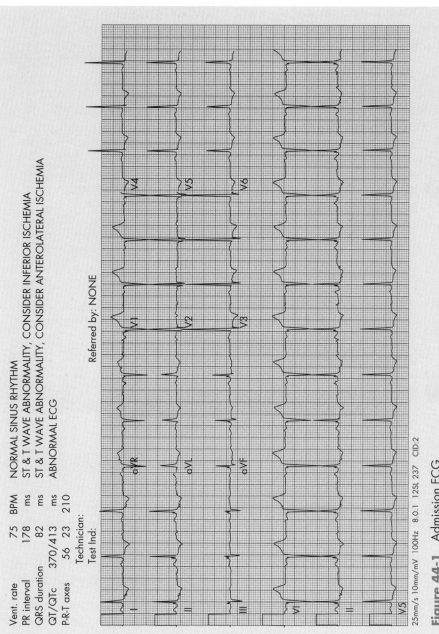

Vent. rate   75   BPM   NORMAL SINUS RHYTHM
PR interval   178   ms   ST & T WAVE ABNORMALITY, CONSIDER INFERIOR ISCHEMIA
QRS duration   82   ms   ST & T WAVE ABNORMALITY, CONSIDER ANTEROLATERAL ISCHEMIA
QT/QTc   370/413   ms   ABNORMAL ECG
P-R-T axes   56   23   210

Technician:
Test Ind:

Referred by: NONE

25mm/s 10mm/mV 100Hz 8.0.1 12SL 237 CID:2

Figure 44-1 Admission ECG.

When he got off the plane, his son noted he was "sweaty" and did not look good, and brought him immediately to the hospital.

His ECG shows sinus rhythm with ventricular rate of 75. ST- and T-wave abnormality in inferior leads, seen in prior ECG from 3 years ago. New ST- and T-wave abnormalities are seen in the anterior/lateral leads including ST-segment depression and T-wave inversion in I and AVL, and V4 through 6. See ECG (Figure 44-1).

His current medication list includes aspirin 81 mg daily, repaglinide 1 mg three times a day with meals, atenolol 50 mg daily, losartan 25 mg daily, and simvastatin 40 mg daily.

❓ What are the pertinent positives from the information given so far?

- Prior cardiac history: MI, cardiac catheterization with PCI
- Cardiac risk factors including: HTN, HLD, DM
- Nitroglycerin use with no relief of chest pain
- The patient is on cardiac medications
- Description of symptoms: increase in severity of chest pain with radiation to jaw, left arm and back, description of symptoms similar to prior acute MI, associated symptoms of dyspnea, diaphoresis
- New ECG changes

❓ What are the significant negatives?

- ECG changes were not indicative of ST-elevation MI
- Absence of COPD, asthma
- Absence of esophageal reflux disease
- No trauma prior to the pain onset

❓ Can the information gathered so far be restated in a single sentence—problem presentation—highlighting the pieces that narrow down the cause?

The problem representation in this case is: a 61-year-old male with significant history of CAD presents with chest pain similar to pain he had with a prior MI.

Case Analysis: The results of his chest x-ray will help rule out some of the pulmonary differential diagnoses. I am less inclined to think this is a pulmonary embolism based on the fact that his pain was initially intermittent and resolved at first with nitroglycerin. However, he did have a period of immobility, the airplane trip, so when I do a review of systems and physical examination, I will check for signs and symptoms of deep vein thrombosis (DVT).

Esophageal rupture or perforated peptic ulcer cannot be definitely ruled out at this point but are unlikely given the chronic recurrent nature of the pain and lack of abdominal distress on current presentation. To further evaluate this, I will collect more information about gastrointestinal symptoms. Because of his extensive cardiac history, risk factors, presentation of symptoms, and ECG changes, the most likely diagnoses are NSTEMI or unstable angina (UA).

There are three main presentations of UA. The first is rest angina, which is defined as pain occurring when the patient is not performing any activities, but is at rest. The next is new onset, severe angina that has started within the last 2 months. The third is increasing angina. This is when the angina has been increasing in intensity, duration, and frequency. The angina is then graded according to the Canadian Cardiovascular Society (CCS) from Class I to IV.[3]

UA/NSTEMI is a clinical subset of the ACS and is defined by ECG changes of ST-segment depression or prominent T-wave inversion and the absence of ST-segment elevation in conjunction with clinical symptoms. UA and NSTEMI are closely related in clinical presentations and frequently indistinguishable at initial presentation but they differ in severity. The primary difference is whether there is sufficient ischemia to cause myocardial damage. The biomarkers of troponin I (TnI), troponin T (TnT), and creatine kinase MB (CK-MB) are the gold standard diagnostic tests for determining if ischemia has progressed to infarction. Two or more samples should be collected at least 6 hours apart. Results of these tests allow the distinction between UA, in which there is no elevation in biomarkers and, transient if any, ECG changes of ischemia, and NSTEMI, in which the biomarkers will show elevations.[2]

Since my patient has increasing angina episodes and is unable to carry on physical activity without discomfort he is classified as CCS IV. His ECG is consistent with either UA or NSTEMI because it shows T-wave inversions in the anterior and lateral leads, suggesting ischemia.

? What diagnostic tests should be done and in what order?

I order stat labs including cardiac enzymes (troponin I) along with chemistries, CBC, CK-MB, PT/INR, brain natriuretic peptide (BNP), and ALT and AST, as patient is on statin therapy.

CASE INFORMATION

Review of Systems

The patient is a Hispanic male, bilingual, who is accompanied by son.
- Allergies: Unable to tolerate angiotensin converting enzyme inhibitors (ACE-I) due to cough.
- Constitutional: + Easily fatigue with exertion.
- Head/eyes/ears/nose/throat: Not pertinent.

- Cardiovascular: + Chest pain/burning which has become more frequent, with severe episode prior to admission. Rated chest discomfort 4/10. + dyspnea on exertion, left arm, jaw and back discomfort. + swelling in lower extremities.
- Pulmonary: Denies cough, wheeze, or pain on inspiration, denies shortness of breath except as noted in cardiovascular review.
- Gastrointestinal: Denies nausea, vomiting, constipation, diarrhea, heartburn or gastroesophageal reflux disease.
- Genitourinary: Not pertinent.
- Musculoskeletal: Denies any pulled muscles or trauma.
- Neurological: Numbness/discomfort left upper arm.
- Psychological: + Episodes of anxiety with chest discomfort.
- Social history: Widower, lives alone in Honduras, visits family in the United States frequently, states he takes his medication "most of the time," but admits to occasional missed doses. Does not follow low sodium diet, nonsmoker, nondrinker, retired laborer.

Physical Examination

- Vital signs: Blood pressure 150/84 mm Hg, heart rate 88 beats per minute, respiratory rate 26/min. Oxygen saturation 89% on room air, weight 152 lb (69 kg), BMI 21.8 kg/m².
- Constitutional: Appears older than stated age, rubbing anterior chest, in mild distress
- Neuro: Alert and oriented × 3, no focal deficits.
- Head/eyes/ears/nose/throat: Pupils equal, round, and react to light, no xanthelasma, + jugular venous distention 5 to 6 cm.
- Cardiovascular: S1, S2 with S3 gallop. Heart rate and rhythm regular. No murmur, rubs.
- Pulmonary: Breathing slightly labored with conversation, + use of accessory muscles, fine rales at bases.
- Cardiovascular: S1, S2 with S3 gallop. Heart rate and rhythm regular. No murmur, rubs
- Gastrointestinal: Abdomen soft, not tender, not distended, + bowel sounds in all four quadrants.
- Extremities: Warm to touch, no cyanosis, no erythema, 1+ ankle edema.
- Psychiatric: Appears anxious.

? Given the new information, what additional pertinent positives and significant negatives can you add to your list?

- **Pertinent positives:** ongoing chest discomfort/symptoms, noncompliance with medications and diet, hypertensive with systolic blood pressure over 140, increased respiratory effort, hypoxemic with oxygen saturation less than 90%, + jugular venous distension, +fine rales at bases, labored breathing with conversation, + lower extremity edema

- **Significant negatives:** heart rhythm regular, no abdominal distention, no murmurs, extremities warm without cyanosis

---

❓ How does the information provided so far affect the list of potential causes?

In evaluating a patient for short-term risk of death or nonfatal MI with UA/NSTEMI, a patient is graded as high risk if he has at least one of the five features. At this point, the patient has the first four of the five listed below.

1. History of accelerating tempo of ischemic symptoms in the preceding 48 hours.
2. Character of pain described as prolonged ongoing (greater than 20 minutes) rest pain.
3. Clinical findings of pulmonary edema.
4. ECG demonstrating transient or new ST-segment changes greater than 0.5 mm.
5. Cardiac markers and abnormal troponin levels.[2]

CASE INFORMATION

Results of Diagnostic Tests Obtained Earlier

The ECG completed on admission (findings listed above and shown in Figure 44-1) is the first priority.

Bloodwork drawn within 10 minutes of admission shows the following:

Troponin I = 0.1 (Normal = <0.01 ng/mL), CK-MB = 18 (Normal = 0–3 ng/mL)

Comprehensive metabolic panel is within normal limits, showing normal kidney and liver function.

Complete blood count is within normal limits, as is the protime and INR.

Brain natiuretic peptide (BNP)=323 (Normal = <100)

Hemoglobin A1c 7.8 (Normal = ≤5.4)

Lipid panel: total cholesterol 210 (Normal = <200 mg/dL), triglycerides 163 (Normal = <150 mg/dL), high-density lipoprotein (HDL) = 41 (Normal = >35), low-density lipoprotein (LDL) = 133 (Normal = 65–180 mg/dL)

Chest x-ray: shows increased interstitial markings consistent with pulmonary edema

Echocardiogram done last admission (3 years ago) at the time of his MI: severe left ventricular dilation, inferior apex is dyskinetic, overall severe decreased left systolic function with ejection fraction 37%, abnormal diastolic filling pattern, normal right ventricular size and function, no aortic stenosis, mild mitral regurgitation, mild tricuspid regurgitation

Diagnosis and Treatment: NSTEMI

Reviewing the patient's labwork, the first set of troponin I is positive, so I can diagnose the patient with NSTEMI. A second set is ordered for 6 hours after the first. An increasing pattern in serial levels best helps determine whether the event is acute, distinct form a previous event, subacute, or chronic. Initial medical therapy is similar to that which is used for acute ST-elevation MI patients, except that acute fibrinolytic therapy is contraindicated for ACS patients without ST-elevation MI. Fibrinolytic agents have not shown significant beneficial effect and actually increased the risk of MI in patients who do not have a ST-segment elevation MI or new bundle branch block.[2]

Since the patient did not take any of his medications this morning before his plane flight, he needs to be treated with dual antiplatelet therapy. He is given aspirin 325 mg to chew and a second antiplatelet agent, ticagelor, is ordered. This medication is preferred for patients that are being treated with early invasive strategies or with medical management.[4] Anticoagulation with intravenous heparin is also started. Supplemental oxygen is ordered for his hypoxemia at 2 liters per minute via nasal cannula. This improves his oxygen saturation to 92%. For the ongoing chest pain, which has persisted despite treatment with nitroglycerin, I will start an intravenous nitroglycerin infusion to be titrated upward to achieve relief of chest pain relief and/or SBP of 90. The infusion is started at 5 µg/min and titrated to 15 µg/min before his chest pain is 0/10. At that level, he is more relaxed and comfortable. Had the pain persisted, I would have given him a dose of morphine 2 to 4 mg intravenously for relief of chest pain and anxiety.

β-Blockers are used in NSTEMI for the benefit of decreasing the cardiac workload and myocardial oxygen demand. I order short-acting metoprolol (Lopressor) 25mg every six hours and will monitor his heart rate continuously on telemetry. In addition, because of his elevated BNP, pulmonary congestion (edema) on chest x-ray and crackles on examination, I order furosemide 40 mg intravenously with orders to monitor intake and output. I will continue his home dose of losartan as this is beneficial in patients with heart failure and offers renal protection in light of his history of diabetes.

A fasting lipid profile should be done on all cardiac patients within 24 hours of admission. My patient's admission LDL is 133, and he is on pravastatin (Pravachol) 40 mg, but reports he is nonadherent. I discontinue the pravastatin and start atorvastatin 80 mg because I want the patient to benefit from initial intensive statin therapy given within 30 days of infarction. This is proven to be more effective than gradual dose titration in the setting of acute infarction.

Electrolytes are monitored closely to keep the potassium ≥ 4.0 mEq/L and a magnesium concentration above 2.0 mEq/L. The risk of arrhythmias is greater in the presence of electrolyte imbalance.[5]

In patients with UA and NSTEMI, a Thrombolysis in Myocardial Infarction (TIMI) risk score accurately risk stratifies patients with undifferentiated chest pain presenting to an emergency department.[6] This score, based on a simple set of seven questions, categorizes a patient's risk of death and ischemic events and provides a basis for therapeutic decision making. One point is given to each positive answer. For example, one question is: Does the patient have at least three risk factors for CAD, such as hypertension or on antihypertensives, current cigarette smoker, low HDL cholesterol, diabetes mellitus, or family history of premature CAD? The score is then added up and correlated to the percentage of risk at 14 days of all causes of mortality, new or recurrent MI, or severe recurrent ischemia. Patients with TIMI scores of 0 to 1 have a 4.7% risk whereas with a final score of 6 to 7, a patient has a 41% risk and should be targeted for early aggressive treatment with antithrombotic drugs and direct triage from the emergency department to specialist cardiology services.

Case Follow-Up

My patient has a TIMI score of 6, warranting early invasive treatment, so he is scheduled for a cardiac catheterization. The results of the cardiac catheterization show two-vessel CAD, with patent intervention sites of the RCA, a 70% lesion to the proximal left anterior descending (LAD), and an 80% lesion to the mid LAD. Two drug eluting stents are placed successfully in the mid- and proximal LAD arteries.

The patient is monitored on telemetry unit overnight after the cardiac catheterization and has no further episodes of chest discomfort. Discharge is planned for the following morning providing the ECG remains unchanged, and labs are normal. This patient requires extensive patient education. He is instructed in his medical management plan, specifically on the purpose, dose, frequency, and pertinent side effects of his medications, especially the new antiplatelet medication, ticagrelor 90 mg, which is taken daily for 1 year . If a patient fails to get this prescription filled, or stops taking it, the risks of recurrent MI, stent thrombosis, or even death are high. His other discharge medications include aspirin 81 mg daily, metoprolol XL 50 mg daily, losartan 25 mg daily, atorvastatin 80 mg daily, nitroglycerin sublingual tablets as needed, and repaglinide 1 mg three times a day. The rationale for these medications and their potential side effects are explained to the patient. The patient is instructed in risk factor modifications such as dietary restrictions, medication adherence, importance of regular medical follow-up, and physical activity. He is educated in detail regarding specific targets for his lipid profile, and blood pressure levels. The diabetes nurse practitioner is consulted to reinforce diabetes management strategies and lifestyle changes. The patient is informed about symptoms of worsening myocardial ischemia and MI and instructed how, and when, to seek emergency care and assistance should they occur.[7]

Instructions are given to both the patient and his son. I ask the son to contact a family and/or friends in Honduras who may be a support to the patient once he returns. A cardiac rehabilitation referral is made. In addition I make a follow-up appointment for my patient with the cardiology interventionist in 1 week, also request that the patient and son contact his physician in Honduras so medical information can be provided, a follow-up appointment made on his return to Honduras, and continuity of care maintained.

References

1. Diagnostic approach to chest pain in adults. UpToDate Web site. 2014. http://www.uptodate.com. Accessed July10, 2014.
2. Anderson JL, Antman EM, Califf RM, et al. ACCF/AHA focused update incorporated into the ACCF/AHA 2007 guidelines for the management of patients with unstable angina/

non-ST-elevation myocardial infarction. ahajournal.org Web site. http://circ.ahajournal.org/content/early/2013/04/29/CIR.0b013e31828478ac.full.pdf. Updated 2012. Accessed July 20, 2014.

3. Canadian Cardiovascular Society Functional Classification. Centre for Evidence Based Physiotherapy Web site. www.cebp.nl/vault_piblic/filesystem/?ID=1267. Accessed July 20, 2014.

4. Amsterdam EA, Wenger NK, Brindis RG, et al. 2014 ACC/AHA guideline for the management of patients with non– ST-elevation acute coronary syndromes: a report of the American College of Cardiology/American Heart Association Task Force on Practice Guidelines. Circulation. 2014;000:000–000.

5. Overview of the acute management of unstable angina and non-ST elevation myocardial infarction. UpToDate Web site. 2014. www.uptodate.com. Accessed July 20, 2014.

6. TIMI Risk Calculator Score. MDCalc Web site. www.mdcalc.com/risk-score-for-uanstemi/. Accessed July 20, 2014.

7. Smith SC, Benjamin EJ, Bonow RP, et al. AHA/ACCF secondary prevention and risk reduction therapy for patients with coronary and other atherosclerotic vascular Disease: 2011 Update. 2011. JACC Journals Web site. content.onlinejacc.org/article.aspx?articleid=1147807. Accessed July 20, 2014.

CASE 45

Sheila Melander

Sheila Melander has practiced as an ACNP in interventional cardiology inpatient and outpatient settings for over 14 years. Dr Melander has also served as faculty in ACNP programs for over 15 years teaching core AG-ACNP courses and is currently on the faculty at the University of Kentucky.

CASE INFORMATION

Chief Complaint

A 75-year-old retired nurse presents with complaints of shortness of breath with exertion and fatigue associated with blurred vision, which has increased over the last month.

❓ What is the potential cause?

The patient's main complaints are fatigue and exertional dyspnea, which in a female patient can be caused by many different conditions. Because she is female, I am particularly concerned about coronary artery disease (CAD), because women with CAD often do not complain of chest pain, but present with atypical constitutional symptoms such as fatigue.

Comprehensive Differential Diagnoses for Patient With Fatigue and Dyspnea[1]

- Cardiac: acute coronary syndrome, myocardial infarction (MI), ST elevation myocardial infarction (STEMI), Non-ST segment elevation myocardial infarction (NSTEMI), unstable angina, Prinzmetal angina, pericarditis, mitral valve prolapse, aortic aneurysm, cardiac arrhythmia, heart failure exacerbation, aortic dissection
- Pulmonary: pulmonary emboli, pneumonia, pleuritis, pneumothorax, pulmonary hypertension, hypoxia, chronic obstructive pulmonary disease (COPD) exacerbation, tracheobronchitis
- Gastrointestinal: esophageal spasm, esophageal reflux, esophageal tear, esophagitis, peptic ulcer disease, gastritis, cholecystitis, pancreatitis
- Musculoskeletal: chest wall injury or strain, rib fracture, cervical or thoracic disk disease, shoulder arthroscopy, costochondritis, trauma
- Neurological: herpes zoster, nerve root compression
- Psychiatric: anxiety, panic disorders, depression, grief, stress
- Endocrine: diabetes, hypoglycemia, thyroid disorder
- Exogenous: insomnia, physical deconditioning, vitamin B or vitamin D deficiency, medication side effect or interaction or withdrawal, drug overdose, carbon monoxide inhalation

CASE INFORMATION

History of Present Illness

A 75-year-old female with a history of ventricular fibrillation requiring car-dioversion and resuscitation comes to scheduled episodic outpatient visit with new symptoms of dyspnea and fatigue. The patient's general survey reveals an alert, appropriate, well-groomed, well-nourished female in no acute distress. In gathering the history of this illness, I initially focus on the shortness of breath and fatigue and ask about the pattern of these symptoms. The patient reports she is very active and volunteers at the hospital and also at the zoo. She is insistent that "I just can't do as much as I need to do daily or what I was able to do 4–6 weeks ago." She denies chest discomfort, and when asked about any other atypical symptoms such as scapular pain, neck, epigastric, or jaw pain, she denies these as well but then states: "It seems strange, but at the times that I am most fatigued, my vision seems altered and almost blurred." She has not previously had any issues with her vision or her eyesight and as we are continuing to talk, she is associating the blurred vision episodes with the exacerbation of the shortness of breath and fatigue. The patient denies a history of cardiac disease but does note that members of her family have had heart trouble, and she believes this was due to cigarette smoking.

Medical History

She denies any previous diagnoses of CAD, stroke, hypertension, lung disease, GI disorders, neurological disorders, diabetes, cancer, or recent injury/physical trauma or mental health conditions. She was seen in the ER approximately 6 years ago in ventricular fibrillation but was resuscitated successfully per the ER records.

Social History

Married, two grown children, social alcohol intake, nonsmoker, exercises regularly, three to four times/week.

Family Medical History

Both parents deceased; father was former cigarette smoker, overweight, and had a myocardial infarction at age 50. One brother and one sister living, brother had myocardial infarction at age 64.

Medications

She uses no complementary medications or alternative therapies. Her cholesterol levels have been increased in the past, but she has chosen to defer any treatment as she has "never been overweight," and she felt that the increases noted in her cholesterol were "negligible" and "nothing to worry about." She denies trying any over-the-counter remedies or any medications for any symptoms discussed.

❓ What are the pertinent positives from the information given so far?

- Increased SOB with activity.
- Dramatic change in ability to complete physically demanding activities.
- Increased fatigue noted with less than normal activity.
- Increased fatigue noted after shortness of breath and blurred vision symptoms.
- Blurred vision noted at times of increased physical activity.
- Blurred vision noted at times of increased fatigue.
- History of high cholesterol levels.
- Positive paternal history premature CAD/MI.
- Positive brother's history of MI.
- Previous history of ventricular fibrillation with resuscitation.

❓ What are the significant negatives from the information given so far?

- The patient is in no acute distress.
- No complaint of chest discomfort.
- No previous diagnosis of any chronic health conditions including cardiac disease, pulmonary disease, or diabetes.
- There is an absence of GI disorders, neurological disorders, or musculoskeletal disorders.

❓ What is the problem representation?

The problem representation is "shortness of breath and fatigue with minimal exertion in a 75-year-old active, physically fit female without previous pulmonary or cardiac comorbidities."

❓ How does this information affect the list of possible causes and what do you need to do now?

I know that women have atypical cardiac symptomology. Exertional dyspnea along with fatigue is a common angina equivalent in women. Combine this information with the fact that she has had a previous ventricular fibrillation episode, a family history of CAD as well as hyperlipidemia, it paints a different and more inclusive picture of possible etiologies. Because rapid diagnosis of CAD enables efficient treatment and lowers morbidity, I will need to rule this out quickly so I order a stat ECG. The other life-threatening items on my differential list, aortic dissection, pneumothorax, pulmonary embolism, and perforated esophagus seem less likely given that she is not in any distress, and these symptoms have occurred for over a month. I do not think this discomfort results from trauma as she denies any history of this. It is also less likely to be the exacerbation of chronic disease process because she has no prior chronic health condition diagnosis.

❓ What diagnostic tests should be done and in what order?

A 12-lead ECG is performed during the outpatient visit and based on the results, a Cardiolite stress test is also ordered and performed in our office.

Further laboratory testing is ordered to determine additional possible etiologies. This includes a complete metabolic profile (CMP), a complete blood count (CBC), a thyroid panel, and a fasting lipid panel to begin addressing the other items on my list. These blood tests will help me determine if the patient has hypothyroidism, anemia, or hyperglycemia that could account for the fatigue and possible dyspnea. Because of her episode of ventricular fibrillation, I also order a magnesium level. She still also complains of occasional blurred vision.

CASE INFORMATION

Review of Systems

The patient is a retired nurse with full mental capacity. She is a very good historian and provides detailed health information.

- Constitutional: Denies fever and chills, denies any changes in weight or changes in appetite. No recent falls or trauma, no problems with sleep.
- Head/eyes/ears/nose/throat: Complains of blurred vision when fatigued and with exertion. Denies discharge from ears, nose, denies cough and denies secretions.
- Cardiovascular: Denies chest pain, palpitations, edema, or orthopnea.
- Pulmonary: Complains of exertional dyspnea with minimal exertion, denies wheezing or coughing.
- Gastrointestinal: Denies nausea and vomiting, denies pain with eating or drinking, denies blood in stool, abdominal pain, or reflux disease.
- Genitourinary: Denies dysuria or hematuria.
- Musculoskeletal: Denies chest wall tenderness or pain with movement, occasional back pain noted "only after lifting or working in the garden," pain is relieved with Advil or Aleve, denies cervical or thoracic disk pain. On further questioning, she notes occasional scapular pain at times although she initially denied this.
- Neurological: Denies headaches, syncope, vertigo, falls, history of stroke, seizure disorder numbness, tingling or weakness in extremities, changes in speech or motor activity.
- Hematology/immunology/oncology: Denies blood clotting abnormalities, easy bruising, infections, or history of previous diagnosis of any type of cancer.

- Endocrine: Denies change in appetite, weight change, excessive thirst or urination, denies history of diabetes or thyroid disorder.
- Mental health: Denies depression, or panic disorders. Married with grown children, volunteers at numerous philanthropic organizations. Alert, interact easily, with appropriate demeanor.

Physical Examination

- Vital signs: Pulse 64, blood pressure 116/68, respiratory rate 20, oxygen saturation 94% on room air.
- Constitutional: 75-year-old Caucasian female, well developed and appears stated age, well groomed, no acute distress.
- Head/eyes/ears/nose/throat: Head symmetrical without lesions or pain, pupils equal, round, reactive to light and accommodation, ear canals with small amount dry cerumen, no nasal deviation or polyps, buccal mucosa moist, oropharynx moist without lesions. Neck: trachea midline, thyroid without palpable masses or enlargement, no palpable lymph nodes, no jugular venous distension.
- Cardiovascular: Normal point of maximal impulse, heart sounds regular without murmurs, clicks, rubs, or gallops.
- Pulmonary: Lungs clear to auscultation, no wheezes, rhonchi, or crackles.
- Gastrointestinal: Abdomen soft, nondistended without tenderness or organomegaly.
- Extremities: Moves all extremities without restrictions, nail beds pink without clubbing, brisk capillary refill.
- Integumentary: Intact, no rashes, lesions, normal skin turgor.
- Musculoskeletal: Active range of motion of all extremities.
- Neurological: Alert and oriented to person, place, and time, no neurological deficits
- 12-Lead ECG: Acute ST elevation in anterior and lateral leads. Evidence of old anterior infarct age undetermined.

? **Given the information to this point what elements of the review of systems and the physical examination should be added to the list of pertinent positives? Which items should be added to the list of significant negatives?**

- **Pertinent positives:** subjective—increased fatigue with minimal exertion; blurred vision associated with increased fatigue and increased dyspnea. Scapular pain as well, unsure of associated pattern. Objective—abnormal changes reflected on the 12-lead ECG performed in the office, old anterior infarct noted, previous history of ventricular fibrillation episode, positive family history of coronary artery disease; social alcohol use, hyperlipidemia.

- **Significant negatives:** the review of systems and the physical examination are both consistent with an adult female in general good health. No previous history pulmonary or endocrine comorbidities. Subjective—the review of systems reveals no localizing complaints such as substernal pain, radiation of pain, diaphoresis, nausea, and vomiting; the review of systems for other pertinent systems such as pulmonary, gastrointestinal, musculoskeletal, and neurological are normal. Objective—the physical examination is essentially normal with the exception the abnormal 12-lead ECG showing acute changes and previous myocardial infarction.

How does this information affect the list of possible causes?

The review of systems and physical examination have helped prioritize the need for additional studies to confirm a possible diagnoses. The positive change on her 12-lead ECG substantiates my concern that these symptoms may be due to coronary artery disease. Because the ECG shows acute changes, stat cardiac enzymes/troponin levels are ordered, along with nuclear stress testing which will help to affirm or negate the 12-lead interpretation. I will also order an echocardiogram to further evaluate her cardiac function.

At this point, evaluating her for coronary artery disease is the highest priority. Her review of systems and physical examination are essentially normal and I doubt that she has a pulmonary or gastrointestinal disorder causing her symptoms. In addition, her symptoms are really too vague to indicate a musculoskeletal cause, and I do not see evidence of an endocrine disorder. She seems to be in excellent mental health but evaluating this is a much lower priority than pursuing her cardiac workup.

At this point do you need to reexamine and restate the problem representation?

After reviewing the data as described above I would state the problem as: "A 75-year-old female with complaints of extreme fatigue, dyspnea on exertion, and scapular pain presents with acute 12-lead ECG changes." Even though ECG changes are noted, she is in no distress and is in stable condition so I will substantiate the 12-lead ECG reading with further testing to validate and confirm cardiac diagnosis.

What additional diagnostic testing should be done and in what order?

Since there is an acutely abnormal ECG, I schedule a nuclear stress test such as a Cardiolite study as soon as possible and an echocardiogram to be done on the same day that I am seeing her in my office. This is possible as we do have ultrasound personnel available daily within our practice suite. As mentioned above, in addition to the stat troponin level, I will need lipid levels and at this point I do not wait for this to be fasting; I request that it is drawn with her other labs. I also proceed with the lab work ordered above, which includes a CMP, a CBC, thyroid studies, and a PT/PTT and INR. I am less concerned about the lab results for my differential diagnosis and more concerned about having the data I need to prepare the patient for a cardiac catheterization, in case this is necessary.

CASE INFORMATION
Results of Initial Diagnostics

- ECG: Acute ST elevation in anterior and lateral leads. Evidence of old anterior infarct age undetermined.
- Labs: CBC is normal; PTT/ PT/INR all are within normal limits. CMP is normal with normal potassium, sodium, and glucose levels; magnesium level is normal. Her normal creatinine, BUN, and GFR are of particular importance as this means the patient can proceed to coronary angiography if necessary. Troponin level is still pending when the echocardiogram was performed.
- Cardiolite treadmill: Results reveal evidence for ischemia at an adequate level of stress; left ventricular ejection fraction (LVEF) is noted at 39% and a large anterior wall scar is noted.

Echocardiogram is performed while still in office and shows ischemic cardiomyopathy with ejection fraction of 35% as well as old anterior wall scar. Left anterior wall is also noted to be sluggish upon echocardiogram review. At this time we decide to admit her for coronary angiography.

Coronary angiography reveals the following:
- Left main coronary artery: Patent without significant disease.
- Left anterior descending artery: There is 100% occlusion of this vessel just distal to the takeoff of the diagonal branch.
- Right coronary tree: This vessel is dominant and widely patent without significant disease.

Successful stenting was performed of the 100% LAD lesion. A Promus drug-eluting stent was deployed in the mid- and distal LAD. No residual stenosis was noted after multiple dilations.

A portable chest x-ray was ordered prior to coronary angiography and was normal.

Other laboratory studies are necessary to rule out some of my lingering diagnoses. The patient's thyroid-stimulating hormone comes back within normal limits, ruling out hypothyroidism. In addition her blood glucose is within normal limits, and normal hemoglobin A1C confirms that she does not have diabetes. Her cholesterol studies come back as follows: total cholesterol 130; LDL-C 55; HDL-C 65; triglycerides 48.

Case Analysis: The results of the diagnostic testing confirmed the diagnosis of coronary artery disease. She underwent successful intervention of stent deployment with reperfusion established. The interesting piece of this case was while the patient was on the cath table, immediately after the stent was deployed into the LAD, her blurred vision completely cleared. This was her main angina equivalent. The coronary angiography confirmed the reduced LVEF at 39%. Prior echocardiogram showed LVEF at 35%.

Treatment of Coronary Artery Disease

Once changes have been identified in ECG, further testing as described above is deemed necessary to substantiate the diagnosis. Once validated, immediate intervention is needed for an acute or evolving myocardial infarction, and that is the first priority.[2-4] Rapid treatment preserves cardiac function. If the patient is having chest discomfort or complains of an alternate angina equivalent such as neck pain, jaw pain, scapular pain, extreme shortness of breath, diaphoresis, fatigue, or in this patients situation, blurred vision, nitroglycerin 0.4 mg sublingual can be administered per protocol, which is usually every 5 minutes $\times$ 3. If pain persists, the patient should call 911 and proceed to the emergency room. If chest pain is present, aspirin should be given and preferably chewed, oxygen administered at 2 liters per nasal cannula, and intravenous access obtained. Strategies for achieving improved cardiac perfusion include stenting and coronary artery bypass grafting. Other strategies to increase function include pharmacological use of nitrate, β-blocker therapy, aspirin therapy, and angiotensin converting enzyme-inhibitor therapy unless contraindicated. Healthy lifestyle choices including diet and exercise should as well be part of the teaching as well as cholesterol and blood sugar control as these all affect cardiovascular health.[2-4]

Once a diagnosis of CAD is confirmed, ongoing medical management is essential to prevent reoccurrence. If no renal artery stenosis is present, angiotensin-converting enzyme inhibitors (ACE-I) or angiotensin receptor blockers (ARBs) should be started. In addition, patients require a β-blocker to reduce cardiac workload, and a statin to treat hyperlipidemia.[5-7] Consideration should also be given to a program of cardiac rehabilitation if patients have experienced a loss of functional status. The recent literature supports rehabilitation efforts in further decreasing morbidity and mortality rates. Following stent placement, patients require dual anti-platelet therapy, usually aspirin and clopidogrel (Plavix). These medications work at different points in the clotting cascade and can both be very beneficial in combination when needed for specific patient populations.[2-4]

Comorbidities are also especially important to keep in mind as treatment regimens are discussed. The diabetic client as well as the patient with chronic pulmonary disease may not be as able to tolerate β-blocker therapy and may need other alternative therapies or closer monitoring. Heart failure combined with CAD requires additional therapeutics such as diuretic therapy that can affect the ACE-inhibitor choice or ARB treatment depending on their potassium levels and renal function as well must be monitored.[2-4]

The 75-year-old female patient in this case was also diagnosed with ischemic cardiomyopathy with an LVEF of 39%. With her combined diagnoses of CAD, ischemic cardiomyopathy, and hyperlipidemia, she was started on the following:

- Valsartan 80 mg, one tablet daily (an ARB)

- Aspirin 81 mg, one tablet daily (for antiplatelet)

- Rosuvastatin 20 mg, one tablet every evening (to treat hyperlipidemia)

- Carvedilol 6.25 mg, one tablet twice daily (a cardioselective β-blocker)

- Clopidogrel 75 mg, one tablet daily (for antiplatelet)

- Fish oil 1200 IU one tablet twice daily

- Nitrostat 0.4 mg SL as needed per protocol, to be taken for blurred vision

Patient Follow-Up: Recurrence 1 Year Later

One year later this same 75-year-old female presented to the office with the same complaint of blurred vision and associated chest discomfort with exertion, exertional dyspnea, and fatigue. The consistent complaint was the blurred vision, and she again stated that this was the most noticeable symptom. ECG was performed, which denoted lateral wall changes once again. Cardiolite stress test was repeated, which showed evidence for ischemia at an adequate level of stress with an LVEF at 51%.

Patient presentation 1 year after initial stenting of LAD was the same as the previous occurrence. ECG changes as well as the Cardiolite results are the same. The patient was taken for coronary angiography where "in-stent restenosis" in the proximal left anterior descending artery stent previously placed 1 year prior was noted. The patient had continued her medications consistently, did not miss any doses of clopidogrel (Plavix), continued the rosuvastatin, and lab results remained within normal limits prior to the restenosis.

Institution on New Methodology

Since the patient adhered to prescribed CAD protocol therapies and still had in-stent restenosis, comprehensive cholesterol consultation was ordered and it was discovered that she had elevated levels of lipoprotein (a) or small LDL. In addition she was a cloprodrigel nonresponder per the *CYP2C19* gene. The *CYP2C19* gene can be measured through genetic cardiac testing and patients can be classified as a responder, or nonresponder to clopidogrel. This had been our mainstay treatment to maintain stent patency. Once it was established that she was not a clopidogrel responder, alterations in therapy become necessary. A consultation was scheduled to discuss the advanced cholesterol testing results and at that time the following was ordered:

- Niaspan 500 mg once daily

- Stop clopidogrel as she was a clopidogrel mid-level responder and start ticagrelor (Brilinta) 90 mg one tablet twice daily

- Continue Omega 3 fish oil tablets

- Continue rosuvastatin 20 mg, one tablet daily

Two and a half years after initial diagnosis: She was seen by her primary care provider for complaints of hip pain and musculoskeletal issues. It was decided by her orthopedic surgeon after testing that she needed to have a hip replacement. Prior to the hip replacement the surgeon requested cardiac risk stratification due to her ECG obtained in his office. She was scheduled and seen in our office where subtle changes were noted in her ECG and she complained of vague fatigue. Due to her history of in-stent stenosis, a coronary angiography was scheduled. The LAD stent was noted to be widely patent. She had done very well once she had been switched from the clopidogrel to ticagrelor.[2–4]

Summary

This case is an excellent illustration of the fact that we cannot be complacent in the presentation of our patients and that we must always be mindful of atypical symptoms. In addition, we also need to be aware of alternative treatments that are available to prevent additional adverse events. The initiation of the advanced cholesterol genetic testing and the *CYP2C19* testing was an example of using an "out-of-the-box" type thinking. By doing so we identified the cause of the in-stent restenosis. This was validated by the fact that after 18 months of treatment on ticagrelor, the stent was widely patent upon angiography. She was discharged with LVEF at 51%, scheduled for hip surgery and discharged from the hospital. She had a successful hip surgery and continues to do very well without blurred vision or cardiac complaints.

References

1. 2013 ACCF/AHA guideline for the management of ST-elevation myocardial infarction: a report of the American College of Cardiology Foundation/American Heart Association task force on practice guidelines. Circulation. http://circ.ahajournals.org/content/early/2012/12/17/CIR.0b013e3182742cf6. citation.

2. 2013 ACCF/ACA guidelines for the ST elevation myocardial infarction. JACC Journals Web site. http://content.onlinejacc.org/article.aspx?articleid=1486115.

3. ACC/AHA guidelines for the management of patients with unstable angina and non-ST elevation myocardial infarctions—executive summary. Circulation. http://circ.ahajournals.org/content/102/10/1193.full.

4. Guidelines for the management of patients with stable ischemic heart disease. American Association of Cardiovascular and Pulmonary Rehabilitation Web site. https://www.aacvpr.org/Portals/0/resources/professionals/2012%20Guidelines_StableIschemicHeartDisease_11-20-12.pdf.

5. NHI guidelines for lipid management. Circulation. http://circ.ahajournals.org/content/early/2013/11/11/01.cir.0000437738.63853.7a.

6. High cholesterol treatment options (beyond the basics). UpToDate Web site. http://www.uptodate.com/contents/high-cholesterol-treatment-options-beyond-the-basics.

7. 2013 ACC/AHA guideline on the treatment of blood cholesterol to reduce atherosclerotic cardiovascular risk in adults. Circulation. http://circ.ahajournals.org/content/early/2013/11/11/01.cir.0000437738.63853.7a.

CASE 46

Helen F. Brown

Helen F. Brown is an NP in an emergency department in Annapolis, Maryland. Helen has extensive critical care and emergency medicine experience. She is also on the faculty of Georgetown University where she teaches in the ACNP Program.

CASE INFORMATION

Chief Complaint

The patient is a 76-year-old female admitted to the medical intensive care unit (MICU) 2 weeks ago with acute respiratory failure and septic shock due to multilobar pneumonia. She has required mechanical ventilation since admission to the unit, and attempts to wean the ventilator have been unsuccessful. I am consulted to evaluate her weaning potential.

❓ What are the potential causes of "unsuccessful weaning attempts?"

Unsuccessful liberation from ventilator support may be the result of an unresolved condition that initially necessitated mechanical ventilation, or may be due to a new complication or iatrogenic condition. In this patient's case, she has been on ventilator support for 2 weeks and has experienced numerous unsuccessful weaning trials despite being hemodynamically stable and having been treated for her pneumonia, respiratory failure, and sepsis.

The requirement for continued mechanical ventilation is not a condition in and of itself, but rather a supportive intervention. The inability to be successfully liberated from the ventilator is likely the result of clinical factors that impede her return to her preadmission baseline health.[1] Reasons for ventilator dependency may be multifactorial and potential causes are numerous.[1] At this point I cannot develop a useful differential until I fully evaluate the patient because "failure to wean" or "unsuccessful weaning attempts" do not point to the associated symptoms or signs that may identify a potential cause.

In order to develop a useful differential for the causes of unsuccessful weaning, I must review her clinical course to date, her laboratory studies and diagnostics, and most importantly I must do a comprehensive history and physical examination (H and P).

CASE INFORMATION

History of Present Illness

This 76-year-old female presented 2 weeks ago to the emergency department (ED) via emergency medical services (EMS), confused, febrile, in acute respiratory distress. Concerned neighbors, having not seen her for 3 days, went to her home to check on her. She was found moaning in bed, hot, flushed, and "talking out of her head." 911 was activated and she was transported to the ED. In the ED she was found to be hypoxemic with oxygen saturation of 83% on room air, her blood pressure was 80/42 mm Hg, and heart rate was 145 beats per minute. A portable chest x-ray revealed a right middle lobe and left lower lobe (RML and LLL) pneumonia. She was intubated and ventilated, with propofol and succinylcholine used for rapid sequence intubation. She received 3 liters (L) of normal saline (NS) and an infusion of norepinephrine at 10 µg/min was started to maintain a mean arterial pressure (MAP) of 65 mm Hg. She was transferred to the medical intensive care unit for further care and management.

In the medical intensive care unit she was effectively treated for her pneumonia, respiratory failure, and septic state with full ventilator support, fluid resuscitation, vasopressors, and antibiotics and became hemodynamically stable. Efforts to wean her from the ventilator began on day 4, with daily evaluations using spontaneous breathing trails (SBT). She was able to tolerate a decrease in ventilator support but reached a plateau on day 8 with minimal progress seen over the last 5 days.

Currently, she is ventilated on pressure support (PS) ventilation of 15 cm H_2O, post–end-expiratory pressure (PEEP) of 8 cm H_2O, and a fraction of inspired oxygen (FIO_2) of 40%. She tolerates these settings with a respiratory rate of 10 to 14/min, tidal volumes (Vt) of 350 mL, and an oxygen saturation of 95%. Attempts to decrease the PS level have caused tachypnea, shallow respirations, accessory muscle use, a decrease in Vt to 200 mL, and a decrease in oxygen saturation to 85%. She also failed a spontaneous breathing trial yesterday.

Past Medical History

Hypertension, probable heart failure (HF) based on review of her home medications

No past surgical history

Social History

Single, lives alone, retired high school English teacher, closest relative is a niece who lives out of state.

Habits

No use of tobacco, alcohol and illicit drug use—per neighbor and niece

Home Medications

Paramedics found two empty prescription bottles, one for lisinopril 20 mg daily and the other for furosemide 40 mg daily.

Hospital Medications (Current and Discontinued)

Current Medications

- Lorazepam 1 mg IV q1hour as needed for agitation, average dose over last 72 hours = 2 to 4 mg/24 hours
- Fentanyl 25 mg intravenously every hour as needed for pain, dose over last 72 hours—25 mg every 8 hours
- Azithromycin 500 mg intravenously every 24 hours
- Ceftriaxone 1 g intravenously every 24 hours
- Heparin 5000 mg subcutaneously every 8 hours
- Ranitidine 50 mg intravenously every 12 hours
- Insulin humalog correctional scale coverage

Discontinued Medications

- Vancomycin 1 g intravenously every 12 hours, discontinued on hospital day 2
- Hydrocortisone sodium succinate (Solu-Cortef) 100 mg intravenously every 8 hours discontinued on hospital day 6
- Regular insulin infusion titrated to keep fingerstick blood glucose— 120 mg/dL. Titrated off on hospital day 8 according to insulin protocol. Has not required any insulin for the last 5 days
- Norepinephrine infusion titrated off on hospital day 5

Review of Systems

The system review is obtained from the patient, her niece at the bedside, and the bedside nurse. Data are obtained by asking the patient yes and no questions and lip reading her responses. I first ask the patient to give the name of her niece and to identify where she is. She answers both questions correctly, though she is not able to identify date or time. Her attempts to write answers are unsuccessful due to weakness and fatigue.

- Constitutional: endorses feeling fatigue, tires very easily, per niece, she was more spontaneous and energetic a week ago
- Head/eyes/ears/nose/throat: endorses throat discomfort due to endotracheal tube.
- Cardiovascular: denies chest pain or palpations
- Pulmonary: endorses shortness of breath with activity and weaning trials (ie, CPAP or PS), denies any pain with breathing
- Gastrointestinal: no abdominal pain, denies nausea
- Genitourinary: no complaints of burning or discomfort

- Integumentary: no complaints of itching or painful spots
- Musculoskeletal: endorses feeling "weak"
- Neurological: denies headaches or feeling she is unable to move extremities although she endorses generalized weakness
- Endocrine: denies feeling cold or hot, denies cramping in extremities
- Psychosocial: reports difficulty sleeping and having "bad dreams"

Physical Examination

- Vital signs: Temperature 96.2°F rectal, pulse 60 beats per minute, respirations 12 breaths per minute, blood pressure 110/60 mm Hg, oxygen saturation 94%, FIO_2 40%, weight 85 kg, height 67 in, BMI 27.
- Constitutional: Hypothermic temperature range 95°F to 97°F, fatigued appearing, edematous female, dozing on ventilatory support, opens eyes when name is called. Weight gain of 5 kg since admission.
- Head/eyes/ears/nose/throat: Head normocephalic, atraumatic, hair dry, and brittle. Pupils equal, round, reactive to light and accommodation (PERRLA), extraocular movements intact (EOMI) conjunctiva pale, loss of lateral eye brows; small bore feeding tube in left nostril, moist mucus membranes, no oral lesions, # 7.5 oral tube, 22 cm at the lip; intact swallow; + 1 facial edema.
- Cardiovascular: Point of maximal impulse at fourth Intercostal space (ICS), mid-clavicular line (MCL), regular rate and rhythm (RRR), no murmur, rub, or gallop, sinus bradycardia on telemetry monitor. No jugular venous distension (JVD), carotid pulse brisk upstroke, no bruit. Nurse notes that blood pressure has decreased over the last several days but MAP has not decreased below 65 mm Hg and she has not required fluid or vasopressor support.
- Peripheral vascular: Radial, posterior tibia, and pedal pulses +2/+4, capillary refill less than 3 seconds, generalized edema—hands, legs, sacrum.
- Pulmonary: Regular, rate 14 breaths per minute on continuous positive airway pressure (CPAP) at 8 cm H_2O, pressure support 15 cm H_2O, FIO_2 40% decreased breath sounds with dullness on percussion at bilateral bases. Rhonchi and crackles noted bilaterally in right middle lobe and left lower lobe to auscultation. Nurse reports small quantity of sputum with suctioning, weak cough. Sputum is white in color.
- Review of data from ventilator, set at PEEP 8, PS 15, and FIO_2 40%.
- Respiratory rate: 10 to 14/min.
- Tidal volume: 250 to 300 cc (predicted 400 cc lean body weight).
- Forced vital capacity: 500 cc (predicted 800 cc lean body weight).
- Minute ventilation: 3.5 L.
- Negative inspiratory pressure: −14 cm H_2O.
- Arterial blood gas: pH 7.34, $PaCO_2$ 48, PaO_2 100.

- Rapid shallow breathing index (RSBI) = 100 (an RSBI of <105 generally indicates readiness to wean).
- Gastrointestinal: Nondistended, normoactive bowel sounds in all quadrants, nontender to palpation, tube feeding off. Nurse reports two episodes of regurgitating "large amount" tube feedings in last 24 hours, no stool in 3 days, no melena, hematochezia, or tarry stools.
- Genitourinary: Normal genitalia, Foley #16, urine clear yellow. Hourly output 50 to 75 mL/h.
- 24-hour intake/output: In 3150 cc, out 1200 cc; 24-hour fluid balance + 1950, + 5 kg since admission.
- Integumentary: Complexion sallow, poor skin turgor with tenting, skin intact, no lesions, rashes, or breakdown to skin or oral or nasal mucosa, #20 Angiocath peripheral IV left forearm, site clean, dressing intact.
- Musculoskeletal: Full range of motion of all joints, uniformly weak muscle strength of all extremities.
- Neurological: Lethargic, arouses to name, fatigues easily but will nod head appropriately to questions, follows commands including lifting head off bed, squeezing hands and releasing, moves all extremities though weakly and slowly, strength is +3 out of 5 throughout, cranial nerves II-VII grossly intact. Difficulty performing pronator drift due to limited ability to extend both arms for 10 seconds, intact symmetrical dermatome sensation to light touch, intact finger to nose but unable to perform heel to shin due to weakness, deep tendon reflexes +2/+4 symmetrical with delayed release ("hung up reflex"), Babinski negative.
- Hematologic: No bleeding or bruising noted.
- Lymphatic: No nodes appreciated.
- Endocrine: Nurse confirms two episodes of hypoglycemia in last 26 hours treated with glucagon, no current use of insulin or oral diabetic medications, hypothermic.

Current Diagnostic Data

- Chemistry: Sodium 128 mEq/L (135–146 mEq/L), potassium 4.5 mEq/L (3.2–5.0 mEq/L), chloride 90 mEq/L (95–112 mEq/L), bicarbonate 29 mEq/L (18–32 mEq/L), BUN 24 mg/dL (5–25 mg/dL), creatinine 1.0 mg/dL (0.5–1.5 mg/dL), glucose 68 mg/dL (70–115 mg/dL).
- Anion gap: 9 (8–12), Serum osmolality 268.7 (285–295 mOsm/kg, creatinine clearance (Cockcroft-Gault) 53.3 mL/min (>60 mL/min).
- CBC: WBC 12,900 cells/μL (4500–10,000), hemoglobin 8.8 g/dL (12–15 g/dL), hematocrit 26.8% (36%–44%), platelets 295 K/μL.
- ABG: pH 7.34, $PaCO_2$ 48 mm Hg, PaO_2 100 mm Hg, HCO_3 26, base excess −0.3.
- Chest x-ray: The admission x-ray demonstrated a right middle and left lower lobe infiltrate consistent with pneumonia, and the current chest

x-ray shows a resolving right middle lobe and left lower lobe pneumonia, hilar engorgement, interstitial edema, cardiomegaly, and an appropriately placed endotracheal tube.

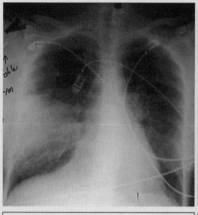

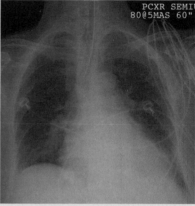

Admission Chest X-ray	Current Chest X-ray
Interpretation: RML and LLL infiltrate	Interpretation: Resolving RML and LLL infiltrates, hilar engorgement interstitial edema, cardiomegaly, appropriate endotracheal tube placement.

• ECG admission: Interpretation—sinus tachycardia otherwise normal ECG.

Review of Medical Record from Admission to Current Date

There is a downward trend in the patient's vital signs. Reviewing the past 8 days revealed this pattern: temperature range was 97.8°F oral and is now 95.2°F, heart rate was 75 to 90 beats per minute and is now 50 to 60 beats per minute, respiratory rate was 18 to 22 breaths per minutes and is now 12 to 14 per minute on CPAP, and blood pressure was 120 to 135/60 to 80 mm Hg and is now 90/50 to 100/75. On review of her current medications, she is not receiving any medications that lower the heart rate or blood pressure.

❓ Given the information obtained so far, what are the pertinent positives and significant negatives?

Pertinent Positives

• Constitutional: Somnolent, fatigued, edematous, unable to sustain spontaneous breathing without ventilator support.

• Cardiovascular: Sinus bradycardia, lower blood pressure off antihypertensive, 5 kg weight gain, +24-hour fluid balance, peripheral edema, chest x-ray with increased pulmonary congestion, interstitial edema, and cardiomegaly.

- Pulmonary: Diminished breath sounds, dullness on percussion of bases. Spontaneous pulmonary parameters all below expected value (ie, tidal volume, minute ventilation, forced vital capacity, negative inspiratory force, and respiratory rate). Accessory muscle use and labored respiratory pattern and dyspnea during spontaneous breathing trials. Slow respiratory rate with hypercarbia on spontaneous breathing mode.

- Pneumonia resolving but hilar engorgement and cardiomegaly slightly increased from admission x-ray.

- Gastrointestinal: Two episodes of regurgitation of tube feedings, tube feeding currently off, no stool for 3 days.

- Musculoskeletal: Generalized decreased muscle strength in all extremities, unable to weight bear for transfer. Generalized anasarca.

- Neurologic: Episodic confusion at night, somnolent, generalized weakness but moves all extremities equally, abnormal deep tendon reflexes (slow with delayed release), exposure to anxiolytics and analgesic medications.

- Endocrine: Hypothermic, two episodes of hypoglycemia requiring treatment and exposure to corticosteroids during the first 6 days of hospitalization, loss of lateral eyebrows, change in skin turgor.

- Metabolic: Hypervolemic hyponatremia, uncompensated respiratory acidosis, anemia, hypochloremia, elevated bicarbonate level.

Significant Negatives

- Constitutional: No fever for over 1 week.

- Neurologic: Normal examination with the exception of weakness and decreased reflexes. Use of anxiolytics and analgesic has been minimal over last several days.

- Cardiovascular: No chest pain, no ventricular dysrhythmia, no jugular venous distension, normal peripheral pulses, normal perfusion.

- Gastrointestinal: No abdominal pain.

- Musculoskeletal: No joint pain/swelling.

- Endocrine: No use of insulin in last 7 days.

- Metabolic: Normal white blood cell count, normal renal function.

Case Analysis: My impression is that this patient has a progressive generalized intrinsic weakness, anasarca, and fatigue and has also experienced some periodic nighttime confusion. Her underlying causes for mechanical ventilation (pneumonia with sepsis) are resolved and there is no indication of a hospital-acquired infection or condition. But she does exhibit many abnormal clinical signs and symptoms. I suspect these abnormal findings are related. A systematic evaluation of my findings may elucidate causes. I start by considering categories that may result in generalized weakness in a critically ill patient.

I will expand my differential to include additional chronic diagnoses if these do not point to a cause.

> ### Differential Diagnoses for Generalized Weakness
> - Cardiovascular: myocardial infarction, dysrhythmias, heart failure, cardiomyopathies, pericardial effusion, and tamponade
> - Neurologic and neuromuscular: stroke, encephalopathies, critical illness myopathies
> - Endocrine/metabolic: syndrome of inappropriate antidiuretic hormone (SIADH), diabetes insipidus (DI), hypoglycemia, thyroid and/or adrenal insufficiency, electrolyte disturbances
> - Medications: paralytics, sedatives, drug interactions, and allergies
> - Hematologic: anemia

I use a system approach to analyze my findings so far.

Neurologic

I have learned that the patient's mental status change is limited to confusion at night, somnolence, and slow responses to verbal stimuli. On clinical examination she has no focal deficits, can move all extremities equally, and responds appropriately to commands and to questions. The most significant neurological finding is her profound generalized weakness, which is symmetrical in distal and proximal muscles. She demonstrates decreased bilateral motor strength of $+3/+5$ in all extremities and her deep tendon reflexes are $+2/+4$ and symmetrical with a delayed release, called "hung up reflex." Hung up reflex is defined as a slow return of the limb to a neutral position following a tap to the tendon. This prolonged relaxation phase is characteristic of reflexes in persons with hypothyroidism and now makes me consider hypothyroidism as a potential cause of her weakness, somnolence, fatigue, and failure to wean. It may also explain her anasarca. I will order thyroid studies to rule this in or out but I still must consider other potential causes.

The patient's neurological findings are normal except for her changes in alertness and overall strength, which have occurred over time, making the likelihood of stroke low on my differential. Other potential causes include cerebral hypoxia, metabolic disturbances, or the toxic effects of medications that have caused her depressed sensorium. Global hypoperfusion due to hypotension in the presence of hypoxemia related to her respiratory failure can produce an anoxic encephalopathy. Encephalopathy may also be related to electrolyte and acid-base abnormalities such as hyponatremia and/or respiratory acidosis, both of which she has experienced. The primary symptom of an encephalopathy is altered mental status and cognitive dysfunction. Other features of encephalopathy include seizures, myoclonus, sensorimotor dysfunction, which she has not experienced. She is somnolent and fatigued but when stimulated she provides appropriate responses and attempts to follow commands. In addition her somnolence and weakness have progressed over time; she was not this way earlier in course of her ICU stay; her symptoms occurred 8 days into her hospitalization. If she sustained an impairment of cerebral perfusion severe enough to cause a stroke or cerebral hypoxia I would expect the abnormal findings to be present earlier in the hospital course. Her history does not bear this out as she was initially improving and progressing as expected and then her progress plateaued. I will consider a head CT should other causes not emerge or should she further deteriorate.

Delirium is common in ventilated patients, especially elderly patients, who are given sedatives for greater than 24 hours.[2] The use of sedatives in this patient has been minimal. There are reports by the nursing staff that she has experienced some confusion at night and this could be delirium but delirium is generally not limited to nighttime episodes. The hallmark findings of delirium are acute mental status changes and disordered thinking. Fatigue and weakness are not typical symptoms associated with delirium and she is alert when aroused, oriented, and appropriate. Delirium is possible but unlikely the cause of her symptoms.

Cardiovascular

The patient has experienced a series of stressful events over the course of her hospitalization but is currently hemodynamically stable and has not required the use of vasopressors, fluids, or inotropes to maintain her blood pressure since the earlier portion of her admission when she was septic. But I must consider a potential cardiac event such as a myocardial infarction (MI) as a reason for her fatigue and failure to wean. Risk factors for a cardiovascular event include her age, hypertension, and septic shock causing hypoperfusion of the myocardium. There is evidence of volume overload and her chest x-ray findings of increased heart size and bilateral infiltrates, and overall weight gain may be related to heart failure. However, there is no JVD, and there were no reported dysrhythmias, until the development of sinus bradycardia which emerged over the last 3 days. The bradycardia may indicate a cardiac event while she was hypotensive and acutely ill or could be caused by a metabolic or endocrine disorder. On review of her current medications, she is not receiving any medicine that causes bradycardia. An additional finding is a gradual trending down of her blood pressure. Although we have limited data regarding her past medical history, there is evidence that she has a history of hypertension so her low blood pressure is unusual. There is no evidence of a perfusion problem, as she has an adequate hourly urine output, skin is warm, with normal capillary refill, and her peripheral pulses are intact. It is possible she sustained a myocardial infarction in the initial phase of her illness or developed a cardiomegaly related to the acute infectious process or myocardial ischemia. Her volume overload may be due to the septic process and related myocardial pump failure, or due to an endocrine or metabolic process such as adrenal insufficiency, hypothyroidism, acidosis, or electrolyte disturbances. Laboratory and other diagnostics will need to be done to confirm or refute these potential conditions.

Metabolic Derangements

Her diagnostic studies reveal a hypervolemic hypotonic hyponatremia, mild anemia, elevated bicarbonate, and an uncompensated respiratory acidosis. These are concerning labs.

Hyponatremia can cause muscle weakness and mental status changes which, as noted previously, may contribute to this patient's failure to progress.[3] A rapid change in serum sodium is more likely to produce symptoms versus a slow chronic change to which the patient can adapt. On review of the electronic medical record the downward sodium trend from 136 to 128 mEq/L occurred over last 6 days. Acute symptomatic hyponatremia will produce mental status changes, seizures, muscle weakness, nausea, vomiting, and fatigue. She has evidence of hypervolemia with edema and a low serum osmolality, which allows me to categorize this hyponatremia as a hypervolemic, hypotonic hyponatremia. The differential diagnosis for this form of hyponatremia includes heart failure and volume overload. Given the pulmonary involvement with multilobar pneumonia and positive pressure ventilation there may be a component of syndrome of inappropriate antidiuretic hormone (SIADH) causing the lower serum sodium. Typically individuals with SIADH as a cause of the hyponatremia are euvolemic. It maybe that this patient's hyponatremia is multifactorial.

Her anemia may be chronic, acute, or simply the result of frequent blood draws in the ICU. The staff did not report any signs of acute bleeding and she has not had evidence of bleeding such as tarry stools or blood in her vomit. While anemia can result in dyspnea during activity, her current hemoglobin of 8.8 g/dL is not excessively low. Regardless I will further explore this by evaluating her CBCs over the course of her MICU stay.

She is mechanically ventilated on CPAP 8 cm H_2O with pressure support of 15 cm, FIO_2 40%. Her electrolyte panel shows an increase in the bicarbonate; her kidneys are reabsorbing bicarbonate. The $PaCO_2$ on the arterial blood gas is elevated, which is unusual since she is spontaneously breathing and should decrease her $PaCO_2$, yet she is not. This is likely due to her generalized weakness. Her ABG indicates an uncompensated respiratory acidosis. Her kidneys are reabsorbing bicarbonate in an effort to compensate for the respiratory acidosis. Metabolic compensation for a respiratory acidosis is a delayed response taking more than 24 hours to respond to the acid-base disturbance. She is also hypochloremic; to compensate for the lower chloride, bicarbonate is reabsorbed by the kidney. Her electrolyte disturbances may be the cause of her weakness but endocrine causes such as adrenal insufficiency and hypothyroidism are emerging as potential causes and fit with the related symptoms as well. I continue to explore other metabolic causes.

She has experienced two episodes of hypoglycemia requiring intervention and her fasting blood sugar is 68 mg/dL. Over the last 6 days the fasting blood sugars have decreased from 95 to 68 mg/dL. She is not receiving a hypoglycemic agent. The normalization of the blood sugar and discontinuation of the insulin infusion occurs with resolution of acute illness. With physiologic improvement there is a decrease in production of stress hormones such as epinephrine, norepinephrine, glucagon, and growth factor and the blood sugar in nondiabetic individual returns to normal. The concern in this patient is the unexplained episodes of hypoglycemia. An endocrine cause again emerges as a potential reason for her symptoms; both adrenal insufficiency and hypothyroidism can result in metabolic disarray such as this patient is experiencing.[3,4]

Endocrine Disorders

There are multiple endocrine findings that I note may be responsible for her weakness and thus the inability to wean. Pituitary and adrenal causes are possible and signs and symptoms seem consistent with the findings discussed above. At this point SIADH does not explain the entire constellation of symptoms noted in this patient. Adrenal insufficiency and hypothyroidism, on the other hand, are potential endocrine abnormalities which may well be the cause of the patient's symptoms.[3,4]

Medications can adversely affect electrolyte balance and adrenal and thyroid functions. Review of the discontinued medication notes the use of hydrocortisone (Solu-Cortef) for the first 6 days of the hospitalization. Adrenal insufficiency can produce hypotension, electrolyte disturbances, hyponatremia, hyperkalemia, hypoglycemia, muscle weakness, and fatigue.[3] Tapering corticosteroids are not deemed necessary if the medication is discontinued within 1 week of initiating the drug. This is true of this patient's situation. Data that support considering this as a potential cause for her failure to wean from the ventilator are the generalized weakness, fatigue, suppressed respiratory parameters, lower blood pressure, hyponatremia, and hypoglycemia.

A second consideration related to the use of steroids is the development of myopathies and neuropathies. Risk factors for developing myopathy of critical illness include prolonged bed rest, mechanical ventilation, corticosteroid exposure, use of neuromuscular blocking agents, and prolonged sedation.[2,5] She meets four of these criteria. During rapid sequence intubation succinylcholine and propofol were administered. There was limited neuromuscular blocker exposure and no exposure to etomidate. Etomidate is implicated in producing adrenal insufficiency in patients with septic shock. Myopathy of critical illness and deconditioning are possible but will be a diagnosis of exclusion if the other conditions on the differential list cannot be validated. There is currently no indication of oversedation as a cause for the weaning failure. Delirium secondary to the use of sedatives early in her course may be a component of the problem, but seems less likely as noted earlier.

Hypothyroidism at this point is highest on my list of differential diagnoses. She has multiple symptoms compatible with this disease including her profound weakness, bradycardia, low blood pressure, hypothermia, hyponatremia, hypoglycemia, mental status changes, myocardial suppression causing heart failure, and bradypnea with development of respiratory acidosis, decreased gastrointestinal motility, anasarca, and mental status changes. In addition, the finding of "hung up reflex" following a tendon tap is a characteristic finding in hypothyroidism. Alteration in thyroid hormone metabolism and utilization is recognized as a component of critical illness but rarely requires treatment. It is unusual for a patient to develop myxedema coma, as a sequel to an acute critical illness. Myxedema coma is the most severe form of hypothyroidism, and can produce a relative adrenal insufficiency as well. I am wondering if she is normally hypothyroid and if there is more to her medical history than we have obtained so far.

Unfortunately there is limited history available on this patient in the electronic medical record, the niece did not report that her aunt suffers from hypothyroidism, and no medication bottles containing thyroid were found in the home by paramedics. However, the symptoms are strongly suggestive of this disease.

Upon completing this analysis, my problem representation is now: "This 76-year-old female requiring mechanical ventilation for a resolved multilobar pneumonia, respiratory failure, and sepsis is failing attempts to successfully wean from the ventilator due to progressive muscle weakness, somnolence, and fatigue potentially due to an endocrine etiology."

At this juncture the differential diagnosis of highest probability appears to be hypothyroidism or adrenal insufficiency with a concomitant cardiomyopathy and potential heart failure. I discuss my analysis with the patient, niece, bedside nurse, and critical care team.

❓ What diagnostic testing should be done and in what order?

My initial intervention is to obtain additional history from the patient, niece, and primary care provider to determine if the patient has other underlying comorbidities such as cardiomyopathy, coronary artery disease, heart failure, or hypothyroidism.

Diagnostics that I order are a TSH, free T4, cortisol level, echocardiogram (ECG), and chest x-ray. The thyroid function studies will determine if she is experiencing a severe hypothyroidism or myxedema. A free cortisol level addresses the concern for adrenal insufficiency. An ECG can be compared to the ECG preformed upon admission, assessing for changes of a myocardial infarction. There would be no benefit in obtaining cardiac enzymes. The echocardiogram will identify wall motion abnormality if she sustained a myocardial infarction, in addition to diagnosing a cardiomyopathy. The chest x-ray will assess improvement in the underlying pneumonia but most importantly will assess for evidence of volume overload or heart failure. A CT scan of the head is not indicated, there is no focal deficit and cognitively her mental status is appropriate. The problem is somnolence and profound weakness.

CASE INFORMATION

Final Lab Results

Contact with the primary care provider revealed a past medical history for hypertension and hypothyroidism. Prior to admission she was taking levothyroxine 0.125 µg daily. Her niece found an empty bottle in her bedside nightstand that the EMS team did not find. But, with input from the pharmacy, it appeared she had not been taking her levothyroxine for at least 2 weeks prior to admission. Withdrawal of the levothyroxine for 1 month plus the stress of a critical illness, exposure to sedatives and analgesics place her at high risk to develop myxedema coma. The results of her laboratory studies revealed TSH level was 35 mIU/L (0.3–4.7 IU/L) and the free T4 was 0.12 ng/dL (0.7–2.2 ng/dL), free cortisol level 6 µg/dL (6–23 µg/dL), ECG shows sinus bradycardia rate of 52 beats per minute, no indication of ischemia, injury, or infarction, and echocardiogram noted global hypokinesis with moderate mitral valve regurgitation.

Myxedema Coma: Diagnosis and Treatment

Myxedema is a severe manifestation of hypothyroidism, which initially presents as mental status changes. The initial symptom is typically confusion and can progress to psychosis, lethargy, obtunded state, and ultimately coma. As the syndrome progresses all systems are affected by the lack of thyroid hormone and cellular metabolic activity cannot be maintained.[4] The clinical presentation pattern is of hypothermia, bradycardia, hypoventilation with carbon dioxide retention and respiratory acidosis, hypotension, hyponatremia, and hypoglycemia. Additional findings include exfoliation of the skin, thick doughy skin, yellow-orange cast to skin, development of pericardial and pleural effusions, and delayed relaxation of the deep tendon reflexes. Risk factors for developing myxedema coma are noncompliance with taking thyroid medication, infection, pneumonia, sepsis, major trauma, surgery, gastrointestinal bleeding, heart failure, cold exposure, and medication related particularly to sedation and analgesia.

Treatment typically requires intubation to correct the hypercarbia and respiratory acidosis. If profoundly hypothermic (generally cooler than 35°C), gradual rewarming is recommended to avoid the associated dysrhythmias and coagulopathies such as disseminated intravascular coagulation that result from being hypothermic. The cornerstone of treatment is to initiate thyroid medications, such as thyroxine 500 µg IV then 75 to 100 µg daily. Alternatively T3 or liothyronine 25 to 50 µg IV can be started with a reassessment in 4 to 12 hours to determine if additional dosing is necessary. Once the thyroid hormone replacement has been started, an improvement in vital signs will occur in approximately 6 hours and mental status changes improve in 24 to 48 hours. There is frequently a concomitant adrenal insufficiency in patients with myxedema. This is attributed to the impaired adrenal cellular response that ensues due to the lack of thyroid hormone which maintains cellular metabolic function. Therefore, corticosteroids in the form of hydrocortisone (Solu-Cortef) are administered every 8 hours. Glucose levels are normalized if the patient is hypoglycemic and dextrose is added to maintenance intravenous fluids. Treatment of hypotension can be difficult, due to a diminished response to vasopressor therapy. Volume resuscitation to support blood pressure must be carefully monitored to avoid volume overload in a patient who may already be experiencing difficulty with fluid volume balance.[4]

Case Follow-Up

Upon receipt of the TSH results the patient was started on intravenous levothyroxine. Within 8 hours her heart rate had increased to 80 to 90 beats per minute and her blood pressure was 130 to 145 systolic/80 to 85 diastolic, and urine output increased. Within 2 days she was alert and participative. She was extubated on the third day following the initiation of thyroid therapy.

References

1. Burns S, Fisher C, Tribble S, Lewis R, Merrel P, Conaway M. Multifactor clinical score and outcomes of mechanical ventilation weaning trails: burns wean assessment program. *Am J Crit Care.* 2010;19:431-439.

2. Kress J, Hall J. ICU-acquired weakness and recovery from critical Illness. *New Engl J Med.* 2014;370(17):1626-1635.

3. Tucci V, Sokari T. The clinical manifestations, diagnosis, and treatment of adrenal emergencies. *Emerg Med Clin North Am.* 2014;32(2):464-484.

4. Hampton J. Thyroid gland disorders and emergencies: thyroid storm and myxedema coma. *AACN Adv Crit Care.* 2013;3:325-332.

5. Schweickert W, Hall J. ICU-acquired weakness. *Chest.* 2007;131:1541-1549.

CASE 47

Nancy Munro

Nancy Munro is the senior ACNP at the National Institutes of Health. She works in the Critical Care Medicine Department and with the Pulmonary Consult Service and is also a part-time instructor at the Georgetown University School of Nursing where she teaches ACNP students.

CASE INFORMATION

Chief Complaint

A 68-year-old male with a history of mucinous adenocarcinoma of the appendix presents with persistent fever and confusion/agitation several days after cytoreductive surgery with hyperthermic intraperitoneal chemotherapy. As part of the critical care team I was asked to evaluate the patient who has been in the intensive care unit (ICU) since the operation (post-op day #9).

❓ What is the potential cause?

There are many causes of fever and it is important to try to refine the list of causes. A careful review of the patient's history of his present illness and a focused physical examination are essential to make a correct diagnosis. While the patient is also confused and agitated, these symptoms are likely to be related to the cause of the fever. I start with a differential for fever.

Differential Diagnoses for Fever of Unknown Origin

This can be a very long differential diagnosis list but may be organized by magnitude of fever and then whether the fever is infectious or non-infectious in nature (Figure 47-1). Since the patient is in the ICU when the fever starts, I can make the analysis faster by narrowing the long differential list to those causes which are associated with ICU admission, including both shock and nonshock states.[1]

Magnitude of Fever

- Fever 38.3°C (101°F) to 38.8°C (101.8°F): can be infectious or noninfectious in nature

- Fever 38.9°C (102°F) to 41°C (105.8°F): usually infectious
- Fever >41.1°C (106°F): usually noninfectious

Infectious

- Ventilator-associated pneumonia (VAP): intubation must be for greater than 48 hours
- Intravascular catheter–associated infection
- Surgical site infection
- Bacteremia
- Urinary catheter–associated infection
- Sinusitis

Noninfectious Causes Without Shock

- Nonhemolytic transfusion fever
- Drug fever
- Acalculous cholecystitis
- Mesenteric ischemia
- Acute pancreatitis
- Deep vein thrombosis (DVT)
- Pulmonary embolism (PE)

Noninfectious Causes With Shock

- Adrenal crisis
- Thyroid storm
- Acute hemolytic transfusion fever

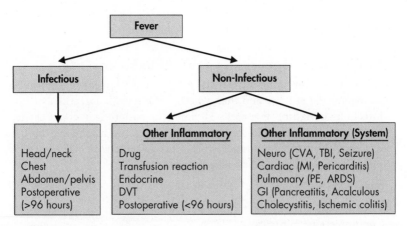

Figure 47-1   Causes of fever. (From Munro N. Fever in acute and critical care: a diagnostic approach. *AACN Adv Crit Care*. 2014;25:238-247.)

Infection is the first cause of fever that should immediately rise to the top of the differential diagnosis list. This patient has many reasons to be infected including cancer (immunocompromised state), recent abdominal surgery, chemotherapy, and age, which are the most obvious causes. Understanding what the surgical procedure entailed and the chemotherapy used is important. Cytoreductive surgery is debulking of the tumor when complete removal is not possible. This technique is performed in order to enhance the effectiveness of chemotherapy. Hyperthermic intraperitoneal chemotherapy (Mitomycin-C and cisplatin) is a localized treatment used during the surgical procedure in order to maximize the beneficial effects of chemotherapy locally, to destroy tumor cells, and to minimize the systemic effects.

CASE INFORMATION

History of Present Illness

The cytoreductive surgery took place 9 days ago, and was successful in achieving reduction in tumor size. The patient returned to the operating room (OR) on postoperative day #2 for a washout and application of biological mesh and wound vacuum dressing application. In discussing the case with the surgical team, I learn that the OR course was unremarkable and there was no obvious suspicion for contamination of the surgical field. Follow-up examinations by the surgical team reveal that he is progressing as expected, has no signs of unusual drainage from the wound vacuum dressing, and has no disproportionate abdominal pain with palpation. He did require 1 unit of packed red blood cells on postoperative day 3 for a hemoglobin of 7 g/dL but he had no sign of transfusion reaction and his hemoglobin has been stable.

The patient was extubated and weaned to room air following the second surgery, and he was alert and oriented for the first few days of his ICU stay. The fever and altered mental state started approximately 6 days postoperatively. Over the past 3 days, his fever has ranged from 38°C to 40.2°C and his agitation has been managed with sedatives, antipsychotics, and analgesics including dexmedetomidine, midazolam, lorazepam, haloperidol, olanzapine, epidural fentanyl with bupivacaine, and as-needed doses of fentanyl and hydromorphone intravenously. The rest of his vital signs including his oxygen saturation remained stable, though he did have one episode of hypotension and tachycardia, which resolved with an intravenous fluid bolus. His lactate level was normal at 0.5 mmol/L (normal is 0–2 mmol/L) after this episode.

I review the patient's record and find that the following diagnostics were completed over the last 3 days in an effort to find a fever source and help explain his altered mental state:

- A computerized tomography (CT) of the head showing no gross cause for the change in level of consciousness such as intracranial bleed or thrombus. In addition air/fluid levels and/or other signs of sinusitis are not seen on the head CT.

- Chest x-ray showing left lower lobe atelectasis with volume loss and displacement of the left pulmonary hila to the left side. There was also elevation of the left hemidiaphragm. No evidence of pneumonia.

- A right upper quadrant ultrasound showing some sludge in the gallbladder, but no other findings.

- Cultures of blood, urine, and sputum have come back negative, and the last set drawn in the last 24 hours is negative so far.

- Laboratory results including amylase and lipase to rule out pancreatitis, lactate level to assess tissue perfusion, serum cortisol and thyroid-stimulating hormone (TSH) to evaluate for an endocrine disorder are all within normal limits. In addition, comprehensive metabolic panels and complete blood counts drawn daily do not show any significant abnormality, other than mild anemia.

? What are the pertinent positives so far?

- Major abdominal surgery with significant debulking of tumor
- Return to OR for washout and placement of mesh and vacuum dressing application
- Hyperthermic intraperitoneal chemotherapy
- Persistent fluctuating fever at high levels for 3 days
- Change in level of consciousness
- Agitation treated with analgesics, sedatives, and antipsychotics
- One episode of mild hypotension resolved with fluids
- Tachycardia
- Right upper quadrant ultrasound found sludge in gall bladder

? What are the significant negatives so far?

- No positive cultures at this point
- No catheter infections (blood or urine)
- No purulent drainage from abdominal wound
- No transfusion reaction

- X-ray demonstrates postoperative atelectasis but no signs of pneumonia
- VAP is unlikely due to intubation for less than 48 hours and rapid progression to spontaneous breathing on room air
- No hypoxia or shortness of breath
- No indication of shock
- No elevation of lactate
- No elevation in amylase or lipase
- No intracranial bleed or thrombus on CT head
- No abnormal TSH or cortisol levels

Case Analysis: The ICU team has completed the initial evaluation for the fever but a more structured approach is needed to try to identify the cause of his fever and confusion. A fever workup is very time consuming and can be quite expensive. A focused approach can lead to a more productive differential diagnostic process. His fever has been in the high range multiple times but even a temperature of 38 C should be considered a fever since he is immuno-compromised.[2] I now consider the information I have obtained and group it into infectious and noninfectious causes.

Infectious Causes

Cultures of sputum, blood, and urine are all negative so far. Though evidence for infection has not emerged, infection continues to remain high on my differential. Infection with an abdominal source still needs to be considered. The surgical wound remains a possible source, though the drainage is not puru-lent and his abdominal examination per the progress notes is not convincing for peritonitis or abscess formation. A pulmonary cause such as pneumonia is ruled out by x-ray. Also, he rapidly progressed to spontaneous breathing on room air, which suggests normal resolution of the atelectasis. So far no pulmo-nary cause for fever is evident. Catheter-related infections are not obvious at this time but culture negative sepsis may be a possible alternative diagnosis. Sinusitis was not seen on the head CT and the short intubation time makes this diagnosis unlikely. The patient may have had a past history of sinus issues since he uses fluticasone nasal spray and fexofenadine at home but imaging does not reveal any current sinus issues.

Noninfectious Causes

To date the patient has not suffered inadequate tissue perfusion from a pro-tracted shock state as the episode of hypotension resolved quickly with flu-ids. Also his normal lactate at that time suggests adequate tissue perfusion. I move mesenteric ischemia lower on my differential now due to the fact that his examination by the team does not suggest it as a reason and his serum lactate is normal. Acalculous cholecystitis is unlikely given the results of his abdomi-nal ultrasound. I also rule out pancreatitis because of his normal amylase and lipase. Endocrine causes such as adrenal insufficiency and a hypothyroidism are ruled out with his normal cortisol and TSH levels.

The combination of tachycardia and fever leads me to always consider deep vein thrombosis (DVT) and/or pulmonary embolism. However, there is no hypoxemia reported and no pulmonary complaints to date. Deep vein thrombus is always a concern, particularly in a patient with cancer who is now immobile. However, he has been on appropriate prophylaxis throughout his hospitalization. While a fever is possible with a DVT, high fevers such as seen in this patient are not usually present. While I cannot rule these out, they are lower on my differential.

The search for a source of infection has not resulted in any positive findings at this point. Although infection remains on the diagnostic list, evaluation of the other symptoms in this patient's presentation, confusion and agitation, may be helpful to consider. The CT of his head ruled out intracranial bleed or thrombus so other reasons for confusion and agitation in the ICU setting need to be considered. ICU delirium is a top consideration and the patient was treated for this condition with a variety of medications such as haloperidol and olanzapine. A common challenge in dealing with the postoperative patient is that agitation can also be an indication that the patient is in pain. Thus, sedatives, anxiolytics, and narcotics are commonly used, often in combination. Drug combinations may be advantageous in some cases but in elderly patients, minimizing the use of sedatives may be more prudent to avoid side effects including agitation and confusion. I consider the possibility that his symptoms may be a reaction to these medications, but there is more for me to evaluate. I turn to his current record to obtain additional pertinent information including past medical history, past surgical history, medications, and allergies, and I also compete a comprehensive history and physical.

CASE INFORMATION

Past Medical History
- Mucinous adenocarcinoma of the appendix; carcinomatosis, hypertension, gastrointestinal esophageal reflux disease (GERD); L1 compression fracture with fall 2013

Past Surgical History
- Appendectomy in 2004; right hemicolectomy in 2004; ventral hernia repair with mesh in 2005; resection of metastatic lesion in right upper quadrant in 2006

Home Medications
- Lisinopril 40 mg daily; hydrochlorothiazide/triamterene 37.5/25 mg daily; aspirin 81 mg daily; simvastatin 20 mg daily at bedtime; omeprazole 20 mg twice daily; fluticasone nasal spray 15 µg each nostril daily; fexofenadine 100 mg daily

Allergies

• Lobster (rash)

Current medications

• Piperacillin/tazobactam 4.5 g IV every 6 hours; vancomycin 1 g IV every 12 hours; micafungin 100 mg IV daily; metronidazole 500 mg IV every 8 hours; meropenem 1 g every 8 hours; linezolid 600 mg IV every 12 hours; levofloxacin 750 mg IV every 24 hours; heparin 5000 units SQ every 8 hours, and pantoprazole 40 mg IV daily

Review of Systems

Since the patient is not verbalizing or speaking, the review of systems information is obtained from the chart, from his initial history and other notes during this hospitalization. The family is not available at the time of my examination. The physical examination below constitutes my examination findings.

• Constitutional: Positive for gradual increase in confusion and agitation over last several days. No documented evaluation for delirium. Required various medications to decrease agitation, negative for increase in fatigue, weight loss, loss of appetite, problems sleeping, recent falls, or trauma prior to hospitalization.

• Eyes/ears/nose/throat: Denies any vision changes, double vision, or eye pain. Positive for intermittent sinus "stuffiness" and runny nose with seasonal allergies; negative for nose bleeds, sore throat, hoarseness.

• Cardiovascular: Negative for shortness of breath, chest pain, palpitations, leg or arm swelling; negative for history of heart attack (but does take a statin and aspirin but no reason documented in chart) or heart failure; positive for history of hypertension.

• Pulmonary: Positive for seasonal allergies to grass; negative for shortness of breath, cough or sputum production (purulent or blood); wheezing; no history of pneumonia, tuberculosis, or blood clot.

• Gastrointestinal: Positive for intermittent left lower quadrant pain and numbness in right lower quadrant, which has been chronic since surgery; positive for indigestion or heartburn especially after meals; negative for nausea, vomiting, diarrhea, constipation, any change in stool character or color, or difficulty in swallowing.

• Genitourinary: Negative for frequency of urination at night; pain on urination; gross blood in urine or foul smelling urine; incontinence or weak stream of urine.

• Neurologic: Positive for recent confusion and muscle rigor; negative for headache, dizziness, change in level of consciousness; numbness, tingling, extremity weakness, tremors; no change in balance or speech; no history of stroke, seizures, depression, anxiety.

• Hematologic: Negative for increase/decrease in thirst, appetite; preference for heat or cold; change in weight; high or low blood pressure or change in blood pressure with position.

- Endocrine: Negative for easy bruising or prolonged or excessive bleeding, history of anemia or need for blood transfusion until this ICU stay.
- Lymphadenopathy: Positive for nodes in groin.

Physical Examination (Current)

- Vital signs: Temperature 38.9°C; heart rate 115 beats per minute; respiratory 22 breaths per minute; blood pressure 160/92 mm Hg; oxygen saturation 98% on room air
- General: Sleeping but arousable with effort, does not speak.
- Head/eyes/ears/nose/throat: Pupils equal, round, reactive to light and accommodation, small but not pinpoint. Extraocular movements: only upward gaze but initial opening of eyes show lateral and inferior gaze. Blinks to threat; corneal reflexes intact. No facial asymmetry. Hearing grossly normal bilaterally as he opens eyes to command; sticks out tongue to command and it is midline and normal. No nuchal rigidity noted. Full range of motion of neck.
- Cardiovascular: S1, S2 normal, 2/6 systolic ejection murmur. Extremities are warm, no mottling; +1 peripheral edema in both lower extremities; dorsalis pedis pulses +2 bilaterally.
- Pulmonary: Regular, symmetrical, unlabored respirations; breath sounds clear bilaterally posteriorly.
- Gastrointestinal: Soft, mild appropriate postoperative discomfort for postoperative day 9; abdominal incision intact without drainage; bowel sounds present; no organomegaly noted with mild palpation.
- Skin: No bruising, no rash.
- Neurological: Opens eyes to command but somewhat difficult to arouse. Looks around for 1 to 2 seconds and then mostly upward gaze. Follows commands with both hands, can show two fingers. Can add two plus two and show the answer with fingers. Moves toes and hands to command. Drowsy and needs to be awakened. Dramatic increase in tone in every muscle group. Clonus of at least 4 to 5 beats. Hyperreflexia. Responds to touch on both sides.

? **What element of the review of systems and the physical examination should be added to the list of pertinent positives? Which items should be added to the list of significant negatives?**

Pertinent Positives

- Currently febrile
- Hypertensive, tachypnea, and tachycardia
- Past abdominal surgery
- Bilateral lower extremity edema
- Lateral and inferior gaze
- Rigid extremities with increased muscle tone with clonus and hyperreflexia

Significant Negatives

- No hypoxia or shortness of breath
- No focal neurological deficits
- Normal abdominal examination for this stage of recovery
- No skin changes

Case Analysis: A systemic infection is not supported by the data at this point but infection is still high on my list as the cause of his symptoms. Considering his altered mental state, a central nervous system infection is possible, though he does not exhibit signs of meningeal irritation such as nuchal rigidity. Seizures are also possible, and some of the antibiotics he is receiving can produce seizures, including the β-lactamases, carbapenems, and quinolones. A significant finding on his physical examination is mild swelling in his lower extremities. Though low on my list, DVT and PE are still in my differential. Additional diagnostics are necessary to determine to cause of this patient's symptoms. Drug fever, often a diagnosis of exclusion, also remains on my differential diagnosis list.

❓ What is the problem representation?

Given what I have learned so far my problem representation is: A 68-year-old male with a history of mucinous adenocarcinoma of the appendix with persistent fever and confusion with agitation 9 days after cytoreductive surgery with hyperthermic intraperitoneal chemotherapy, which may be related to a central nervous system infection, seizures, DVT with PE, or drug fever.

❓ Given the information obtained so far what additional diagnostics are necessary at this time?

The combination of fever and change in level of consciousness leads to a concern for meningitis or encephalitis, and the best initial assessment to determine this diagnosis is a lumbar puncture (LP). I confer with the ICU team and recommend that an LP be performed immediately. Because there is still concern for a DVT with PE, I also order bedside Doppler ultrasound of the lower extremities.

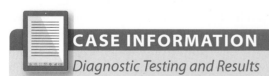

CASE INFORMATION
Diagnostic Testing and Results

Lumbar Puncture Results

- Cerebral spinal fluid (CSF) is clear (appearance: clear, colorless)
- CSF total protein: 16 mg/100 mL (normal 15–60 mg/100 mL)

- CSF glucose: 80 mg/100 mL (normal 50–80 mg/100 mL, or greater than 2/3 of blood sugar level)
- Serum glucose: 120 mg/100 mL
- CSF cell count: WBC 1; RBC 2 in the first tube (0–5 white blood cells—all mononuclear), and no red blood cells)[3]
- Lower extremity ultrasound: negative for deep vein thrombosis

Case Analysis: These results quickly confirm that a central nervous system (CNS) infection is unlikely. Signs of CNS infection include a cloudy appearance of the fluid and a high total protein; both of which are absent in this case. I would also expect an elevated white blood cell count because of the presence of the infecting organism, and CSF glucose level that is lower than the serum glucose. Normally the CSF glucose is at least 2/3 of the serum level. If the CSF glucose is lower, infecting organisms are thought to be consuming the glucose in the CSF to maintain their cellular integrity. The red blood cell count is slightly elevated most likely due to a traumatic puncture and is not a significant sign of infection. Further imaging can be considered such as MRI of the head to assist in the diagnostic process but other diagnoses, especially seizure or drug fever, require further evaluation first. The negative Doppler rules out DVT and makes PE less likely.

A more detailed neurologic examination is performed and the abnormal preferential gaze and increased extremity muscle tone were more noticeable and constant in nature. The physical examination findings are dramatic and redirect diagnostic thinking. This is a concerning finding since seizures now need to be considered urgently. He did not have any trauma or hypoxic episodes that may result in seizure activity. I review the patient's medication list. There are multiple medications that could result in seizure activity and fever especially the β-lactamases (piperacillin/tazobactam), the carbapenems (meropenem), and the quinolones (levofloxacin) (Table 47-1). These drugs can produce fever but do not cause the extremity rigidity and gaze issues. As I was considering seizures as a diagnosis, I recognized that my examination, and others, consistently demonstrated the ability of the patient to perform higher-level cognitive functions such as two-step commands and correctly perform math questions even if he does not verbalize his thought processes. This significant finding does not correlate with seizures. If seizures were present the patient would not be able to perform these functions. However, I called a neurology consult to confirm my thoughts and to request an electroencephalogram (EEG) if necessary. The neurology consult service agreed with my evaluation above and did not do an EEG. Seizure as a diagnosis is eliminated from the differential diagnosis list.

The combination of fever (hyperthermia), muscle rigidity, and lateral/inferior gaze now narrows the diagnosis to possible drug-induced fever

Table 47-1   Drugs That Cause Fever

Antimicrobials especially β-lactam drugs

Antiepileptic drugs especially phenytoin

Antiarrhythmics especially quinidine and procainamide

Antihypertensives especially methyldopa, hydralazine

H_1- and H_2-blocking antihistamines

Iodides

Anti-Parkinson drugs

Phenothiazines

Butyrophenones especially haloperidol

Thyroxine

Drugs producing cytokine storm especially monoclonal antibodies

Penicillins

Antimalarials

Source: From Munro N. Fever in acute and critical care: a diagnostic approach. *AACN Adv Crit Care.* 2014; 25:238–247.

syndromes including neuroleptic malignant syndrome (NMS). The patient received antipsychotics including haloperidol and olanzapine, which traditionally are implicated in this syndrome. He is given bromocriptine 2.5 mg per nasogastric tube twice daily for only 3 days and his neurologic clinical presentation returned to baseline. This was a short course for this drug, which is recommended to be given for up to 10 days depending on clinical findings. The patient is transferred to the floor on postoperative day 12, 3 days after my consult, and discharged home 2 weeks later.

Neuroleptic Malignant Syndrome: Pathophysiology, Diagnosis, and Management

Neuroleptic malignant syndrome is not completely understood but it is thought to be the result of the disruption in the thermoregulatory process in the brain. The body tries to maintain a temperature near a set point, which is thought to be 37°C. The preoptic region in the brain is where temperature control is directed and it is a balance between heat loss responses (vasodilation and sweating) and heat generation response (shivering). The process is complex but the body is usually able to maintain tight control of body temperature to deal appropriately with fever.[4] Hyperthermia is a pathologic state where the thermoregulatory mechanism is bypassed and heat production becomes uncontrolled or heat dissipation is not adequate.[5] Clinical hyperthermia can be defined as a temperature between 39°C and 40°C, and if sustained, can cause cellular damage.[6] The clinical parameters used to assess this damage are creatine kinase (CK) and lactate dehydrogenase (LDH). Antipsychotic medications are thought to interfere with thermoregulation because they have an antagonistic effect on dopamine receptors, leading to increased muscle activity. Normally dopamine receptor agonism in the preoptic area leads to increased heat loss.[6]

For this patient, his clinical presentation seems to conform to many of the pathogenesis processes. It is important to know that his CK and LDH values were within normal limits but that may be related to the fact that his hyperthermia peak was only reached one time. The confirmation of the diagnosis of NMS was the administration of bromocriptine. The other clinical diagnoses to consider in this category are malignant hyperthermia (MH) and serotonin syndrome (SS). Both can lead to hyperthermia but MH occurs almost immediately after administration of anesthesia agents and this can be ruled out in this patient since he was postoperative day #9. Serotonin syndrome is associated with excessive stimulation of the 5-hydroxy-tryptamine 1A receptors, which leads to increased muscle activity, and is more twitchy in nature.[4] His presentation was muscle rigidity.

This case follows a classic presentation of NMS, which was easily recognized once the diagnostic reasoning process eliminated the more common diagnosis of infection. The frequent use of antipsychotic drugs in ICU especially haloperidol and olanzapine can be very helpful in controlling patient agitation but it is imperative that the clinician always keep in mind the side effects of all drugs that are given because important diagnoses like NMS may be missed.

References

1. MacLaren G, Spelman D. UpToDate Web site. http://www.uptodate.com/contents/fever-in-the-intensive-careunit?source=machineLearning&search=differential+diagnosis++fever&selectedTitle=3%7E150&sectionRank=1&anchor=H3#H3. Accessed November 15, 2014.
2. O'Grady NP, Barie PS, Bartlett JG, et al. Guidelines for evaluation of new fever in critically ill adult patients: 2008 update from the American College of Critical Care Medicine and the Infectious Diseases Society of America. *Crit Care Med*. 2008;36:1330-1349.
3. Johnson KS, Sexton DJ. UpToDate Web site. http://www.uptodate.com/contents/cerebrospinal-fluid-physiology-and-utility-of-an-examination-in-disease states?source=search_result&search=lumbar+puncture+results&selectedTitle=1%7E150#H17. Accessed December 2, 2014.
4. Munro N. Fever in acute and critical care: a diagnostic approach. *AACN Adv Crit Care*. 2014; 25:238-247.
5. Rehman T, deBoisblanc BP. Persistent fever in the ICU. *Chest*. 2014;145:158-165.
6. Gillman PK. Neuroleptic malignant syndrome: mechanisms, interactions and causality. *Move Disord*. 2010;25:1780-1790.

CASE 48

Janie Heath

Dr Heath is Dean and the Warwick Professor of Nursing at the University of Kentucky in Lexington. For the past 30 years Janie has been a national leader for tobacco control and advanced practice nursing where she has directed academic programs and practiced as an ACNP in South Carolina, Washington DC, Georgia, and Virginia.

CASE INFORMATION

Chief Complaint

A 32-year-old white female is brought to the emergency department at 6 AM via ambulance for intractable nausea and vomiting.

❓ What is the potential cause?

Nausea and vomiting are common symptoms with a wide range of conditions that may be chronic, acute, or emergent. In a young adult female, the symptoms raise concern for an emergent state requiring urgent intervention. While some conditions are more likely to cause the presenting symptoms, I must consider others that may be life threatening or threatening to the patient's functional status. Acute gastrointestinal conditions such as gastric outlet/intestinal obstruction, cholecystitis, ischemic bowel, or pancreatitis require immediate attention. In addition, disorders outside the gastrointestinal system such as cerebral hemorrhage, stroke or meningitis, myocardial infarction, volume depletion with shock, and adrenal insufficiency can also present with nausea and vomiting and require immediate intervention. Although these etiologies are all possible, nausea and vomiting also occur in common benign conditions such as a stomach virus, pregnancy, or food poisoning.

Comprehensive Differential Diagnoses for Patient With Nausea and Vomiting[1]

- Gastrointestinal etiology: peptic ulcer disease, gastric outlet obstruction, mesenteric ischemia, intestinal obstruction, colonic obstruction, choledocholithiasis, cholecystitis, acute pancreatitis, peritonitis, gastritis, acute gastroenteritis, chronic postviral nausea and vomiting, post-op surgery sequelae, bariatric surgery sequelae, malignancy
- Cardiac etiology: acute coronary syndrome, myocardial infarction, postural orthostatic tachycardia syndrome

- Neurological etiology: acoustic neuroma/vestibular disorder, traumatic brain injury, meningitis, brain abscess, cerebrovascular event (embolic/ischemic/hemorrhagic), CNS tumor, migraine, motion sickness, benign paroxysmal positional vertigo
- Mental health etiology: anorexia nervosa, bulimia nervosa
- Metabolic etiology: diabetes, heat stroke, adrenal insufficiency, hypercalcemia, hypopituitarism, thyroid disorder
- Renal etiology: uremia, nephrolithiasis, malignancy
- Exogenous etiology: medication side effect or interaction or withdrawal, alcohol induced, drug induced, cannabinoid hyperemesis, food poisoning, pregnancy

CASE INFORMATION

General Survey and History of Present Illness

In this case, a general survey of the patient yields the following: a well-developed, young woman, in no acute distress but who appears unkempt, agitated, and exuding a fishy odor. The emergency room (ER) staff recognizes her as a "frequent flyer" for alcohol-related incidents. When asked what happened, she states: "I have no clue; that is why I called 911. I've been in my house watching TV for the past 2 days. I fell asleep around midnight and woke up this morning sick as a dog." The emergency medical technicians (EMTs) report they found her in an air conditioned home sitting on the couch vomiting into a trash can. They also report seeing an empty quart bottle of vodka on the coffee table and a broken 30 mL bottle of peach schnapps flavored e-cigarettes with several e-cigarette cartomizers on the floor. The patient looks at the EMTs and says: "Is that the thanks I get for trying to quit smoking? So I had a little to drink but at least give me some credit for using e-juice and not smoking cigarettes." When asked about the content in the broken bottle of "e-juice," one of the EMTs replies, "From my own personal experience I can tell you this brand of e-juice has nicotine in it but these things are not regulated so, who knows what the heck we are consuming?" The EMTs then report that the patient's vital signs were stable throughout transport; they started oxygen at 2 L/min, began intravenous fluids at 85 mL per hour, and initiated continuous cardiac monitoring. The emergency room provider then continues the assessment between the patient's bouts of retching and/or vomiting clear phlegm.

The patient describes "feeling like a dog" means she woke up nauseated and thought her heart was racing away and within a few minutes started vomiting undigested food. This lasted for an hour and was accompanied by a pounding headache. She states the headache resolved after drinking some water and her heart "settled down" after vomiting but she became worried when the vomiting reoccurred and she experienced waves of nausea when standing up. She reports her last meal, left over pizza, was probably about 10 PM the prior evening, and she denies eating fish. She denies abdominal pain, chest pain, diaphoresis, shortness of breath, seizures, or vertigo. When asked about her emesis, she denies blood or feces and reports it is non-projectile and "nonstop" for approximately 2 hours. She also denies diarrhea, dysuria, or fever. She complains of having a burning sensation in her left arm that was worse when she first woke up but improved since EMTs arrived. She attributes the sensation to falling asleep on it. She admitted drinking vodka while "vaping her e-cigs." She denies using any illegal substances or using any other tobacco products while using e-cigarettes.

Past Medical History

When asked about her past medical history the patient states she was told she has a drinking and smoking problem so she decided to tackle one addiction at a time. A friend at the women's shelter told her about electronic cigarettes so she bought them and has not smoked cigarettes for 2 months. She denies a history of heart disease, stroke, lung disease, GI disorders, neurological disorders, diabetes, cancer, or recent injury/physical trauma or mental health conditions. She reports having a history of recurrent pelvic inflammatory diseases and was told she could never get pregnant.

Review of the emergency room's electronic medical record shows that she was admitted to the ER three times over the last 2 months each time via ambulance. The first time was for a head laceration from a fall, the second time was for a syncopal episode at the women's shelter, and the third time was for a motor vehicle accident. She does not have a primary care provider and states: "You guys do a good enough job. Why do I need a private doc?"

Social History

She admits to drinking a pint of vodka daily for the past 5 years and smoking 1 pack of cigarettes a day for 10 years. When asked about her e-cigarette use, she states she goes through a bottle of e-juice every 10 days because she cannot get the "same buzz" as her cigarettes. She has not been in a sexual relationship for the past 6 months, reports she is divorced, lives alone, and has no children. She has an associate degree in business from a local community college, previously employed as a cashier at a retail store but quit because of "differing views on health benefits." Currently receives income from unemployment check and family support, and is dependent on others for transportation.

Family Medical History

Both parents alive and healthy; no siblings; no children.

Medications

She has no allergies and denies taking any medications, including birth control or over-the-counter products.

❓ What are the pertinent positives from the information given so far?

- The patient consumed a quart of vodka and inhaled an unknown quantity of liquid nicotine before nausea and vomiting began.
- She has a diagnosis of alcohol and tobacco abuse.
- She presents with an unkept appearance and fish odor.
- She is a frequent visitor to the ER for alcohol-related incidents.
- She is of childbearing age and does not use birth control.
- She has emesis, which is now the consistency of clear phelgm.
- She had a headache and heart palpitations, which have now resolved.

❓ What are the significant negatives from the information given so far?

- The patient is in no distress and vital signs reported as stable.
- She currently denies abdominal pain, chest pain, and headache.
- She denies chronic health problems such as heart disease, pulmonary disease, metabolic conditions such as diabetes, gastrointestinal disorders, neurological disorders, or musculoskeletal disorders.
- There is no evidence of recent injury or trauma.
- The patient reports that she has not been sexually active.
- No reported hematemesis, fecal emesis, or projective vomiting.
- No reported diarrhea, dysuria, or fever.

❓ Given the current information what is the problem representation in this case?

I state the problem representation as "a 32-year-old white female alcoholic with suspected nicotine toxicity presents with severe nausea and vomiting."

❓ How does this information affect the list of possible causes?

The patient's overall stable condition, age, and lack of pain make the following diagnosis less likely: acute abdomen, myocardial infraction, or cerebrovascular event. In addition, the general survey shows that the patient is well developed, which makes an eating disorder or trauma/recent injury less likely, while the unkept grooming appearance makes a mental health issue a moderate to high probability. Her benign past medical history makes health problems such as diabetes, adrenal insufficiency, and thyroid disorder less likely to be the cause of this presentation, although the patient does not receive regular outpatient medical care and therefore may have chronic health problems that are not diagnosed. The possibility of a dehydrated state from continuous emesis is highly probable; however, she spent most of the last 48 hours in an air conditioned environment, making heat exhaustion or heat stroke less likely. Pregnancy is a possibility especially if she is not accurately reporting her sexual activity. The recent use of electronic cigarettes and the knowledge that they are unregulated make a toxic exposure high on the list of suspected causes of this patient's symptoms but I need to proceed with a full history and physical to further sort my differential.

CASE INFORMATION

Review of Systems

The patient appears to be a good historian although she admits to heavy alcohol use prior to ER admission, which may affect her recall of recent events.

- Constitutional: Denies fever, malaise, fatigue, upper respiratory infection symptoms, or recent travel; reports weight stable and appetite good; denies recent falls or trauma.
- Cardiovascular: Denies chest pain, edema, palpitations, or orthopnea.
- Pulmonary: Denies dyspnea or cough.
- Gastrointestinal: Denies pain with eating or drinking, reports regular bowel movements that are soft and firm, denies blood in stools, abdominal pain, or reflux; reports this is the first time she has had continuous nausea and vomiting.
- Genitourinary: Denies dysuria or hematuria; reports menstrual cycle regular and last menses approximately 30 days ago; states uses "self-control" for birth control; denies ever being pregnant. Denies vaginal discharge or odor.
- Musculoskeletal: Reports left arm burning and tingling as a first time occurrence; denies history of muscle or joint pain.
- Neurological: Denies vertigo, syncope, tremors, hyperactivity, falls, history of seizure disorder or stroke, numbness, tingling or extremity weakness, change in speech; denies history of headaches or migraines.
- Endocrine: Denies polyuria, polydipsia, and polyphagia.
- Hematology/immunology: Denies blood disorders or viral infections such as herpes zoster.
- Psychiatric: Denies suicidal ideation, depression, or panic disorders, states, "I am struggling to get my life in order. I know I drink more than I should but my women's group is helping me learn new coping skills like vaping instead of smoking cigarettes"; admits to driving under the influence twice but without arrests/court charges.

Physical Examination

- Vital signs: Pulse 88 beats per minute, blood pressure 110/80 mm Hg, respiratory rate 16/min, and oral temperature 97.5°F
- Bedside monitoring: Oxygen saturation by pulse oximeter 97% on room air, breath carbon monoxide 4 parts per million, 12-lead ECG and continuous cardiac monitoring—sinus rhythm no ST elevation or depression.
- Constitutional: 32-year-old white female, well developed and appears stated age, poorly groomed, clothes wrinkled, stained with food, has odor of fish, no acute distress but appears agitated, maintains eye contact and communicates effectively.
- Head/eyes/ears/nose/throat: Head symmetrical without lesions or pain, pupils equal, round, reactive to light and accommodation, ear canals clear, no nasal deviation or polyps, buccal mucosa pale and dry, oropharynx pink and dry without lesions.
- Neck: Trachea midline and freely movable, thyroid without masses or enlargement, no palpable lymph nodes, no jugular venous distension.
- Cardiovascular: No heaves, lifts, or thrills; S_1, S_2 regular rate and rhythm; no murmurs, gallops, or rubs; no edema; pulses intact 2+, no carotid or abdominal bruits. Nail beds pink without clubbing, brisk capillary refill.
- Pulmonary: Regular and symmetrical, lungs clear to auscultation and resonant to percussion.
- Gastrointestinal: Nondistended, hyperactive bowel sounds, tympanic on percussion, abdomen soft without tenderness, no organomegaly, emesis guaiac negative.
- Genitourinary: External genitalia unremarkable without lesions or discharge or odor, cervical os small, round, and slightly pink, no cervical motion tenderness or masses, rectum intact, and stool guaiac negative.
- Integumentary: Overall skin intact but with poor skin turgor. There is a circular area, approximately 2 inches in diameter, "oily" red, with small fluid filled vesicles on her left forearm.
- Neurological: No focal neurologic deficits, face symmetric, speech clear, upper and lower extremities strength intact, cranial nerves II-XII intact.

? **What elements of the review of systems and the physical examination should be added to the list of pertinent positives? Which items should be added to the list of significant negatives?**

- **Pertinent positives:** subjective—history of loss of job, history of pelvic inflammatory disease, reports stable weight and appetite, reports regular menstrual cycles and regular bowel movements; objective—fishy odor, localized "oily" rash on left forearm with small fluid filled vesicles, dry mucosa oral membranes, overall poor skin turgor, hyperactive bowel sounds.

- **Significant negatives:** The review of systems and the physical examination are reassuring in suggesting a nonemergent cause of her symptoms. The review of systems reveals no significant constitutional signs or localizing complaints to suggest an acute process. The physical examination, including stable vital signs as well as an afebrile state, is essentially normal with the few exceptions of the left forearm rash and skin turgor noted above.

? How does this information affect the problem representation and the list of possible causes?

An acute abdomen etiology, such as gastric outlet/intestinal obstruction, cholecystitis, pancreatitis, or bowel obstruction or ischemia, is very unlikely given the patient's stable condition and normal abdominal examination. The negative review of symptoms and physical examination also rules out life-threatening conditions such as cerebral hemorrhage, stroke, meningitis, myocardial infarction, or adrenal insufficiency. Migraine and benign positional vertigo are less likely causes since she does not report a history of migraines, is not in a state of distress, and is not dizzy upon standing up. The report of regular menses and the negative pelvic examination make pregnancy less likely, but a test is needed to confirm this. In addition, the history of alcohol use makes further testing of liver function warranted. The odor of fish in combination with the left forearm rash is suspicious for a liquid nicotine spillage incident, resulting in systemic toxicity from skin absorption. The bedside carbon monoxide of 4 parts per million reassures me that within the past 4 to 6 hours combustible tobacco products have not been consumed along with the e-cigarettes.

At this point it is important to reexamine the problem representation. The new problem representation currently reads: "a 32-year-old white female alcoholic with suspected nicotine toxicity presents with severe nausea and vomiting." From my perspective, there is enough evidence to support, with a high probability that the broken liquid nicotine bottle (e-cigarette refill) spilled on the patient's left forearm resulting in a localized rash and systemic absorption effects. When exposed to warm air, liquid nicotine has a fish odor, thus accounting for that clinical manifestation. The heavy use of alcohol makes the patient incapable of recalling the incident to determine if she was indeed refilling her e-cigarette with the liquid nicotine and "passed out." Thus further diagnostic testing is needed to confirm the suspected etiology.

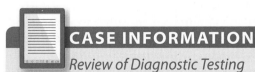

CASE INFORMATION
Review of Diagnostic Testing

The immediate evaluation of oxygenation and cardiac function, as well as the carbon monoxide level, shows nonsignificant findings. Labs ordered at the same time of the initial ECG including a comprehensive metabolic panel shows a mildly elevated blood urea nitrogen (BUN) at 22 mg/dL, normal creatinine, normal blood glucose, normal electrolytes, normal bilirubin, mildly elevated GGT at 53 units/L, normal troponin, and the remaining liver enzymes and albumin levels are normal, indicating normal synthetic function. The mildly elevated BUN is likely related to the continuous emesis and subsequent dehydration but no other significant renal condition. A complete blood count shows a normal white blood cell count, red blood cell count, hemoglobin, hematocrit, and platelet count. Her blood alcohol level is 0.10 mg/dL. A urinalysis for microscopy and urine pregnancy test are both negative. A urine drug screen is negative for tetrahydrocannabinol (THC) and positive for cotinine of 8000 ng/mL (cotinine is a metabolite of nicotine). Although unnecessary to narrow my diagnosis, a serum cotinine level is ordered. Serum measurements of cotinine are more specific and sensitive than urine samples.[2]

At this point I ask my patient additional questions about the number of e-cigarettes she used and the timing, which proved informative. The patient believes that over a 24-hour period approximately 5 e-cigarettes were smoked, equivalent to 100 cigarettes or 5 packs of cigarettes.[3] In addition, an unknown amount of liquid nicotine was spilled during an attempt to refill the cartridge. The diagnosis of intractable nausea and vomiting induced by nicotine poisoning via skin and inhaled absorption is established and falls in the category of "exogenous etiology," which is among one of my top differentials.

Liquid Nicotine Poisoning

Diagnosis and Treatment

E-cigarettes, also known as electronic nicotine delivery systems (ENDS), are battery-operated devices that, when filled with liquid nicotine, flavorings or other chemicals such as ethylene glycol (chemical in antifreeze) produce a vapor which the user inhales. A diagnosis of liquid nicotine poisoning can be made with the presence of symptoms and significantly elevated cotinine levels.[4] In this case, the combination of multiple "hits" of e-cigarettes with the spilled liquid nicotine caused the poisoning symptoms of nausea and vomiting.

The Centers for Disease Control and Prevention reports dramatic increases in electronic cigarette–related calls to poison control centers with one call per month in September 2010 to 215 calls per month in February 2014.[5] While the majority of ENDS do contain nicotine, the exact content is not known.[3,6] Currently the refillable liquid nicotine bottles are not regulated to require an OSHA Personal Protective Equipment Standard to prevent harm and promote safety nor are they required to report the nicotine levels.[5] Most refillable solutions contain nicotine levels in the 1.8 to 2.4 mg/mL range; however, some are as high as 87 mg/mL.[2,3] On average, when a smoker consumes one cigarette, 1 mg of nicotine is absorbed and it is reported that 60 mg can cause death for a 150-lb adult.[6,7]

Nicotine is a colorless to pale yellow oily liquid that turns brown on exposure to air or light. It is a naturally occurring toxic chemical found in tobacco plants and has a fishy odor when warm. Nicotine can be absorbed into the body by inhalation, ingestion, skin contact, and mucous membranes.[5] In this case, nicotine was consumed by both inhalation and skin contact.

Once absorbed, nicotine is metabolized to an alkaloid, cotinine, which is used as a biomarker for exposure to tobacco. Typically, cotinine has an in vivo half-life of approximately 20 hours. Depending on the type of measurement used (Table 48-1), cotinine is detectable from 1 to 7 days after nicotine is consumed.[8]

Table 48-1   Nicotine Metabolite (Cotinine) Measures[4,8]

Type	Exposure Time	Range of Values	Comments
Hair	30 to 90 days post-nicotine/ tobacco exposure if hair collection sufficient (0.5–1.5 in from the shaft)	<0–7 ng/mg of hair[a]	Most expensive; used predominantly for passive smoke/second-hand smoke analysis; used predominantly with neonates and children; technically noninvasive; specimen collection test specific and cannot be combined for other analysis; difficult to tamper with specimen[b]; no rapid tests; results may take days to weeks
Saliva	1 to 2 days post-nicotine/ tobacco exposure	<2 ng/mg[a]	Least expensive; noninvasive; specimen collection test specific and cannot be combined for other biometric analysis; difficult to tamper with specimen[b]; rapid tests available
Serum	Up to 7 days post-nicotine/ tobacco exposure	200 ng/mL to 800 ng/mL (peak level)[a]	Considered the gold standard for direct exposure analysis; invasive; can be collected for other biometric analysis; difficult to tamper with[b]; no rapid tests; results may take days to weeks
Urine	4 to 7 days post-nicotine/ tobacco exposure	1000 to 5000 ng/mL (peak level)[a]	Mostly obtained as noninvasive but may require invasive method; can be collected for other biometric analysis; easy to tamper with[b]; rapid tests available

[a] Values may vary depending on collection procedures, gender, age, ethnicity, and exposure history.
[b] Degree of tampering (if easy) may render a false-negative result.
Data from Alere quit for life—nicotine testing guideline. New Line Medical Web site. http://www.newline medical.com. Accessed July 5, 2014; and Salimetrics guidelines for interpreting cotinine levels: United States. Salimetrics Web site. http://www.salimetrics.com/assets/documents/Spit_Tips_-_Cotinine_Guidelines.pdf. Accessed July 5, 2014.

There is a spectrum of clinical features from nicotine poisoning (ingested and/ or inhaled) that include early phase clinical manifestations of headache, nausea, vomiting, tachycardia, hypertension, confusion, and agitation to late phase clinical manifestations of diarrhea, hypoventilation, hypotension, bradycardia, shock, coma, and death. In this case, recognizing that nontobacco users with no passive exposure to tobacco smoke would have a urine cotinine <5.0 ng/mL, the accumulation of nicotine metabolite is significantly high (8000 ng/mL) with clinical manifestations more consistent with early phase nicotine poisoning. It is important to consider the time lapse between specimen collection and the patient's hits of the e-cigarette and the exposure to liquid nicotine so that the patient's nicotine poisoning can be appropriately managed.

Usually, early phase symptoms of nicotine poisoning occur within 15 minutes to 1 hour of ingestion, and late phase poisoning symptoms occur within 30 minutes to 4 hours. The duration of symptoms is approximately 1 to 2 hours following mild exposure and up to 18 to 24 hours following severe exposure.[5] In this case, with the exception of the significantly high nicotine metabolite, the clinical manifestations do not match with the timing of symptoms. This is because the clinical symptoms are more consistent with an early phase nicotine poisoning, yet these symptoms are occurring more than 4 hours after exposure.

Treatment of nicotine poisoning aims to address both the long- and short-term consequences. Guidelines typically recommend administration of activated charcoal to decrease the absorption of nicotine and recommend that any significant cholinergic response effects are treated. In this case, much of the nicotine has been eliminated, based on the time that has elapsed. Since arriving in the ER, the patient is stable, and the nausea and vomiting are resolving. The overall prognosis of nicotine poisoning is typically good when the exposure or ingestion is eliminated, and when the patient presents with early phase symptoms.[5] However, observation over the next 12 hours is warranted to ensure that the patient does not experience metabolic, neurological, or cardiac adverse effects. I order the following: intravenous fluids of normal saline at 125 mL per hour, continuous oxygen per nasal prongs to maintain an O_2 saturation of >95%, and continuous cardiac monitoring. In addition, I order advance diet as tolerated and a repeat chemistry panel and ECG in 6 hours, serial troponin levels, orthostatic vital sign checks in 4 hours and 6 hours, thorough rinsing of left forearm with cool normal saline and thin application of 1% hydrocortisone ointment.

Case Follow-Up

Additional interventions provided in this case include substance abuse counseling as well as teaching the patient about the dangers associated with the doses of nicotine in unregulated e-cigarettes and the potential hazards of improper refilling. When confronting the patient about "health goals" the question was raised about which was more important, to quit alcohol or quit tobacco. I reinforced that this is a personal decision, that many patients make the decision to do both simultaneously while others elect to address one addiction at a time. In my patient's case, this was the fourth alcohol-related ER admission via ambulance. Although initially argumentative stating, "but my diagnosis is nicotine poisoning," I reminded her that the poisoning occurred as a direct result of alcohol consumption, causing her to inadvertently spill the liquid nicotine, increasing her exposure.

Questioning her level of readiness to quit smoking on a scale of 0 to 10 with "0" representing not ready and "10" representing highly ready, the patient reported a "10." Recognizing that smokers are highly motivated to quit after a near death episode[9] the five Rs (relevance, risks, rewards, roadblocks, and repetition) are reviewed.[10] This is repeated for quitting alcohol and the same response is given.

Further exploration of her smoking history reveals a moderate Fagerström test for nicotine dependence level of 6/10 with "10" representing highly dependent. I recommend that she use FDA-approved medications for quitting versus e-cigarettes. To that end, I order a 24-hour release nicotine replacement therapy (NRT) patch 21 mg, with NRT gum/lozenge 2 mg every 2 to 4 hours for breakthrough cravings.[10]

A CAGE (cut down, annoy, guilty, eye opening) assessment is obtained to determine her degree of concern about alcohol use. Her CAGE screening indicates high alcohol dependence with "all four" items responses "yes." The four CAGE questions are: (1) Do you ever feel like you should cut down? (2) Do you get annoyed when people talk to you about your drinking? (3) Do you ever feel guilty about how much you drink? (4) Do you ever need a drink in the morning to get you going?

During her observation unit admission she remains in normal sinus rhythm, the repeat ECG is normal as are the troponin levels, her chemistry panel is normal, vital signs remain stable with an O_2 saturation of 98% on room air, and breath CO was 0%.

Later that evening, the patient is discharged from the observation unit in the care of a staff member from the women's shelter. She is provided a prescription of 1% topical hydrocortisone ointment to apply to left forearm three times a day and follow-up appointments with a primary care provider, a social worker, a nicotine specialist, and an AA sponsor. A note is dictated to the new PCP and the tobacco cessation specialist, including a reminder to draw a follow-up serum cotinine level.

References

1. Epocrates essentials 2014—Disease management module—acute abdominal pain. Epocrates Web site. http://www.epocrates.com/products. Accessed July 5, 2014.
2. Flouris AD, Chorti MS, Poulianiti KP, et al. Acute impact of active and passive electronic cigarette smoking on serum cotinine and lung function. *Inhal Toxicol.* 2013;25(2):91-101.
3. Cheng T. Chemical evaluation of electronic cigarettes. *Tob Control.* 2014;23(2):ii11-ii17.
4. Alere quit for life—nicotine testing guideline. New Line Medical Web site. http://www.newline medical.com. Accessed July 5, 2014.
5. The National Institute for Occupational Safety and Health (NIOSH). Nicotine: systemic agent. Centers for Disease Control and Prevention (CDC). http://www.cdc.gov/niosh/ershdb/Emergency ResponseCard_29750028.html. Updated June 18, 2013. Accessed July 5, 2015.
6. Centers for Disease Control and Prevention (CDC). Notes from the field: calls to poison centers for exposures to electronic cigarettes—United States, September 2010-February 2014. *MMWR,* 63(13):292-293. http://www.cdc.gov/mmwr/preview/mmwrhtml/mm6313a4.htm. Accessed July 5, 2015.
7. Bayer B. How much nicotine kills a human? Tracing back the generally accepted lethal dose to dubious self-experiments in the nineteenth century. *Arch Toxicol.* 2014;88:5-7.

8. Salimetrics guidelines for interpreting cotinine levels: United States. Salimetrics Web site. http://www.salimetrics.com/assets/documents/Spit_Tips_-_Cotinine_Guidelines.pdf. Accessed July 5, 2014.

9. Katz DA, Vander MW, Holman J, et al. The Emergency Department Action in Smoking Cessation (EDASC) trial: impact on delivery of smoking cessation counseling. *Acad Emerg Med.* 2012;19(4):409-420.

10. Fiore MC, Jaén CR, Baker TB, et al. *Treating Tobacco Use and Dependence: 2008 Update. Clinical Practice Guideline.* Rockville, MD: US Department of Health and Human Services. Public Health Service; 2008.

CASE 49

Elizabeth S. Gochenour

Elizabeth S. Gochenour is an ACNP on the Wound Ostomy Care team at the University of Virginia Medical Center in Charlottesville.

CASE INFORMATION

Chief Complaint

This is an 81-year-old man transferred from a local skilled nursing facility to the emergency department (ED) for changes in mental status.

History of Present Illness

Mr W is an 81-year-old man with a history of coronary artery disease (CAD), peripheral artery disease (PAD), hypertension (HTN), diabetes mellitus (DM), end-stage renal disease (ESRD), and dementia. He is dialyzed 3 days per week at a local hemodialysis facility. He was seen by the vascular clinic 2 months ago for a nonhealing right toe wound and underwent an above-knee to below-knee popliteal artery bypass with a right reversed greater saphenous vein.

The patient resides at a local skilled nursing facility. The nursing staff reports that he was in his usual state of health this morning, ambulated to the dining hall, ate breakfast, and then returned to his room. When the nursing staff went to wake him for lunch, he was difficult to arouse, and did not follow commands. His vitals at that time were temperature of 101.8°F oral, heart rate of 101 beats per minute, respiratory rate of 22 breaths per minute, blood pressure 120/84 mm Hg, and oxygen saturation 93% on room air. Per nursing staff he is usually alert and oriented to person, pleasantly confused, able to recognize family members and follow commands; however, he is not oriented to place or time. Because of his altered mental status and vital signs, the staff called 911 to transfer him to the ED.

On arrival to the ED, his initial triage survey triggers the "sepsis alert" for a heart rate greater than 100 beats per minute and temperature greater than 40°C. He has an episode of hypotension in the ED of 80/35 mm Hg but this resolved spontaneously. He is somnolent, a notable change from his baseline mental state, so a "stroke alert" is also called. The neurology team orders a stat computed tomography (CT) scan of his head, which shows no acute abnormalities. He is empirically started on vancomycin and piperacillin/tazobactam for sepsis of unknown origin and given IV fluids to maintain his blood pressure. Baseline laboratory tests are drawn including blood cultures. The ED provider examines him to look for a potential sepsis source and identifies heel ulcers and a toe on his right foot that looks abnormal.

The ED team then calls a consultation with the wound care team to evaluate, what they refer to as "Mr W's chronic diabetic toe and heel ulcers." At this point the source of his sepsis is as yet unclear.

❓ What is the potential cause?

The patient's initial problem triggering his transfer to the ED was "mental status changes," but on further evaluation the ED team has diagnosed sepsis. It is likely the septic state is related to the new mental status changes. Because his CT does not demonstrate any emergent neurologic conditions that may explain his mental status, it is essential that I look for a source of infection. As the ACNP called to consult on his toe and heel ulcers, I already have a high index of suspicion that they will be the source of his sepsis. However, I must also consider other potential sources so start with a differential diagnosis organized by system. I will expand this differential if I do not quickly identify a source of infection.

Initial Differential Diagnoses

- Pulmonary: pneumonia
- Genitourinary: urinary tract infection, pyelonephritis
- Integumentary: infected diabetic foot ulcer, cellulitis
- Musculoskeletal: osteomyelitis
- Cardiovascular: blood stream infection from AV fistula used for dialysis
- Gastrointestinal: abdominal abscess, peritonitis
- Dehydration from unknown cause

With all of these possible causes in mind, I start to narrow down my list by gathering data and eliminating some of these diagnoses.

CASE INFORMATION

General Survey

I begin with a general survey of the patient. He appears to be well nourished and well developed. He does not appear to be in any distress and shakes his head "no" when I ask if he is having any difficulty breathing or if he is in any pain. He is somnolent but will rouse to my voice and answer simple questions with yes or no. When I ask, "can you tell me where you are?" he does not answer. Generally he is slow to answer and follow commands. He says "no" when I ask if it hurts when he voids or if he has the need to urinate frequently. He tells me he is tired, and he sleeps when not being stimulated. There is no family present and I am unable to obtain a history or review of systems. At this time I continue to gather information for the history of present illness. I know that I cannot rely on a full patient history or review of systems but will gather data as quickly as I can. A thorough examination and analysis of his toe and heel are especially important, as I have been called specifically as a consultant for these findings.

? Given the information provided so far, what are the pertinent positives and significant negatives?

Pertinent Positives

- Baseline dementia but decreased mental status from baseline, somnolent
- +Fever
- +Tachycardia
- Presence of wounds on toe and heels
- One episode of hypotension (resolved spontaneously)

Significant Negatives

- No acute process on head CT
- No apparent distress or pain or respiratory distress
- Well nourished and well developed
- Denies pain
- Denies shortness of breath
- Denies polyuria, dysuria

? Can the information gathered so far be restated in a single sentence highlighting the pieces that narrow down the cause? How does this information affect the differential diagnosis?

The problem presentation in this case may be: "An 81 year old man presenting with decreased mental status, increased somnolence, and a septic picture the origin of which is unknown."

While I am a consultant in this case, it is likely that the patient will be transferred to the medicine service and I will work closely with the medicine team to care for him. I must evaluate his toe and heels but must also continue to consider other causes of potential infection so we do not lose time while we wait for transfer. I review what has been done already.

? What diagnostics are important to order?

Because Mr W is unable to give me much information, I order a chest x-ray since sepsis from pneumonia is high on my differential. I also order a clean catch urine specimen or an "in and out" sterile specimen if he is unable to get a clean catch (which he is likely unable to do). I check to ensure that labs including blood cultures, complete blood count with differential, blood urea nitrogen and creatinine, electrolytes, lactic acid, and coagulation studies are all ordered. I suspect he is dehydrated so order 1 L of 0.9% NS to infuse at 75 mL/h. I also ensure that the renal team is involved and will have a blood culture sent from his AV fistula when it is accessed for hemodialysis to rule out an infected fistula.

CASE INFORMATION

Obtained From the Electronic Medical Record

- Additional past medical history: significant for prostate cancer and cirrhosis, heart failure, degenerative joint disease, and glaucoma
- Past surgical history: hemicolectomy, prostatectomy, coronary angioplasty with stent placement, AV fistula placement, right leg above the knee arterial bypass surgery (popliteal to popliteal bypass)
- Family history: unable to be assessed secondary to patient's mental status
- Review of systems: unable to obtain
- Medications: per documentation from nursing facility
  Acetaminophen 650 mg by mouth every 4 hours as needed pain
  Amlodipine 5 mg by mouth daily
  Aspirin 81 mg by mouth daily
  Atorvastatin 80 mg tablet daily by mouth
  Gabapentin 100 mg two times daily
  Glimepiride 5 mg daily
  Xalatan 0.005% ophthalmic solution
  Lisinopril 10 mg by mouth daily
  Effexor 75 mg by mouth daily
  Loratadine 10 mg by mouth daily
  Carvedilol (Coreg) 6.25 mg by mouth daily
- Allergies: none known

Physical Examination

- Vital signs: Blood pressure 129/60 mm Hg, heart rate 90 beats per minute, temperature 36.6°C (97.8°F) orally, respirations 18 breaths per minute, SpO$_2$ 94% on room air. Weight 75 kg (164 lb) body mass index 24.9. Blood glucose by fingerstick 131 mg/dL.
- Constitutional: Lying in bed sleeping, wakens briefly when stimulated by touch or voice, no apparent distress.
- Head/eyes/ears/nose/throat: Head: normocephalic, atraumatic. Eyes: extraocular movements normal, pupils equal, round, reactive to light, no injection or scleral icterus. Nose: dry mucous membranes, no exudate. Throat: no oral erythema, lesions, or exudate. Neck: Supple full range of motion without pain.

- Cardiovascular: Regular rate and rhythm, no murmurs, rubs, or gallops. No edema, distal pulses intact and equal bilaterally. AV fistula in right arm with bruit and thrill, no redness or swelling.
- Pulmonary: Breathing pattern symmetrical and eupneic appearing, no accessory muscle use, clear bilaterally to auscultation.
- Gastrointestinal: Abdomen obese, positive bowel sounds in all quadrants, soft, nontender, nondistended. No rebound or guarding.
- Musculoskeletal: Moves all extremities, strength 4/5 in all extremities, no edema.
- Neurological: Arouses to voice, however, falls back to sleep after a brief time. He is able to state his first name. Follows simple commands such as "squeeze my hand", "wiggle your toes". Facial features symmetrical, grips equal, sensation intact.
- Integumentary: Skin warm and dry, no rashes or bruising. There is a large misshapen toenail on the right great toe that extends onto the tip wrapping around posteriorly. I cut the toenail and the calloused area on the tip was disrupted, causing purulent matter to pour from the wound (see Figure 49-1). I am able to probe directly to the bone, and express a moderate to large amount of purulent matter. He also has a large black eschar on his right heel. There is no erythema, fluctuance, or induration noted. This eschar is stable. The left foot does not have any wounds.
- Genitourinary: Anuric; dialysis dependent.

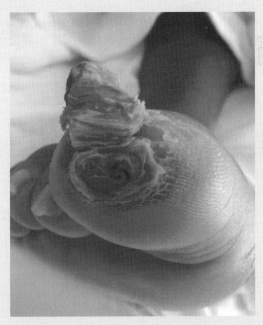

Figure 49-1 Right great toe with misshapen toenail and callous formation.

What elements of the history and physical examination should be added to the list of pertinent positives? Which items should be added to the list of significant negatives?

Pertinent Positives

• Purulent drainage from toe wound, tracks to the bone
• Heel eschar noted but no signs of infection

Significant Negatives

• Lungs clear
• Normal cardiac examination
• Abdominal examination benign
• No focal neurological deficits

 How does this new information affect the potential causes?

The finding of purulent drainage from the patient's toe wound is evidence of infection, and the fact that the wound reaches the depth of the bone suggests possible osteomyelitis. He does have an eschar on his heel but it appears stable and not infected. No other potential sources are obvious in the examination as all systems are relatively normal. The exception is his baseline dementia and his somnolence that I attribute to his infection, fever, and septic state. It is possible that there are other sources but for now, I must focus on treating this patient's wounds immediately. I will review his diagnostics when they return. His most recent vital signs reveal him to be normotensive and I must be cautious with fluids as he has significant chronic cardiac and renal conditions. His bedside glucose is normal; I will have a Hemoglobin A1c drawn during this admission to assess his overall glucose control.

CASE INFORMATION

Laboratory Results

• Complete blood count with differential: hemoglobin 11.5 g/dL (normal = 14–18), hematocrit 35.6 (normal = 40%–52%), white blood cell count 9.19K/µL (normal = 4–11K/µL) with 85% neutrophils
• Electrolytes: within normal limits with the following exceptions: glucose 134 mg/dL (normal = 74–99), sodium 129 g/dL (normal = 136–145), creatinine 3.6 (normal = 0.7–1.3 mg/dL)
• Albumin: 2.7 g/dL (normal = 3.2–5.2)

- Anion gap: normal—no gap
- Calculated glomerular filtration rate (GFR): 15 (mL/min/1.73 m^2)
- Coagulation studies: normal
- Chest x-ray: mild cardiomegaly, no acute cardiopulmonary disease
- Urinalysis: in and out cath for scant amount dark urine—on dipstick +protein, but negative for ketones, leukocytes, and nitrates
- Blood cultures: pending

Case Analysis: The lab results confirm his chronic anemia, likely due to his renal disease, and the elevated neutrophils support the presence of an active infection. His elevated creatinine is consistent with his renal failure as is his low GFR. His low albumin suggests he is somewhat malnourished, which affects his ability to heal. His urinalysis and chest x-ray rule out sepsis of urinary origin and pneumonia as causes of his altered mental state, fever, and tachycardia. I am still awaiting blood cultures and results will likely not return for 24 to 72 hours.

At this point I diagnose the patient with osteomyelitis of the right great toe and initiate a plan of care to address that. While the appearance of pus suggests cellulitis, soft tissue infection, or osteomyelitis, wounds that probe all the way to the bone, as this one did, are assumed to be osteomyelitis until proven otherwise.[1] There should be no delay in initiating treatment once osteomyelitis is suspected. Because the bone is avascular, infection of the bone is very difficult to treat, requiring long-term antibiotic therapy and often surgical intervention. Further testing to confirm the diagnosis can be ordered along with appropriate antibiotics and consultations to address osteomyelitis.

? Given the information obtained so far, what additional diagnostics are necessary to obtain?

In most cases a magnetic resonance image (MRI) and bone biopsy are the definitive diagnostic tests to identify osteomyelitis. MRI and bone scintigraphy have improved diagnostic accuracy and the ability to identify infection as they provide views of the bone and surrounding tissues and help differentiate between cellulitis and osteomyelitis. Bone biopsy along with blood cultures or cultures of wound drainage are essential to identify the specific organism causing infection, which dictates appropriate antibiotic therapy.

Additional testing to consider includes an ankle-brachial index test or a lower extremity arterial Doppler ultrasound to evaluate perfusion to the affected limb and the ability of the limb to heal. Transcutaneous oxygen measurements (TcPO$_2$) also assess the adequacy of tissue perfusion for and the degree of tissue ischemia. The values obtained from the TcPO$_2$ are predictive of the healing potential of the lower limbs.[2] These values may help determine the need for a vascular intervention, hyperbaric oxygenation to treat the wound, and if necessary, amputation. If amputation is the treatment of choice, the data obtained with $TcPO_2$ may assist in deciding between above the knee versus a below the knee amputation (AKA vs BKA).

CASE INFORMATION

Because I was able to access the patient's bone directly with my probe, other definitive tests as described above were not required. A culture of the purulent drainage was sent to the lab for Gram stain and culture. I also ask the primary team to consult the vascular surgery and orthopedic surgery services for their input on revascularization procedures and surgical interventions including amputation.

The following day, Mr W's blood cultures show *Proteus mirabilis* and *Morganella morganii*. The infectious disease consult team is contacted and based on their recommendations his antibiotic regimen is adjusted to vancomycin, meropenem, and cefepime. I also continue local management of the wound with daily dressing changes and an antimicrobial packing. The vascular team and the orthopedic team evaluate the patient and amputation is discussed while further vascular interventions are not considered based on his recent femoral-popliteal bypass.

Osteomyelitis: Diagnosis and Treatment

When osteomyelitis is suspected an MRI should be done to confirm the diagnosis. Once confirmed, a bone biopsy and culture are needed to determine the causative organism. Management requires placement of a long-term intravenous access, such as a peripherally inserted central catheter (PICC) and 6 weeks of intravenous antibiotics.[3] Local wound care should also be provided. Packing the wound with an antimicrobial wound packing such as a packing strip impregnated with silver is one technique.

Surgical intervention to treat osteomyelitis includes debridement of the affected bone, drainage, and possibly placement of a soft tissue graft or muscle flap.[4] In addition, osteomyelitis occurring in the presence of rods or other hardware requires removal of all hardware as the infection is likely to become chronic if left in place. In some cases amputation is the treatment of choice, particularly when the affected individual has severe peripheral vascular disease, impairing the ability to heal following a debridement and drainage. The rationale for amputation is to remove not only the infected bone, but also the surrounding areas of poor perfusion that pose a high risk for recurrent infection. Amputations in diabetic patients account for more than 50% to 80% of the estimated 120,000 amputations in the United States, not related to trauma.[1]

One approach to determining the treatment of osteomyelitis is a staging system that considers not only the degree of infection but also the state of the affected individual. By staging the disease and the host, providers can determine who will benefit from surgery and correctly identify situations in which a conservative approach is more appropriate. An otherwise healthy individual may derive a clear benefit from surgical intervention even for less invasive disease, whereas in a compromised host, the risk of surgery may outweigh the risk posed by a severe case of osteomyelitis.[4]

Whenever amputation is considered, quality of life and baseline mobility should be assessed. The patient's ability to participate in postoperative rehabilitation, the burden that the symptoms of the osteomyelitis poses, and the preferences of the patient and family are all key considerations. The impact of surgical amputation extends beyond the patient and includes his or her caregivers and family members. When possible, input from all affected should be included in the decision-making process.

Case Follow-Up

On hospital day 5, Mr W's mental status cleared to his baseline level and he told nursing staff that he did not want an amputation and "had enough and wanted to die." The primary team, the patient, and his family had a "goals of care" discussion. Given the nature of his severe bacterial infection, poor circulation, chronic diseases, and baseline dementia, as well as his stated desire not to have an amputation, the major goal of care was agreed to be Mr W's comfort. Over the next several days Mr W decided to stop dialysis and antibiotics and to return to the nursing facility. He passed away 3 weeks later.

References

1. Krasner DL, Rpdemjeaver G, Sibbald RG. *Chronic Wound Care: A Clinical Source Book for Healthcare Professionals*. Wayne, PA: HMP Communications; 2001.
2. Moosa HH, Makaroun MS, Peitzman AB, Steed DL, Webster MW. TcPO2 values in limb ischemia: effects of blood flow and arterial oxygen tension. *J Surg Res*. 1986;40(5):482-487.
3. Bryant RA. *Acute & Chronic Wounds: Nursing Management*. St Louis, MO: Mosby, Inc; 2000.
4. Kishner S. Osteomyelitis. Medscape Web site. http://emedicine.medscape.com/article/1348767-overview. Updated August 15, 2014. Accessed April 16, 2015.

CASE 50

Elizabeth W. Good

Elizabeth Good works with hepato-pancreato-biliary surgical oncology patients at the Emily Couric Clinical Cancer Center at the University of Virginia Health System, Charlottesville.

CASE INFORMATION

Chief Complaint: "I am yellow and feel lousy"

A 70-year-old Caucasian male is brought to the emergency room by his wife with complaints of jaundice, fatigue, nausea, diarrhea, and weight loss. He is admitted to an acute inpatient unit for evaluation. He recently retired to the area and has not yet established any local health care providers.

❓ What is the potential cause?

Jaundice is indicative of liver or biliary tract dysfunction or injury. It is an uncommon presenting complaint, and consequently, I prioritize this above the other complaints of nausea, diarrhea, and weight loss, all of which are common and nonspecific presenting symptoms. While it is possible that these symptoms are unrelated and of separate significance to jaundice, my initial presumption is that they are a related cluster of symptoms until the etiology of the jaundice is determined.

Jaundice in the adult patient can result from a benign or deadly disorder. Listing the potential causes of jaundice as prehepatic, hepatic (intrahepatic), and posthepatic (extrahepatic) helps me efficiently organize my diagnostic approach and management of this patient.[1]

Differential Diagnoses for a Jaundiced Patient (With Presumed Hyperbilirubinemia)

- Prehepatic: hemolytic anemias, hemolysis from autoimmune disorders/medications/defects in hemoglobin or thalassemias, genetic syndrome, hematoma reabsorption
- Hepatic: viral or alcoholic hepatitis, autoimmune disorders, toxins/medications, sarcoidosis, primary biliary cirrhosis, primary sclerosing cholangitis
- Posthepatic: cholelithiasis and choledocholithiasis, cholangitis, biliary tract tumors, gallbladder cancer, stricture from previous surgery, cholangiocarcinoma, pancreatitis, pancreatic tumor/cancer

These differential diagnoses can be further characterized by distinguishing between unconjugated (indirect) hyperbilirubinemia and conjugated (direct) hyperbilirubinemia. Bilirubin is a brown-yellow substance that comprises bile and results when the liver breaks down old red blood cells. It is excreted in feces and accounts for the brown color of stool. Unconjugated bilirubin is insoluble and transforms to conjugated bilirubin in the liver, which is soluble. If the liver is not working, this bilirubin transformation cannot occur, resulting in higher than normal unconjugated bilirubin levels. Excess conjugated bilirubin levels result when the liver is working appropriately but the body is unable to excrete the byproduct via the usual pathways. Knowing this difference, I can reorganize and classify the differential diagnoses into either grouping. I adapted the following groupings and subcategories from UptoDate tables.[2] Here is how it looks:

Unconjugated (indirect) hyperbilirubinemia: increased bilirubin production—hemolysis, extravasated blood, defective erythrocyte development; impaired hepatic bilirubin uptake—medications; impaired bilirubin conjugation either inherited or acquired—Gilbert syndrome (inherit); Crigler-Najjar syndrome (inherit); liver diseases (acquired) including chronic hepatitis, cirrhosis, Wilson disease

Conjugated (direct) hyperbilirubinemia: extrahepatic cholestasis or biliary obstruction—choledocholithiasis, tumor of pancreas, gallbladder, bile duct environs; primary sclerosing cholangitis, acute/chronic pancreatitis, localized strictures from the previous procedure or surgery, parasitic infections; intrahepatic cholestasis—hepatitis (viral, alcoholic, chronic), drug toxicity, primary biliary cirrhosis, primary sclerosing cholangitis, infiltrative disease—lymphoma, sarcoidosis, amyloidosis; end-stage liver disease

Of note, elevations in both unconjugated and conjugated bilirubin is often termed conjugated hyperbilirubinemia even though both are higher than normal. This occurs with hepatocellular disease, impaired excretion of bilirubin, or biliary obstruction.

With all possible causes in mind, my next step is to begin to gather data and narrow down the list. My initial goal is to broadly define the cause of his jaundice as an impairment of bilirubin production, conjugation, or uptake, or as a result of hepatic inflammation/hepatocellular disease or biliary blockage. Another more basic way to think about this is to define the causative agent of his jaundice as autoimmune/hereditary, toxin or medication, infection, or mass/malignancy until I am able to gather more data.

I start with a thorough and detailed patient history before proceeding with my physical examination. I do have a few strategic inquiries foremost in my mind that I hope will help me confirm or eliminate potential causes quickly as the patient shares his story of how he came to the hospital with his current signs and symptoms. The first key question I hope to answer is whether or not he is experiencing any abdominal pain. Is he demonstrating painless jaundice or painful jaundice? I am also keen to learn whether all of his presenting signs and symptoms came on suddenly/acutely, have ever previously presented and resolved, or whether they presented in an insidious and progressive nature over time. Another essential question is whether or not he began taking any new medications in the past few weeks or months that maybe the causative agent for his jaundice.[3,4] My remaining questions are related to his bodily exposures. Has he traveled outside the United States in the past year? Has he been exposed to a work toxin recently or in the past? Does he take acetaminophen for arthritis or daily pain management? Does he consume alcohol in excess? Has he ever been involved in a car accident, for example, or a fall that resulted in abdominal harm?

CASE INFORMATION

History of Present Illness

"My wife and daughter noticed I was yellow, I didn't see it at first but I do now especially in my eyes." He reports a week long history of progressive jaundice, pruritus, dark or tea-colored urine. He has a back scratcher device that he uses frequently and states it "never leaves my side." These signs and symptoms have never occurred before, in him or anyone in his family. His appetite is fair and has been "off" for months and associated with early satiety and bloating. He has lost about 25 lb over 2 months and associates this with his intention to lose weight; however, he admits he has lost the weight more easily than he anticipated. He reports new onset of nausea over the past 2 to 3 days. He has never had emesis although has come close on a few occasions. He is fatigued and this has become more pronounced. He was walking on a treadmill and lifting weights two to three times a week until a month ago when he quit due to fatigue. He is having mild epigastric "aching" radiating to his back; he takes no pain medications. The discomfort was initially intermittent and has become more constant in the past 2 weeks. The pain is not associated with food intake or bowel movements. His bowel movements vacillate between constipation and diarrhea. Currently he is experiencing loose stools, up to five a day, sometimes clay colored. He takes a pill for his diabetes but this medication and his other current medications have not changed for more than a year. He has never taken weight loss or herbal supplements. He has never traveled outside the United States or experienced abdominal trauma from a fall or motor vehicle accident.

Allergies

• No known allergies.

Medications

• Benazepril (20 mg)-hydrochlorothiazide (25 mg) tablet, take one tablet daily; glimepiride 2 mg tablet, take one tablet every morning (before breakfast); rosuvastatin 20 mg tablet, take one tablet daily; sitagliptin

(50 mg)-metformin (1000 mg) tablet, take one tablet two times a day (with meals).

Past medical history

• Hypertension; coronary artery disease; hyperlipidemia; diabetes mellitus (for 5+ years); benign prostatic hypertrophy. He denies any history of gall-bladder disease, pancreatic disease, or liver problems.

Past surgical history

• Rotator cuff repair/right; leg surgery for trauma injury/right; coronary angioplasty (PCI) with stent ×2 (4 years ago).

Family History

• The patient's family history was reviewed and negative for GI malignancy, pancreatic disease, and liver disease. Heart disease and hypertension are prevalent in both his maternal and paternal families.

Social History

• He is a retired insurance agent. He denies history of exposure to noxious chemicals or toxins. He has been married for over 40 years. He reports his alcohol consumption as "never." He smokes cigarettes "some days" but not every day, previously smoked one pack per day for 25 years. He denies current and previous illicit, recreational, or intravenous drug use.

❓ What are the pertinent positives from the information given so far?

• Progressive and insidious onset of symptoms including:

  • Jaundice.

  • Itching.

  • Tea-colored urine, indicates presence of excess conjugated bilirubin or bilirubinuria. Bilirubin is normally absent from urine but is present in urine when excess conjugated bilirubin is present in the body.

  • Fatigue that now inhibits his ability to exercise.

  • Weight and appetite loss with early satiety and bloating.

  • Variable stool consistencies. A pale, clay color, or acholic stool is a distinct finding and indicative of a common bile duct obstruction, that is, absence of bile pigments or bilirubin breakdown in the stool. A brown stool color represents the presence of bile or bilirubin. A pale or clay-colored stool means that the liver is not producing enough bile or there is a blockage of bile flow, resulting in the absence of brown stool.

- Some abdominal pain, his subacute pain has evolved to a constant epigastric and mid-back aching.

❓ What are the significant negatives from the information given so far?

- Taking no new medications or herbal supplements
- Taking no pain medications including non-steroidal anti-inflammatory drugs (NSAIDs) or acetaminophen
- Never traveled outside the United States
- No previous exposure to noxious chemicals or toxins
- No recent or previous abdominal trauma from an accident or fall
- No history of liver disease or hepatitis, however, but unknown if he has been tested for hepatitis in the past
- No history of autoimmune disorders
- No history of gallbladder problems or cholecystectomy. His gallbladder has never been removed
- No history of acute or chronic pancreatitis
- No history of current or previous alcohol or intravenous drug use

❓ Can the information obtained so far be summarized into a single sentence, a problem representation?

The problem representation in this case might be: "a 70-year-old diabetic male presents with jaundice, worsening fatigue, nausea, and weight loss. His other signs and symptoms include tea-colored urine, clay-colored stools, early satiety, abdominal bloating, and constant epigastric/mid-back aching."

Case Analysis: I answered my intended questions and learn that the patient is experiencing mild pain with his jaundice. His signs and symptoms evolved over time and progressed to encompass a cadre of clinical complaints. He does not drink alcohol, and he is not taking any new medications, acetaminophen, or herbal supplements toxic to the liver. He has not traveled outside the United States to areas of the world endemic with parasites and infections that may result in jaundice. With these pertinent positive and significant negative findings, the notion of toxins or drugs as the cause of his jaundice is unlikely.

I can also rule out hemolysis as the cause of this patient's jaundice. The clay-colored stool and tea-colored urine demonstrate the presence of conjugated hyperbilirubinemia, not unconjugated hyperbilirubinemia. With this information, the differential shifts more toward a cholestasis or an obstructive process. This leaves the remaining categories of autoimmune/hereditary, infection, or mass/malignancy as causes for his jaundice. An autoimmune or hereditary etiology is less likely for this patient given his age and lack of familial autoimmune history or hereditary malady. Autoimmune hepatitis, for example, is unlikely as it is associated more with young women. Autoimmune pancreatitis is a subset of chronic pancreatitis and remains a possibility. This disorder occurs more often in men and presents with jaundice, weight loss, and mild pain; severe abdominal pain is unusual.

An infectious etiology for the patient's jaundice seems unlikely, as the patient is without fevers, acute pain, and general malaise (other than fatigue). Additionally, he presents with weight loss and itching, which are not usually seen with an infectious process. While I cannot rule out cholangitis, cholelithiasis, and choledocholithiasis, they are lower on my differential at this point. Generally, gallstone obstruction resulting in jaundice is quite painful especially with a large impacted stone, and this patient's pain is troubling but not severe. Applying Charcot's triad of fever, jaundice, and right upper quadrant pain, which indicates cholangitis, this patient has only one out of the three of those symptoms. Primary sclerosing cholangitis is more prominent in men and often associated with inflammatory bowel syndrome. Primary biliary cirrhosis usually presents in middle-aged women, so that is less likely to be present in this patient.

He has no hepatitis history that he is aware of but viral testing for this is warranted when I begin diagnostic testing. I will also need to order amylase and lipase to evaluate for pancreatitis, which I cannot completely rule out at this time. Pancreatitis is most often caused by gallstones or alcohol and can lead to obstruction of the common bile duct because of compression by the inflamed pancreas. I can best rule out gallstones with ultrasound, which is another diagnostic test I will likely need to order, as gallstones play a role with cholelithiasis, choledocholithiasis, and gallstone pancreatitis.

Based on the information I have so far, malignancy is high on the differential and is the most probable at this time. The insidious and progressive nature of his symptoms, the associated weight loss, and the changes in stool and urine indicating a conjugated hyperbilirubinemia all suggest a malignant process. Gallbladder cancer usually presents with jaundice, hepatomegaly, and a mass in the right upper quadrant. Cholangiocarcinoma manifests as jaundice, pruritus, weight loss, and abdominal pain. Pancreatic malignancy also commonly presents with pain, jaundice, and weight loss.

Prior to beginning my complete review of systems and physical examination, I order some preliminary lab work which will help me quickly rule out certain diagnoses.

❓ What preliminary laboratory tests should be obtained at this time?

I start with a complete blood count (CBC), basic metabolic panel (BMP), hepatic panel which includes a conjugated (direct) bilirubin, amylase, lipase, protime, urinalysis (UA) with reflex culture, and viral hepatitis screen. Further lab work will be dictated by the findings on examination of the patient.

CASE INFORMATION

Review of Systems

- Constitutional: Endorses fatigue, weight loss, loss of appetite, early satiety
- Denies fever, chills, diaphoresis, malaise.
- Head/ears/nose/throat: Denies hearing loss, trouble swallowing, congestion, rhinorrhea.
- Eyes: Endorses scleral icterus. Denies itching, pain, redness to eyes, or visual disturbances.
- Cardiovascular: Denies chest pain, leg swelling, or difficulty breathing when lying down.
- Pulmonary: Denies shortness of breath, cough, snoring/apnea when sleeping.
- Gastrointestinal: Endorses constant nausea, epigastric aching, abdominal bloating, loose stools (<5 per day) and pale/clay colored. Denies emesis.
- Genitourinary: Endorses nocturia. Denies hematuria, dysuria, urgency, incontinence.
- Integumentary: Endorses jaundice, generalized pruritus. Denies rash or skin infection.
- Musculoskeletal: Endorses mid-back aching. Denies arthritis, myalgias, or gait difficulties.
- Neurological: Denies weakness, numbness/tingling in extremities, headache, dizziness, change in speech, tremors, seizures.
- Endocrine: The patient is not sure of his diabetes control, he does not check blood glucose by fingerstick. Denies polyuria, polydipsia.
- Psychiatric: Endorses nervous/anxious about diagnosis. Denies sleep disturbance, depression, agitation, confusion.

Physical Examination

- Vital signs: Blood pressure 108/60 mmHg; temperature 37.4°C (tympanic); respirations 20/min; oxygen saturation by pulse oximeter is 98% on room air; BMI 28.
- Constitutional: He appears his stated age. He is well developed and well nourished. He is cooperative.
- Head/eyes/ears/nose/throat: Head: normocephalic and atraumatic. Uvula is midline, oropharynx is clear and moist and mucous membranes are normal. Eyes: scleral icterus. Conjunctivae, extra ocular movements and lids are normal. Pupils are equal, round, and reactive to light. Neck: normal range of motion and phonation. No tracheal deviation present. No mass and no thyromegaly present. Neck is supple. Carotid bruit is not present.

- Cardiovascular: Normal rate, regular rhythm, normal heart sounds, and intact distal pulses. Examination reveals no gallop or friction rub. No murmur. No pedal edema, capillary refill brisk.
- Pulmonary: Effort normal and breath sounds normal. No respiratory distress. He has no wheezes. He exhibits no tenderness. No CVA tenderness. No scapular pain, negative Boas sign.
- Gastrointestinal: Soft. Normal appearance and bowel sounds. He exhibits no distension and no mass. No abdominal hernia present. Negative Murphy sign. There is no hepatomegaly. There is no splenomegaly. There is no tenderness. No abdominal hernia present. There is no rebound, no guarding.
- Integumentary: Jaundiced. Skin is warm and dry. Scratches and excoriation primarily present on back, and bilateral arms. No lesions or rash. No clubbing, no cyanosis.
- Musculoskeletal: Normal range of motion. He exhibits no edema and no tenderness.
- Neurological: He is alert and oriented to person, place, and time. He has normal strength. No cranial nerve deficit or sensory deficit.
- Lymphatic: No cervical or supraclavicular adenopathy. No inguinal adenopathy present.
- Psychiatric: He has a normal mood and affect. His speech is normal and behavior appropriate. Judgment and thought content normal.

ECOG score[5] = 1: Restricted in physically strenuous activity but ambulatory and able to carry out work of a light or sedentary nature, for example, light house work, office work (see Box 50-1).

Results of Preliminary Laboratory Tests

- Complete blood count: normal white blood cell count, normal platelet count, hemoglobin 12 (14.0–18.0 g/dL), hematocrit 35 (40%–50%), RBC 4.0 (4.6–6.2 M/μL)
- Basic metabolic panel: normal with the exception of glucose of 350 (74–99 mg/dL)
- Hepatic panel: Total bilirubin 19 (0.3–1.8 mg/dL); direct (conjugated) bilirubin: 15 (0.0–0.20 mg/dL); alkaline phosphatase 390 (40–150 U/L); AST (SGOT) 150 (<35 U/L); ALT (SGPT) 440 (<55 U/L); and albumin is normal
- Amylase and lipase within normal limits
- Protime/INR normal
- UA: positive trace ketones; large bilirubin; negative nitrites, bacteria, white cells
- Hepatitis screen: negative

BOX 50-1   ECOG Performance Status

These scales and criteria are used by doctors and researchers to assess how a patient's disease is progressing, assess how the disease affects the daily living abilities of the patient, and determine appropriate treatment and prognosis. They are included here for health care professionals to access.

ECOG Performance Status[a]	
Grade	**ECOG**
0	Fully active, able to carry on all predisease performance without restriction
1	Restricted in physically strenuous activity but ambulatory and able to carry out work of a light or sedentary nature, eg, light house work, office work
2	Ambulatory and capable of all self-care but unable to carry out any work activities. Up and about more than 50% of waking hours
3	Capable of only limited self-care, confined to bed or chair more than 50% of waking hours
4	Completely disabled. Cannot carry on any self-care. Totally confined to bed or chair
5	Dead

[a]Used with permission from Oken MM, Creech RH, Tormey DC, et al. Toxicity and response criteria of the Eastern Cooperative Oncology Group. *Am J Clin Oncol.* 1982;5:649-655. http://www.npcrc.org/files/news/ECOG_performance_status.pdf.

The ECOG Performance Status is in the public domain therefore available for public use. To duplicate the scale, please cite the reference above and credit the Eastern Cooperative Oncology Group, Robert Comis M.D., Group Chair.

> **What elements of the review of systems and the physical examination should be added to the list of pertinent positives? Which items should be added to the list of significant negatives?**

- **Pertinent positives:** Icteric sclera, skin excoriation. Nocturia. Hyperglycemia. Elevated conjugated bilirubin and liver function tests. Trace ketones, bilirubin in urine.

- **Significant negatives:** Abdominal examination normal, specifically no hepatomegaly, no right upper quadrant or abdominal tenderness with palpation or percussion, and negative Murphy sign. He denies fever, chills, and diaphoresis. His vital signs are stable, and he is not febrile at the time of presentation to the ED. Normal hepatitis panel, normal amylase and lipase, he is not anemic, he does not have leukocytosis, his PT, INR, and albumin are normal. His intrinsic liver function appears to be intact based on the normal INR and albumin levels.

Case Analysis: This additional information adds some key pieces to the puzzle. While the nocturia is likely related to his ongoing benign prostatic hypertrophy and perhaps his hyperglycemia, it is unlikely to be related to his other presenting symptoms. His excoriated skin and icteric sclera, however, are signs of jaundice. Based on his lab results, I confirm that he has conjugated hyperbilirubinemia. (Note: Total bilirubin and conjugated bilirubin levels are derived from serum or blood measurement. The difference of the total bilirubin level from the conjugated level equals the unconjugated bilirubin level.) To further support this, the patient is not anemic so he is not undergoing hemolysis that would contribute to unconjugated hyperbilirubinemia. From his hepatitis screen, I know he has not been exposed to viral hepatitis. The patient's normal abdominal examination along with his normal white blood cell count makes infection, such as cholecystitis or cholangitis, less likely. Acute and chronic pancreatitis is ruled out by the normal amylase and lipase levels; however, autoimmune pancreatitis remains a possibility.

The patient's profound fatigue, jaundice, elevated transaminases, and bilirubinuria are all definitive signs and symptoms of cholestasis and an obstructive process. His intrinsic liver function is intact, indicated by the normal protime and albumin.

❓ How does the additional information affect the problem representation?

I reexamine my problem representation and determine the following: "a 70-year-old diabetic male presents with jaundice, worsening fatigue, nausea, and weight loss. Early satiety, abdominal bloating, and epigastric/mid-back aching are also present. He denies fever or chills. His WBC is not elevated. He reports tea-colored urine and acholic stools. He complains of pruritus and skin excoriation. His liver enzymes are elevated and bilirubin is 19, consistent with cholestasis and obstruction." I believe that a malignancy or the blockage of the common bile duct and/or pancreatic duct with a mass is highly probable. Further diagnostic testing is essential to proceed with confirming or refuting my assumption.

❓ Given the new information what diagnostic testing should be done and in what order?

His obstructive jaundice remains the immediate problem and in conjunction with his subacute abdominal discomfort warrants diagnostic imaging and additional laboratory studies.

I must decide if a transabdominal ultrasound or CT scan should be ordered. In this case, he has no acute pain per se or clear-cut clinical signs directing me toward cholecystitis, cholangitis, or gallstones. Nevertheless, the presence of epigastric discomfort, jaundice, and my inclination that a mass may be present necessitates imaging. Acute right upper quadrant abdominal discomfort, clinical signs and symptoms indicative of gallbladder concerns including a positive Murphy sign, and/or an elevated white blood cell count denote the need for an abdominal ultrasound to evaluate for cholecystitis. Cholecystitis is best imaged by ultrasound and hepatobiliary iminodiacetic acid (HIDA) scanning. The HIDA scan though sensitive has low specificity and utilizes ionizing radiation; it is best utilized in addition to ultrasound when findings are unclear for cholecystitis. For jaundice, the transabdominal ultrasound can identify biliary tract dilation, area of obstruction, and pancreatic masses. It can further characterize the cholestasis as intrahepatic or extrahepatic. CT is also a possibility; however, it exposes the patient to unnecessary radiation. The safest and most cost-effective initial study for acute cholecystitis and jaundice is a transabdominal ultrasound. A CT scan and/or MRI can be ordered based on results of the ultrasound.

CASE INFORMATION

His ultrasound reveals a discrete pancreatic mass and ductal dilation (extra-hepatic cholestasis), and no gallstones or gallbladder abnormalities were visualized. Based on these results, a triphasic or pancreatic protocol CT scan is ordered to provide detailed cross-sectional imaging and evaluation of surrounding vasculature and possible invasion. This course of imaging in comparison with non-pancreas protocol CT scans has resulted in disease staging and patient management modifications.[6]

The scan demonstrates hydropic or watery fluid around the gallbladder, which is generally the consequence of chronic obstruction or narrowing of the cystic duct. Both the common bile duct and pancreatic duct are dilated and there is an ill-defined 3 × 2 cm solid mass at the pancreatic head. The mass effect of the tumor is causing dilation of the ducts and subsequent jaundice. No hepatic metastases or lymphadenopathy is present, and the pancreas appears normal in size and shape. The mass appears to be involved with aspects of the surrounding vasculature.

Case Analysis: Based on these imaging studies, the differential diagnosis is now narrowed to include pancreatic cancer, pancreatic neuroendocrine tumor, autoimmune pancreatitis, and rarely lymphoma or a metastatic cancer. I previously ruled out acute/chronic pancreatitis with normal amylase and lipase results; however, autoimmune pancreatitis does not always demonstrate these elevations. This is an important distinction to make as autoimmune pancreatitis can present as a pancreatic mass or obstructive jaundice, which can result in the erroneous presumption of pancreatic cancer. The treatments and prognosis are divergently different; the gold standard for a potential cure for pancreatic cancer is surgery and the recommended treatment for autoimmune pancreatitis is glucocorticoids. The radiologic feature of autoimmune pancreatitis on CT is the diffuse yet distinct "sausage" shape enlargement of the pancreas. The parenchyma of the pancreas on his CT scan is normal other than the presence of the mass. The presumption of a malignancy is even higher on my differential. I can order serum IgG subclasses to ensure there is no IgG4 elevation, which would be indicative of autoimmune pancreatitis. Pancreatic lymphoma is rare, but to further rule this out, I can order a lactic dehydrogenase (LDH), anticipating that this would be elevated in the presence of lymphoma. I doubt this mass represents metastasis as the patient has no prior history of cancer, but there could be an undiagnosed primary site. Pancreatic metastases are rare and most often result from a renal malignancy but can occur as a consequence of colorectal, melanoma, breast, or lung malignancy.[7] At this point, I strongly suspect this mass is primary pancreatic cancer or a pancreatic neuroendocrine tumor which seems less likely based on the imaging appearance and characteristics.

Diagnosis and Management: Pancreatic Head Mass With Obstructive Cholestasis

A mass at the head of the pancreas requires further testing and evaluation to direct treatment, including possible surgical intervention. Cancer markers including carbohydrate antigen 19-9 (CA 19-9) and carcinoembryonic antigen (CEA) help determine the nature of this mass. While CA 19-9 and CEA are both antigens and so may or may not be elevated in pancreatic cancer, they can play a role in evaluating and monitoring the patient's response to chemotherapy, chemoradiation, or surgery. They serve to help detect disease, inform about prognosis and recurrence, and predict treatment response.[8] Neither antigen can be used alone to diagnose or screen for pancreatic cancer as there are noncancerous conditions that can result in elevations of these levels. I will also check hemoglobin A1C (HgbA1C) because he does not routinely check his blood sugars and his glucose level was significantly elevated on the BMP.

After obtaining these additional lab studies, the next step is an endoscopic retrograde cholangiopancreatography (ERCP), which has both therapeutic and diagnostic rationale. During this procedure, a stent can be placed in the common bile duct to relieve the obstruction and allow the flow of bile, improving symptoms of jaundice and pruritus. In addition, ductal brushings are collected for biopsy. A fine-needle aspiration (FNA) of the mass can be performed with endoscopic ultrasound guidance. This is the preferred approach because percutaneous FNA carries the risk of peritoneal seeding, and because the endoscopic ultrasound allows evaluation of the size and position of the mass, nearby blood vessels, and anatomic structures.[9] These findings in conjunction with the pancreatic protocol CT determine the surgical resectability of the mass. The type and degree of the tumor involvement locally and regionally, and in particular with respect to surrounding vasculature, are key considerations.

The National Comprehensive Cancer Network (NCCN) has specific guidelines for hepatobiliary cancers, pancreatic adenocarcinoma, and neuroendocrine tumors of the pancreas.[10-12] In actuality, NCCN guidelines recommend pancreatic protocol CT or MRI as preferred imaging for pancreatic adenocarcinoma workup, or both CT and MRI in high-risk patients for additional assistance in staging. The guidelines also include recommendations for multiphasic contrast-enhanced CT or MRI for pancreatic neuroendocrine tumors. Once biopsy results are available, an institution's tumor review board can offer additional guidance for treatment. While surgical resection is the gold standard for potential cure of pancreatic cancer, patients may require early treatment with chemotherapy or radiation before surgery. Only a small proportion of diagnosed patients are eligible for surgery. Some may be unresectable.

Case Follow-Up

His lab results show a normal CEA level (0.0–2.5 ng/mL nonsmoker; 0.0–5.0 ng/mL smoker), but an elevated adjusted CA 19-9 level of over 250 U/mL (normal is <37 U/mL). This value is adjusted for jaundice by dividing the reported value by the serum bilirubin. Levels greater than 100 U/mL have been linked with higher probability of advanced disease.[13] His IgG4 level is normal at 61.0 (2.4–121 mg/dL) and this in conjunction with previous CT imaging rules out autoimmune pancreatitis.

He undergoes endoscopic retrograde cholangiopancreatography (ERCP) with stent placement to relieve his ductal obstruction, and fine-needle aspiration samples are obtained with endoscopic ultrasound (EUS) from the observed 3.3 cm mass in the head of his pancreas. These results show adenocarcinoma of the pancreas, which confirms that this mass is not lymphoma, neuroendocrine tumor, or a metastasis from another site. He is deemed borderline resectable because of the degree of vasculature involvement. His case is presented and discussed at the multidisciplinary gastrointestinal tumor board and chemoradiation with capecitabine is recommended prior to undergoing surgery. The patient and family meet with the hematology oncology and radiation oncology services while in the hospital and agree to this plan.

Prior to discharging him home, there are three essential considerations. First, I ensure that he has follow-up care that includes checking his liver function tests and bilirubin. These values should return to normal over time now that the stent is in place. He recently retired to the area and has not yet established any local health care providers, so a referral and an appointment with a primary care provider are made for him.

The second issue with this patient is his diabetes. While new onset diabetes or a sudden change in previously well-managed diabetes may be signs of pancreatic cancer, he fits neither category; he has been a diabetic for over 5 years and chosen not to routinely check his blood sugars. Evaluating his diabetes is vital as we consider future surgery, since this impacts his risk for infection and potential for delayed wound healing. His hemoglobin A1c is 9.9%, indicating an average blood glucose of 240 mg/dL, and well above the goal of 7% or less set by the American Diabetes Association.[14] I need to help him better manage his blood glucose and encourage him to do so. The third consideration is boosting his nutritional intake and stabilizing his weight loss. His presenting signs and symptoms of nausea and loose stools have lessened or resolved since the stent placement. His bowel movements are transitioning to a brown color, and he does not require pancreatic enzyme supplementation for steatorrhea. I order a nutrition consult prior to discharge and he is scheduled for further follow-up by phone as an outpatient for guidance and assistance. Again, this is particularly important in preparation for potential surgery.

He has a restaging abdominal scan (CT or MRI) 4 weeks following the completion of his chemoradiation. He meets with me and our surgery team and we discuss the findings of his MRI. The tumor is deemed resectable and pancreaticoduodenectomy or Whipple procedure is recommended. Following verbal and written consent for surgery and preoperative clearance with cardiology, he proceeds to complete screening and evaluation with the preanesthesia team. His chest x-ray is with negative findings and his laboratory results and ECG are unremarkable. Fatigue is his primary complaint and this is common in patients with his diagnosis; he reports no other health status changes or decline. His functional or ECOG status (=1) remains consistent. He undergoes diagnostic laparoscopy to evaluate for possible subradiologic metastases, and assuming there is no evidence of advancing malignant disease, he then undergoes pancreaticoduodenectomy or Whipple procedure including vein excision and repair.

References

1. Roche SP, Kobos R. Jaundice in the adult patient. *Am Fam Physician.* January 15, 2004; 69(2):299-304. http://www.aafp.org/afp/2004/0115/p299.html.
2. Diagnostic approach to the adult with jaundice or asymptomatic hyperbilirubinemia. UpToDate Web site. http://www.uptodate.com/contents/diagnostic-approach-to-the-adult-with-jaundice-or-asymptomatic-hyperbilirubinemia. Updated January 29, 2014. Accessed September 27, 2014.
3. Chalasani NP, Hayashi PH, Bonkovsky HL, Navarro VJ, Lee WM, Fontana RJ. ACG clinical guideline: the diagnosis and management of idiosyncratic drug-induced liver injury. *Am J Gastroenterol.* 2014;109:950-966. doi:10.1038/ajg.2014.131.
4. US National Library of Medicine/National Institutes of Health. Medications that cause abnormal liver tests. http://livertox.nlm.nih.gov. Updated November 4, 2014. Accessed November 10, 2014.
5. Oken MM, Creech RH, Tormey DC, et al. Toxicity and response criteria of the Eastern Cooperative Oncology Group. *Am J Clin Oncol.* 1982;5:649-655. http://www.npcrc.org/files/news/ECOG_performance_status.pdf.
6. Walters DM, Lapar DJ, de Lange EE, et al. Pancreas-protocol imaging at a high-volume center leads to improved preoperative staging of pancreatic ductal adenocarcinoma. *Ann Surg Oncol.* 2011; 18:2764-2771. http://www.ncbi.nlm.nih.gov/pubmed/21484522.
7. Sperti C, Moletta L, Patane G. Metastatic tumors to the pancreas: the role of surgery. *World J Gastrointest Oncol.* October 15, 2014;6(10):381-392. doi: 10.4251/wjgo.v6.i10.381.
8. Morris-Stiff G, Taylor MA. CA 19-9 and pancreatic cancer: is it really that good? *J Gastrointest Oncol.* 2012;3:88-89. http://www.ncbi.nlm.nih.gov/pubmed/22811875.
9. Karachristos A, Scarmeas N, Hoffman JP. CA 19-9 levels predict results of staging laparoscopy in pancreatic cancer. *J Gastrointest Surg.* 2005;9:1286-1292. http://www.ncbi.nlm.nih.gov/pubmed/16332484.
10. National Comprehensive Cancer Network. NCCN guidelines version 2.2014: hepatobiliary cancers. http://www.nccn.org/professionals/physician_gls/pdf/hepatobiliary.pdf. Published April 1, 2014. Accessed September 29, 2014.
11. National Comprehensive Cancer Network. NCCN guidelines version 2.2014: pancreatic adenocarcinoma. http://www.nccn.org/professionals/physcian_gls/pdf/pancreatic.pdf. Published May 27, 2014. Accessed September 29, 2014.
12. National Comprehensive Cancer Network. NCCN guideline version 1.2015: neuroendocrine tumors of the pancreas. http://www.nccn.org/professionals/physician_gls/pdf/neuroendocrine.pdf. Published November 11, 2014. Accessed December 2, 2014.
13. Micames C, Jowell PS, White R, et al. Lower frequency of peritoneal carcinomatosis in patients with pancreatic cancer diagnosed by EUS-guided FNA vs. percutaneous FNA. *Gastrointest Endosc.* 2003;58:690-695. http://www.ncbi.nlm.nih.gov/pubmed/14595302.
14. American Diabetes Association. Standards of medical care in diabetes—2014. *Diabetes Care.* 2014;37(suppl 1):S14-S80. doi: 10.2337/dc14-S014.

CASE 51

Theresa R. (Roxie) Huyett

Theresa R. (Roxie) Huyett is an ACNP in a 12-bed cardiothoracic postoperative ICU at the University of Virginia. Roxie has more than 30 years of experience in caring for the critical care cardiac surgery population.

CASE INFORMATION

Chief Complaint

A 34-year-old female on veno-venous extracorporeal membrane oxygenation (V-V ECMO) for severe hypoxic respiratory failure due to influenza A develops sudden onset of hypotension, hypothermia, and leukocytosis.

Differential Diagnoses for ICU Patient With Hypothermia, Hypotension, and Leukocytosis[1]

Most Common Infectious Causes

- Bacterial: bacteremia, intravascular catheter–related infection, surgical site infection, ventilator-associated pneumonia, sepsis of urinary origin, abdominal or pelvic abscess, *Clostridium difficile* infection, endocarditis, sinusitis, dental abscess
- Viral: HIV, hepatitis, cytomegalovirus, Epstein-Barr virus
- Fungal or parasitic: fungemia, toxoplasmosis, *Giardia*
- Infectious complications of postpartum state: breast abscess, pelvic inflammatory disease, tubo-ovarian abscess

Common Noninfectious Causes

Acalculous cholecystitis, adrenal insufficiency, hypothyroidism, deep vein thrombosis, medication side effect, pancreatitis, thyroid storm or hypothyroidism, pheochromocytoma, transfusion reaction, leukemia, lymphoma, metastatic carcinoma, lupus, rheumatoid arthritis, sarcoidosis

---

CASE INFORMATION

History of Present Illness

This is a 34-year-old female, current smoker, who was discharged home after a C-section delivery of a healthy infant. This was her first pregnancy and it was complicated by preeclampsia. No surgical complications were noted and full and complete removal of the placenta was accomplished.

On her third postpartpartum day she began experiencing symptoms of an upper respiratory infection and presented to an outside hospital's emergency room with shortness of breath. Her chest x-ray showed diffuse bilateral alveolar infiltrates and her PaO_2/FiO_2 was ≤100, which meets the Berlin criteria definition of severe acute respiratory distress syndrome (ARDS).[2] She was intubated and admitted to the intensive care unit. Supportive care with mechanical ventilation and 3 days of prone positioning was provided but her hypoxemia did not improve. She was transferred to our university medical center for the purpose of providing extracorporeal membrane oxygenation (ECMO) for her severe ARDS. I assumed care of the patient upon admission to the thoracic-cardiovascular unit.

On the day of admission she was sedated and paralyzed and ECMO was initiated. Multiple vasopressors were required to support her blood pressure. Baseline admission labs including blood cultures were drawn and a chest x-ray obtained. She was in anuric renal failure and was started on continuous renal replacement therapy (CRRT). On the second day, she required transfusion of packed red blood cells, platelets, cryoprecipitate, and fresh frozen plasma and was empirically started on intravenous steroids for potential adrenal insufficiency. The referring hospital reported that her influenza A test had come back positive. On day 3 of veno-venous ECMO (V-V ECMO), she became more hypotensive, requiring increasing doses of vasopressors. She was also hypothermic, tachycardic, and her white blood cell count (WBC) showed a new leukocytosis. These signs were concerning as I recognized that, in combination, they meet the definition of septic shock (ie, systemic inflammatory response syndrome [SIRS] + presumed source of infection + organ dysfunction, hypotension, or hypoperfusion).

Past Medical History

The patient's record from the outside hospital shows that the family reports no history of diabetes, heart disease, cancer, or lung disease. They are not aware of any autoimmune disorders, kidney disease, or liver disease. She was in good health except for a pregnancy complicated by preeclampsia. The patient's family also denies any surgical procedures, prior to the C-section. The only prescribed medication she was taking prior to admission was a prenatal vitamin.

Social History

The patient does have a history of smoking. Previously she was smoking 1 pack per day but cut back to several cigarettes per day during her pregnancy. The family reports no alcohol or illicit substance use. She lives with her spouse and has no prior pregnancies.

Medication List

• Ipratropium bromide/albuterol inhaled (Duoneb) every 6 hours through endotracheal tube

- Methylprednisolone sodium succinate (Solu-Medrol) 10 mg continuous IV infusion over 24 hours (first day of admission to unit)
- Heparin IV infusion at 1500 U/h
- Hydromorphone (Dilaudid) 4 mg/h continuous IV infusion
- Ketamine 0.4 mg/kg/h continuous IV infusion
- Midazolam (Versed) 12 mg/h continuous infusion
- Rocuronium 4 µg/kg/min
- Intravenous vasopressors: norepinephrine and vasopressin titrated to achieve mean arterial blood pressure (MAP) of 60 to 70. Epinephrine added on hospital day 3 due to low blood pressure

Case Analysis: Signs of septic shock, such as the ones present in this patient, are particularly confounding in a paralyzed and sedated patient because any subjective data such as a complaint of pain, which may help sort the differential diagnosis, are absent. Thus I must carefully proceed through a list of possible conditions, taking into consideration both the most likely causes and the most life threatening.

Given the complexity and unstable nature of this young V-V ECMO patient, it is critical to intervene as quickly as possible. After initiating fluid resuscitation to maintain her blood pressure and decreasing the rate of her CRRT so the additional volume is retained, I begin gathering data to address the differential diagnosis. In this situation, despite my ongoing familiarity with all details of this complex patient, my first step is to perform a new, meticulous comprehensive, physical examination. No physical finding can be assumed to be unchanged, and any objective information that suggests a change in her condition is of greater importance since I do not have any subjective data I can apply. With a thorough physical examination, even tiny variations can present new and important findings, leading to diagnostic clues. In addition, a review of all current laboratory and imaging data is essential.

CASE INFORMATION
Physical Examination

- Vital signs: Pulse is 120 beats per minute, BP is 96/50 mm Hg, respiratory rate is 20 breaths per minute, which is the set rate on the ventilator, temperature is 35.2°C (95.3°F), oxygen saturation by pulse oximeter is 100% (ECMO and mechanical ventilation), fingerstick blood glucose is 130.

- Constitutional: Caucasian female who appears her documented age. Eyes closed, not moving. Facial features are symmetric. She appears well nourished, markedly flushed in face and upper torso.
- Head/eyes/ears/nose/throat: Head normocephalic with normal hair distribution. #7.5 Endotracheal tube in oral position. Native dentition. Moist buccal mucosa. Review of nursing notes shows that oral care consistent with guidelines for preventing ventilator- associated pneumonia is documented. Head of bed cannot be elevated due to the unstable status of the patient and presence of ECMO catheter which is positional. To minimize aspiration, reverse Trendelenburg position is used, maintaining a 30° head of bed elevation equivalent.
- Cardiovascular: Heart rate regular, tachycardia. No murmurs, rubs, or gallops. Trace edema equally present in ankles bilaterally. V-V ECMO as above, via right internal jugular extracorporeal bicaval dual lumen catheter with pulmonary artery catheter, intravenous infusions, and fluid resuscitation in left jugular vein. Right femoral arterial line. CRRT piggybacked to ECMO circuit, running to maintain hourly output even with intake.
- Extremities: 2+ palpable pulses—dorsalis pedis and posterior tibial bilaterally. Nail beds pink. Skin warm and dry.
- Pulmonary: On V-V ECMO 100% FiO_2. On pressure-regulated, volume-controlled mechanical ventilation, settings are FiO_2 = 100%, PEEP = 10, tidal volume = 6 mL/kg for lung protection. On auscultation, diffuse crackles without wheezes or rhonchi throughout lung fields bilaterally.
- Gastrointestinal: Tube feedings at goal with small-bore nasojejunal feeding tube. Abdomen soft and round, absent bowel sounds. No palpable masses, no palpable uterine fundus. No diarrhea.
- Genitourinary: Foley catheter with a scant amount of dark yellow urine, on CRRT, no vaginal discharge.
- Breast examination: No breast swelling, no masses, no areas of redness or warmth noted.
- Integumentary: Multiple access lines as above, no redness, warmth, or discharge at insertion sites, sterile dressings clean dry and intact, and in date. Abdominal surgical wound—well approximated, no drainage, staples in place, surrounding skin is pink, cool to touch, no redness, no swelling.
- Neurological: Chemically paralyzed and sedated. Bispectral index (BIS) sensor on forehead; BIS score 40. Train of four elicits two out of four muscle twitches. Pupils 2 mm and sluggishly reactive bilaterally.

Review of Diagnostic Testing Results—Day 3

Chest x-ray done on morning of day 3: bilateral alveolar infiltrates unchanged from admission, consistent with severe ARDS.

> *Laboratory Results (Morning of Day 3):*
> - Sodium: 137 mEq/L (135–147 mEq/L)
> - Potassium: 3.9 mEq/L (3.5–5.2 mEq/L)
> - Chloride: 101 (95–107 mEq/L)
> - Carbon dioxide: 26 mEq/L (23–28 mmEq)
> - Blood urea nitrogen (BUN): 16 mg/dL (7–20 mg/dL)
> - Creatinine: 1.6 mg/dL (0.5–1.4 mg/dL)
> - Total bilirubin: 1.8 mg/dL (0.1–1.2 mg/dL)
> - Alkaline phosphatase, alanine aminotransferase, aspartate aminotransferase all within normal limits
> - Amylase: 44 U/L (normal 25–125 U/L), lipase: 124 U/L (normal 8–78 U/L)
> - Complete blood count (CBC) within normal limits except white blood cell count (WBC) of 14,000 cells/µL (4,500–10,000 cells/µL)
> - Repeat CBC and coagulation studies drawn every 4 hours, values varied but were consistent with a patient on ECMO receiving ongoing blood products in the presence of full systemic heparinization to prevent clotting of ECMO circuit
> - Blood cultures drawn on admission are negative to date

? What are the pertinent positives that help sort out the potential causes of this patient's hypotension, hypothermia, and leukocytosis?

- Recent pregnancy
- Recent abdominal surgery (C-section)
- Chest x-ray shows ARDS pattern
- Lab: positive for influenza A
- Presence of multiple large-bore invasive arterial and venous lines, as well as Foley catheter and endotracheal tube, V-V ECMO
- Received packed red blood cells, platelets, cryoprecipitate, and fresh frozen plasma within last 48 hours
- Mechanically ventilated
- Elevated WBC
- Elevated total bilirubin, creatinine, and lipase

? What are the significant negatives?

- Chest x-ray shows no new changes, making new pneumonia or pleural effusions less likely

- No indications of vaginal or breast infection
- Blood cultures drawn at the outside facility and on admission to my facility are negative to date
- No obvious skin interruption except invasive lines (limited to anterior of body due to inability to turn)

❓ Can the information gathered so far be restated in a single sentence highlighting the pieces that narrow down the cause?

The problem representation in this case is: A critically ill 34-year-old post-partum female on ECMO for severe ARDS develops new signs of septic shock.

Case Analysis: Although the physical examination does not indicate a source of infection, my findings along with my review of recent diagnostics do help me quickly prioritize the diagnostic studies I need to obtain. The most likely sources of infection include line-related bloodstream infection, sepsis of urinary origin, or pneumonia from intubation and mechanical ventilation. These items are the first to rule out, both because they are most likely and they are life threatening. The gold standard for the diagnosis of bacterial infection is identification of organisms by culture, usually blood, urine, and sputum.[4] These cultures can take up to 72 hours before they are fully grown and read, but a positive result is sometimes available sooner. Given the severity of this patient's illness, I immediately order new percutaneous blood cultures, which is the preferred method of obtaining cultures at my institution. I also request a urine culture from her Foley catheter. The chest x-ray does not show evidence of a new pneumonia; however, radiographic changes can lag behind changes in the patient's clinical condition. After discussion with the ICU team, a diagnostic bronchoscopy is performed, a bronchoalveolar lavage (BAL) is done and samples are sent for culture to rule out a respiratory infection. It is possible that she has a postinfluenza, aspiration, or ventilator-associated pneumonia and this will help identify the causative organisms.

In addition to common sources of infection in ICU patients, I must also consider infections related to her recent pregnancy and C-section. These include vaginal, breast, or intraoperative site infections. Because her C-section was accomplished without intraoperative complications, the possibility of infection from retained remains of the placenta is low. Potential infections such as mastitis or a vaginitis are not supported by her examination. Her C-section incision shows no signs of redness or swelling. These sources of infection cannot be eliminated but are lower on my differential at this time. Regardless, if I cannot identify an actual source of infection, I will consult obstetrics/gynecology to help me further evaluate her gynecologic status. I am also concerned with her elevated lipase and total bilirubin, both of which can be elevated with cholecystitis. I will keep this on my differential.

Empiric antibiotic coverage is appropriate in a patient with hemodynamic instability while awaiting culture results. After blood, urine, and sputum cultures are obtained, I order broad-spectrum antibiotic coverage: vancomycin 1 g intravenously, dose to be adjusted based on trough levels, to cover

Staphylococcus including MRSA, and piperacillin/tazobactam 3.375 g intravenously every 6 hours, to cover gram-positive and gram-negative organisms, specifically *Pseudomonas*. Once I receive the culture results, I can narrow or broaden the antibiotic regimen to specifically cover the source of her infection.[4] To address her hemodynamic instability, I continue fluid resuscitation in accordance with the guidelines of the Society of Critical Care Medicine[3] and ensure that the CRRT is running to maintain an even intake and output.

While infection is my chief concern, there are other potential noninfectious causes for the changes in the patient's condition that I must consider and that are on my differential. I will focus initially on the ones that are most likely and emergent. Potential adrenal insufficiency was treated with steroids on day 1 of admission to our unit and there was no positive response. Deep vein thrombosis is possible and may need to be further evaluated with Doppler ultrasound but is less likely given her state of anticoagulation. Pancreatitis is generally identified by the patient's complaints of abdominal pain and an elevated amylase and lipase. Her lipase is elevated so this is higher on my differential list now until I can eliminate it with additional diagnostic studies.[4]

Another noninfectious cause is a delayed atypical transfusion reaction. Generally these reactions are more mild than an immediate acute hemolytic transfusion reaction (AHTR) response and may be identified by elevations in LDH and bilirubin, and a positive direct antiglobulin test. Because she was recently transfused, this may represent a delayed, atypical transfusion reaction but signs are often subtle and due to her sedated and paralyzed state will be difficult to determine. I will consider this possibility, however, as I quickly try to move through other likely causes. Transfusion-related acute lung injury (TRALI) is a possible reason for her pulmonary condition but the ARDS diagnosis emerged at the referring hospital prior to the transfusions. While either diagnosis could contribute to her current deterioration, her lung status is severe but stable.

The patient could also have more than one condition causing her symptoms; for instance, the leukocytosis may be a side effect of starting her on methylprednisolone (Solumedrol) and her hypothermia could be the result of a hypothyroid state. I cannot eliminate either possibility yet. At this point, based on her age and history, I am less concerned about a malignant process or an autoimmune process.[4] These conditions tend not to present emergently and are less likely than septic shock in an ICU patient. I must look for a source of infection so I can treat appropriately and quickly as she is very ill.

❓ What diagnostic tests would be done next and in what order?

In determining additional diagnostic testing and interventions, the severity of the patient's illness is a key consideration. For instance, ordinarily, a patient with evidence of septic shock undergoes replacement of existing invasive lines because these lines are so frequently the source of infection. In the case of this patient, she cannot tolerate this procedure because it would require stopping the V-V ECMO and the CRRT for the duration of the line change. Similarly

I would normally consider a computed tomography (CT) scan of her abdomen, which would rule out, or rule in, several of the diagnoses on my list including colitis, ischemic bowel, and abdominal/pelvic abscess. However, in this patient, I have to weigh the risks and benefits of sending her off the unit for further diagnostic imaging. Though transporting an ECMO patient to the radiology department is possible, the safety of transporting an unstable patient with an enormous amount of equipment is weighed against the benefit of doing so. I determine the risk to be high and I do not pursue CT imaging at this time. I do order a bedside echocardiogram (ECHO) to rule out endocarditis; the risk-benefit ratio favors doing this test. The ECHO has few risks because it does not require stopping any of her current therapies and the benefit of diagnosing and treating endocarditis is high. Similarly I order a right upper quadrant ultrasound to check the patient's gallbladder, as cholecystitis is high on my list. The risks of doing this test are very low as it is noninvasive and can be done at the bedside.

I also repeat a metabolic profile, CBC with differential, and a lipase since it was slightly elevated on day 3 and at this point we have no explanation for why this may be. Possible reasons for elevated lipase include pancreatitis, tumors of the pancreas or stomach, a gallbladder infection, and in some cases kidney failure. Because lipase is generally very high in acute pancreatitis I am keeping this diagnosis on my list along with gallbladder disease, but at this point will just trend it with serial labs. I also order hemolysis labs (LDH, direct antiglobulin test, and haptoglobin) to rule out transfusion reaction.

CASE INFORMATION

Results of Diagnostics

The echocardiogram shows no signs of valve disease or vegetation that would indicate endocarditis. The right upper quadrant ultrasound shows a patent biliary tree and no evidence of sludge or gallbladder disease. While both the initial and subsequent cultures drawn at my facility continue to be free of growth, I receive a call from the outside hospital and learn that cultures drawn there show growth of yeast in one bottle out of four. This level of growth may represent contamination of the sample and not true infection; however, I start micafungin because I have not identified an alternative source of infection and the patient is extremely unstable.

The patient's hypothermia is managed by warming the ECMO and CRRT circuits and by placing a continuous airflow warming system blanket over her. She continues on vasopressors and fluid resuscitation to support her blood pressure. Laboratory findings are unremarkable (CBC stable; WBC, lipase, and total bilirubin all still elevated at previous levels; hemolysis labs negative, negative Coombs).

CASE INFORMATION

Over the next 2 days, with the interventions described above and empiric broad-spectrum antibiotic coverage, her temperature and blood pressure stabilize and her cultures, including blood, urine, and BAL, remain negative for any growth. I consult obstetrics/gynecology and am assured based on their assessment that the patient is not experiencing postpartum complications such as breast abscess or a tubo-ovarian abscess.

On day 6 of her admission, 72 hours after the start of broad-spectrum antibiotics, and 48 hours after starting antifungal therapy, the patient's WBC further rises to 21.4. The WBC differential is as follows:

Neutrophils 68.2% (54%–62%), lymphocytes 10.9% (24%–44%), monocytes 6.9% (3%–6%), eosinophils 1.0% (0%–3%), basophils 1.0% (0%–1%).

Differential absolute: neutrophil 11.5 cells/µL (normal 1.8–8 cells/µL), lymphocyte 1.84 cells/µL (1.0–5.0 cells/µL), monocyte 1.17 cells/µL (0–1.0 cells/µL), eosinophil 0.17 cells/µL (0–0.6 cells/µL), bands 12.6% (0–7).

Case Analysis: I return to my original differential because this patient's elevated WBC with a shift to the left leads me to believe that there may be a diagnosis I have missed. Her monocytes are slightly elevated. Generally elevations of monocytes are due to chronic infections. There is no change in either basophils (which are elevated with anaphylaxis) or her eosinophils (which elevate with allergic reactions). But bacterial infections cause neutrophilia with bandemia, which she now exhibits.[4] Based on the negative cultures, I do not believe she has a bacterial blood infection, sepsis of urinary origin, pneumonia, or even an atypical lung infection since her BAL was negative. Other sources of bacterial infection, such as dental abscess or sinusitis, ought to improve after 72 hours of treatment with broad-spectrum antibiotics. I doubt she has *Clostridium difficile* given the absence of any diarrhea. A new viral infection seems less likely, as her lymphocyte count is normal but she had a positive influenza A (H1N1) lab result at the other hospital and may still be experiencing the effects of the flu. She is on treatment for a fungal infection and is not improving. Persistent signs of infection when the most common sources are ruled out warrant an abdominal CT scan, and possibly a lumbar puncture depending on the symptoms the patient reports. However, this patient cannot report any symptoms and is too unstable to undergo abdominal CT scan, and her ECMO catheter will not function if she is repositioned for a lumbar puncture. So I will hold on pursuing these tests at present.

Looking at the noninfectious items on my list again, I can rule out adrenal insufficiency as the cause of her hypotension as her blood pressure actually dropped further after starting on steroid therapy. I can also rule out leukocytosis as a side effect of steroids because the level of elevation (ie, 21.4) is generally higher than seen with steroids alone and has not decreased since the discontinuation of the steroids following the initial infusion. Pheochromocytoma usually causes elevations in blood pressure, not a drop, and her relatively stable heart rate makes thyroid storm less likely. Persistence of her symptoms 4 days after transfusion and her negative hemolysis and immune reaction studies (negative Coombs) make transfusion reaction unlikely.[1]

While it will not yield the same level of detail that a CT scan can provide, an abdominal ultrasound is a safer alternative; it can be done at the bedside without stopping any of the treatments the patient is currently receiving. The abdominal ultrasound can yield additional information to rule out cholecystitis and possibly pancreatitis. I can also do blood work very easily and safely on this patient so I order thyroid studies and a repeat amylase and lipase to address the remaining noninfectious items on my differential, hypothyroidism and pancreatitis. If these tests are unrevealing and the symptoms persist, I may reconsider doing an abdominal CT scan.

CASE INFORMATION

Additional laboratory testing done on day 6 shows normal thyroid function but an elevated amylase and lipase, at 200 and 115 U/L, respectively. Prior to these study results, her lipase was just slightly elevated and her amylase was normal. A STAT abdominal ultrasound shows a diffusely enlarged pancreas with poor echogenicity, consistent with a diagnosis of pancreatitis.

Both amylase and lipase trended sharply upward with peaks of amylase 669 U/L and lipase of 653 U/L 3 days later.

Case Analysis: While the actual reason for this patient's septic shock is unclear, my patient is requiring extremely aggressive interventions to keep her alive. She may have had a fungal infection or a worsening of her flu; both possibilities are reasonable explanations for her critical state. And whether her newly diagnosed acute pancreatitis is the cause of her septic shock state or a complication of another condition that was not identified may continue to be a mystery. However, Akbar et al have reported on a phenomenon described as ECMO-related ischemic pancreatitis.[5] So, it is possible that the application of this technology is responsible for this patient's pancreatitis and the reason for her further deterioration on day 3. Regardless, she is still very unstable and must remain on ECMO for now.

Often the care of severely ill patients requires reasoned but extreme measures, some of which are not fully supported in the literature. The inherent instability of the patient's condition precludes many diagnostics (CT, MRI, etc), and thus hindered our ability to accurately determine the cause of her symptoms. Regardless, evidence-based guidelines such as those for the management of septic shock help ensure supportive measures are maximized.[3] With the new information confirming that this patient now has an acute pancreatitis, management will focus on ensuring that evidence-based interventions for the treatment of acute pancreatitis are accomplished.

Management of Sepsis and Acute Pancreatitis

Initial management of the patient with acute pancreatitis consists of supportive care with fluid resuscitation, pain control, and nutritional support. In the first 12 to 24 hours of acute pancreatitis, fluid replacement has been associated with a reduction in morbidity and mortality.[3,6] In this patient, fluid management is completely controlled via V-V ECMO with piggybacked CRRT. In addition, unlike the typical patient with pancreatitis, this patient has ARDS and avoiding excessive fluid, which would increase her pulmonary capillary leak, is the suggested strategy. However, her low blood pressure despite treatment with high-dose epinephrine at 15 µg/min, norepinephrine at 15 µg/min, and vasopressin at 0.12 U/min suggests the need for aggressive fluid resuscitation. I need to monitor her blood pressure, oxygen saturation, central venous pressure, and arterial blood gases closely as her fluid balance is really a dynamic process, and will require frequent adjustment of the CRRT.

This patient, like many ICU patients, is already on continuous infusions of a narcotic and a benzodiazepine to ensure that she is comfortable and to reduce oxygen demand. This patient also has a large ECMO catheter/cannula in the right internal jugular vein, requiring that the patient not move or be moved at all. For unknown reasons, this small adult female is requiring enormous amounts of narcotic, benzodiazepine infusions, and ketamine to maintain a BIS score of 40 to 60 (which is our unit guideline requirement for a chemically paralyzed patient). Based on the levels of pain medication dosages and her BIS score, I believe her pain control was adequate.

Nutrition support options for patients with pancreatitis are enteral feedings or parenteral nutrition.[7] Parenteral nutrition was the standard of nutritional management for nearly four decades based on the concept of "pancreatic rest" (ie, to decrease pancreatic activity and allow for recovery). However, critics argued that, in addition to cost and catheter-related sepsis, parenteral nutrition can lead to electrolyte and metabolic disturbances, as well as gastric mucosal barrier alteration, and increased intestinal permeability. Despite the benefit of enteral over parental nutrition in reducing the risk of infectious complications and mortality, the exact mechanism of its favorable effect remains unclear. Enteral nutrition may prevent or attenuate the mucosal barrier breakdown and subsequent bacterial translocation that plays a pivotal role in the development of infectious complications in the course of severe acute pancreatitis. The most notable and consistent improvement in outcomes over the last decade has come from the use of enteral nutrition in patients with acute pancreatitis. Eight randomized, controlled trials between 1997 and 2010 comparing total parental nutrition and total enteral nutrition in patients with severe acute pancreatitis demonstrated the benefits of enteral over parenteral nutrition.[7] With the benefits of enteral nutrition apparent, one of the unanswered questions is: What is the optimal site for tube placement during feeding administration? The options are prepyloric (bolus or continuous gastric feeding) or postpyloric (continuous feeding into the duodenum).[7] Postpyloric feedings may reduce the risk of aspiration, but placement of a postpyloric tube is more complicated and may delay the start of nutritional support.

My patient already has a postpyloric nasogastric small bore tube in place although her feedings are on hold due to her high vasopressor requirements and instability. The plan is to restart tube feeds when vasopressor requirement decreases.[7,8] Nasojejunal tube feedings beyond the ligament of Treitz are an acceptable option in acute pancreatitis.[7,8]

Case Follow-Up

We continued supportive care of this patient, allowing time for her pancreatitis to resolve. Twenty-four hours after the diagnosis was made and following increased fluid resuscitation, we were able to wean her high-dose vasopressors and initiate enteral tube feeding. Tube feedings were provided via nasojejunal small-bore feeding tube. Her serum amylase slowly trended down over a 10-day period. Her interstitial pulmonary edema due to ARDS resolved slowly over several weeks, and she was successfully weaned off V-V ECMO after 23 days of support. She was discharged to a long-term acute care hospital (LTAC) 3 months after admission, on minimal mechanical ventilator support. On discharge to the LTAC, her iatrogenic narcotic dependence was managed with enteral agents.

Prior to 2013, there is no report in the literature of ECMO-induced pancreatitis.[5] Due to timing and previous stability despite being on ECMO in this patient, there does appear that a cause-effect relationship exists between this patient's ECMO support and the development of acute pancreatitis. As a result of our experience and the report by Akbar et al, our unit does closely monitor (daily) amylase/lipase levels on all ECMO patients. Subsequent to our experience with this patient, a second patient developed pancreatits after initiating ECMO therapy. In this case the discovery of acute pancreatitis without the benefit of subjective reporting from the paralyzed/sedated patient was a diagnostic victory. The happy ending to our patient's story is that she was successfully discharged from the hospital to a long-term acute care hospital, and then discharged home 8 weeks later. Recently she walked into our ICU with her baby to visit those who had cared for her.

References

1. Fever in ICU. UpToDate Web site. http://www.uptodate.com/contents/fever-in-the-intensive-care-unit?source=machineLearning&search=fever+in+ICU&selectedTitle=1%7E150&sectionRank=1&anchor=H3#H3. Accessed September 19, 2014.
2. ARDS Definition Task Force. Acute respiratory distress syndrome. The Berlin definition. *JAMA.* 2012;307:2526-2533.

3. Dellinger RP, Levy MM, Rhodes A, et al. Surviving sepsis campaign: international guidelines for management of severe sepsis and septic shock. *Crit Care Med*. 2013;41:580-637.

4. Clinical presentation of leukocytosis. Medscape Web site. http://emedicine Medscape.com/article/956278-clinical. Accessed January 1, 2015.

5. Akbar A, Baron TH, Freese DK. Severe ischemic pancreatitis following the use of extracorporeal membrane oxygenation. *J Pediatr Gastroenterol Nutr*. 2013;55(6):144.

6. Clinical manifestations and diagnosis of acute pancreatitis. UpToDate Web site. http://www.uptodate.com/contents/clinical-manifestations-and-diagnosis-of-acute-pancreatitis?source=machineLearning&search=diagnostic+evaluation+of+acute+pancreatitis&selectedTitle=1%7E150&sectionRank=1&anchor=H26225963#H26225963.

7. Petrov, M. Nutrition, inflammation and acute pancreatitis. *ISRN Inflamm*. 2013, Dec 29;2013:341410. doi: 10.1155/2013/341410.

8. Management of acute pancreatitis. UpToDate Web site. http://www.uptodate.com/contents/management-of-acute-pancreatitis?source=machineLearning&search=managment+of+acute+pancreatitis&selectedTitle=1%7E150&sectionRank=2&anchor=H20#H20. Published September 2014. Updated April 8, 2014.

CASE 52

Donna Charlebois

Donna works in an electrophysiology clinic, Cardiology Urgent Clinic, as well as a cardiology interventional procedural unit.

CASE INFORMATION

Chief Complaint

A 54-year-old male presents to cardiology clinic with a chief complaint of worsening shortness of breath. He also notes fatigue and leg and abdominal swelling.

? What is the potential cause?

Dyspnea can be the presenting symptom for a long list of etiologies, from a life-threatening acute illness to an exacerbation of an ongoing chronic disease. As dyspnea can signify a life-threatening health crisis, I need to quickly evaluate and provide immediate intervention to ensure a positive outcome.

Differential Diagnoses for Life-Threatening Causes of Dyspnea

Pulmonary Causes
- Pulmonary embolism
- Chronic obstructive pulmonary disease (COPD)
- Asthma
- Pneumothorax or pneumomediastinum
- Pulmonary infection
- Adult respiratory distress syndrome
- Direct pulmonary injury

Cardiac Causes
- Acute coronary syndrome (ACS)
- Acute decompensated congestive heart failure (CHF)
- Flash pulmonary edema
- High-output heart failure
- Cardiomyopathy
- Cardiac arrhythmia
- Valvular dysfunction
- Cardiac tamponade

Neurological Causes
- Stroke
- Neuromuscular disease

Toxic and Metabolic Causes
- Poisoning
- Sepsis
- Anemia

CASE INFORMATION

History of Present Illness

J is a 54-year-old male with atrial fibrillation, a remote history of mediastinal seminoma and thyroid cancer treated with radiation, and a recent hospital admission with pericardial effusion who presents to the cardiology urgent clinic with worsening shortness of breath associated with new onset fatigue, leg swelling, and abdominal bloating. He reports the symptoms have developed over the past 3 days. His most concerning symptom is not being able to sleep due to increased dyspnea when lying on his left side or on his back. The dyspnea is also worse when he leans forward. He has no chest pain, pressure, or discomfort. He states that as soon as he closes his eyes the "air shuts off." He also feels like his body has been "heating up" and he wakes up diaphoretic when he does fall asleep. He reports bendopnea (shortness of breath when bending over). He states he has not had palpitations, racing heart, chest pain, nausea, vomiting, chills, light-headedness, or dysuria. He has had diarrhea, which he attributed to the colchicine prescribed following his recent hospital admission.

I review the medical records from the recent hospitalization and learn that he presented with chest pain and palpitations and had a preexisting diagnosis of pericarditis and pericardial effusion from an outside hospital. A transthoracic echocardiogram showed a moderate circumferential pericardial effusion and borderline tamponade with a normal ejection fraction of 55% to 60%. He was treated with colchicine 0.6 mg once a day and ibuprofen 600 mg three times a day. A computed tomography scan of the chest showed a large left pleural effusion and he underwent a thoracentesis. Fluid studies revealed that this was a transudative effusion, negative for malignant cells. See Table 52-1 for a discussion of analysis of pleural fluid to determine if it is a transudate or exudate. Cultures of the fluid were also negative. He was discharged home 8 days ago on colchicine and ibuprofen.

Table 52-1   Analysis of Pleural Effusion to Determine Transudate or Exudate

Pleural fluid is sent for LDH, total protein, cell count and differential, Gram stain, and cultures. Depending on the patient's risk factors and immune status, it may also be appropriate to send pleural fluid for *Mycobacterium* and fungal cultures and analysis for the presence of cancer cells.

Serum LDH and protein are drawn close to the time of the thoracentesis, as the analysis includes comparison with serum levels. Fluid is considered an exudate if analysis meets one or more of Light criteria.

Light criteria are highly sensitive for identifying an exudative pleural effusion, but less specific. Up to 20% of transudative effusions may be mislabeled as exudates so correlation with the clinical picture is essential.

Visual inspection of pleural fluid during paracentesis is helpful to identify hemothorax (fluid appears bloody), empyema (fluid appears purulent), or chylothorax (fluid is milky white).

Type of Effusion	Characteristics	Causes
Exudate	One or more of Light criteria: • Fluid LDH is ≥two-thirds the serum LDH • Ratio of fluid protein to serum protein is ≥0.5 • Ratio of pleural LDH to serum LDH is ≥0.6 Other characteristics: fluid total protein is ≥3 and serum protein-pleural fluid protein is ≤3.1	Infections such as pneumonia, TB, viral infection, HIV Inflammatory disorders including sarcoid, rheumatoid arthritis, SLE Cancer Pulmonary embolism Uremia Diaphragmatic abscess Medication side effect Pancreatitis Esophageal rupture
Transudate	Fluid analysis does not meet Light criteria If clinical suspicion for transudate is high and pleural fluid does meet Light criteria then: Calculate the difference between serum total protein and fluid total protein (serum total protein-pleural fluid total protein). If the difference is ≥3.1 g/dL, the fluid is transudate.	Heart failure Cirrhosis Hypoalbuminemia Nephrotic syndrome Hydronephrosis Constrictive pericarditis Atelectasis

Data from Pleural effusion. The Merck Manuel Professional Edition.http://www.merckmanuals.com/professional/pulmonary_disorders/mediastinal_and_pleural_disorders/pleural_effusion.html Updated October 2014. Accessed April 3, 2015.

Past Medical History

• Mediastinal seminoma, treated in 1980s with radiation
• Thyroid cancer—treated with radiation
• Atrial fibrillation

Denies chronic health issues including diabetes, coronary artery disease (CAD), chronic obstructive pulmonary disease (COPD), asthma, or congestive heart failure (CHF); no lung disease or heart disease until recent hospital admission

Family and Social History

- No family history of heart disease
- Nonsmoker
- Denies illicit drug use

Medication List

- Ibuprofen 600 mg three times a day for recent diagnosis of pericarditis
- Colchicine 0.6 mg once a day for recent diagnosis of pericarditis
- Amiodarone 200 mg once a day for atrial fibrillation
- Aspirin 81 mg once a day for prevention of cardiovascular disease
- levothyroxine 125 mcg once a day for thyroid replacement

❓ What are the pertinent positives obtained from the information obtained so far?

- Dyspnea, orthopnea, and bendopnea
- Recent diagnosis of cardiac tamponade
- Recent pleural effusion treated with thoracentesis
- History of cancer with radiation treatment
- History of atrial fibrillation

❓ What are the significant negatives obtained from the information so far?

- No palpitations
- No chest pain or pressure
- No history of CHF, COPD, asthma, or CAD
- Nonsmoker

Case Analysis

Based on the information I have so far, I am most concerned that this patient has recurrent pericardial effusion, or recurrent pleural effusions. Of course I cannot rule out other life-threatening illnesses, such as acute coronary syndrome (ACS), without more information. I need to quickly and efficiently obtain the key data to begin narrowing down the above differential list and initiate appropriate treatment. Using my expertise in the assessment of cardiopulmonary issues, I will prioritize my assessment findings. My immediate approach is a general survey of the patient, followed by a focused history and physical examination.

CASE INFORMATION

General Survey

The patient is a well-nourished normal-weight 54-year-old male who appears his stated age, is in mild distress, has an anxious facial expression and a mildly elevated respiratory rate. He is sitting on the examination table and as he is wearing shorts and I can immediately see lower extremity edema, estimated at 2-3+. I ask that the nurse obtain vital signs and prepare to do a 12-lead ECG while I conduct a focused history and physical.

Review of Systems

- Constitutional: As noted in HPI, poor appetite, unable to sleep, night sweats, no fevers, denies recent weight gain or weight loss.
- Head/eyes/ears/nose/throat: Noncontributory.
- Cardiovascular: Denies any history of coronary artery disease in self or family, denies chest pain, pressure, or discomfort and palpitations. Endorses edema and shortness of breath as noted in history of present illness.
- Pulmonary: Endorses shortness of breath, worse with laying or bending, denies cough, denies wheezing, denies any history of pulmonary disease including asthma, emphysema, or bronchitis.
- Gastrointestinal: Denies abdominal pain, reflux, nausea, vomiting, constipation. Endorses diarrhea, two to three episodes each day which he attributes to the colchicine prescribed during his recent admission. Denies blood in his stools.
- Genitourinary: Denies pain with urination, blood in urine, prostate disease, urinary frequency.
- Musculoskeletal: Denies weakness, joint pains, muscle aches, denies any falls or recent injury.
- Neurological: Denies headache, denies any recent change in speech or strength.
- Endocrine: Denies a history of diabetes, takes a thyroid pill since radiation therapy over 20 years ago, and follows up with PCP every 6 months to evaluate his thyroid function.

Physical Examination

- Nurse obtains vital signs: Blood Pressure 140/80 mm Hg, heart rate 76 beats per minute, respiratory rate 22 breaths per minute, oxygen saturation by pulse oximeter 95% on room air, temperature 36.8°C, weight 158 lb.

- Constitutional: Awake, appropriate, uncomfortable but in no apparent distress. Well groomed, well nourished.
- Cardiovascular: Jugular venous distension immediately apparent to jaw line. No bruit in bilateral carotids, carotid upstrokes faintly palpable. Heart tones muffled, normal S1, split S2, friction rub heard. Despite presence of compression stockings, patient has 3+ pitting edema bilaterally, pulses are palpable 1+.
- Pulmonary: Mild tachypnea, diminished breath sounds, worse on the left, no crackles or wheezes.
- Gastrointestinal: Normoactive bowel sounds, abdomen distended, firm but nontender to palpation.
- Skin: Cool dry and intact.
- Neurological: Moves all extremities equally, face symmetrical, clear speech, no facial droop.
- The ECG shows normal voltage, no electrical alternans, no arrhythmia, old right bundle branch block, sinus rhythm, no ST elevation or depression, or T-wave abnormalities.

❓ What are the pertinent positives obtained from the information obtained so far?

- Patient's dyspnea is worsening and he is notably uncomfortable at rest.
- He has new onset of bilateral lower leg edema with abdominal bloating.
- Physical examination reveals jugular venous distension and bilateral lower extremity edema indicating fluid volume overload.
- He has a pericardial friction rub.
- He has diarrhea, which may be due to medication side effect.

❓ What are the significant negatives obtained from the information so far?

- He has no chest pain.
- The patient has no facial droop or slurred speech or other focal neurological signs/symptoms.
- The patient has stable vital signs with normal oxygen saturation.
- He has no fever and no productive cough.
- ECG is negative for ACS, no ECG evidence of cardiac tamponade, no evidence of arrhythmia.
- No recent injuries or falls.

? Can the information gathered so far be restated in a single sentence highlighting the pieces that narrow down the cause?

The problem representation in this case might be: "A 54-year-old male with a recent history of pericarditis and pericardial and pleural effusions presents with new onset heart failure symptoms."

Case Analysis

From my focused physical examination, I am less concerned about a neurological etiology for the patient's symptoms. He has no signs of weakness or focal deficits consistent with neuromuscular disease or cerebrovascular accident. A pulmonary disorder is also less likely as he has no fever or cough to suggest a pulmonary infection, and no history of lung disease to suggest an acute exacerbation of an underlying chronic pulmonary disorder. I cannot definitively rule out a pulmonary embolism without more testing, but based on the diagnosis made during his recent hospital stay, his current symptoms are far more likely to be the result of a cardiac disease process.

Despite his tachypnea, his blood pressure, heart rate, and oxygen saturation are stable at this time and the ECG shows no sign of acute coronary syndrome so there is no need for immediate transport to the emergency room. The fact that the ECG shows normal voltage and no electrical alternans (alternating voltage across the precordial leads) is helpful information for ruling out acute pericardial effusion with tamponade. There is no arrhythmia on ECG; his review of systems describes an absence of symptoms such as racing heart or palpitations so I do not think his dyspnea is due to uncontrolled atrial fibrillation or other arrhythmias. I decide to gather more information with additional diagnostic testing to include a troponin level to assess for myocardial infarction, a complete blood count to determine if he is anemic, and to further rule out an infectious process, and a comprehensive metabolic panel, to evaluate his intravascular fluid status, given that he has signs of volume overload on my examination. My main priority is to obtain an echocardiogram and a chest x-ray as my leading concerns are acute heart failure, recurrent pleural effusions or worsening of his pericardial effusion.

 CASE INFORMATION

His blood work shows a mild anemia with hemoglobin 13 g/dL (normal range 14–18 g/dL), hematocrit 39.2% (normal range 40%–52%). His comprehensive metabolic panel is normal except for a low sodium at 135 mmol/L (normal range 136–145 mmol/L). His troponin is normal at 0.01 µg/L (normal range is less than or equal to 0.01 µg/L). The chest x-ray shows bilateral pleural effusions obscuring the heart borders; lung parenchyma is normal. A transthoracic echocardiogram reveals normal left ventricle size and wall thickness, with an ejection fraction of 60% to 65% (normal is 55%–65%). Global and segmental wall motion is within normal limits. There is a trivial circumferential pericardial effusion, much smaller than found on the study done 3 weeks prior. There are new large bilateral pleural effusions.

❓ What elements from the additional diagnostics should be added to the list of pertinent positives or significant negatives?

- **Pertinent positives:** slightly low sodium, mild anemia, worsening pleural effusions
- **Significant negatives:** normal ejection fraction, trivial circumferential pericardial effusions.

❓ How does the information affect the list of possible causes?

As stated above, an acute coronary syndrome such as ST elevation myocardial infarction or non-ST elevation myocardial infarction is unlikely based on his ECG findings, the absence of chest pain, and his normal troponin. His blood work revealed hyponatremia. Low sodium can be indicative of many conditions. In this patient with his lower extremity edema, abdominal fullness, and bilateral pleural effusions, the diagnosis is most probably acute heart failure, with preserved ejection fraction (EF). Like most other causes of hyponatremia, heart failure impairs the ability to excrete ingested water by increasing antidiuretic hormone levels. When cardiac output and systemic blood pressure are reduced, "hypovolemic" hormones, such as renin (with a subsequent increase in angiotensin II formation), antidiuretic hormone (ADH), and norepinephrine, respond, resulting in retention of fluid.[2]

The patient's recent diagnosis of pericarditis and his remote history of radiation therapy to his mediastinum due to his mediastinal seminoma, both suggest that chronic constrictive pericarditis is the most likely cause of his acute heart failure. The patient's acute pericarditis was appropriately treated with anti-inflammatory medications, ibuprofen and colchicine; however, he now presents with volume overload, suggesting that his acute pericarditis is actually a chronic process, impacting his diastolic filling pressures and cardiac output.[3] Following my assessment, I determine that the patient needs to be at a higher level of care and I arrange for him to be directly admitted from my clinic to the acute cardiology service for further investigation of his pericarditis and the etiology of his heart failure symptoms.

Chronic Constrictive Pericarditis: Treatment and Management

Often pericarditis, an inflammation of the sac surrounding the heart, is an acute, self-limiting disorder and, though the pain can be significant, it usually responds to anti-inflammatory medications.[3] This patient presents pain free, which may be due to use of round-the-clock ibuprofen. Pericarditis can occur as a complication of myocardial infarction, autoimmune disorders such as rheumatoid arthritis, and rarely, malignant disorders. Idiopathic cases of pericarditis are probably due to a viral infection and account for a large percentage of cases. Infectious pericarditis due to bacteria or *Mycobacterium*, such as tuberculosis, carries a significant risk of mortality. While controlling inflammation is a key component in the management of pericarditis, it is also essential to identify and treat the underlying cause if possible.[3]

Most cases of pericarditis present as chest pain as this patient did on his first hospital admission. The fact that he returns for care with signs of acute heart failure suggests that his disease is actually chronic constrictive pericarditis. In some cases, pericardial inflammation leads to fibrosis and thickening of the pericardium, significant enough to constrict diastolic ventricular filling, leading to venous engorgement and ultimately affecting cardiac output. Constrictive pericarditis causes symptoms of acute heart failure.

In the past, differentiating constrictive pericarditis from restrictive cardiomyopathy (RCM), due to conditions such as amyloidosis, required surgical intervention and biopsy. Both conditions cause diastolic dysfunction, or impaired ventricular filling, which leads to symptoms of acute heart failure. However, the disorders differ significantly in their response to treatment; RCM has few treatment options while urgent surgical intervention can result in significant improvement in patients with constrictive pericarditis. The unique features of these disorders are not consistently apparent on routine imaging, though echocardiogram sometimes shows abnormal myocardial texture suggestive of amyloidosis, and a chest x-ray may reveal pericardial calcification, which strongly suggests constrictive pericarditis. On cardiac catheterization, diastolic filling pressures tend to be equal or differ by a value of less than 5 mm Hg in constrictive pericarditis while the difference is usually greater than 5 mm Hg in patients with restrictive cardiomyopathy. Further research is needed but cardiac MRI may offer key diagnostic information in distinguishing these two conditions.[4]

In the case of this patient, I had a high suspicion for chronic pericarditis due to his history of mediastinal seminoma in the 1980s. At that time, patients received large amounts of therapeutic radiation. Irradiation of a substantial volume of the heart at sufficiently high doses can damage virtually any component of the heart, including the pericardium. Pericarditis is the typical acute manifestation of radiation injury, while chronic pericardial disease can manifest years or decades after the original treatment.[4,5] These complications can cause significant morbidity or mortality.

Case Follow-Up

To further delineate the diagnosis and degree of pericarditis (constrictive vs restrictive or a combination), the patient underwent a right heart catheterization following admission to the acute cardiology service. Patients with constrictive pericarditis have elevated left- and right-sided filling pressures, often of equal magnitude to within 5 mm Hg, and usually have normal systolic ventricular function.[6] The right heart catheterization revealed an elevated right atrial pressure. All other pressures were normal. Cardiac output and the initial wedge pressure were both normal. These values indicate a chronic pericarditis without a significant constrictive element.[6]

Transthoracic echocardiogram completed during his last admission and redone during this admission shows bilateral pleural effusions. The pleural effusions are not significant enough to require drainage and so are managed with gentle diuresis. The patient is given intravenous furosemide initially then changed to oral furosemide. His edema in his lower extremities improved with this therapy. His clinical symptoms of dyspnea also improved significantly. He was discharged on oral furosemide with close follow-up.

References

1. Pleural effusion. The Merck Manuel Professional Edition.http://www.merckmanuals.com/professional/pulmonary_disorders/mediastinal_and_pleural_disorders/pleural_effusion.html. Updated October 2014. Accessed April 3, 2015.
2. Leier CV, Dei Cas L, Metra M. Clinical relevance and management of the major electrolyte abnormalities in congestive heart failure: hyponatremia, hypokalemia, and hypomagnesemia. *Am Heart J.* 1994;128(3):564.
3. Imazio M. Contemporary management of pericardial diseases. *Curr Opin Cardiol.* 2012;27:308.
4. Parks JL, O'Brien TX, Lange R. Constrictive pericarditis workup. Medscape Web site. http://emedicine.medscape.com/article/157096-workup#aw2aab6b5b8. Updated December 23, 2014. Accessed April 29, 2015.
5. Yusef SW, Sami S, Daher IN. Radiation-induced heart disease: a clinical update. *Cardiol Res Pract.* 2011. http://dx.doi.org/10.4061/2011/317659.
6. Little WC, Freeman, GL. Pericardial disease. *Circulation.* 2006;113:1622.

CASE 53

Brian Widmar

Brian Widmar works in a CVICU in Nashville, Tennessee. Dr Widmar also is an Assistant Professor of Nursing and teaches ACNPs in the intensivist subspecialty program at Vanderbilt University School of Nursing.

CASE INFORMATION

Chief Complaint

SB is a 65-year-old man who was admitted to the cardiovascular intensive care unit (CVICU) 3 days ago, and is now postoperative day 2 from a coronary artery bypass grafting (CABG) of the left internal mammary artery (LIMA) to the left anterior descending artery (LAD) and a reverse saphenous vein grafting to the left circumflex coronary artery (LCx). He is reporting that his "chest hurts" and, per his bedside nurse, administration of intravenous morphine sulfate has been ineffective in relieving his pain.

❓ What is the potential cause?

When a patient recovering from cardiac surgery complains of chest discomfort, my immediate thought is that postoperative pain management is inadequate. Even though that seems pretty straightforward, given this patient recently had a coronary revascularization, it is prudent to see the patient and speak with him about the nature of his chest discomfort. There are many other potential etiologies that need to be considered before developing a management plan. A focused history, physical examination, and review of available diagnostic data are essential to narrowing down the differential diagnosis list, and to figuring out the most appropriate course of action to treat this patient's pain.

> **Comprehensive Differential Diagnoses for a Patient With Chest Pain**
>
> - Cardiovascular: myocardial ischemia (angina, myocardial infarction, coronary vasospasm, increased metabolic demand secondary to tachycardia, anemia, hyperthyroidism), pulmonary embolism, aortic dissection, pericarditis, cardiomyopathy, myocarditis, mitral valve prolapse, aortic insufficiency, pulmonary hypertension
> - Pulmonary: pneumonia, pleuritis, pneumothorax

- Gastrointestinal: esophageal rupture, gastroesophageal reflux disease (GERD), peptic ulcer disease, cholecystitis, pancreatitis
- Musculoskeletal: costochondritis, cervical or thoracic disk disease, sternal/sternotomy pain, mediastinitis, chest wall tumor
- Other potential causes: anxiety/panic attack, herpes zoster

Since this patient was originally admitted and treated for myocardial ischemia that presented as chest pain, the history of that illness is really important. I will need to compare his current report of pain with his reported preadmission chest pain and to monitor him for recurring myocardial ischemia (especially secondary to graft failure, vasospasm, or demand ischemia due to postoperative blood loss and anemia). Pericarditis, pulmonary embolism, and tension pneumothorax are also potential postoperative complications that lead to chest pain and need to be diagnosed or ruled out quickly to ensure appropriate treatment. I will use supportive history and physical examination data and diagnostic tests to narrow down this differential list and plan the appropriate course of action.

CASE INFORMATION

History of Presenting Illness

SB has a past medical history of morbid obesity, hypertension (HTN), hyperlipidemia (HLD), and type 2 diabetes mellitus (T2DM). On admission, he reported a 2-day duration of progressively worsening chest discomfort. He notified emergency medical services (EMS) after experiencing a crushing chest pain of 10 out of 10 pain scale severity, localized mostly in the mid-sternal region, with some radiation to his right arm and shoulder. He noted nausea and shortness of breath, and none of these symptoms improved with lying down. EMS took SB immediately to the emergency department (ED) for further evaluation.

While in the ED, cardiac markers and routine laboratory testing were completed. A 12-lead electrocardiogram (ECG) revealed ST-segment depression in leads V3 through V6 and delayed repolarization, suggesting anterolateral ischemia. His troponin level peaked at 6.15 ng/mL. He was taken urgently to the cardiac catheterization laboratory (CCL), and angiography revealed an 80% occlusive lesion to the distal left main coronary artery (LMCA), and a 90% occlusive lesion to the distal left circumflex artery (LCx). Ejection fraction was 60%. He was referred to cardiac surgery for urgent coronary revascularization and underwent CABG that day. He was transferred to the cardiovascular intensive care unit and his postoperative recovery has thus far been unremarkable: he was extubated successfully and is no longer requiring supplemental oxygen, his vasoactive medications have been weaned off, and central venous lines, chest tube drains, and urinary catheter have all been removed.

He notes that his current chest pain started about 2 to 3 hours ago, and really has not improved much with oral hydrocodone or intravenous morphine sulfate. He describes the chest pain as sharp, and a 7 out of 10 scale severity. The pain is localized in the sternum and left chest and seems to radiate to the left side of his middle back. Exertion or rest does not impact the pain. He has asked me to raise the head of bed because he is more uncomfortable lying flat. He denies palpitations, nausea, and shortness of breath, but he states that it is difficult for him to take a deep breath as the pain is worse with deep inspiration.

? What are the pertinent positives from the current information?

- Relatively sudden onset of chest pain (about 2 to 3 hours ago).
- Pain is described as sharp and is localized to the middle sternum and left chest. The pain radiates to the middle left side of the patient's back.
- Pain is exacerbated by lying flat and by deep inspiration.
- The patient is post-op day 2 following cardiac surgery, a preoperative enzyme leak (troponin-I 6.15 ng/dL) and 12-lead ECG consistent with non-ST-segment elevation myocardial infarction.
- Pain has not been adequately relived with narcotics (hydrocodone by mouth and morphine sulfate by IV).

? What are the significant negatives from the current information?

- The nature of his current chest pain is different than the chest pain that prompted his initial hospital admission (currently reported as "sharp" vs a "crushing" chest pain; pain is not reported as a "tearing" or "ripping" sensation).
- Pain is not worsened by exertion.
- Pain does not radiate as it did prior to admission.
- The patient is alert and oriented, denies previously associated symptoms (nausea and shortness of breath), and remains off of vasoactive medications.

? Can the information gathered so far be restated in a single sentence highlighting the pieces that narrow down the cause?

SB is a 65-year-old man with a past medical history of obesity, HTN, HLD, and T2DM who is now postoperative day 2 from CABG × 2 who now complains of sharp, mid-sternal/left chest pain, which radiates to his middle left back region and worsens with inspiration and when lying supine.

❓ How does this information affect the list of possible causes?

The information gathered in the HPI helps me sort out my differential list and prioritize those diagnoses according to what I think is most likely. Based on his past medical history, identified risk factors, and recent operative procedure, inadequate postoperative pain management is still high on the differential list, though I need to first rule out the life-threatening cardiovascular and pulmonary disorders on my list. His current chest pain is significantly different from the chest pain he reported upon admission so I am not convinced that myocardial ischemia is the culprit. In addition to the difference in symptom presentation, he is alert and oriented, remains off of oxygen and vasoactive medications, which is reassuring. I will need to order a 12-lead ECG and compare it to preadmission before I can positively rule out ischemia. I am also planning a careful pulmonary assessment and possibly a stat portable chest x-ray to rule out pneumothorax and pneumonia and to evaluate mediastinal width.

CASE INFORMATION

Social History

Habits

- Exercise: Walks 1 to 2 miles two to three times a week.
- Caffeine intake: One cup of black coffee each morning and one diet soda daily at lunch.
- Alcohol intake: Denies.
- Illicit substance use: Denies.
- Tobacco use: Has a remote smoking history, he reports he quit 30 years ago. Smoked one pack per day but cannot recall duration.
- Sleep patterns: Reports sleeping 6 to 7 hours per night.
- Current occupation: He is a retired electrician.
- Living situation: Lives in a home with his wife of 41 years. Has four children and six grandchildren who visit often.

Current medications

- Enteric coated aspirin 81 mg by mouth daily
- Metoprolol 25 mg by mouth twice daily; hold for heart rate <60 or for systolic blood pressure <100
- Furosemide 2 mg by mouth twice daily
- Potassium chloride sustained—release tablet 20 mEq by mouth twice daily
- Captopril 6.25 mg by mouth every 8 hours, hold for systolic blood pressure <110
- Calcium citrate two tablets by mouth twice daily with meals

- Esomeprazole 40 mg tablet by mouth once daily
- Gabapentin 300 mg by mouth every 8 hours
- Clopidogrel 75 mg by mouth daily
- Citalopram 40 mg by mouth daily
- Insulin-aspart sliding scale subcutaneous with meals and at bedtime for blood glucose:
  - 0 to 60: give 1 amp $D_{50}W$ and notify house officer
  - 61 to 160: nothing
  - 161 to 200: give 2 units
  - 201 to 250: give 4 units
  - 251 to 300: give 6 units
  - 301 to 350: give 8 units
  - 351 to 400: give 10 units
  - >400: give 12 units and notify house officer
- Dextrose 50% in water: $D_{50}W$ 50 mL IV; give as directed
- Hydrocodone-acetaminophen 5 mg/325 mg one tablet by mouth every 4 hours as needed for pain (give for pain scale <5)
- Hydrocodone-acetaminophen 5 mg/325 mg two tablets by mouth every 4 hours as needed for pain (give for pain scale 6–10)
- Hydromorphone injection 0.25 mg every 3 hours intravenously as needed for pain (may give if pain not relieved by hydrocodone)
- Docusate sodium 100 mg by mouth twice daily
- Bisacodyl 10 mg suppository per rectum as needed for constipation

Review of Systems (ROS)

- Constitutional: Denies history of fever or chills, no recent weight loss or weight gain.
- Cardiovascular: See HPI regarding history of chest pain. Denies history of palpitations, lower extremity edema, and dyspnea on exertion, paroxysmal nocturnal dyspnea, or orthopnea. Lying down worsens chest pain. No history of claudication or deep vein thrombosis.
- Pulmonary: Denies shortness of breath, cough, wheezing, hemoptysis. No history of pneumonia, pulmonary embolism, or recurring upper respiratory tract infections.
- Gastrointestinal: Denies abdominal pain, nausea, or vomiting. No history of peptic ulcer disease or gastroesophageal reflux disease. No bowel movement since surgery, but reports one bowel movement daily prior to hospital admission. Denies melena or hematochezia.
- Genitourinary: Currently voids per urinal. No history of urgency, hesitancy, frequency, dysuria. Denies urinary tract infections or benign prostatic hypertrophy.

- Musculoskeletal: Takes ibuprofen as needed for arthritis pain in hands and knees on occasion. Denies muscle trauma or injury. No report of muscle weakness, joint edema, or erythema.
- Integumentary: Denies history of skin rash, lumps, or pruritus.
- Neurological: Denies history of seizures, syncope, falls or stroke, numbness, or extremity weakness.
- Psychiatric: Denis history of substance abuse, depression, or anxiety.
- Endocrine: No intolerance to heat or cold, no excessive thirst, urination, or hunger.
- Hematologic/lymphatic: Denies easy bruising, bleeding, or enlarged/tender lymph nodes. No history of blood transfusion prior to cardiac surgery.
- Allergic/immunologic: Denies fever/chills, history of immunosuppression, or frequent infections.

Physical Examination

- Vital signs: Temperature is 98.4°F (oral), pulse is 75 beats per minute, blood pressure is 138/78 mm Hg (left arm), 140/76 (right arm), and respiratory rate is 17/min. Oxygen saturation is 98% on room air. Fingerstick blood glucose is 110 mg/dL. Weight 230 lb. BMI 33 kg/m^2.
- Constitutional: Well-developed, well-nourished man who is sitting upright and in moderate discomfort. He is alert, oriented, and cooperative.
- Cardiovascular: Regular rate and rhythm. S1 and S2 obscured by a two-part scratching sound best heard at the left sternal border and at the fifth intercostal space at the midclavicular line. No S3, S4 or murmurs appreciated. No heaves or lifts noted upon palpation. No JVD noted with head of bed at 45°. Bilateral lower extremity edema 1+. Capillary refill is <3 seconds in upper and lower extremities bilaterally. Radial, dorsalis pedis, and posterior tibial pulses are 2+ and equal in quality bilaterally. No cyanosis, clubbing, or claudication. No carotid bruits appreciated. Bilateral carotid pulses are smooth and regular.
- Pulmonary: Trachea midline. Chest expansion is symmetrical with regular rate and rhythm. No accessory muscle use. Bilateral breath sounds are clear to auscultation in all lung fields.
- Gastrointestinal: Abdomen appears soft and protuberant. Bowel sounds normoactive in all four quadrants. Nondistended, nontender to palpation. Tympanic to percussion throughout.
- Genitourinary: Voids clear yellow urine per urinal.
- Musculoskeletal: No tenderness upon palpation of extremities. Sternum is without fluctuance to palpation.
- Integumentary: Midline sternotomy incision is open to air, without drainage. Minimal erythema. There is a clean bandage covering old central

venous line insertion site. Old chest tube insertion sites covered with clean gauze. Venous harvest sites on right lower leg are open to air, have minimal erythema and no drainage. Epicardial pacing wires are taped to the anterior chest wall.

- Neurological: Alert and oriented × 3. No focal neurological deficits. PERRLA 3 mm bilaterally. Strength is 5/5 throughout. Speech is clear.
- Psychiatric: Calm with appropriate affect and behavior. Thought processes are logical and speech is clear and easily understandable. Converses appropriately.
- Hematologic/lymphatic/immune: No signs of occult bleeding. No petechiae or purpura. Wound dressing sites are all clean and intact. No lymphadenopathy.

❓ What are the pertinent positives and significant negatives found in the review of systems and physical examination?

Pertinent Positives

- S1 and S2 are obscured by a scratching sound best heard at the left sternal border and cardiac apex.

Significant Negatives

- SB has a negative ROS and PE for all remaining systems.
- There is no difference in blood pressure between right and left arms.
- There is no difference in breath sounds or lung expansion bilaterally.
- There is no decrease in bilateral pulse quality, capillary refill, urine output, or in overall neurological status.

❓ How does this information affect the list of possible causes?

Based on the information gathered so far, I think I am able to rule out more diagnoses and can begin to prioritize my top causes of his chest pain. Given the only significant examination finding is that of a friction rub, my primary concern at this point is acute pericarditis. I am less concerned about myocardial ischemia because he shows no evidence of cardiac insufficiency or hemodynamic instability: his blood pressure is acceptable on no vasoactive medications, and pulse rate and quality, capillary refill, mentation, and urine output are all acceptable. These findings also make pericardial effusion with tamponade very unlikely. Similarly, aortic dissection is less likely given the equal blood pressures in both arms and the nature of the patient's chest pain.

The patient is oxygenating well on room air and bilateral breath sounds are even and clear to auscultation, which makes pneumonia or pneumothorax less likely. The abdominal examination is essentially benign, although the examination is challenging given the patient's body habitus.

At this point, I am confident that my areas of focus remain the evaluation of the patient's current pain management plan, the potential for myocardial ischemia, and the potential for acute postoperative pericarditis.

❓ What diagnostic testing should be done and in what order?

Because my primary concerns are myocardial ischemia and pericarditis, I think a 12-lead ECG should be the first test I order. I can compare this new 12-lead ECG to the baseline ECG completed upon admission, and that may identify patterns of myocardial ischemia, either new or recurrent. ST-segment changes on a 12-lead ECG will support the diagnosis of pericarditis, particularly in light of his history and examination findings.

Increases in serum cardiac biomarkers such as troponin-I also occur in the setting of pericarditis.[1] As myocardial ischemia is also a concern in this case, I will also order a CK-MB and troponin-I. Though troponin levels are very sensitive to myocardial injury, it is difficult to interpret their significance in the postoperative cardiac surgery patient, as average values may range anywhere from 6 to 18 ng/mL.[2]

CASE INFORMATION
Diagnostic Testing Results

The new ECG, when compared to the one done immediately after surgery, shows diffuse ST-segment elevation and PR-interval depression. These changes are pervasive across almost every lead. In addition, SB's CK-MB was 8.59 ng/mL (normal range <6.00) and troponin-I was 2.37 ng/mL (actually down from initial peak of 6.15 ng/mL).

A widely accepted definition of perioperative MI is an elevation of biomarkers to greater than five times the 99th percentile of the normal reference range during the first 72 hours after CABG, plus new pathological Q waves or left bundle branch block on ECG, new graft or native coronary occlusion seen on angiogram, or imaging evidence of new loss of viable myocardium.[2] Given the nature of the patient's chest pain and physical examination, cardiac insufficiency secondary to myocardial ischemia is unlikely, and at this point, I am ready to list acute postoperative pericarditis as my primary diagnosis (Figures 53-1 and 53-2).

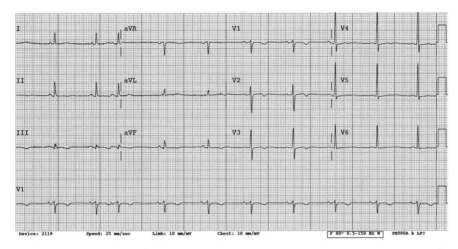

Figure 53-1 Initial 12-lead ECG taken during the immediate postoperative period.

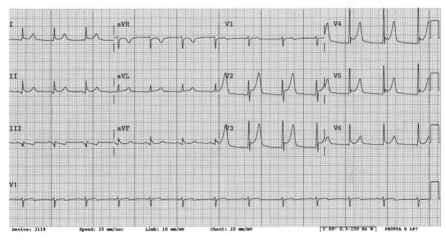

Figure 53-2 12-lead ECG taken after report of new-onset postoperative chest pain.

Acute Pericarditis: Diagnosis and Treatment

The patient with pericarditis usually has a sternal or precordial chest pain that is described as a sharp or stabbing quality.[3] The pain associated with pericarditis can be confused with pleuritic pain because it worsens with inspiration. Patients typically have some relief when sitting upright and leaning forward; pain is worsened when lying supine. Precordial chest pain requires careful assessment to differentiate pericarditis from unstable angina and acute myocardial infarction.

The pericardial friction rub can help differentiate pericarditis from a pleuritic chest pain: the friction rub can be clearly heard when the patient holds their breath.

The rub sound can have from one to three components: a systolic sound, an early diastolic sound, and a late diastolic sound.[3]

The 12-lead ECG is vital in differentiating between pericarditis and myocardial ischemia. In the early phase of acute pericarditis, diffuse concave up elevation of the ST segment can be seen in almost all leads except rarely in V1 and V2; reciprocal ST depression can be seen in leads aVR and V1. PR-interval depression may also be seen. These changes are seen because of ventricular and atrial current of injury associated with epicardial inflammation.[1] Because ST-segment elevation is seen globally, reciprocal changes often seen with myocardial infarction are often not present, helping differentiate between pericarditis and acute MI.

Treatment of acute pericarditis is targeted toward the underlying etiology, and most patients can be managed effectively with medical therapy alone.[4] Patients who have hemodynamic compromise secondary to pericardial effusion and tamponade or constrictive pericarditis should be evaluated for more invasive therapy.[4] If invasive therapies are not indicated, as is the case for SB, the goals of therapy are relief of pain and reduction of inflammation. Primary medical therapy includes the use of nonsteroidal anti-inflammatory drugs (NSAIDs) such as ibuprofen, indomethacin, or aspirin. In patients with ischemic heart disease or a new MI, higher-dose aspirin may be an appropriate choice.[3] For patients without a contraindication, duration of treatment with NSAIDs is based on the persistence of symptoms, usually a 1- to 2-week duration, for initial occurrence followed by a taper over the next 1 to 2 weeks.[4] An individualized approach to dosing and tapering is done based on resolution of symptoms and normalization of C-reactive protein levels.[5] In patients intolerant to NSAIDs or higher-dose aspirin, colchicine or corticosteroids may be used. In patients with STEMI, the use of NSAIDs, ibuprofen, and corticosteroids in the treatment of pericarditis are potentially harmful and have been associated with an increased risk of reinfarction, cardiac wall rupture (due to thinning of myocardial scarring), renal insufficiency, and heart failure and are contraindicated in the STEMI patient population.[3]

Due to concerns of GI upset with high-dose aspirin, SB was treated with colchicine 0.5 mg twice daily, and pain management was supplemented with opioid analgesics as needed. He continued colchicine therapy for the following 2 to 3 months, and was followed and tapered off of therapy in the outpatient setting.

References

1. Imazio M. Pericardial diseases. In: Kathleen S and David LB, eds. *Evidence-Based Cardiology Consult.* London: Springer; 2014:79-89.
2. Bojar RM. *Manual of Perioperative Care in Adult Cardiac Surgery.* 5th ed. Hoboken, NJ: Wiley-Blackwell; 2011.
3. Jacobson C, Marzlin K, Webner C. Inflammatory cardiovascular diseases: diseases involving the pericardium, myocardium and endocardium. In: Jacobson C, Marzlin K, Webner C, eds. *Cardiovascular Nursing Practice: A Comprehensive Resource Manual and Study Guide for Clinical Nurses.* 2nd ed. Burien, WA: Cardiovascular Nursing Education Associates; 2014.
4. Imazio M, Bobbio M, Cecchi E, et al. Colchicine in addition to conventional therapy for acute pericarditis: results of the COlchicine for acute PEricarditis (COPE) trial. *Circulation.* 2005;112(13):2012-2016.
5. Imazio M, Spodick DH, Brucato A, Trinchero R, Adler Y. Controversial issues in the management of pericardial diseases. *Circulation.* 2010;121(7):916-928.

CASE 54

David V. Strider, Jr

David V. Strider, Jr. is an ACNP for the vascular surgery patient population at the University of Virginia Medical Center. Dr Strider provides inpatient and outpatient support for adult patients with a wide variety of vascular conditions. He also serves as clinical instructor for the ACNP Program at the University. He has a vast background in critical care nursing with an emphasis on cardiothoracic ICU care.

CASE INFORMATION

Chief Complaint

A 57-year-old cattle farmer, BJ, arrives at the emergency department at 6 PM, stating, "I just cannot take this pain in my leg anymore. It has been hurting bad since lunchtime, and got out of control when I was feeding the cattle this afternoon. This leg (he points to his right leg) almost gave out on me. Can you please do something to help my pain?"

❓ What is the potential cause?

I need to obtain more information and will do so with a complete history and physical but in the meanwhile I start by considering a comprehensive differential diagnoses list for leg pain.

Differential Diagnoses for Leg Pain

- Peripheral arterial disease
- Peripheral venous disease (venous insufficiency) or deep venous thrombosis
- Osteoarthritis or rheumatoid arthritis
- Sciatica
- Peripheral neuropathy
- Gout
- Previous hip fracture
- Trauma
- Spinal cord invasion by a neoplasm
- Lumbar spinal nerve root degeneration
- Insect bite (such as the brown recluse or black widow spider, or the deer tick)

CASE INFORMATION

History of Present Illness

The patient tells me that he has had right calf pain for 6 months but only when climbing a flight of stairs or walking at a brisk speed. Today, he tells me that his pain has increased so that it is bothering him at rest. He rates his leg pain as 4 to 5 on a scale of 0 to 10. The way that he is grimacing, it looks as if his pain may be a bit higher than that, but we will go with a "4 to 5" rating. BJ states that his pain starts in his lower thigh and runs down the back of his calf to his ankle and the top of his foot. He also says that his right foot has been very cool for the last few days. He adds that he can now only walk 150 ft before his right calf starts to throb. He notes that the pain gradually improves after he sits down for 10 to 15 minutes. Cold temperatures and elevation of his right leg make the pain worse, whereas hanging his foot over the sofa or bed consistently improves the pain. He denies left leg pain. He states he has not had any skin color or texture changes or swelling in his right leg and he denies any falls, injury or bug bites to his right leg. BJ adds that he has cut back on his cigarettes since his heart attack 6 months ago.

Past Medical History

Per patient report and review of electronic medical record:
- Myocardial infarction, 6 months ago, after which he was hospitalized for 3 days, and underwent coronary catheterization and stent placement in his left anterior descending artery.
- High blood pressure.
- Diabetes mellitus, type 2.
- One episode of gout with swollen left great toe, 3 years ago, with no recurrence.
- Chronic kidney disease, stage 3.
- Asthma, worse in the spring and in the fall, uses inhaler with relief.
- Motor vehicle accident in 1994, tree versus car. He sustained three fractured ribs, a pneumothorax, and a lacerated spleen. He underwent splenectomy.

Surgical History

- Elective tonsillectomy in 1965
- Open reduction and internal fixation of the left mid-tibial fracture, 1968
- Splenectomy in 1994
- Resection of ingrown toenail (right great toe)—2012

Social History

BJ is married and in a monogamous relationship. He smokes 3/4 pack of cigarettes per day, and one case (10 packs/case) may last him for 2 weeks.

He smokes cigarettes all the way down to the filter. He denies any tobacco chewing. He used to drink beer but he quit because he no longer has a "taste" for it. He denies taking any illegal drugs or herbal supplements; however, he did take ginseng for approximately 6 months. BJ drinks up to six cups of coffee per day.

Family History

BJ has two children, a 28-year-old son and a 24-year-old daughter, both of whom are in good health. His mother died at the age of 72 from a myocardial infarction and his father died in a car accident at the age of 68. His father had high blood pressure. BJ has three siblings. One brother has diabetes mellitus, one brother had an abdominal aortic aneurysm repair, and his sister has asthma. All three stopped smoking in the last 3 years.

Current Medications

- Allopurinol: 100 mg twice a day, by mouth
- Lisinopril: 10 mg by mouth, once per day
- Amlodipine: 5 mg by mouth, once per day
- Simvastatin: 20 mg by mouth, once at bedtime
- Metformin: 500 mg by mouth, twice per day
- Singulair: 10 mg by mouth, once per day
- Cromolyn sulfate: two sprays in each nostril, three times per day
- Albuterol inhaler: two puffs every 6 hours, as needed, for wheezing
- Clopidogrel: 75 mg by mouth, once per day
- Aspirin: 81 mg by mouth, once per day (patient stopped 3 months ago)

Immunizations

BJ had his influenza shot this year, and he received haemophilus, meningococcus, and pneumococcal vaccinations in 1994, following splenectomy.

Allergies

BJ is allergic to penicillin, states his reaction is rash and trouble breathing.

❓ What are the pertinent positives from the information given so far?

- Painful right leg when walking, progressively worse, to now having pain at rest
- Pain is worse with elevation, and relieved with sitting in dangling position
- Right foot is cool
- Coronary artery disease with recent MI
- Diabetes mellitus and hypertension

- Current smoker
- History of gout
- First-degree relative with abdominal aortic aneurysm
- Chronic obstructive pulmonary disease
- Asplenia
- Chronic renal insufficiency
- Caffeine abuse (excessive coffee)

❓ What are the significant negatives from the information given so far?

- No trauma to his right leg
- No swelling in the leg
- No exposure to insects that patient is aware of
- No history of cancer or hypercoagulopathy

❓ Can the information gathered so far be restated in a single sentence highlighting the pieces that narrow down the cause?

The problem representation in this case might be: "This 57-year-old male presents with a chief complaint of worsening right calf pain, that is exacerbated by walking, and improves with rest."

❓ How does the information collected so far affect the differential diagnoses?

At this point I will review my differential list of potential causes as some of the information I obtained may help rule out, or rule in, some of the diagnoses. Since his right leg pain is worse with elevation and with exercise, I do not think it is related to venous insufficiency. His description of the pain does not fit with a diagnosis of sciatica, since it does not radiate from his back or buttocks and is not aggravated by sudden position changes. He denies any history of trauma so I am less concerned about a hip fracture, compression fracture, or other traumatic injury.

Osteoarthritis and rheumatoid arthritis usually result in bilateral pain and this patient presents with unilateral pain. In addition, arthritis pain is usually in the joints and not necessarily in the calf or thigh. Given the sudden onset of severe pain over the last few hours, I am less convinced that arthritis is the primary cause of his pain. He does report a history of gout, but the pain from gout is usually localized to the toe, knee, or more rarely a joint in an upper extremity. Gout pain tends to begin in the night, and worsen to a point of extreme sensitivity to even light touch, and that is not the pattern of this patient's pain.

I also need to consider a spinal cord tumor, which is less likely to occur but requires rapid intervention. The symptoms of a tumor are often bilateral and would not cause coolness of the foot or worsening of pain with exercise. I am still thinking about a possible insect bite, but he did not mention any event of this kind. The indigenous insects that could incur considerable lower extremity pain include the brown recluse, black widow, hornets, wasps, and ticks. He is wearing boots, which makes me speculate that he is less susceptible to a tick bite or a snakebite (copperheads, cottonmouth, and rattlesnakes are indigenous to this area.)

Reviewing the patient's past medical history, he has multiple risk factors for peripheral arterial disease, including diabetes, hypertension, smoking, and coronary artery disease. Patients with one form of vascular disease are more likely to have other forms. In addition, his family history, remarkable for coronary artery disease and abdominal aortic aneurysm, suggests that he may have a predisposition to vascular disease along with his existing risk factors. He is prescribed aspirin and clopidogrel, which would offer some protection against a DVT or an arterial embolism, but I am not sure how well he has adhered to that regimen.

At this point, I strongly suspect that the patient's right leg pain is due to severely limited arterial blood flow to his right foot. The area of most significant arterial blockage is usually found one "joint" above the region of the affected limb, so in this case we need to think about possible right thigh arterial blood vessels that may be significantly blocked. Some of these arteries include the external iliac, the femoral artery, and the popliteal artery. Reduced blood flow in any one of the above arteries would result in the right calf exercise–induced pain and cool foot that BJ is experiencing. I will gather more information in my review of systems and physical examination, to help me rule in or out other diagnoses on my list.

CASE INFORMATION

Review of Systems

- Constitutional: Denies fevers, chills, or unexpected weight gain or loss.
- Head/ears/eyes/nose/throat: Denies headaches, earache, hearing deficit, nasal congestion, any new visual deficits, and trouble swallowing. He states he has regular dental care.
- Cardiovascular: Denies chest pain, palpitations, nausea, and shortness of breath when at rest.
- Pulmonary: No hemoptysis, dyspnea at rest, or prolonged coughing. Endorses occasional cough with white phlegm and "wheezing" at times, which resolves with two puffs of his inhaler. He sleeps on two pillows at night. He tells me that his wife has stated that he "snores loudly at night when asleep." The patient denies any pneumonia.
- Gastrointestinal: Denies stomach pain, diarrhea, constipation, nausea, and denies any previous history of pancreatic or liver disease.

- Genitourinary: Denies urinary tract infections, hematuria, dysuria, hesitancy, or frequency, and states his doctors are concerned about his "weak kidneys."
- Musculoskeletal: Denies upper extremity, neck and back pain, denies arthritis, endorses leg pain per HPI.
- Neurological: Denies history of stroke, seizure, spinal cord injury, and migraine headaches. He notes that he has persistent tingling in his right foot.
- Hematological: Denies easy bruising, denies history of cancer.
- Psychiatric: Denies depression, anxiety, hallucinations, or schizophrenia.
- Integumentary: Denies any skin infections, rashes, severe itching, or skin discoloration.
- Endocrine: No history of thyroid, pituitary, or adrenal disease. He does not check blood sugar.
- Glucose by fingerstick: He states his last "diabetes number" at his primary care provider's office was normal.

Physical Examination

- Vital signs: blood pressure: right arm 155/82 mm Hg, left arm 125/74 mm Hg, heart rate 70 to 75 beats per minute, with up to 10 premature beats auscultated per minute, respirations 18 breaths per minute, at rest, temperature 35.9°C oral, oxygen saturation on room air 93%, weight 167.2 lbs (76 kg) with height of 5 ft 9 in (175 cm), slender body habitus
- Constitutional: Well nourished, appropriately groomed, appears stated age. The patient is engaged in examination, very forthcoming with information, in moderate distress from the right leg pain.
- Head/eyes/ears/nose/throat: Head: atraumatic, male patterned baldness. Eyes: no discharge or conjunctival erythema. No papilledema or nicking noted with ophthalmoscopic examination. No peripheral field visual deficits. Ears: Moderate cerumen in the left ear, tympanic membrane is easily visualized in both ears. Nose: Septum appears to be deviated slightly to the right, scant clear exudate. Mouth: The tongue, mucosa, and posterior pharynx are normal. The teeth are discolored but no loose teeth and gums are intact.
- Cardiovascular: His overall color is pale. He has a regular-irregular pulse with multiple premature beats and a grade IV/VI systolic murmur, which is loudest over his right sternal border. The patient has bilateral carotid bruits, rated as III/VI. (I am wondering if the carotid bruits are due to actual carotid artery stenosis or due to radiation of his rather loud cardiac murmur.) The peripheral pulse examination is as follows:

Peripheral Pulse Examination

Site	Femoral	Popliteal	Dorsalis Pedis	Posterior Tibial	Radial	Ulnar
Right	1+	0	0	0	2+	1+
Left	2+	1+	2+	1+	1+	0

(Key: 0 unable to palpate, 1+ faint palpable pulse, 2+ easily located/palpated, 3+ bounding pulse)

The right popliteal pulse and left ulnar pulse had monophasic Doppler signals. The right foot is markedly cooler and paler than the left foot. There is no hair on the lower half of the right calf, and the right mid-calf is 1.5 cm shorter in circumference than the left leg mid-calf. There is 4-second capillary refill in the right foot and 2-second capillary refill in the left foot and in both hands. I perform ankle brachial indices on the right foot, using a manual blood pressure cuff, and measure an opening pressure on the right arm of 155 mm Hg, and then opening pressure of the right PT as 52 mm Hg. The resultant ankle brachial index is obtained with the following formula: opening pressure of foot/ open pressure brachial. For this patient, 52/155, which is 0.33. This is very low and is consistent with impending limb ischemia.

- Pulmonary: Breath sounds are symmetric with marked inspiratory and expiratory wheezes bilaterally. He becomes slightly tachypneic with minimal exertion, getting up from the stretcher to stand.

- Gastrointestinal: The abdomen is soft, rounded, and with normoactive bowel sounds in all four quadrants. The liver inferior border is percussed to just 0.5 cm below the right costal margin. There is no flank tenderness on light palpation. There is a pulsatile, nontender mass noted on deep palpation just above and 1 cm to the left of the umbilicus. There is no evidence of any ventral or inguinal hernia when the patient does vagal maneuvers.

- Neurological: BJ is alert, oriented to person, place, and time, with 4/5 grips bilaterally. Gait is normal but slow, due to his right leg pain. He has strong dorsal and planter flexion bilaterally, at 5/5. He has loss of sensation with scratch test, on the soles of both feet. He has intact cranial nerves II-XII and his deep tendon reflexes are intact. His Romberg sign is negative.

- Integumentary: Scar on the left lateral lower quadrant was dry and completely healed. There is an incision on the lower left leg that is well healed. Thickened fingernails and toenails bilaterally. No petechiae on the lower extremities. No sign of rash or puncture wound to suggest a spider or snake bite.

❓ What are the pertinent positives and significant negatives from the review of systems and physical examination?

Pertinent Positives

- Tingling in the right foot, cooler right foot, pain in the right calf and foot
- Absent DP and PT pulses in the right leg, loss of hair in the right lower calf, and delayed capillary refill in right foot.
- Irregular heart rhythm, with frequent premature beats, tachypnea on exertion
- BJ has other examination findings to suggest vascular disease including carotid bruits, upper extremity blood pressure discrepancies, heart murmur, and small abdominal pulsatile mass (possibly and aortic aneurysm or arterio-venous fistula)

Significant Negatives

- The review of systems and the physical examination are both negative for any focal neurologic deficits, evidence of insect bites, evidence of chemical or traumatic injury to the leg, no swelling or discoloration, no associated back pain or radiation of pain

Case Analysis

With this additional information, I can sort the differential more as follows:

BJ definitely has decreased arterial flow to his right lower leg, as noted by the color, temperature, capillary refill, loss of right lower leg hair, and attenuation of his pulses. In addition, the ankle-brachial index of 0.33 suggests impending limb ischemia. The next step is an arteriogram to determine the location of the blockage and possibly treat the reduced arterial flow with a catheter-based intervention. Additional imaging such as a computed tomography (CT) scan is not necessary because the arteriogram is the gold standard for diagnosing peripheral arterial disease and offers the opportunity to both confirm the diagnosis and intervene to correct the pathology at the same time. The arteriogram includes infusion of contrast dye, which can cause kidney injury so I order a chemistry panel to evaluate his renal function. This is particularly important as the patient's diabetes puts him at high risk for renal insufficiency.

I also order telemetry monitoring and an ECG, to be done prior to the arteriogram. His irregular heart rhythm with frequent premature beats is concerning for atrial fibrillation, which can lead to a left atrial or ventricular thrombus, and subsequent embolization to the lower extremity. The ECG will tell me about the patient's baseline heart rhythm, but I will need ongoing telemetry monitoring to evaluate for paroxysmal atrial fibrillation. To rule out an existing thrombus in the left side of his heart, I will need to order an echocardiogram but this can be done after the arteriogram is completed.

CASE INFORMATION

Diagnostics: Results

Lab results (blood sent as part of emergency room routine admission)

Complete blood count including hematocrit, hemoglobin platelets and white blood cell count is within normal limits

BUN = 36 mg/dl (normal 7–20), creatinine = 1.5 mg/dl (normal 0.5–1.4), GFR = 45 mL/min/1.73m^2, glucose (random) = 286 mg/dL (normal 70–140 mg/dL), Sodium, chloride, potassium bicarbonate and magnesium are all within normal range. HgbA1C = 12.2 (normal < 5.5)

Uric acid = 4.5 (normal range = 2.4–7.5). Thyroid-stimulating hormone (TSH) = 6.5 (normal range 0.3–3.0)

Prothrombin INR = 1.2, partial thromboplastin = 31

Troponin = < 0.02 (within normal limits)

Twelve-lead electrocardiogram: There are Q waves noted in leads V1–V4, with unifocal wide complex premature beats noted. There is evidence of left anterior fascicular block (eg, left axis deviation of 45°, qR I lead I and in lead AVL).

Transthoracic Echocardiogram (TTE)

Left ventricular ejection fraction is calculated at 35% to 40%. There is moderate aortic stenosis. There is no regurgitation or stenosis noted in the mitral, pulmonic, and tricuspid valves. There is no pericardial effusion. There is no dissection in the aortic root (max diameter = 2.9 cm) or in the ascending aorta (max diameter = 2.1 cm). There is moderate hypokinesis noted in the anterior and inferior wall, and there is moderate right ventricular hypertrophy. There are no thrombi noted in the cardiac chambers.

Case Analysis

The lab profile shows that BJ is a poorly controlled diabetic, with moderate renal insufficiency, resulting in mild hyperkalemia and elevated BUN and creatinine. His normal WBC count argues against any active infection in his leg at this point. His uric acid is normal, suggesting he does not have active gout. Of note, he does have an elevated TSH, suggesting hypothyroidism, which can be further evaluated as an outpatient. He has no evidence of myocardial ischemia, as troponin is normal and there are no ST changes on his 12-lead ECG.

The 12-lead ECG demonstrates cardiac muscle scarring from a previous myocardial infarction. The left anterior block suggests there is extensive disease in the intraventricular conduction tissue, and the PVCs represent an alternative conduction pathway in the heart that may be chronic in nature. The heart rate is 80 to 85 beats per minute. BJ has extensive myocardial muscle damage from a prior infarction, but does not appear to have any acute myocardial ischemia. The patient's TTE rules out intracardiac thrombi, as a source of right leg arterial embolization. The depressed LV ejection fraction translates to lower cardiac output, which will be important when optimizing the fluid status and perfusion to the distal extremities.

CASE INFORMATION

BJ proceeds to angiography. His left groin is cannulated and a guidewire is placed cephalad into his distal abdomen. Findings with this arteriogram include:

- 3.5 max diameter infrarenal abdominal aortic aneurysm, stable, no evidence of leak.
- Left renal artery stenosis, approximately 60%.
- Focal, 2 cm, area of high-grade stenosis in the right proximal superficial femoral artery (SFA), with reconstitution of flow below the stenosis. There is a 45 mm Hg gradient across the blockage. Vascular surgery and radiology review the images and agree to intervene on the right SFA segment. The patient consents for this procedure, and a wire is successfully passed across the tight SFA region, followed by balloon angioplasty to open the stricture and placement of a covered stent to maintain patency.

This diagnostic test merged into an intervention, since there was a focal stenotic area in the right SFA that directly correlated with the patient's signs and symptoms. The high-grade 2-cm-long stricture in the proximal right SFA most likely accounted for the coolness, pain, loss of hair, and diminished pulses in the right calf and foot.

Following the procedure, BJ is admitted to the vascular service for an overnight observation stay. Orders are placed for bedrest and monitoring of the left groin puncture site and right foot pulses, as well as intravenous normal saline at 75 cc per hour to prevent acute kidney injury, from the contrast. He is given a bolus of IV heparin and then started on a continuous infusion, titrated to keep PTT between 60 and 80 to prevent thrombus formation in the new SFA stent. His blood glucose is managed with sliding scale insulin as his metformin is held for 48 hours after the procedure. In addition, labs are ordered to determine if he has an underlying condition leading to hypercoagulopathy (protein C or protein S deficiency, factor V Leiden mutation, cardiolipin antibodies).

Twelve hours after the procedure, his kidney function is reassessed with a repeat basic metabolic panel, and repeat testing of his ankle brachial index is done to ensure that his leg perfusion has improved.

Prior to discharge, BJ is scheduled in the vascular clinic for a follow-up appointment 4 weeks after the day of discharge to evaluate his right lower extremity perfusion with noninvasive pulse volume recordings and to undergo ultrasound of his carotid arteries. He is also given an appointment with his PCP to take place 2 weeks after discharge so that his renal function can be reassessed. A dictated letter is sent to the PCP describing the events of this admission.

His discharge medications include aspirin, clopidogrel, and simvastatin, which the patient was previously taking because of his recent MI, and which will also help treat his PAD.[1,2] His lisinopril is also continued but the patient is cautioned to follow a low potassium diet with this medication.[3,4] He is started on levothyroxine at 0.25 mg per day, and encouraged to follow up with his primary care doctor about the dosing of this medication. Inhalers and singular for COPD are continued and the patient is advised to resume taking his metformin 1 day after discharge.[5] His allopurinol is discontinued as he reports only a single episode of gout.

Case Follow-Up

Discharge teaching for BJ includes emphasis on the importance of smoking cessation and written information about existing resources to assist him (current strategies include nicotine patch, bupropion hydrochloride, varenicline, and hypnosis).[6,7] Prior to discharge, he is seen by the diabetic educator and instructed on monitoring his blood glucose and maintaining a log book to take with him to his PCP and endocrinology appointments.[8,9] She also provides information on food choices and portion sizes, as well as foot care, and the patient is given additional written information on these topics. For activity, he is encouraged to walk three times a day for at least 15 minutes to enhance arterial collateral circulation. Finally, he is given information about the PAD support group. BJ is advised to be seen by a health care provider immediately or come to the emergency room if his symptoms reoccur.

References

1. Coffer-Chase L. Changing paradigms for the prevention of cardiovascular events. *J Nurse Pract.* 2014;10(5):293-301.
2. Scordo K. Managing hyperlipidemia. *Nurse Pract.* 2014;39(7):28-32.
3. Caboral-Stevens M, Rosario-Smi M. Review of the Joint National Committee's Recommendation for management of hypertension. *J Nurse Pract.* 2014;10(5):325-330.
4. Scordo K, Picket K. Hypertension in 2014: making sense of the guidelines. *Nurse Pract.* 2014;39(6):19-23.
5. Bull A. Primary care of chronic dyspnea in adults. *Nurse Pract.* 2014;38(8):34-39.
6. McGrath C, Zak C, Baldwin K, Lutfiyya M. Smoking cessation in primary care: Implementation of a proactive telephone intervention. *J Am Assoc Nurse Pract.* 2014;26(5):248-254.
7. Clearing the air: quit smoking today. National Cancer Institute. National Institutes of Health. http://www.cancer.gov. Published August 2011.
8. Dlugasch L, Ugarriza D. Self-monitoring blood glucose experiences of adults with type II diabetes. *J Am Assoc Nurse Pract.* 2014;26(6):323-329.
9. Zitkus B. Update on the American Diabetes Associations standards of medical care. *Nurse Pract.* 2014;39(8):22-31.

CASE 55

Julie K. Armatas

Julie Armatas works in Vascular and Endovascular Surgery at the University of Virginia in Charlottesville. She cares for patients with both venous and arterial disease in an inpatient setting as well as an outpatient setting.

CASE INFORMATION

Chief Complaint

A 68-year-old female presents to the clinic with complaints of worsening right leg edema and pain over the last several months.

There are numerous etiologies for lower extremity edema, especially in women, but the vast majority is secondary to venous insufficiency. Idiopathic edema is the most prevalent cause of lower extremity swelling in premenopausal women.[1] Systemic disease, trauma, or malignancies may also play a role. Edema as a presenting complaint therefore may be difficult to diagnose. Initially categorizing edema into unilateral or bilateral, as well as acute or chronic, will help organize the differential. Etiologies may fit into any or all categories at different stages of the disease process.

Differential Diagnoses: Unilateral Versus Bilateral

Unilateral edema is frequently associated with obstructive disorders, injuries, infection, or lymphatic disease. Venous insufficiency, however, remains the most common etiology and is always first on my differential list. I have a low threshold for ordering a D-dimer and ultrasound to rule out a deep venous thrombosis (DVT), as they are noninvasive, inexpensive, and because missing a diagnosis of DVT could have deleterious consequences.

Bilateral edema is generally chronic and systemic in nature. Patients with cardiac or hepatic disease commonly have lower extremity dependent edema and it is important to distinguish this from an acute exacerbation of the underlying disease process. Assessing for systemic symptoms, such as shortness of breath (SOB), chest pain, or palpitations, will help determine the severity. Less concerning etiologies for bilateral edema are idiopathic edema, pregnancy, lymphedema, drugs, dependent edema, and venous insufficiency.

Differential Diagnoses: Acute Versus Chronic

In my clinic, I define acute edema as "onset of edema within 2 weeks from the time of presentation," although much of the literature defines acute edema as less than 72 hours. Acute edema is the most worrisome and may be associated with life-threatening conditions, such as a DVT. Ruling this out quickly is of utmost importance. Acute edema may be unilateral or bilateral and etiologies are frequently associated with obstructive, traumatic, musculoskeletal, or venous origins.

Edema derived from systemic conditions, such as cardiac, hepatic, or renal disease may present acutely, but is more commonly chronic in nature. Although not as common, pulmonary hypertension and early heart failure may cause chronic leg edema prior to becoming clinically obvious.[1] This should be considered when no other cause is found. Other contributors to chronic edema are the use of certain medications, lymphedema, and venous disease.

Table 55-1 outlines and categorizes common etiologies for edema.

Table 55-1   Common Etiologies of Lower Extremity Edema[1,2]

Unilateral		Bilateral	
Acute	**Chronic**	**Acute**	**Chronic**
DVT	Venous insufficiency	Idiopathic	Venous insufficiency
Musculoskeletal	Secondary lymphedema (tumors, radiation, surgery, external compression of lymph system, reflex sympathetic dystrophy)	Worsening pulmonary hypertension	Secondary lymphedema (tumors, radiation, surgery, external compression of lymph system, reflex sympathetic dystrophy)
Ruptured medial head of the gastrocnemius muscle	DVT/postphlebitic syndrome	Worsening heart failure	Pulmonary hypertension
Compartment syndrome	Primary lymphedema (Rare)	Worsening hepatic disease	Heart failure
Cellulitis	Congenital venous malformation (rare)	Worsening renal disease	Hepatic disease
Ruptured Baker cyst	May-Thurner syndrome (rare)	Inferior vena cava (IVC) obstruction	Renal disease
		Bilateral DVT	Pregnancy
		Drugs	Drugs
			Hypoalbuminemia
			Obesity
			Inferior vena cava (IVC) obstruction
			Dependent edema
			Premenstrual syndrome
			Idiopathic

Identifying several key variables during the history and physical examination will help prioritize the differential diagnosis list and assessment:

- What is the duration of symptoms? Determining acute versus chronic will narrow the differential by 50%.
- Unilateral or bilateral edema is easily identified on physical examination.
- Is there a family history of venous disease?
- What medications does the patient take that may contribute to edema? Calcium channel blockers and nonsteroidal anti-inflammatory drugs (NSAIDs) are medications known to cause lower extremity edema.[1]
- Is the condition painful? In general, DVTs are painful, venous insufficiency causes mild aching, and lymphedema and dependent edema are painless.
- Is there a known history of DVT? DVTs promote the development of postphlebitic syndrome, which may occur soon after a DVT, or years later.
- Is there a history of cardiac, renal, or hepatic disease? An exacerbation of any of these medical conditions may contribute to edema. A thorough history and physical examination are necessary to rule in or rule out systemic disease.
- Is there a history of cancer, radiation, or abdominal surgeries? Pelvic tumors or scar tissue secondary to previous surgery or radiation may contribute to venous outflow obstruction.
- Is there a history of obstructive sleep apnea (OSA) or daytime somnolence? OSA may contribute to pulmonary hypertension, a frequently overlooked etiology for lower extremity edema.
- Does the edema stop at the ankle or extend over the dorsum of the foot and toes? Venous edema stops at the ankle, while lymphedema extends across the dorsum of the foot and into the toes ("boxcar toes").
- Does the patient wake with edema? Venous edema generally subsides overnight while lymphedema may not.

CASE INFORMATION

General Survey

The patient is a 68-year-old female who is obese for her short stature. She otherwise appears healthy and walks with ease. She does not appear short of breath or uncomfortable, and has a calm demeanor.

History of Present Illness

The patient reports that she first had lower extremity swelling during pregnancies, over 40 years ago. With each pregnancy, she developed noticeable varicose veins on her legs, as well as edema, pain, and pressure in her legs during the third trimester. The symptoms resolved spontaneously after each pregnancy. Over the years, however, she has had occasional bouts of bilateral swelling and discomfort, usually in the summers and always worse in the right leg. A few years ago, she began having daily swelling in her right ankle along with aching, pressure, and tightness as the day progressed, at times necessitating rest with elevation of the extremity, which seemed to improve the symptoms. Occasionally, she has itching in the late evening around the ankle, so much so that she has difficulty falling asleep. The symptoms are gone in the morning, and return shortly after rising. Six months ago she began to notice a slight darkening of the skin around the medial right ankle. It has continued to darken over the last several months to the point that she is now alarmed by the appearance. She has been wearing a light grade compression sock at the recommendation of her primary care physician, but it does not seem to be helping.

Past Medical History

The significant past medical history is borderline hypertension, although she has not required medication. She has arthritis in her hands, knees, and hips, treated with occasional NSAIDs. Swimming in warm water seems to help. There have been no recent accidents or falls, changes in medication, or any recent hospitalizations or surgeries. She has no history of DVT or thrombophlebitis. She has no history of cardiac, renal, pulmonary, or hepatic disease.

Past Surgical History

Past surgical history includes a left knee replacement 6 years ago. She needs to have her right knee replaced, but she is waiting for resolution of the edema.

Social History

She is a lifelong nonsmoker and reports she does not drink alcohol. For the past year, she has been careful about her diet, has been exercising more, and trying to lead a healthy life. She is widowed and lives alone.

Family History

Her mother had a DVT in her 60s, ultimately requiring vein stripping. Additionally, two sisters have large varicose veins with daily pain.

Medication List

Her medication list is mostly comprised of supplements and one prescription medication. She takes a multivitamin, vitamin D, vitamin E, and a statin (she is not aware of hypercholesterolemia as a current diagnosis, but states her doctor wanted her on a statin), and NSAIDs as needed.

Case Analysis

It is clear from her history that she has struggled with venous disease for many years. Knowing that venous insufficiency is the most common etiology for lower extremity edema in women over the age of 50,[3] it is at the top of my differential. However, I still break this down into acute or chronic, and unilateral or bilateral.

In this particular case, the patient states she first developed leg edema with her pregnancies many years ago, and over the last 2 years her symptoms have worsened, indicating chronic disease. Another sign of chronic disease in this patient is the skin darkening on the right lower medial leg. Hemosiderin deposition (Figure 55-1) arises from the breakdown of the red blood cells releasing protein and iron into the tissue. It usually evolves over several years as a result of the overburdened venous system. Given the years of edema and hemosiderin staining, it is safe to say this patient has chronic lower extremity edema.

Now I determine if her edema is chronic unilateral or chronic bilateral. In chronic unilateral disease, we would expect venous insufficiency, lymphedema, or chronic DVT as the etiology. This patient, however, reports edema in both legs, worse on the right. Although she has edema bilaterally, the

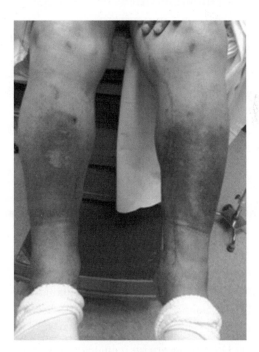

Figure 55-1   Example of advanced hemosiderin staining (notice the hemosiderin deposition has a distinct line of demarcation representing the area of increased venous pressure).

identifying variable is the distribution of the edema. Systemic disease contributes to bilateral edema with an even distribution. The fact that there is a discrepancy in her leg size makes systemic disease less likely. Venous insufficiency and lymphedema, however, often present with swelling that is worse in one leg. Based on the fact that her symptoms are present in both legs, albeit in different degrees, and that they have been present for many years, I have determined that she has chronic bilateral edema, currently worse on the right. From Table 55-1, I know that the most likely diagnoses for chronic bilateral edema are venous insufficiency, bilateral DVTs, secondary lymphedema (tumor burden, pelvic radiation, surgery, external compression of the lymphatic system), pulmonary hypertension, heart failure, renal failure, hepatic failure, pregnancy, drugs, hypoalbuminemia, obesity, IVC obstruction, dependent edema, and idiopathic edema. This may seem like a long list; however, most of these can be eliminated with a thorough history and physical examination.

So, to narrow the differential even further, I look at the pertinent positives and significant negatives from the data I have acquired so far.

❓ What are the pertinent positives from the patient's history thus far?

- 68-year-old female (venous insufficiency is the most common cause of edema in women over the age of 50[3])
- Strong family history of varicose veins (a positive family history, multiparity, female sex, and obesity are all risk factors for venous insufficiency[3])
- Varicose veins during pregnancy
- NSAID use (calcium channel blockers result in edema in up to 50% of patients; however, NSAIDs result in edema in only 5% of users[1])

❓ What are the significant negatives from the patient's history?

- Healthy diet and non-smoker
- Walks easily and swims for exercise
- Hypertension (HTN) is mild and controlled without medication
- No history of heart, pulmonary, renal, or hepatic disease
- No history of DVT or thrombophlebitis
- No history of OSA (less concern for pulmonary hypertension)
- No history of cancer
- No recent trauma, accidents, or falls

CASE INFORMATION

Review of Systems

- Constitutional: denies fever or chills, stable weight, good appetite
- Cardiovascular: denies chest pain, palpitations, or paroxysmal nocturnal dyspnea (PND)
- Pulmonary: denies cough, wheezing, shortness of breath, or obstructive sleep apnea
- Gastrointestinal: denies nausea, vomiting, diarrhea, abdominal pain, and has normal bowel movements
- Genitourinary: denies pain with voiding, reports normal urine output
- Musculoskeletal: endorses knee, hip, and hand pain that is chronic in nature and exacerbated by activity in the early morning (treated with NSAIDs and warm water exercises), endorses an ache, pressure, swelling, and heaviness in the right leg that worsens as the day progresses
- Integumentary: endorses the development of red/brown skin discoloration in her right ankle/lower right leg over the past 6 months and itching in her legs that is worse later in the day
- Neurological: no complaints of dizziness, confusion, trouble walking, falls, or numbness and tingling in her extremities
- Endocrine: not pertinent

Physical Examination

- Vital signs: Pulse is 76 beats per minute, blood pressure is 142/86 mmHg, respiratory rate is 16 breaths per minute, and temperature is 98.6 F oral. Weight is 182 lb and height is 5 ft 4 in (BMI 31.2).
- Constitutional: Well-developed obese female who is well groomed, appears stated age, and in no acute distress.
- Head/ears/eyes/neck/throat: Unremarkable.
- Cardiovascular: Regular rate and rhythm, no extra systolic beats, no murmur or gallop, no jugular venous distension (JVD), strong radial, femoral, posterior tibial and dorsalis pedis pulses bilaterally, 3 + edema in right lower leg from ankle to tibial tuberosity, 1+ edema of left ankle, no edema in feet.
- Pulmonary: Lungs clear in all fields, no accessory muscle use, and good air movement noted.
- Gastrointestinal: Abdomen large, nontender on palpation, unable to palpate liver or spleen borders, normoactive bowel sounds.
- Genitourinary: Normal.
- Neurological: Alert and oriented ×3, moves all extremities, strength 5/5 in all extremities, sensation intact to lower extremities bilaterally.
- Extremities: Right lower extremity with a large 4 to 5 mm varicosity that is first noted at the anterior shin just a few inches proximal to the dorsum

of the foot, it extends caudally, traversing the anterior-medial shin and continues to travel across the medial thigh, finally disappearing in the proximal anterior thigh. There are several notable 2 to 4 mm secondary veins scattered on the posterior thigh, medial thigh, and lateral side of the calf. There is 3+ pitting edema from the ankle to the tibial tuberosity and the dorsalis pedis pulse is easily palpable. The foot is unremarkable. The left leg has 1+ edema distally and a few scattered varicosities, the dorsalis pedis pulse is easily palpable. The foot is unremarkable.

- Skin: Right lower extremity is warm and the medial malleoli has hemosiderin deposition, there is mild dermatitis on the medial distal surface, thickening of the skin marks the area of discoloration and the beginning of lipoderma-tosclerosis, the left lower leg has mild edema and no skin changes.

❓ What elements of the review of systems and physical examination should be added to the pertinent positives list? Which items should be added to the list of significant negatives?

- **Pertinent positives:** pitting edema, aching, heaviness, and fatigue in the leg that worsens as the day progresses, hemosiderin staining, large varicose veins, lipodermatosclerosis, itching in the evenings after the veins become engorged

- **Significant negatives:** no shortness of breath, paroxysmal nocturnal dyspnea, obstructive sleep apnea, or palpitations, no cough, no abdominal distention, nausea, vomiting, or diarrhea, normal urine output, stable weight, no evidence of altered mental status (AMS) or anxiety

❓ How does this list affect all possible causes?

I know that she has chronic bilateral edema, so now I will review my list of differential diagnosis and narrow it using the information I have acquired.

- Premenstrual syndrome: She is postmenopausal.
- Pregnancy: She is not pregnant.
- Heart disease: She has no known diagnosis of heart disease; however, it could be a new diagnosis. During my examination, I have determined that she has no chest pain or shortness of breath, paroxysmal nocturnal dyspnea (PND), crackles, or jugular venous distention (JVD) to suggest cardiac disease, so I rule it out. If I were concerned, I would proceed with a B-type natriuretic peptide (BNP), electrocardiogram (ECG), echocardiogram (echo), and chest x-ray.
- Hepatic and renal disease: There is no known history and she exhibits no disease-specific symptomatology such as jaundice, ascites, spider hemangiomas,

altered mental status, anasarca, or decreased urine output. If I were concerned I would order a liver function panel, hepatitis screening, blood urea nitrogen, creatinine, electrolytes, renal duplex, abdominal duplex, or abdominal CT scan.

- Pulmonary hypertension: Once again, there is no history of pulmonary hypertension or obstructive sleep apnea, and no shortness of breath, chest pain, JVD, or other systemic symptoms to support a diagnosis of pulmonary hypertension. An echo could easily rule this out.

- IVC obstruction: If this were acute, she would have rapid onset of bilateral leg edema, and any chronic IVC obstruction would already be a known diagnosis and presented in the history of present illness or past medical history. Additionally, an IVC obstruction would cause uniform bilateral edema. I think it is safe to rule this out.

- Obesity: Obesity contributes to leg edema by impeding venous return due to excess fat compressing on the pelvic and abdominal venous system. Although she is in the obese category, she stays very active walking and swimming. Exercise promotes venous return and I doubt her weight is contributing to her edema. If it is, it is not the primary cause.

- Dependent edema: Likewise, she would not have dependent edema as this arises from a sedentary lifestyle and limited use of the *calf muscle pump*, which when contracted, propels venous blood back toward the heart. It is commonly seen in stroke patients who are confined to a wheelchair.

- Medications: While she does take NSAIDs as needed for arthritic pain, only 5% of users report edema.[1] It is much more common in daily NSAID users and I have a low index of suspicion for this given that her use is occasional. If all other possibilities were to be ruled out, I could stop the NSAIDs for 1 month to see if this helps alleviate the edema.

- Hypoalbuminemia: She exhibits no signs of malnutrition such as muscle wasting, so I have removed this from my differential. When in doubt, check an albumin level.

- Secondary lymphedema: This is due to impedance of lymphatic drainage. Common reasons are tumor burden in the abdomen or pelvis, previous trauma, radiation, or abdominal surgeries that damage lymphatic vessels, or reflex sympathetic dystrophy (RSD). She has had no radiation or surgeries, and reflex sympathetic dystrophy is unlikely as her condition has been chronic and is not associated with severe burning pain as is seen in RSD. If I were concerned about a tumor burden I would order a CT scan. Additionally, edema develops on the dorsum of the foot in both primary and secondary lymphedema and she has no pedal edema.

- Idiopathic edema: This is edema that occurs in young women during menses so it can easily be ruled out.[1]

- Venous insufficiency: The hallmark signs of venous insufficiency are leg edema, aching, heaviness, fatigue, itching, and in the chronic later stages, hemosiderin staining, skin thickening (lipodermatosclerosis), and venous stasis ulcers. Other than ulceration, she has all of these.

Simply put, almost everything one needs to know in order to diagnose limb edema can be gathered from the history and physical examination prior to ordering any diagnostic tests. Testing is therefore useful to confirm a diagnosis and guide treatment, but is not always necessary in making a diagnosis. Looking again at this patient, she has no other systemic symptoms to suggest a systemic disorder as the cause of her edema. She had no trauma, surgeries, cancers, radiation, or previous DVTs to raise concern for obstructive etiologies such as lymphedema, malignancy, or IVC obstruction. She has no acute flare of edema, as one would expect with a DVT, cellulitis, musculoskeletal injury, or compartment syndrome. Instead, she presents with classic venous insufficiency symptoms of aching, heaviness, edema, itching, and the associated skin changes of hemosiderin deposition and lipodermatosclerosis. She also notes her symptoms worsened as the day progresses. This is a classic sign of venous disease as gravity in combination with incompetent valves allows blood to reflux down the leg, resulting in engorgement of the veins. Though I am confident that my patient has venous insufficiency, I reevaluate my remaining differential diagnoses to ensure that I do not miss anything.

❓ What diagnostic tests should be done and in what order?

Some tests, such as CT scans and echocardiography, may take several days to obtain. Considerations are given to whether or not the patient's condition warrants quicker evaluation or if she is stable enough to wait for testing. With a low suspicion for systemic disease or malignancy, I refrain from ordering any labs or CT scans.

As mentioned before, if I have any suspicion for a DVT, I order a D-dimer and a venous duplex DVT ultrasound. This is an easy and inexpensive way to avoid a potential catastrophe such as pulmonary embolism arising from undiagnosed and untreated DVT. Any systemic cause of edema should be further evaluated with basic laboratory work such as a complete blood count, comprehensive metabolic profile, liver function test, urinalysis, blood sugar, thyroid-stimulating hormone, and albumin level. Additionally, a chest x-ray, electrocardiogram, echocardiogram, and B-type natriuretic peptide are useful in identifying cardiac, renal, pulmonary, or hepatic involvement. Any patient with daytime somnolence, loud snoring, and a neck circumference of >17 inches should have a sleep study and echocardiogram to rule out OSA and pulmonary hypertension.[1] This association is frequently overlooked and should always be considered part of the differential until otherwise ruled out. CT scan of the abdomen and pelvis is useful with a suspected malignancy. Likewise, CT angiography and/or venogram can be obtained to look specifically for venous obstruction and/or anatomical abnormalities, as is seen with a venous thrombosis or May-Thurner syndrome (compression of the left iliac vein by the right iliac artery). Lastly, venous duplex ultrasound is the gold standard for diagnosing venous disease. It is an easy and noninvasive way to assess the degree of venous reflux and amenability to interventions.

I order a venous duplex to rule out DVT, which is negative. Since I have a high suspicion for venous insufficiency, I also order a venous reflux study to be done at the same time as the DVT study. Reflux studies look at the deep and superficial venous systems even though there are currently no surgical treatments for defects of the deep venous system. The reflux study confirms my suspicion that she has severe reflux in the greater saphenous (superficial) veins bilaterally, worse on the right. She has moderate reflux of the deep venous system and no reflux in the small saphenous (superficial) veins. With this knowledge, I can forgo all other tests and focus on treatment options for venous insufficiency of the greater saphenous vein of the right leg.

Diagnosis and Treatment: Chronic Venous Insufficiency

The Society for Vascular Surgery (SVS) and the American Venous Forum (AVF) have developed clinical practice guidelines for the care of patients with varicose veins of the lower limbs and pelvis. Diagnosis of chronic venous disease should be based on a thorough history and physical examination as well as a duplex ultrasound of the deep and superficial veins.[3] The standard initial treatment for venous insufficiency is compression hose, rest with elevation, moderate activity, and over-the-counter (OTC) pain medications, such as acetaminophen or ibuprofen. Symptomatic patients should be instructed to wear 20 to 30 mm Hg compression hose. Higher compression, such as 30 to 40 mm Hg, is warranted in the presence of hemosiderin staining or venous ulceration. Activity is important as the calf muscle pump helps mobilize fluid out of the leg. One should alternate activity with periods of rest and leg elevation higher than the level of the heart. For most people with mild to moderate disease, this regime of compression, elevation, activity, and OTC medication is adequate. For people with more severe disease, however, this may not be enough.

Medication management alone has not proven to be effective in the treatment of venous disease. There are those who advocate for the use of venoactive drugs such as diosmin, hesperidin, rutoside, sulodexide, micronized purified flavonoid fraction, or horse chestnut extract.[3] These are not all readily available in the United States, however, and those that are available do not have enough supporting research to warrant their use. They should only be used as part of a comprehensive treatment program that combines medication with compression and elevation. It is not uncommon to see prescription diuretics given to patients with venous disease. While spironolactone is an acceptable treatment for idiopathic edema,[1] diuretics in general have little utility in the treatment of venous disease. I do not routinely prescribe diuretics for my patients with chronic edema associated with venous disease. If I do, it is because I suspect a combination of venous and chronic systemic disease.

Over time, venous insufficiency may worsen, leading to hemosiderin staining, skin thickening, and ulceration. When symptoms from saphenous insufficiency become disruptive to daily activity and quality of life, there are a number of surgical interventions that are safe and effective. A referral to a vascular surgeon or vein specialist is necessary for surgical treatment.

Vein ligation and stripping (surgical removal of the vein), once the gold standard treatment for varicose veins, has been widely replaced by newer less invasive laser techniques. Surgical treatment requires the use of general anesthesia in the outpatient surgery center, is far more painful, and the recovery longer than for laser treatment. Phlebectomy (removal of the secondary veins by making a small stab incision and pulling the vein out) is commonly done in conjunction with vein stripping.

Endovenous laser ablation and endovenous radiofrequency ablation are now the mainstay of treatment in the majority of patients with saphenous insufficiency. The procedure is done in the office setting with the use of conscious sedation. A catheter is inserted in the saphenous vein from the level of reflux to the junction with the deep system, and the vein is ablated (burned). This causes the vein to collapse and shut down. Patients are then instructed to walk frequently and may return to work the very next day. There are no incisions, only one puncture site to access the vein, and patients generally have mild to moderate pain.

Last, sclerotherapy is the injection of a sclerosing agent into a vein to scar the vein wall and permanently collapse the vein. This is usually performed for cosmetics, or for aching small to moderate sized veins that persists following laser ablation.

CASE INFORMATION

The duplex ultrasound on this patient confirmed severe reflux in the deep and superficial veins of the right leg. There are no surgical procedures available for deep veins; however, she was offered a laser ablation of the right greater saphenous vein, which she tolerated well. After the procedure she was instructed to walk hourly and she was able to return to usual activity the next day. She was placed in waist high compression hose, 30 to 40 mm Hg, to aid in closure of the vein. She returned in 1 week for a post-procedure duplex ultrasound, which confirmed the vein was closed and she had no DVT (a potential, yet rare complication of the procedure). Her symptoms of heaviness, aching, fatigue, itching, and edema had all greatly subsided. Given the presence of deep reflux, she is at greater risk of developing new symptoms over time. I encouraged her to continue to wear knee high compression hose daily as a preventative measure.

Summary and Recommendations

When evaluating a patient for leg edema, first rule out those conditions that pose a greater risk for adverse outcomes, such as acute DVT. A duplex ultrasound study is quick, noninvasive, and should be ordered with even a small suspicion for DVT, because of the potential for life-threatening complication with pulmonary embolism. If the patient has no signs or symptoms, such as shortness of breath, JVD, crackles, ascites, or murmurs, then systemic disease can be ruled out. If it is unclear, laboratory tests can easily be done to rule out most systemic causes. Question each patient to determine if their edema is unilateral or bilateral, or acute or chronic, to help narrow the differential. If the edema is chronic, and the patient has no systemic disease, venous insufficiency is the most likely diagnosis and can easily be evaluated with a venous reflux study. Initial treatment for venous disease is compression hose, rest, and elevation. For a more definitive treatment, patients who remain symptomatic may be treated with vein ligation and stripping, phlebectomy, endovenous laser ablation, or local sclerotherapy, by a qualified vascular surgeon.

References

1. Ely J, Osheroff J, Chambliss ML, Ebell MH. Approach to leg edema of unclear etiology. *J Am Board Fam Med.* 2005;19(2):148-160. doi: 10.3122/jabfm.19.2.148.
2. Smith D. *Field Guide to Bedside Diagnosis.* 2nd ed. Philadelphia, PA: Lippincott Williams & Wilkins; 2007: 51-52, 69-70.
3. Gloviczki P, Comerota A, Daising M, et al. The care of patients with varicose veins and associated chronic venous disease: clinical practice guidelines of the Society of Vascular Surgery and the American Venous Forum. *J Vasc Surg.* 2011;53(5 suppl):2s-48s. doi: 10.1016/jvs.2011.01.079.

CASE 56

Sheryl Hollyday

Sheryl Hollyday specializes in Palliative Care in both inpatient and outpatient settings at St Vincent's Medical Center. She is an end-of-life care trainer who provides support and education to patients, family members, and professionals.

CASE INFORMATION

Chief Complaint

An 82-year-old female, Martha, comes to the emergency department, brought in from home by a family member who reports she has altered mental status. This case is initially evaluated in the emergency department with subsequent admission to a medical unit.

? What is the potential cause?

In the assessment of an elderly patient, there are multiple conditions that can present with an altered mental status. The key in determining a course of action is the patient's past medical history, current health issues, and functional status. My first priorities include assessment of the patient's physical status and interviewing the patient and family members.

Comprehensive Differential Diagnoses for Patient With Altered Mental State.[1]

- Neurologic: acute stroke (embolic or hemorrhagic), traumatic head injury, seizure with postictal state, seizure, brain tumor, meningitis, delirium
- Cardiovascular: myocardial infarction, cardiac arrhythmia, congestive heart failure (CHF) exacerbation, hypertensive encephalopathy
- Pulmonary: hypoxia, carbon monoxide poisoning, pulmonary embolism, pneumonia, chronic obstructive pulmonary disease (COPD) exacerbation
- Gastrointestinal: ischemic bowel, cholecystitis, appendicitis, diverticulitis, constipation, gastritis, colitis
- Genitourinary: urinary tract infection, urinary retention or obstruction, acute renal failure/azotemia
- Musculoskeletal: fracture
- Endocrine: adrenal insufficiency, myxedema, thyrotoxicosis, diabetes insipidus, syndrome of inappropriate anti-diuretic hormone (SIADH)

- Psychiatric disorder: depression, new onset or exacerbation of bipolar disorder, psychosis
- Metabolic: dehydration, electrolyte imbalance, hyperglycemia, hypoglycemia, hypernatremia, hyponatremia, hepatic encephalopathy, metabolic encephalopathy
- Exogenous: medication side effect or interaction or withdrawal, drug overdose, alcohol intoxication or withdrawal

CASE INFORMATION

History of Present Illness

There are a multitude of differential diagnoses for a patient presenting with an altered mental status. The medical history of a patient is the most useful and important element in making an accurate diagnosis. Prior to my interview and physical assessment, I review the patient's electronic medical record, which delineates three admissions to the medical center over the past 5 months and two to an extended care facility (ECF). The reasons for the admissions to the medical center were as follows: the first due to a fall with subsequent admission to an ECF for rehabilitation, the second a urinary tract infection (UTI). Four weeks ago, after admission for pneumonia and a stage II sacral decubitus ulcer, Martha went to an ECF for rehabilitation purposes and was discharged to home 9 days ago.

According to review, the patient does have a primary care provider, but has not seen her in more than 5 years. Her past medical history is significant for an 8-year history of dementia and asthma. She takes no medications on a regular basis. She is a widow, has no children and has lived with her sister in the home they grew up in for more than 10 years following the death of her husband.

After introducing myself to the patient's sister who is at her side, my general assessment begins. Martha is asleep. She is frail, has positive bitemporal wasting and alopecia. Her skin is clean with no odor appreciated. I am able to awaken Martha to ask her questions. She stares at me cautiously and has a flat affect. She will not answer my simple questions. Her sister Ann begins to speak on her behalf. She tells me that over the past 6 months she has noticed some changes in Martha's behavior. Ann says, "Everything has gone downhill since she fell about 5 months ago. She has always been pretty healthy, but now she doesn't seem to be getting better like I thought she would. When she fell, she bruised her hip, so after staying in the hospital they sent her to rehab. She came back home after about two weeks, but she really wasn't eating very much. She never ate much anyway, look at her." Ann estimates that Martha has lost 15 lb over the last 5 months. I then ask Ann about the more recent discharge to the ECF after being treated for pneumonia and the decubiti. "The antibiotics they gave her cleared the pneumonia up, but that ulcer is still there and we have the visiting nurses coming out to fix that." Ann tells me that "Martha knows who I am, on most days, but is confused around other people and can't remember their names." She can transfer from her bed to the chair, but has not walked on her own for the last 3 months. She no longer bathes, dresses, or feeds herself and relies on others for all of her physical care. She sleeps for much of the day, approximately 10 hours and then seems to be awake more during the night. She does not initiate conversations and generally answers "yes or no" to questions that are asked of her. She eats pureed food, drinks water when offered, but does experience "quite a bit of coughing" while she is eating.

Medical History

Ann reports the patient has no history of diabetes, heart disease, stroke, or cancer. She reports that the patient has been forgetful for the last 8 years, but more confused over the past 5 months. The electronic medical record confirms a history of asthma and dementia, no surgical history.

Family History

Mother died age 85 of stroke. Father died age 79 from sudden cardiac death, also had a history of dementia, unsure of age of diagnosis.

❓ What are the pertinent positives from the information given so far?

- History of fall
- Three admissions during the last 5 months
- Known history of dementia but has not had regular medica. care
- Sleeping hours are more than hours awake
- Mental status deterioration (reason for admit)
- Eating less—mostly pureed, and coughs after eating, cachexia, and 15 lb weight loss over the last 5 months
- Decreased activity level
- Known decubiti

❓ What are the significant negatives from the information given so far?

- The patient appears comfortable.
- No history of heart disease, heart failure, stroke or seizures.

? **Can the information gathered so far be restated in a single sentence highlighting the pieces that narrow down the cause?**

The problem representation in this case might be: "an 82-year-old with a known history of dementia presenting with an altered mental status and overall decline in health; failure to thrive."

CASE INFORMATION

Review of Systems

The patient is unable to participate with interview questions; her family member is able to share some information regarding her health status.

• Constitutional: At home, Ann was unable to take her temperature, but said her skin felt very warm last night. She refused breakfast this morning and had only eaten a small amount of breakfast yesterday. Sleeping approximately 18 hours out of the past 24 hours. No recent falls, less verbal over the past week, and was not able to recognize family members who visited 3 days prior to this admission.

• Cardiovascular: No complaints of chest pain or palpitations.

• Pulmonary: Complaints per sister of rapid breathing at times and trouble catching her breath even with turning in bed. Nonproductive cough following feeding and after drinking fluids.

• Gastrointestinal: Incontinent of stool for more than 5 months. + Constipation, no blood noted in stool.

• Genitourinary: Incontinent of urine for more than 5 months. No change in smell, frequency, or amount noted.

• Musculoskeletal: Generalized pain demonstrated by moaning and facial grimacing when sitting in a chair for prolonged periods of time.

• Neurological: Baseline is confusion. Per Ann, does not initiate conversations with family members anymore. No longer recognizes most family members.

• Endocrine: No issues.

Physical Examination

• Vital signs: Pulse is 94 beats per minute, blood pressure in 160/90 mmHg, respiratory rate is 24 breaths per minute, temperature is 100.6 F rectally, oxygen saturation on room air is 89%, increased to 91% on 2L nasal cannula, calculated BMI is 17.

- General: Chronically ill appearing, asleep at present. She awakens to voice but is unable to participate in interview. She appears frail and cachectic. Sleeping, no indication of pain or discomfort as evidenced by lack of moaning, grimacing, or distress.
- Neurological: Unable to assess as patient is nonverbal at present. Per family, this is her baseline.
- Head/Eyes/Ears/Nose/Throat: Normocephalic, anicteric, bitemporal wasting, missing dentition including two upper canine and two lower bicuspids, dry oral mucosa. Pupils equal and reactive to light.
- Cardiovascular: S1, S2, regular rate and rhythm, no murmurs, rubs, or gallops appreciated; trace edema noted in bilateral lower extremities; ankles and feet. An ECG done in the ED shows no ischemic changes or arrhythmias.
- Pulmonary: Tachypnea—rate 25, slightly labored respiratory effort at rest, with use of accessory muscles. Decreased breath sounds bilaterally, with rhonchi at right lower lobe.
- Gastrointestinal: Normoactive bowel sounds, nontender to gentle palpation.
- Genitourinary: Incontinent small amounts of urine.
- Integumentary: Warm to touch, frail, pale skin, poor turgor. Stage II decubiti ulcer sacral area. Her fingernails are long as are her toenails.

? Given the new information, what additional pertinent positives or significant negatives may be added to your list?

- **Pertinent positives:** chronically ill appearing, lethargic, labored breathing, oxygen saturation 89% on room air, decreased breath bilaterally with right lower lobe rhonchi, trace lower extremity edema, poor skin turgor, missing teeth.
- **Significant negatives:** the review of systems and physical examination reveal no signs of acute pain, her ECG is essentially normal, and cardiac examination normal.

? How does this information affect the list of possible causes?

According to the past medical history and the family reports, the patient has had dementia for at least 8 years, which has worsened over the last 5 months, and most acutely in the last 4 weeks. While dementia is a chronic and terminal condition, an acute change in mental status may be due to a reversible cause. While I suspect this change in mental status may have a treatable cause, it may also be part of a gradual decline in the patient's condition, resulting in a failure to thrive presentation. Regardless, it is important that I consider potential etiologies for the patient's acute mental status changes. I do this by carefully considering my differential by system.

- Neurologic: As I review the differential diagnoses for altered mental status, I am fairly confident that Martha has not had a neurological event such as an acute stroke as evidenced by my examination findings and her known history. Meningitis is possible but I would expect the patient to be much more ill than she currently appears. She has had no injuries to her head and her examination is benign, thus I consider a subdural hematoma very unlikely. Brain tumor and seizures are possible, but again unlikely as her neurologic findings are not focal, no seizure activity has been noted, and neurological changes to date are more consistent with her underlying disease. Because delirium and dementia often coexist, the diagnosis of delirium is high on my differential. A helpful mnemonic as to the most common causes of delirium is DELIRIUMS. Most of these are considered already on my differential and include: Drugs (anticholinergics, neuroleptics, long-acting benzodiazepines, others), Emotional (mood disorder, loss), Low PO_2 (hypoxemia from pneumonia, chronic obstructive pulmonary disorder, pulmonary embolus), Infection (urinary tract, respiratory tract, others), Retention of urine or feces, Ictal or postictal state, Under nutrition (protein/caloric malnutrition, vitamin B_{12} or folate deficiency, dehydration), Metabolic (thyroid, diabetes mellitus), and Subdural hematoma.[2] I continue to evaluate my patient by system as all these potential causes of delirium are accounted for in my comprehensive differential.

- Cardiac: I do not believe that she has had a cardiac event. There are no complaints of chest pain and her ECG is normal. Her heart rate is mildly elevated but she does have a temperature, which can be the cause of the tachycardia. The ED bedside monitor shows normal sinus rhythm at 101 with rare PVCs.

- Gastrointestinal: She is in no acute distress to indicate that she has a gastrointestinal issue, her gastrointestinal examination is benign, and her caregivers report no changes in her usual bowel patterns.

- Pulmonary: Because she has had a fever and currently has right lower lobe rhonchi in addition to hypoxemia on admission, a pulmonary cause such as pneumonia is high on my list of reasons for her decline. In addition, her history of coughing with eating and drinking makes aspiration pneumonia very likely. Exposure to carbon monoxide is not supported by any of her history, she does not have chronic obstructive pulmonary disease (COPD), and while pulmonary embolism as a cause cannot be eliminated, it is lower on my list for now.

- Genitourinary: Elderly women with incontinence have a high risk of urinary tract infections and they commonly result in associated mental status changes. This diagnosis remains a potential cause of her fever and malaise and must be evaluated further.

- Musculoskeletal, psychiatric, and endocrine: These systems are low on my list of potential causes of her decline. No obvious changes in her musculo-skeletal system are present and she has not experienced additional falls or injuries. She shows no physical signs of distress or discomfort with movement or examination. Drug toxicity is not on my differential as she does not take any medications nor have any new drugs been added. And, while she has poor skin turgor, her intake, per Ann, has been decreased and is likely the cause. No other signs of metabolic etiologies are evident in her history or examination. At this point the most likely cause of her recent mental status decline is aspiration pneumonia but focused diagnostic testing is necessary to confirm the diagnosis and definitively rule out other potential causes.

❓ What diagnostic testing should be done and in what order?

Diagnostic testing should be focused in order to reveal a causal etiology for potentially reversible conditions. As a baseline for all patients with changes in mental status, laboratory work should include blood urea nitrogen (BUN), creatinine, glucose, sodium, hepatic enzymes, vitamin B_{12}/folate, thyroid, rapid plasma regain (RPR), complete blood count with white blood count differential, urinalysis (UA), urine culture with sensitivities, ECG, and chest x-ray. The following diagnostic testing can be considered if history and physical, known risk factors, and presentation findings suggest that they are needed: brain imaging (computed tomography vs magnetic resonance imaging), positron emission tomography (PET) scan, toxicology screen, erythrocyte sedimentation rate (ESR), human immunodeficiency virus (HIV).[3]

With the history presented by the family as well as the review of prior medical records, I do not order all the labs that I listed above, as not all are indicated in this case. Instead I have carefully selected the following diagnostics to assess my patient:

- Imaging: Chest x-ray anterior/posterior and lateral.

- Labs: I order a basic metabolic panel, complete blood count with differential, UA, urine culture and sensitivities, and sputum culture. Because of her low BMI, I suspect protein calorie malnutrition. To that end I also check a prealbumin, albumin, vitamin D, and B_{12}. Because she is hypoxemic and in mild respiratory distress, I order an arterial blood gas.

I explain to Ann why the tests will be done and how they will help the care team determine the ongoing plan of care. I also tell Ann why it is important that I admit her sister to the medical floor and that antibiotics will be initiated based on the results of the chest x-ray.

CASE INFORMATION

Diagnostic Results

Chest x-ray: Right lower lobe infiltrate, likely pneumonia.

Labs: The labs show an increased sodium level of 146 mEq/L (normal 135–145 mEq/L) as well as a slightly elevated BUN of 31 mg/dL (normal 7–18 mg/dL) and creatinine 1.7 mg/dL (normal 0.5–1.5 mg/dL), which suggests pre-renal failure likely due to dehydration. The hemoglobin and hematocrit are normal but the white blood cell count is elevated at 18,000 cells/µL (normal 5000–10,000 cells/µL), suggesting an infectious process. The urine culture and sensitivity is negative, and the sputum culture and sensitivity shows gram-positive *Staphylococcus*. Sputum Gram staining and culture are helpful in ascertaining the pathogen in fewer than 50% of persons with health care–acquired pneumonia (HAP.) Most often, the sputum specimen is inadequate, coming from the oropharynx rather than the chest. Clues to an inadequate specimen are the presence of a large number of epithelial cells with few white blood cells. Conversely, if a large number of white blood cells and few epithelial cells are found, the specimen is from the airways or lungs. Because definitive identification of the organism is unlikely, the choice of antimicrobial agent for the treatment of pneumonia is largely empirical, directed at the most likely causative organism in view of patient characteristics, such as age, comorbidities, exposure to hospital-acquired organisms, and aspiration.[4]

The arterial blood gas results on 2 L nasal cannula are as follows: pH 7.47, $PaCO_2$ 30 mm Hg, PaO_2 88, bicarbonate 25 mEq/L, which indicates an uncompensated respiratory alkalosis. Vitamin D 30 ng/mL (normal 30–100 ng/mL), albumin 2.7 (normal 35–50 g/L), pre-albumin 15 mg/dL (normal 18–36 mg/dL), and B_{12} 150 pg/mL (normal >200 pg/mL) are abnormally low, which indicates malnutrition. These along with the history provided confirms my suspicions of failure to thrive. At this point in the assessment, I do not feel further testing such as brain imaging is necessary or appropriate.

❓ How does the additional information obtained affect your problem representation?

The problem representation in this case now is as follows: an 82-year-old female with 8-year history of dementia presents with further decline in mental status, fever, cough with eating and drinking, and probable aspiration pneumonia. Given the progressive decline of the patient, my diagnosis is aspiration pneumonia secondary to end-stage dementia.

? What treatments for the patient are necessary on the medical floor? What other issues related to long-term management are necessary to consider and discuss with the family?

There are goals to be addressed with family members that will require time and effort on the part of the practitioner managing the patient. Aspiration pneumonia can be treated with antibiotics. However, the difficulty with this treatment is that the underlying problem, her dementia and aspiration risk, cannot be fixed. This is a terminal diagnosis in regard to an end-stage dementia patient. The patient will continue to aspirate her oral secretions, so that even if a percutaneous endoscopic gastrostomy (PEG tube) is placed for nutrition purposes, aspiration will continue to occur. End-state dementia is characterized by severe short-term and long-term memory loss, inability to communicate and ambulate, and complete dependence on others to perform the activities of daily living. Frailty, delirium, falls, and urinary incontinence are common symptoms in end-stage dementia.[5] Aspiration of food as well as salivary secretions is an indicator in assessing if a patient has progressed to what can be considered "end-stage dementia."

The discussion with family members may be challenging depending on the practitioner's level of confidence in discussing such sensitive topics such as inability to feed, comfort measures, hospice care, and end-of-life issues. Until I can have these discussions with the family, I order a 7-day course of intravenous antibiotics, which is the mainstay of medical therapy for bacterial pneumonia. First-line antimicrobials for *S pneumoniae*, the most prevalent cause of bacterial pneumonia, are for the penicillin-susceptible form of the bacterium, penicillin G, and amoxicillin. For the penicillin-resistant form of *S pneumoniae*, first-line agents are chosen on the basis of sensitivity.[6] Because of Martha's recent hospital and extended care facility visit, I treat this pneumonia as a health care–acquired (HCA) pneumonia and will prescribe Cefepime 1 g IV every 8 hours. Clindamycin can also be added for coverage if there is evidence of oral abscesses, an implanted prosthetic device, or high suspicion of aspiration of saliva.

I initiate intravenous (IV) hydration therapy with dextrose 5% in water with 0.45% normal saline (D5W1/2NS) at 84 mL/hour because she is dehydrated. There are applications available via the Internet that will help determine maintenance IV therapy. I have found the following formula helpful, and it compares to the results I have found online: add 40 to the patient's weight in kilograms to determine initial maintenance IV fluids. Example: Martha's weight is 43.6 kg. 43.6 + 40 = 83.6. Because of her dysphagia, I have ordered that she not have anything by mouth until a bedside swallow evaluation can be completed by the speech therapist. I have continued her orders for nasal cannula oxygen at 2 liters per minute.

I have also spoken with Ann regarding resuscitation status. All practitioners should be able to thoughtfully talk to patients and family members about this topic. It is important that we never say: "Do you want us to do everything?" "Everything" is never appropriate. All hospitals are required by Medicare to inquire on admission if the patient has a living will, also known as an advanced directive (AD). This is an opportunity to ascertain whether or not this document exists and/or is available to review. Because state laws vary, as does the language within the AD, it is important to clarify what the patient/ family members understand about the written directive. For instance, many directives state, "If I am in a persistent vegetative state, or terminal condition." This is easily misunderstood and deserves clarification. In Martha's case, she does not have any written documents about her wishes, but after talking with Ann about what Martha would want or not want done, I complete an order for no CPR as well as no intubation for respiratory distress.

The speech therapist performs a bedside swallow evaluation on hospital day 2. Martha is more awake than upon admission and is cooperating with the evaluation. Unfortunately, after multiple attempts with various food consistencies, Martha is unable to safely swallow without showing signs of aspiration. Her respirations are less labored, her heart rate is now 75 but she continues to sleep much of the day with very little interaction with her sister or the staff.

My plan during this admission is to involve the palliative care team in assisting the patient's sister to understand that this is terminal diagnosis. Palliative care should not be utilized simply to "get a code status." Palliative care physicians, advanced practice registered nurses, nurses, and social workers meet with patients and family members to determine what the future goals of care are for a patient with a chronic and/or terminal disease. The ability to involve palliative care early in the admission is preferred. This allows the team members to develop a relationship with the patient/family.

On hospital day 2, the palliative care nurse practitioner meets with Ann and discusses goals of care for Martha. Because Martha has "failed" the swallow evaluation, meaning that she cannot safely eat or drink fluids without aspirating, the discussion focuses on allowing a natural death for Martha. It is not appropriate to offer a percutaneous endoscopic tube (PEG tube) in this case, as Martha is now deemed end stage, and terminal in regard to her dementia.

Artificial Nutrition for Patients With Advanced Dementia and Adult Failure to Thrive

There is strong evidence that feeding tubes do not help patients with advanced dementia or adult failure to thrive and expert opinion recommends they not be offered.[7] Studies have definitively demonstrated that such therapy does not prolong life, nor does it decrease the risk of pneumonia. In addition such feedings do not improve wound healing and patients do not gain weight, strength, or functional ability (ie, walking or self-care).[8] Patients with advanced dementia also frequently pull at their tubes, causing them to be dislodged. Unfortunately this results in the use of physical restraints, such as tying their wrists to the bed, in an attempt to keep this from happening. Tube feeding, like all medical treatments, can be declined or stopped, especially in the setting of a terminal illness where its use will not alter the ultimate outcome.

Case Follow-Up

Martha's diagnosis makes her eligible to receive services from a hospice agency. Hospice is a philosophy of care and not necessarily a place. Medicare has criteria for patients that determine eligibility. A key factor in initiating the hospice benefit is the diagnosis of a terminal condition with a prognosis of 6 months or less of life if the illness runs its normal course and further curative treatment for the terminal illness is discontinued. In Martha's case, that would be antibiotic therapy. Each hospital has its own policy about eligibility for hospice within the hospital. In general, if death is imminent (less than 48 hours) the patient may remain in the hospital under hospice care. If the patient's prognosis, as evidenced by vital signs, urine output, and mental status, is thought to have a longer time frame for the expected death, the patient may be moved to an inpatient hospice facility, ECF with hospice support, or the patient's home with support from visiting nurses through an outpatient hospice program.

The palliative care NP and I meet with Ann to provide her with the options for hospice. This type of meeting may be quite lengthy so it is essential to allow adequate time to have a thoughtful and meaningful conversation. Family will never forget the provider and the team that handles this transition well; they will never forgive those who handle it poorly. Hospice is sometimes described as an alternative in which less care is given because curative measures are discontinued. In fact, a better explanation emphasizes the many interventions that the hospice benefit does cover. In the case of Martha, we explain to Ann the specifics of comfort-focused care that Martha will receive as part of the hospice benefit, including bathing, treating fevers, managing anxiety and pain, frequent oral care, and frequent turning and positioning as appropriate. We ask Ann if Martha ever expressed an opinion on the setting of her death, and Ann states her view that her sister would want to die at home. To honor this wish, arrangements are made with the local visiting nurse agency/hospice agency for a hospital bed and oxygen equipment to be delivered to the home that afternoon with transport planned for the next day. I discontinue Martha's antibiotics and the IV hydration, as these are no longer indicated as part of Martha's comfort focused care. Ann expresses some concern about Martha being hungry or thirsty and I reassure her that if Martha requests food or fluid, it will be provided. With time, family members of dying patients often find that their loved one no longer desires or requests these items, as decline in appetite is a natural part of end of life.

Martha's obituary was seen 4 days later in the local paper. It stated, "Martha died peacefully in her home surrounded by her family."

References

1. Epocrates Web site. http://www.epocrates.com. Accessed. August 2, 2014.
2. Fitzgerald MA. *Nurse Practitioner Certification Examination and Practice Preparation*. 2nd ed. Philadelphia, PA: FA Davis Company; 2005.
3. Lab values, normal adult. Medscape Web site. http://emedicine.medscape.com/article/2172316-overview. Accessed December 1, 2014.
4. *Nursing Review and Resource Manual Family Nurse Practitioner*. 3rd ed. Silver Spring, MD: The Institute for Credentialing Innovation; 2009:301.

5. Harrington CC. Clinical considerations in end-state dementia. *Adv NPs PAs*. September 2013;4(9):18-23.
6. Bacterial pneumonia. Medscape Web site. http://emedicine.medscape.com/article/300157-overview. Accessed August 2, 2014.
7. High short-term mortality in hospitalized patients with advanced dementia. JAMA Internal Medicine. http://archinte.ama-assn.org/cgi/content/abstract/161/4/594. Accessed August 2, 2014.
8. Feeding tubes in patients with severe dementia. http://www.drplace.com/Feeding_Tubes_in_Patients_with_Severe_Dementia.16.28273.htm. Accessed August 2, 2014.

CASE 57

Kelly Wozneak

Kelly Wozneak is an ACNP in the Medical Intensive Care Unit at the University of Virginia Health Sciences Center in Charlottesville.

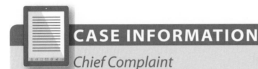

CASE INFORMATION

Chief Complaint

A 60-year-old male presents with shortness of breath progressively worsening over the last 2 weeks and accompanied by increasing production of yellowish/greenish sputum.

❓ What is the potential cause?

Shortness of breath is a nonspecific symptom with a broad differential diagnoses list. I need to review the list of differential diagnoses starting with the most life threatening and working my way down to the least life threatening. In the medical intensive care unit (MICU), our patients are not only very sick, but often have multiple comorbidities. I need to quickly determine if my patient's worsening dyspnea is caused by a pulmonary embolism, a myocardial infarction, or a pneumothorax, as these are diagnoses that require immediate intervention to ensure a successful outcome.

Comprehensive Differential Diagnoses for Patient With Acute Dyspnea[1]

Respiratory
- Chronic obstructive pulmonary disease (COPD) exacerbation
- Asthma exacerbation
- Respiratory airway obstruction, such as a mucous plug or a foreign body (food, pills, etc)
- Spontaneous pneumothorax: in a COPD patient could be from a bleb rupture (also, but less likely, hemothorax possibly from rib fracture or hepatohydrothorax)
- Respiratory infections, pneumonia and bronchitis, viral, bacterial, or fungal
- Pulmonary tumor
- Pleural effusion

Cardiovascular

- Pulmonary embolism or other type of embolus (air, fluid, fat) to an artery in the lungs.
- Acute coronary syndrome (unstable angina or myocardial infarction)
- Congestive heart failure (CHF) resulting in pulmonary edema
- Cardiac arrhythmia
- Valve disease

Neurologic

- Stroke
- Guillain-Barre syndrome
- Myasthenia gravis
- Amyotrophic lateral sclerosis
- Respiratory muscle deficiency

Other

- Noncardiogenic pulmonary edema (adult respiratory distress syndrome).
- Carbon monoxide poisoning.
- Severe allergic reaction: angioedema secondary to allergic reaction can cause airway compromise.
- Ascites
- Gastroesophageal reflux disease
- Acute renal failure
- Anxiety

With all these possible diagnoses in mind, I begin gathering and organizing data to rule out some of the possible life-threatening causes and move other, more likely, choices higher in my differential.

CASE INFORMATION

History of Present Illness

I begin with a general survey of the patient: he is a thin, but not cachectic, well-developed appropriately groomed male appearing moderately distressed as he is tachypneic and wearing oxygen via nasal cannula. He is able to move all extremities. When asked why he came in, he says with minimal eye contact, "My breathing was getting worse and the oxygen wasn't helping enough." The patient denies associated chest pain but does note that his usual productive cough now brings up yellow/green sputum. He denies fevers, chills, night sweats, recent sick contacts, recent trauma, or any falls. He first noticed increased shortness of breath on exertion about 2 weeks ago, and his breathing became increasingly difficult over the last 3 days.

He normally wears oxygen only at night but over the last 3 days he is wearing it all the time, though this did not give him much relief. The patient's son, John, is next to his dad and says, "I brought my dad to the ER because he hasn't been eating much and is wearing his oxygen all the time now instead of just at night and we both agreed his breathing seemed to be getting worse and that we should just go ahead and come to the hospital. He really didn't want to and I kind of had to talk him in to it." The son tells me that his dad has been through so much with his illnesses and seems so tired of all of it at this point, to which the patient said, "You got that right."

Past Medical History (From the Patient's Son and Confirmed by Electronic Health Record)

- Chronic obstructive pulmonary disease (COPD), Pulmonary function tests 5 years ago: chronic obstructive pulmonary disease, FEV_1 65% predicted, Arterial blood gas 7.37, $PaCO_2$ 55 mm Hg, bicarbonate 30 mEq/L, PaO_2 70 mm Hg on RA
- Rheumatoid arthritis (RA)
- Hypertension
- Lung cancer: diagnosed 1 year ago, now status post right upper lobe lobectomy, radiation, and chemotherapy. Biopsy results in the electronic health record show mixed squamous cell and adenocarcinoma
- Community acquired pneumonia: treated by his primary care provider 6 months ago
- The patient denies any history of heart disease or diabetes

Surgical History

- Bilateral cataract removal 5 years ago
- Right upper lobectomy for cancer 1 year ago

Social History

- Smoked 1.5 packs per day for 44 years until diagnosis with lung cancer 1 year ago
- Widower, lives alone, his son lives nearby and helps him out, sees him daily
- Allergies: Arava (leflunomide) caused angioedema (tongue swelling)

Current Medications

- Budesonide-formoterol fumarate (Symbicort): 160 to 4.5 µg/ACT inhaler; two puffs inhaled into lungs two times a day
- Ciprofloxacin 0.3% ophthalmic solution: one drop into both right and left eye four times daily
- Folic acid tablet 1 mg: one tablet by mouth daily
- Hydroxychloroquine (Plaquenil) 200 mg tablet: one tablet by mouth two times daily

- Losartan-hydrochlorothiazide (Hyzaar) 50 to 12.5 mg tablet: one tablet by mouth daily
- Montelukast (Singulair) 10 mg tablet: one tablet by mouth nightly
- Naproxen sodium (Anaprox) 550 mg tablet: one tablet by mouth two times daily with food
- Prednisone (Deltasone) 1 mg tablet: take four tablets (4 mg) by mouth daily
- Tiotropium (Spiriva Handihaler) 18 µg capsule: inhale one capsule via device into lungs daily

Allergies

None known.

What are the pertinent positives from the information given so far?

- The patient has increasing dyspnea starting about 2 weeks ago and worsening over the last 3 days.
- The patient has a history of smoking and significant COPD requiring O_2 at night.
- He has a history of lung cancer treated with surgery, radiation, and chemotherapy.
- The patient has a history of RA and is on hydroxychloroquine, prednisone, and naproxen sodium for treatment.
- The patient was treated for community acquired pneumonia in January.
- He has increased cough and sputum production with color change to darker yellowish-green.
- Increased oxygen requirement over past 3 days.

What are the significant negatives from the information given so far?

- He does not have a history of coronary disease or congestive heart failure.
- No fever, no chills, night sweats.
- No sick contacts.
- No recent history of trauma or falls.
- No history of asthma.
- No history of neurological disease, diabetes.

Given the information obtained so far, what might the problem representation be?

The problem representation in this case is: "a 60-year-old male with hypertension, RA, COPD requiring oxygen at night, history of lung CA and RUL lobectomy presents with increasing shortness of breath and cough over the past 2 weeks with acute worsening in the past 3 to 4 days."

Case Analysis

At this point, COPD exacerbation due to a respiratory infection is my number one suspicion in this older adult with known COPD. The pattern of gradually worsening dyspnea makes pulmonary embolism, myocardial infarction, and pneumothorax—the three diagnoses of greatest concern—less likely. These disorders generally cause an acute onset of severe symptoms and this patient describes a more gradual course. In addition, there is often pain associated with these conditions and this patient denies chest pain. The fact that he has concomitant green sputum production is not associated with these conditions but is consistent with a bronchial or lung infection. But I cannot rule out these critical pathologies without gathering more information. I also am aware that myocardial infarction in particular could have occurred as a result of his greatly increased work of breathing.

His history of lung cancer with surgery, radiation, and chemotherapy raises concern for possible recurrence of his cancer or treatment-related complications such as postsurgical or postradiation obstruction. These conditions would be more likely to cause the gradual progression of symptoms that this patient describes. Severe anemia combined with chronic lung disease could also cause shortness of breath but this would not explain his productive cough. The cough with purulent sputum and the absence of any history of neurological disease make me less concerned about that category of disorders, but I plan to further assess his neurological status when I do my physical examination.

Prior to doing a full history and physical, I order a stat chest x-ray (CXR) that will help me diagnose pneumonia, atelectasis, pneumothorax, pulmonary edema, and pleural effusion. I will also obtain a stat ECG in case this is his first presentation with a cardiac arrhythmia or coronary artery disease. I also order an arterial blood gas (ABG) to assess his degree of hypoxemia and hypercarbia, a complete blood count with differential to evaluate for anemia and leukocytosis due to infection, a basic metabolic panel to evaluate his renal function, and a lactic acid as this is a marker for sepsis. Along with the ECG, I order troponin levels, which can rule out non-ST-elevation myocardial infarction (NSTEMI). The patient does not have a cardiac history but in some patients, shortness of breath is actually a symptom of angina and if this patient is experiencing acute coronary syndrome, time is of the essence. I ask the nurse to place the patient on a monitor so we can watch for any sign of arrhythmia. I also order a type B natriuretic peptide (BNP) to evaluate for cardiac stretch from heart failure or from right ventricular strain. I consider ordering a D-dimer to rule out a pulmonary embolism (PE) but this is not a useful test to rule out PE in patients with cancer and the Wells score for predicating DVT is also less useful in the setting of cancer.[2] I may need to order a cat scan pulmonary angiogram (CTPA) to definitively rule out a PE but based on the information I have so far, a COPD exacerbation seems much more likely so I will proceed with the review of systems and physical examination first while I wait for the results of my diagnostic tests.

CASE INFORMATION

Review of Systems

- Constitutional: Denies fever, chills, reports his appetite is usually "pretty good" but has not eaten well over the last 3 to 4 days due to shortness of breath. Has not experienced any recent falls or trauma. Endorses generalized weakness and fatigue that has worsened over the past few days, and weight loss of 10 lb over the last couple of months. Has not taken any new medications in the past week.
- Cardiovascular: The patient denies chest pain but endorses occasional chest pressure with a deep chest ache; he attributes this to his lung disease and notes that this is not a new symptom. The pressure gets worse with coughing and better when he coughs less, and sometimes he feels pressure in his chest when his breathing becomes "short." Denies leg swelling, or difficulty breathing when lying down.
- Pulmonary: The patient endorses worsening shortness of breath over the last 2 weeks. A month ago he could climb the stairs and in the past couple of days he says he gets short of breath just moving around in the bed. He also endorses changes in sputum production including increased thickening, increased amount, and a change in color to dark yellow with a greenish tint. He denies chest trauma and denies carbon monoxide exposure.
- Gastrointestinal: The patient denies nausea/vomiting, reports he had a bowel movement this morning, denies blood in his stools.
- Genitourinary: The patient denies blood in his urine, pain with urination, change in urine smell, frequency, or amount, or difficulty initiating a stream.
- Musculoskeletal: Endorses chronic joint pain he attributes to his rheumatoid arthritis, which he feels is fairly well controlled with his current regimen.
- Neurological: Endorses generalized weakness, denies headache, falls, loss of consciousness, history of seizure disorder or stroke, numbness, tingling in extremities.
- Endocrine: Denies increased hunger, thirst, or urination.
- Integumentary: Denies itching, rash, open sores.
- Lymph: Has not noticed any nodes.
- Psychiatric: Endorses nervousness and anxiety, which is not usually a problem and he feels it coincides with his increased work of breathing.
- Exposures: He denies exposure to carbon monoxide, second-hand smoke or chemical fumes in the recent past.

Physical Examination

- Vital signs: Pulse is 108 beats minute, blood pressure is 138/78 mm Hg, respiratory rate is 28 breaths per minute, and temperature is 96.8°F axillary, oxygen saturation by pulses oximeter is 95% on 6 L/min O_2 via nasal cannula at rest, and a fingerstick blood glucose is 98 mg/dL.

- Constitutional: Thin male, appears stated age, anxious and in moderate distress, tachypneic, sitting in tripod fashion, wearing nasal cannula at 6 L per minute.
- Head/eyes/ears/nose/throat: Pupils are equal, round, reactive to light, buccal mucosa dry, white patches on tongue. No swelling of lips or tongue. No jugular venous distension noted.
- Cardiovascular: Tachycardia, rhythm regular, no murmurs, no gallops, no ankle edema.
- Pulmonary: Tachypneic with use of accessory muscles, lungs with end-expiratory wheezes bilaterally but diminished to auscultation most notably in right lower lobe, dullness to percussion on the right, no egophony appreciated. Desaturation of SaO_2 noted with coughing/exertion in bed down to low 80s. Sputum is thick and greenish-yellow.
- Gastrointestinal/genitourinary: Normoactive bowel sounds, tympanic on percussion, abdomen soft with no tenderness to palpation. Normal genitalia, no CVA tenderness.
- Extremities: Nail beds are pale with thickened nails, mild clubbing, skin cool to touch, brisk capillary refill, no calf tenderness, no edema.
- Integumentary: Intact, extensive dark brown/red skin discoloration over bilateral forearms up to mid-biceps.
- Hematologic/lymphatic: No evidence of bruising or bleeding. No lymphadenopathy.

Diagnostic Results

- ECG: sinus tachycardia, unchanged when compared to the ECG from January—no ST elevation or depression
- Chest x-ray: awaiting radiology reading with comparison to prior films but on my reading of the x-ray it shows a small right pleural effusion, a small right lower lobe infiltrate which is consistent with pneumonia or atelectasis, a narrow mediastinum and flat diaphragm consistent with COPD, no pneumothorax, no hilar engorgement or edema

---

❓ What elements of the review of systems and the physical examination should be added to the list of pertinent positives? Which items should be added to the list of significant negatives?

- **Pertinent positives:** his oxygen requirement is now 6 L/min at all times and previously he was using 2 L/min at night only. He reports chest pressure that gets worse when he coughs. He is using accessory muscles to breathe and sitting in a tripod fashion. His oxygen saturation drops when he turns in bed or coughs. He is tachycardic and tachypneic. Chest x-ray has right lower lobe infiltrate consistent with pneumonia or atelectasis and a small right-sided pleural effusion. He is anxious. He is thin and has lost 10 lb in 2 months. He has white patches on his tongue, which appear to be oral thrush.

- **Significant negatives:** the history and physical are negative for fever, chills or night sweats, calf tenderness, orthopnea, lungs are free of crackles or edema. No carbon monoxide exposure. He does not presently have a fever. There is no facial swelling. The physical examination as it pertains to his cardiac, gastrointestinal and neurologic systems is normal. His ECG shows no arrhythmia, and no sign of ischemia.

Case Analysis

The chest x-ray and clinical signs and symptoms are consistent with a possible pneumonia resulting in an exacerbation of his COPD. I will initiate empiric antibiotics immediately and ensure that he is given bronchodilator treatments. But I am still concerned that something else is going on with my patient. His 10-lb weight loss is significant and he does appear quite ill. While therapies are initiated to treat his dyspnea, I quickly review the differential to ensure I consider all potential causes of his symptoms.

Based on the additional information from the review of systems, physical examination, and chest x-ray, I can rule out pulmonary edema and the x-ray also rules out pneumothorax and hemothorax. New congestive heart failure with exacerbation is unlikely in the setting of weight loss (not weight gain), the absence of jugular venous distension, and the absence of edema or enlarged heart and hilar engorgement on x-ray. I think large airway obstruction is not the cause of his symptoms although he is producing large amounts of sputum; this is magnifying his airflow limitation secondary to his baseline obstructive disease and may be due to bronchitis. The chest x-ray does show a right lower lobe infiltrate and is possibly consistent with pneumonia or atelectasis. I will need additional diagnostics, such as a computed tomography (CT) scan or magnetic resonance images (MRI) to determine if there is another cause for atelectasis, such as a mass or airway obstruction. The patient is afebrile and did not experience rigors or chest pain which are very common with pneumonia but I know that the elderly do not always mount a fever (often they are hypothermic) in the setting of infection. Still his history is concerning as he did not experience a typical infectious response.

Carbon monoxide poisoning is ruled out by his lack of recent exposures to chemicals/gases. Allergic reaction is unlikely given the gradual progression of symptoms and the absence of facial swelling, stridor to suggest airway swelling, and report of no new exposures. Based on his normal neurologic examination and the abundance of pulmonary symptoms, I am not concerned that his shortness of breath is due to a central nervous system or neuromuscular pathology. The patient does not have ascites and his description of a deep chest ache is not likely to be gastroesophageal reflux disease. The chest pressure is concerning, however, as this may be cardiac pain. So while the most likely diagnosis is COPD exacerbation, I will plan to continue cardiac monitoring and repeat the ECG and troponin levels to rule out a myocardial infarction.

I explain what I have found so far and my plan of care to the patient and his son. We will admit him to treat his severe dyspnea most likely due to COPD exacerbation due to infection and complete his workup to rule out other problems. I am able to reassure the patient's son that he did the right thing bringing him in, and then proceed to order further diagnostic testing.

? What diagnostic testing should be done and in what order?

At this point, I need to look back at the most life-threatening conditions on my differential list. I have ruled out STEMI and I am awaiting a troponin level to rule out an NSTEMI. A large PE is unlikely given that this would cause hypoxemia, hypotension, and more severe symptoms at rest than he is experiencing. While the patient is requiring 6 L/min of oxygen by nasal prongs to maintain an oxygen saturation of 95%, he is normotensive and not in extremis. Cancer is associated with increased clotting, so he may have a smaller PE, or potentially be seeding his pulmonary vasculature from small shower emboli, but his presentation is much more consistent with a COPD exacerbation. Regardless, I cannot exclude PE yet from my differential diagnoses.

His risk of PE is not high enough to warrant the exposure to radiation and contrast that a CTPA (a definitive diagnostic test for PE) would require. Plus, my patient would not be able to lie flat for the scan. However, I will order a bedside Doppler ultrasound of his lower extremities to look for a potential DVT. If positive I will start anticoagulation.[3]

I do think this patient's presentation warrants an echocardiogram, a non-invasive test requiring no radiation exposure and providing key information about the patient's heart function, including valve disorders and an estimation of right heart pressures. Patients with PE can have changes on echocardiogram consistent with increased right ventricular dysfunction, right ventricular bowing, and increased pulmonary artery pressures, and by ordering an echocardiogram I can also rule out several cardiac diagnoses.[3]

I order a sputum culture, as he reports a change in sputum color and consistency. In addition his current arthritis therapies make him more immunocompromised, which can lead to infection with opportunistic organisms. A sign of this is his oral thrush, which I will treat. I also must consider infection with tuberculosis and consider skin testing if other data do not result in a diagnosis. Reviewing his results so far, it is noted that he meets criteria (HR >90, RR >20, T <96.8°F) for systemic inflammatory response syndrome (SIRS), a hallmark for impeding or actual sepsis. I will order blood and urine cultures to look for sources of infection. In addition I will order antibiotics according to the sepsis guidelines.[4] Lastly, I will order urine testing for *Streptococcus pneumoniae* and *Legionella* antigens to help diagnose possible pneumonia causes and guide our antibiotic tailoring if needed later.

CASE INFORMATION

Lab results thus far:

Troponin 0.024 ng/mL (normal = 0.01), lactic acid 2.6 (normal = 0.7–2.1), Na 134 mg/dL (normal = 135–147 mEq/L), BUN 7 (normal = 7–20 mg/dL), glucose 98 mg/dL (normal = 60–110), chloride 96 mEq/L (normal = 95–107), serum CO_2 23 mmol/L (normal = 22–32), BNP 189 pg/mL (normal < 100), WBC 5,000 cells/μL (normal = 4,500–10,000), H/H 8.4 g/dL/24.9% (normal = 13.5–16.5/41%–50%).

Blood, sputum, and urine cultures: no growth to date

Blood gas on 6 L nasal prongs: pH 7.31 (normal = 7.35–7.45), $PaCO_2$ 60 mm Hg (normal = 35–45), PaO_2 68 mm Hg (normal = 80–100), HCO_3 = 25 (normal = 22–28)

ECHO: Estimated PA systolic pressure 42, no RV strain, mild RV dilatation, left ventricular ejection fraction = 55%.

Doppler ultrasound of bilateral extremities: no signs of DVT

Case Analysis

The troponin drawn in conjunction with the ECG is normal, which rules out acute coronary syndrome. His ABG varies from his PFTs obtained 5 years ago. The current results demonstrate a respiratory acidosis with moderate hypoxemia. If he were not on O_2 his current PaO_2 would be severely low. His bicarbonate is normal but I suspect that it is much higher normally to compensate for a baseline hypercarbia due to his COPD. His lactic acid (a marker for sepsis) is only mildly elevated at 2.6, which may reflect his increased work of breathing and is not convincing for sepsis. It may be due to hypoxemia experienced during activity and prior to increasing his inspired O_2. I will continue to monitor ABGs and lactic acid. A comprehensive metabolic panel shows mildly decreased sodium, normal creatinine and low BUN, normal blood glucose and chloride. The serum CO_2 (bicarbonate) on the panel correlates with his ABG bicarbonate. A complete blood count shows mild anemia with a normal white count. The BNP does not reflect significant heart failure, and the echo showed no right ventricular strain (mild pulmonary hypertension in COPD is normal) and his Doppler studies are negative. PE is much less likely at this point.[3]

❓ What treatment should be given?

At this point I am still thinking the patient is suffering from a pulmonary infection and consider a therapeutic plan to address key components.

It is easy to forget, but oxygen is a medical therapy and needs to be monitored closely. My patient is on continuous pulse oximetry to ensure he maintains adequate oxygenation and I will do serial blood gases as needed to assess any changes in his ventilation, specifically his CO_2 and subsequently his pH.

With COPD exacerbations caused by infection, hypoxemia and hypercapnia are likely to worsen if not treated. Respiratory failure ensues due to respiratory muscle fatigue.

While the initiation of aggressive oxygen therapy can result in hypercapnia, apnea, and death, it is essential for survival and should be provided in acute respiratory failure to attain an oxygen saturation of at least 90%. End organs fail when hypoxia ensues. This patient is tolerating the oxygen but should he increase his CO_2 (and subsequently increase his acidosis), ventilatory support (noninvasive or invasive may be necessary). I will monitor him carefully.

An essential second step is to "unload" the respiratory muscles by ensuring maximum bronchodilation. To that end short-acting β-agonists (eg, albuterol) and concomitant anticholinergics (eg, ipratropium) improve dyspnea and the associated work of breathing. I order both medications to be given concurrently via nebulizer every 2 hours as needed. Inhaled corticosteroids do not have a role in treating an acute COPD exacerbation; however, systemic corticosteroids decrease the rate of treatment failure, shorten hospital stays, and improve hypoxemia and forced expiratory volume in 1 second (FEV_1). I order methylprednisolone sodium succinate 125 mg intravenously every 6 hours.[5,6]

Empiric antibiotics are advised in a patient presenting with COPD exacerbation with purulent sputum. Antibiotic choice is guided by patient allergies, interactions with other medications, renal function, suspected organisms, and local patterns of antibiotic resistance. In this case, the patient has no known allergies, normal renal function, and my suspicion is that he has a community-acquired pneumonia (CAP). Typical CAP pathogens include *Streptococcus pneumoniae* (most common), *Moraxella catarrhalis* (frequent in COPD exacerbations requiring hospitalization), influenza (less likely in my patient as we are seeing him in the summer), and *Staphylococcus aureus*. Combination antibiotic therapy is recommended and includes ceftriaxone for the typical pathogens, and the accepted treatment for atypical causes of CAP is azithromycin for a 3-day course. I will use this drug because his pleural effusion may represent an extrapulmonary manifestation of a *Legionella* infection.[7] I review doses with our hospital pharmacist and order these antibiotics for intravenous administration due to the severity of his illness.

Case Follow-Up

This patient was admitted to a general medicine unit and treated for COPD exacerbation secondary to pneumonia. However, he did not improve and in fact began to deteriorate further. He was transferred that evening to the MICU for noninvasive positive pressure ventilation therapy (ie, bilevel positive airway pressure). The next morning he continued to require noninvasive ventilation and his CXR showed further extension of his RLL infiltrate. At this point, due to his accelerating severity of illness a CTPA was done to rule out PE and to further evaluate his infiltrate. This ruled out a PE but showed possible aspiration bronchiolitis, new nodules up to 8 mm in size suspicious for new metastases, and severe stenosis of his right bronchus at the operative anastomosis. After consultation with the thoracic surgery service, we offered the patient the option of a stent in the right bronchus to improve his oxygenation and ventilation. The risks of this procedure including erosion to the large vasculature or the esophagus were explained to the patient. The patient decided not to pursue this treatment and decided to transition to palliative care.

At the beginning, this case looked to me like a classic COPD exacerbation from a probable infection such as pneumonia. Because it is easy to accept the first "most likely" condition as the diagnosis, this case illustrates how complicated patients can be and why considering a comprehensive differential is so important. In addition, his history did have other "red flags," which suggested this was not simply a pneumonia (eg, weight loss, gradual symptoms with no "typical" signs of infection such as rigors or fever).

If this were a more typical case study with a clear diagnosis such as a CAP, the description of the management required would be more straightforward. COPD exacerbations due to pneumonia or bronchitis are managed with antibiotics, systemic corticosteroids, and bronchodilator nebulizer treatments as discussed above. We monitor to ensure oxygen requirements return to baseline and once improved the steroids are converted to an oral prednisone taper over a 1- to 2-week period, and the patient is discharged. Usually these patients are managed well by their PCPs, but occasionally they require hospitalization and more aggressive care. If they have never had PFT testing, we always try to schedule the tests after discharge to help guide future care and treatment. And last we ensure that they have a follow-up appointment with our pulmonary clinic for pulmonary rehabilitation if they are amenable to the idea.

References

1. Ahmed A, Graber MA. Evaluation of the adult with dyspnea in the emergency department. In: Grazel J, Hockberger R, eds. *Up To Date Web site*. Waltham, MA. http://www.uptodate.com/con tents/evaluation-of-the-adult-with-dyspnea-in-the-emergency-department Accessed October 19, 2015.
2. Geersing GJ, Kearon C, Anderson DR, et al. Exclusion of deep vein thrombosis using the Wells rule in clinically important subgroups: individual patient meta-analysis. *BMJ*. 2014;348:g1340.
3. Agnelli G, Becattini C. Acute pulmonary embolism. *N Engl J Med*. 2010;363(3):266-274.
4. Surviving sepsis campaign. International guidelines for management of severe sepsis and septic shock. http://www.sccm.org/Documents/SSC-Guidelines.pdf. Published 2012. Updated 2012. Accessed August 7, 2012.
5. Evensen A. Management of COPD exacerbations. *Am Fam Physician*. 2010;81(5):607-613.
6. Walters JA, Gibson PG, Wood-Baker R, Hannay M, Walters EH. Systemic corticosteroids for acute exacerbations of chronic obstructive pulmonary disease. *Cochrane Database Syst Rev*. 2009;(1):1-14.
7. American Thoracic Society. Guidelines for the management of adults with hospital-acquired, ventilator-associated, and health-care associated pneumonia. *Am J Respir Crit Care Med [Practice Guidelines]*. 2005;171:388-416.

CASE 58

Nancy Munro

Nancy Munro is a senior ACNP at the National Institutes of Health. She works in the Critical Care Medicine Department and with the Pulmonary Consult Service and is also a part-time instructor at the Georgetown University School of Nursing where she instructs and teaches ACNP students.

CASE INFORMATION

Chief Complaint

An 88-year-old Caucasian male comes to the pulmonary clinic with complaints of 2 months of cough and shortness of breath when walking. He is accompanied by his daughter.

? What is the potential cause?

When I encounter a patient who presents with symptoms that may have many causes, I need to prioritize my approach. The patient tells me that he decided to come to the clinic because his shortness of breath and cough, especially when walking, have not improved even after seeing his primary care physician (PCP) and taking a course of azithromycin. His symptoms developed over 2 months, which suggests that the pathologic process is chronic in nature. If the process were acute, I would expect a more symptomatic presentation especially considering his age. Regardless, I will monitor his heart rate and pulse oximetry continuously during his clinic visit to observe his response when talking with me, and as he is examined. Using a systematic approach will lessen the possibility of missing the diagnosis. Even though the patient is not in acute distress, a review of all the potential causes of his symptoms is needed. I will first address potential life-threatening causes but also consider other serious acute and emerging conditions.

> ### Differential Diagnoses for Nonproductive Cough and Increasing Dyspnea on Exertion[1]
>
> - Upper airway causes including tracheal foreign objects, angioedema, anaphylaxis, infection of the pharynx or neck, airway trauma
> - Pulmonary causes including pulmonary embolism, chronic obstructive lung disease (COPD), asthma, pneumothorax and/or pneumomediastinum, pulmonary infection, noncardiogenic pulmonary edema, direct pulmonary injury, idiopathic pulmonary fibrosis

- Cardiac causes including acute coronary syndrome, acute decompensated congestive heart failure, flash pulmonary edema, high output failure, cardiomyopathy, cardiac dysrhythmia, valvular dysfunction, cardiac tamponade
- Toxic and metabolic causes including poisoning (especially carbon monoxide or salicylate), sepsis, diabetic ketoacidosis, toxin-related metabolic acidosis, anemia, acute chest syndrome
- Neurologic causes including stroke, neuromuscular disease
- Miscellaneous causes including lung cancer, pleural effusion, intra-abdominal processes, ascites, obesity, hyperventilation, and anxiety

CASE INFORMATION

General Survey

Although this list may seem intimidating, I can quickly rule out many of these causes with my general survey, a quick assessment of the patient's physical presentation. I spend a few minutes observing the patient from a distance so the patient is not aware that I am watching him. Since his primary complaint is pulmonary, I focus on his breathing patterns, inspiratory and expiratory times, use of accessory muscles, how he positions himself, and his ability to converse with others. He has a small frame, is not overweight, has a strong voice, and seems to be able to talk with his family without difficulty. He is not tachypneic and does not have a prolonged expiratory time. Life-threatening causes on my differential such as airway, cardiac, neurologic, toxic/metabolic issues seem unlikely since he is not demonstrating any acute symptoms. Even the serious pulmonary conditions can be eliminated with the exception of pulmonary infection, pulmonary embolism, and exacerbation of COPD or asthma. I will focus on these diagnoses as well as cancer and pleural diseases as I continue to evaluate my patient. I start by obtaining a history of his illness.

Observing the patient helps me formulate my questions when I talk with him and his daughter about the course of his illness and as I complete a comprehensive history and physical examination. I notice that when he is speaking, his SpO_2 on room air decreases to 90% with a good waveform. A pulmonary condition is emerging as the likely cause of his current symptoms so I will carefully focus my questions and examination to reveal essential information to help me further rule in, or out, specific pulmonary diagnoses. However, other potential causes in other systems like the heart must still be considered. To that end I know my continued evaluation must be comprehensive.

History of Present Illness

The "story" about how the patient's condition has evolved is very important. He states that he has no chronic health problems and was in relatively good health until about 2 months ago when he noticed that he needed to stop more frequently to catch his breath while walking. He did not think he had a fever at that time but he does remember waking up several times at night and being very sweaty. He saw his primary care provider after 1 month of these symptoms and was prescribed azithromycin for a presumed pulmonary infection. He felt better for a few days but then returned to his current clinical presentation. He is very active for his age. He walks daily, works out with his personal trainer, and swims one to two times per week. Prior to a hospitalization 2 years ago for malaise and newly diagnosed renal dysfunction, he was an avid scuba diver and went on diving trips as well as diving weekly in a local aquarium to feed the fish. He was advised to stop diving by his PCP after the hospitalization. Currently he states he can no longer swim due to acute shortness of breath and can only walk about 50 ft before stopping. He notes that he has a nonproductive cough, no purulent or bloody sputum and he has never felt like he had a fever. He sleeps with two pillows and does have night sweats. He has never smoked and has had limited second-hand smoke exposure in his home and work environment. He is a retired executive who worked for an engineering consulting firm. He has an extensive foreign travel history and the last country that he visited was Ireland approximately 4 years ago. He and his wife travel to Florida in the winter and 3 months ago they went to Ohio.

Past Medical History

He has been in good health for the majority of his life. He reports a vague history of asthma and/or allergies related mostly to seasonal changes especially in the spring. He says that these are associated with sneezing and sinus congestion and can persist for several weeks. These complaints have never been formally evaluated. He thinks he was told he has arthritis and he used to take ibuprofen for joint pains. This practice led to acute kidney injury (AKI) approximately 2 years ago, requiring hospitalization for an elevated creatinine. No major intervention was required and he no longer takes ibuprofen but will carefully use aspirin. This is the only medication he takes including any over-the-counter preparations or herbal preparations. He does not have any past surgical history. His family history is positive for hypertension and diabetes but he denies both.

Exposure History

I also explore any environmental exposures, which can contribute to pulmonary symptoms. He reports that he hired a landscaping company to complete a garden project last month but he has not had any exposure to construction at home or at his previous work environments. He cares for his daughter's dog and in the past had exposure to various marine animals in the aquarium.

? What are the pertinent positives so far?

- Progressive shortness of breath
- Persistent nonproductive cough
- Hypoxemia when talking
- Orthopnea
- Night sweats early in the course of his illness
- Past medical history of AKI due to excessive dosing of nonsteroidal anti-inflammatory medications
- Probable arthritis (but not formally diagnosed)
- Travel to Florida and Ohio
- Exposure to dog and marine animals

? What are the significant negatives so far?

- No acute distress on my general survey
- No major pulmonary event including pneumothorax, noncardiogenic pulmonary edema
- No acute cardiac, neurological, or metabolic events
- No history of pulmonary or cardiac disease
- No tobacco use and minimal secondary smoke exposure

Case Analysis

From the information I have obtained so far, a pulmonary cause continues to be the focus of my inquiry. Infection is at the top of my differential list because of the persistent dyspnea on exertion and cough (although nonproductive) and the hypoxemia with talking. Idiopathic pulmonary fibrosis is also a possibility but this is often a diagnosis of exclusion. Thus I will continue my evaluation starting with infectious causes.

When evaluating a patient for a pulmonary complaint, it is imperative to carefully explore all parts of the social history. Common infections in Ohio include histoplasmosis and MRSA while Florida infections include aspergillosis. Pulmonary bacterial infections progress quickly while viral and fungal pulmonary infections can take time to develop. These timelines are helpful when determining what type of infection may be present.[2] MRSA pneumonia seems unlikely because it would likely have a more symptomatic presentation with hemodynamic deterioration. This patient's timeline favors a viral or fungal infection. His animal exposures are also a consideration because animals can be a source of allergic reactions but he denies any symptoms associated with the dog. Animals also carry various microbes and even though marine animal exposure was remote, it is also a potential source of infection.

Pulmonary embolism cannot be eliminated. However, his activity level makes the diagnosis less likely. In my further examination of the patient, I will assess for any type of discomfort in his lower extremities and any asymmetry or swelling of his legs. Lung cancer cannot yet be ruled out, but he does not have a smoking history and has had minimal second-hand exposure. Cardiac causes for DOE need to be considered especially given his age as he may well have some degree of diastolic dysfunction. Careful questioning when reviewing the cardiac system is essential for eliminating this system as a source of this patient's problem. The main complaint of dyspnea needs to be analyzed carefully. Quantifying distance and how the exertion is tolerated can help determine the severity of the dyspnea. The review of systems as well as precise physical examination can reveal details of this case that can lead to an accurate diagnosis.

CASE INFORMATION

Review of Systems

- Constitutional: positive for increase in fatigue; denies recent weight loss, loss of appetite or problems sleeping; no overt fever or rigors but he does report night sweats earlier in this illness; no recent falls or trauma or any new masses
- Eyes/ears/nose/throat: denies any vision change, double vision, eye pain. Positive for intermittent sinus "stuffiness" and runny nose (drainage clear and does not change color); denies nose bleeds, sore throat, hoarseness
- Cardiovascular: positive for shortness of breath especially with walking; denies chest pain, palpitations, leg or arm swelling; denies calf pain, denies history of heart attack or heart failure, denies history of high blood pressure
- Pulmonary: positive for shortness of breath especially with walking or exertion; has to stop to rest after about 50 ft or when climbing more than six to seven stairs; positive for cough without sputum worse in the morning; sleeps with head elevated (uses two pillows); denies wheezing although he thought he was told he had asthma but never had pulmonary function tests; denies history of pneumonia, tuberculosis, or blood clot
- Gastrointestinal: positive for indigestion or heartburn especially after meals; denies nausea, vomiting, diarrhea; denies any change in stool pattern, character or color; denies abdominal pain or cramping; denies any problems with swallowing
- Genitourinary: positive for frequency of urination at night (two to three times); denies pain on urination; denies gross blood in urine or foul-smelling urine; denies incontinence or weak stream of urine
- Musculoskeletal: positive for some joint discomfort especially knees; denies weakness or limited range of motion

- Neurological/psychiatric: denies headache, dizziness, change in level of consciousness; numbness, tingling, extremity weakness, tremors; denies change in balance or speech; denies history of stroke, seizures, depression, anxiety
- Endocrine: denies increase/decrease in thirst, appetite; preference for heat or cold; change in weight
- Hematological: denies easy bruising or prolonged or excessive bleeding; denies history of anemia or need for blood transfusion
- Lymphadenopathy: denies noting any nodes or swelling

Physical Examination

- Vital signs: Temperature 37°C; heart rate 85 beats per minute; respiratory rate 28 breaths per minute; blood pressure 135/76 mmHg; oxygen saturation = 94% on room air at rest and 90% when talking.
- General: Frail, mildly dyspneic when talking.
- Head/eyes/ears/nose/throat: cranial nerves II-XII and extraocular movements grossly intact. Trachea midline.
- Cardiovascular: S1, S2 regular rhythm, 2/6 systolic ejection murmur. Extremities are warm, dry, no mottling; no edema; no clubbing; dorsalis pedis pulses +1 bilaterally.
- Pulmonary: Regular, symmetrical, mild labored respirations but able to speak in full sentences. Intermittent nonproductive cough; breath sounds with fine inspiratory crackles in upper lobes bilaterally.
- Gastrointestinal: Soft, nontender; bowel sounds present; no gross organomegaly.
- Integumentary: No bruising.
- Neurological: Glasgow coma scale =15; no gross focal deficits; 5/5 strength in all muscle groups.

? **What elements of the review of systems and the physical examination should be added to the list of pertinent positives? Which items should be added to the list of significant negatives?**

Pertinent Positives

- Hypoxemia (decreasing SpO_2 with activity or talking)
- Night sweats earlier in course of illness
- Bilateral crackles in upper lobes
- Possible asthma history
- History of sinus congestion with seasonal allergies
- Possible gastroesophageal reflux disease (GERD)

Significant Negatives

- No chronic pulmonary disease such as COPD
- No smoking history
- Normal cardiac examination
- No leg swelling or calf pain

❓ Based on this information, what is the problem representation for this patient?

Given what I have learned so far my problem representation is: This is an 88-year-old Caucasian male with a possible history of asthma who presents at the pulmonary clinic with complaints of nonproductive cough and increasing dyspnea on exertion over the last 2 months.

My review of systems and physical examination confirms my initial finding that a pulmonary process is the most likely cause of his symptoms. Given his normal cardiac and neurological examinations, I can cross disorders in those systems off my list. He is afebrile; however, patients at this age can have an infection without a fever, and he does report night sweats so an unusual pulmonary infection is still on my list. Malignancy is still on my differential, particularly given his age; I will need further diagnostics to rule this out. I doubt that this is a pulmonary embolism at this point given his chronic presentation and the absence of leg swelling or calf pain to suggest a deep vein thrombosis. The majority of pulmonary emboli arises from lower extremity clots. The option exists to do a Doppler ultrasound of his lower extremities to confirm the absence of a clot but given the data that support a primary pulmonary process, including hypoxemia with talking, dyspnea on exertion and crackles on lung auscultation, I will focus my diagnostic testing on the pulmonary system.

❓ What diagnostics are needed at this time?

Immediate diagnostics for my patient include arterial blood gases (ABG), complete blood count (CBC) with differential, electrolytes, ECG, and a chest x-ray. I may also obtain a chest-computed tomography (CT) scan to further delineate specific findings on the x-ray.

CASE INFORMATION

Diagnostic Testing Results

- ABG: pH = 7.32 (7.35–7.45); $PaCO_2$ = 48 mm Hg (35–45 mm Hg); PaO_2 = 50 mm Hg (75–100 mm Hg); SaO_2 = 92% (90%–100%) HCO_3 = 28 mEq/L (22–26 mEq/L).
- His basic metabolic panel is normal except for an elevated blood urea nitrogen (BUN) at 26 mg/dL (normal is 7–20 mg/dl) and a borderline creatinine level of 1.48 mg/dL (normal is 0.5–1.5 mg/dL).

- CBC with differential: His hemoglobin, hematocrit, and platelet counts are all normal, as is his white blood cell count at 7,400 cells/µL; (normal is 5000–10,000 cells/µL); the differential is notable for eosinophils 9.7% (normal is 0%–5%) with an absolute eosinophil count = 718 cells/µL (normally less than 350 cells/µL).
- ECG: Sinus rhythm with no acute changes.
- Chest x-ray: Because the patient has an existing x-ray from a month ago I review it. It shows diffuse bilateral interstitial infiltrates, predominantly in the upper lobes.
- Chest CT: Bilateral ground-glass opacities predominantly in the upper lobes.

❓ Does the information from the diagnostics change your differential?

The ABG reveals a mild respiratory acidosis with hypoxemia, which is not surprising. The resulting alveolar-arterial (A-a) gradient is 40 (on room air and corrected for age), which is a slightly higher gradient than the expected gradient of 29. A bigger gradient indicates worse oxygenation. While his gradient is not severe, trending the gradient over time is useful to assess oxygenation status.

The respiratory acidosis and the elevation of the bicarbonate imply that this process is chronic in nature and correlates with his clinical presentation. The only abnormal values in the electrolytes are an elevated BUN and a borderline high creatinine. His past history of AKI 2 years ago may have led to chronic renal dysfunction, which is exacerbated by his age.

The CBC with differential results is surprising. I was expecting an elevated WBC because I thought infection was a likely cause of the patient's symptoms. Instead I found an elevated eosinophil count, an unusual finding. Eosinophils are white blood cells that combat inflammation but when higher values are discovered, it may be an indication of dysfunction. The elevated peripheral eosinophil levels are important because eosinophils can produce cytokines including interleukins (IL-3 and IL-5) and granulocyte macrophage–stimulating factor, which can cause destruction of local tissues and produce a diffuse infiltrative interstitial pattern as seen in the chest x-ray.[3] Eosinophilic pneumonia presents with dyspnea on exertion and a nonproductive cough with fever and night sweats, very similar to this patient's presentation. With this information, I now put eosinophilic pneumonia at the top of my differential diagnoses list. Causes of eosinophilic pneumonia, which are particularly noteworthy as they appear in this patient's history, include drugs such as nonsteroidal anti-inflammatory agents and exposure to microbes, including *Aspergillus*, which can be found in soil.[3]

Imaging is the next important step to determine the cause of this patient's symptoms. Because the patient is in our system already, I was able to review his chest x-ray from about a month ago. This radiograph is significant for diffuse interstitial bilateral infiltrates, which are predominantly in the upper lobes. Another chest x-ray would not be helpful in the diagnostic process but I do order a chest computerized tomography (chest CT) to further delineate the location and characteristics of the infiltrative process. The findings reveal bilateral ground-glass opacities predominantly in the upper lobes. Of interest, these findings correlate with my physical examination findings of crackles in the upper lobes. This type of presentation is classified as interstitial lung disease and can be challenging to diagnose.

Interstitial lung disease encompasses a large number of disorders and its nomenclature continues to evolve. Experts now prefer the term diffuse parenchymal lung disease because the diffuse scarring process or fibrosis involves all components of the alveolar wall not just certain cells.[3] The pathogenesis includes (1) initiation of an inflammatory process by antigens or toxins and (2) propagation of the inflammatory process with inflammatory cells leading to (3) fibrosis.[3] Interstitial parenchymal lung disease can have many causes including sarcoidosis, histiocytosis (large number of tissue macrophages), idiopathic pulmonary fibrosis, tumor (lymphangitic), asbestosis and other dusts, collagen vascular disease, and drugs. The drugs that can cause this fibrotic process are numerous. NSAIDs are included in this list and this patient used ibuprofen extensively in the past. His age puts cancer or disseminated carcinoma higher in my differential diagnosis and these conditions can present as interstitial patterns on x-ray and CT, so cancer remains on my differential for now.

His cough is considered chronic since he has had it for more than 3 weeks and may be a component of the inflammatory process of diffuse parenchymal lung disease but other causes should also be considered. The more common causes of chronic cough include upper airway cough syndrome, asthma, and GERD.[4] All three of these diagnoses may be a possible cause of the patient's cough. Further testing may be helpful in discerning the reason for the cough but with the radiological findings, history of his presentation, and the high eosinophil counts, eosinophilic pneumonia and its associated cough is the most likely cause.

❓ What additional diagnostic testing is needed at this time and in what order?

The next decision is how to proceed with the further testing. I consider the following additional diagnostics:

- Pulmonary function tests (PFTs)
- Six-minute walk test
- Bronchoscopy with bronchoalveolar lavage (BAL)
- Echocardiogram
- Blood work: sedimentation rate and C-reactive protein (although not specific these do suggest inflammation if elevated)

Because of his age and mild distress, I admit this patient for a short hospitalization to obtain PFTs and a 6-minute walk as well as to perform a BAL. The PFTs detect categories of abnormal lung function such as obstruction, restriction, or diffusion. I suspect that this patient's diffusing lung capacity for carbon monoxide (DLCO) will be low because the fibrotic process and inflammation cause a diffusion barrier for gases, leading to hypoxemia. The PFTs may also reveal airway resistance as the fibrotic process proliferates and can cause narrowing of the small airways. PFTs can identify asthma (an obstructive disease), which may respond to bronchodilators. The criterion for obstructive lung disease using PFTs is either a 12% or 200 mL increase in either functional vital capacity (FVC) or forced expiratory volume in 1 second (FEV_1) as a response to bronchodilators.[5] This is considered a positive response, which may signify reversible reactive airway disease or asthma. A 6-minute walk test is necessary to try to determine his exercise tolerance. The greater the distance the patient can walk without desaturation, the better the exercise tolerance.

With the diffuse infiltrates on chest x-ray and bilateral opacities on the chest CT, infection as a cause must be ruled out. The best test available to do so is a BAL. Because his oxygenation status is tenuous, it is important that this patient be observed closely after the procedure. A BAL can produce an inflammatory reaction and a resultant need for supplemental oxygen. A Gram stain of the BAL fluid may provide some initial insight into the diagnosis. A diagnosis of eosinophilic pneumonia is confirmed when the eosinophils in either the lavage or the tissue sample exceed 25%.[1] This patient has had possible exposure to infection with his travel history as well as the gardening project. Performing a BAL does put the patient at some risk since he is hypoxemic and could potentially result in the need for intubation, and the patient must be informed of this risk. If tissue is biopsied, the risk of pneumothorax is also included in the discussion with the patient.

Although the sedimentation rate and C-reactive protein are not specific inflammatory markers, they can be trended to identify any change in the inflammatory state. The echocardiogram will help determine if heart failure has played a role in this patient's symptoms. The chest CT did not reveal the usual pattern for heart failure and there were no pleural effusions but confirmation of the absence of cardiac abnormalities will be helpful.

CASE INFORMATION

Diagnostic Test Results and Diagnosis

The patient's BAL results reveal an eosinophil count of 27% in the lavage. Thus the final diagnosis is eosinophilic pneumonia but the etiology of this diagnosis remains unclear. A tissue biopsy was deferred due to increased risk. There is no evidence of bacterial infection in the lavage with a negative Gram stain and culture. The viral polymerase chain reaction (PCR) testing is also negative as are tests for fungal infection. The airways are unremarkable in appearance and there are no purulent or bloody secretions.

His PFT results demonstrate a restrictive pattern without a significant response to bronchodilators so asthma is less likely but cannot be ruled out. Further PFT testing is needed. His 6-minute walk results are significant as he was only able to walk 500 ft without desaturation. This finding correlates with his increasing DOE. The echocardiogram shows some diastolic dysfunction with an ejection fraction of 53% but no other findings to indicate a cardiac cause for his presentation. The serum inflammatory markers are slightly elevated and will be trended.

Management of Eosinophilic Pneumonia

Treatment for diffuse parenchymal lung disease or eosinophilic pneumonia includes the use of corticosteroids to control the inflammatory process. The recommended prednisone dosing is 0.5 mg/kg daily.[1,3] These diseases can be acute and chronic in nature. An acute process may be responsive to a shorter course of steroids (months) but if the process is thought to be chronic, treatment may be needed for extended time periods (years). When lung and blood eosinophils return to normal and symptoms improve, the condition has resolved. Other types of immunosuppressive agents may be used including cyclophosphamide, which has a side effect of pulmonary fibrosis, further confusing the diagnostic process.[3]

The patient's exercise tolerance did improve within a month after starting steroids. The steroids will be continued and may be weaned slowly in the future but that decision will be dependent on his clinical course. This patient will be followed closely and instructed to contact the primary care provider or other health care provider if symptoms become worse. It is important to know that the ability to determine the cause of diffuse parenchymal lung disease such as found in this patient is challenging and a final answer may never be reached.

References

1. Brown K, King T. Treatment of eosinophilic pneumonia. http://www.uptodate.com/contents/treatment-of-chronic-eosinophilic-pneumonia?source=machineLearning&search=eosinophilic+pneumonia&selectedTitle=2%7E104&sectionRank=2&anchor=H7#H7. UpToDate Web site. Updated September 19,2012. Accessed November 17, 2014.
2. Mandell, Douglas and Bennett. *Principles and Practice of Infectious Diseases.* 7th ed. Philadelphia, PA: Elsevier; 2010.
3. Weinberger SE, Cockrill BA Mandel J. *Principles of Pulmonary Medicine.* 6th ed. Philadelphia, PA: Elsevier-Saunders; 2014.
4. Irwin RS, Baumann MH, Bolser DC, Boulet LP, Braman SS, Brightling CE, et al. Diagnosis and management of cough executive summary: ACCP evidence-based clinical practice guidelines. *Chest.* 2006;129(1 suppl):1S-23S.
5. Pellegrino R, Viegi G, Brusasco V, Crapo RO, Burgos F, Casaburi R, et al. Interpretive strategies for lung function tests. *Eur Respir J.* 2005;26(5):948-968. doi: 10.1183/09031936.05.00035205.

CASE 59

Carol K. Thompson

Carol is a Professor in the AG-ACNP Program at the University of Kentucky. Dr Thompson was one of the first 100 certified ACNPs and is currently a member of an all NP intensivist team at the University Hospital, Lexington, KY. She was the first ACNP to become President of the Society of Critical Care Medicine and continues to lead internationally.

CASE INFORMATION

Chief Complaint

A 65-year-old male admitted to the hospital 2 days ago with community-acquired pneumonia develops new onset confusion, chest pain, and increased shortness of breath.

❓ What is the potential cause?

Pulmonary diagnoses must be high on my differential list since the patient was admitted with pneumonia. While his symptoms may not be related, given his pneumonia it is likely that they are. However, cardiac causes and age-related comorbidities must also be considered. A comprehensive differential diagnoses is helpful as I further evaluate the patient and sort data to quickly consider the cause and determine treatment.

Comprehensive Differential Diagnoses for Patient With Confusion/Agitation, Chest Pain, and Increased Shortness of Breath

- Cardiac: heart failure, arrhythmias, myocardial infarction/ischemia, shock
- Pulmonary: pulmonary emboli, pneumothorax, hemothorax, acute respiratory distress syndrome (ARDS), pulmonary edema, pleural effusion, asthma exacerbation, worsening pneumonia
- Neurologic: hypoxia, stroke, cerebral bleed, shock, delirium, dementia, and anxiety
- Renal: renal insufficiency/failure, electrolyte imbalance, acidosis, and drug reaction
- Infection: sepsis, urinary tract infection
- Gastrointestinal: gastrointestinal bleed, kidney stone
- Liver: liver failure, alcohol withdrawal

CASE INFORMATION

General Survey and History of Present Illness

The bedside nurse calls me to see the patient, whom she describes as agitated, unstable, and appearing to have labored breathing. I walk into the room and see that he is a thin man with a barrel chest, pale, with blue lips. He is tachypneic at 30 breaths per minute with a prolonged expiratory phase, has an audible wheeze mid-late expiration, and is using his sternocleidomastoid and intercostal muscles. This is extreme respiratory distress. He is nonverbal, trying to climb out of bed, pulling at his intravenous line, and has pulled off his nasal cannula. His behavior is frantic. A tissue box is at the bedside and multiple tissues are in the wastebasket so significant secretion production may be compromising his airway. I greet the patient, give my name, and state: "Your nurse and team asked me to come help you. What's wrong?" I replace the nasal cannula but he does not say anything nor change his behavior. The nurse is in the room so I ask her how he has changed since admission and during her shift. The nurse states he was admitted with a new community-acquired pneumonia and was cooperative and calm at the beginning of the shift 2 hours ago. I ask for a pulse oximeter reading and continue to evaluate the patient.

❓ What are the pertinent positives from the information given so far?

- Tachypnea with wheezing, prolonged expiratory phase, accessory muscle use
- Blue lips indicating cyanosis and pulling off nasal cannula
- Barrel chest consistent with chronic obstructive lung disease (COPD)
- Pulmonary secretions
- Community-acquired pneumonia
- Hospitalized 2 days
- Behavior change/agitation occurring in the past 2 hours
- Nonverbal

❓ What are the significant negatives from the information given so far?

- Mobile, moving all extremities
- Purposefully pulling at IV and removing cannula in preparation for getting out of bed
- No prior behavior change in the last 2 days

❓ What is the problem representation?

I state the problem as: "A 65-year-old male hospitalized with pneumonia develops sudden onset of respiratory distress and agitation."

❓ How does this information affect the list of possible causes and what do you need to do now?

The onset of the patient's symptoms is sudden so the differential is initially narrowed to emergent and life-threatening problems. With the focus of airway, breathing, and circulation as my first priorities, I first must consider pulmonary embolus, pneumothorax, and cardiac causes such as myocardial infarction or arrhythmias as potential causes of his dramatic and severe status change. I order a stat portable chest-x ray, arterial blood gas, bedside cardiac and pulse oximeter monitoring, and a stat 12-lead ECG because these diagnostics will help me quickly rule out or in life-threatening conditions that require immediate treatment. I also order intravenous access, the bedside ultrasound, and the code cart with intubation equipment to the room.

CASE INFORMATION

I need to quickly gather as much information as I can but for now can only do a focused cardiac and pulmonary examination. I will complete a full evaluation when the patient's condition is less emergent. A pulse oximeter is placed on his finger and his oxygen saturation is 72% on 2 liters nasal cannula. I immediately put him on a 100% nonrebreather and check the electronic medical record to determine his code status. I am considering instituting life support in the form of mechanical ventilation, and I want to follow his wishes regarding this kind of care. The medical record and the bedside nurse confirm he does not have a do-not-resuscitate or do-not-intubate order, and therefore should undergo full resuscitative effort. I proceed with a focused cardiac and pulmonary examination.

Focused physical examination

- Vital sign: temperature 100°F oral, pulse 128 beats per minute, respirations 34 breaths per minute and labored, blood pressure 180/102 mm Hg, pulse ox 72% on 2 L nasal cannula, now saturation is 87% on 100% nonrebreathing mask
- General: 65-year-old Caucasian male is in severe distress
- Cardiac: tachycardic at 128 beats per minute rhythm irregular with II/VI systolic ejection murmur
- Pulmonary: tracheal deviation to the left, percussion—tympanic over right upper lobe, auscultation—mid-late end-expiratory wheezing in left lung and distant breath sounds in the right upper lobe

❓ What new pertinent positives or significant negatives might you add to the previous list?

Pertinent Positives

- Tracheal deviation to the left
- Percussion notes tympanic in right upper lobe
- Diminished breath sounds in right upper lobe, wheezing bilaterally
- Systolic ejection murmur
- Hypertensive and tachycardiac
- Some improvement in oxygenation on 100% nonrebreather

Significant Negatives

- There is not a "do not resuscitate order" present in chart

Case Analysis

At this point, the most likely diagnosis for his severe pulmonary compromise is a pneumothorax. He has a tracheal shift to the left and tympanic percussion tones in the right upper lobe, which are consistent with a right pneumothorax. His oxygen saturation has improved somewhat on the 100% nonrebreather mask. My goal is an oxygen saturation of at least 90% while I use the bedside ultrasound to evaluate his lung status. I do not know the patient's usual PaO_2, but an oxygen saturation of 72% on 2 L of O_2 is severe hypoxemia (the equivalent of a PaO_2 of approximately 38–40 mm Hg) requiring emergent intervention. At this level of severe hypoxemia he may sustain multisystem insults such as a cardiac arrest and permanent neurologic damage. It is likely that severe hypoxemia is the cause of his mental status changes. Based on his general appearance, I suspect the patient has COPD, and provision of high levels of oxygen to patients with COPD sometimes causes respiratory depression. Regardless, this degree of hypoxemia is much more dangerous and must be treated aggressively. I monitor him closely and will intubate him if necessary.

CASE INFORMATION

Emergent Treatment

The bedside pulmonary ultrasound confirms a right side pneumothorax. I attempt to talk to the patient about needle decompression and chest tube insertion, but he continues to be agitated and confused; he is not able to make decisions at this time. A needle decompression of the right pneumothorax is done per hospital protocol.

Following the procedure, his agitation decreases rapidly. I realize that this may be an improvement due to an increased oxygen level secondary to decompression of the pneumothorax. But it may also mean a worsening in his level of consciousness for other reasons. I will explore this as soon as he is stabilized.

Needle decompression of a pneumothorax is an important immediate step but the patient needs a chest tube inserted since it may take days for the pneumothorax to resolve. A chest tube is inserted without complications and is placed on water seal with suction. Air bubbles are noted on expiration only so the seal is intact. There is no fluid drainage confirming this is pneumothorax not hemothorax. However, fluid of any sort is gravity dependent. An x-ray will be needed to evaluate his pneumothorax (and determine if there is a concomitant hemothorax or pleural effusion), check chest tube placement, and evaluate for other potential conditions. The formal ECG is in the process of being done and an ABG is drawn.

His oxygen saturation is now 90% and his respiratory rate has decreased to 28/min. I hear bilateral breath sounds on auscultation and he appears more comfortable. I will check the chart for his previous diagnostic findings, such as pulmonary function tests and arterial blood gases, as they will help me determine his baseline oxygenation and carbon dioxide level. If his baseline oxygen values are higher than 90% it is likely that there is another reason for his current low oxygenation. Perhaps his pneumonia is worse, he has a pulmonary embolism, or there is a concomitant cardiac cause. I have also not ruled out additional causes for his change in mental status although hypoxia is the likely cause. I will monitor his neuro status carefully.

I arrange for transfer to the medical intensive care unit so his respiratory status can be closely monitored and mechanical ventilation initiated if needed. I can now perform a thorough evaluation including a history and physical and a review of the diagnostic testing I have ordered, to determine if the patient has another pathophysiology contributing to this acute presentation.

History of Present Illness (Obtained From Medical Record)

The patient has emphysema and was admitted by his primary care provider for community-acquired pneumonia. The patient believes the source of his infection was contact with his grandson who had a fever. He presented to the hospital with a 4-day history of increased cough, productive of thick green secretions. He has felt ill and unable to independently do activities of daily living for the last 3 days. Upon admission 2 days ago, he was started on oxygen 2 liters by nasal cannula and treated with ceftriaxone, azithromycin, and methylprednisolone intravenously, as well as inhaled ipratropium and albuterol every 4 hours by nebulizer. According to the last progress note, he showed only marginal improvement on this regimen.

Past Medical History (Obtained From Record)

Hypertension, cerebral vascular accident (CVA) 6 years ago with residual right arm weakness, emphysema diagnosed 6 years ago, α_1-antitrypsin deficiency negative. A blood gas drawn 2 years ago showed: pH 7.34, $PaCO_2$ 57 mm Hg, bicarb 30, PaO 68 mm Hg, and O_2 saturation 91% on room air.

Past Surgical History

No prior surgery.

Social History

Widower, lives alone in a two-story home which he owns. His two sons live out of town and visit during holidays. He was a smoker, 3 packs per day for 40 years, but quit 1 year ago. He drinks a 6 pack of beer once a month with his poker group. He denies illicit drug use.

Family History

His father and sister died of strokes. His father had a myocardial infarction and hypertension. Both sons are alive and well. He denies a family history of cancer, anemia, and clotting disorders.

Medication List (During Hospital Admission)

- Albuterol, metered dose inhaler: Two puffs every 4 hours as needed for shortness of breath (has been taking every 4 hours since sick)
- Ipratropium, metered dose inhaler: Two puffs every 4 hours
- Prednisone 40 mg/day for 5 days
- Azithromycin 500 mg by mouth daily
- Moxifloxacin 400 mg by mouth daily
- Cefotaxime 1 g intravenously every 8 hours
- Aspirin 80 mg by mouth daily
- Hydrochlorothiazide 12.5 mg by mouth daily

Review of Systems (Obtained From Medical Record)

- Constitutional: Felt increasingly unwell over the 4 days prior to admission, denies subjective fever or weight loss.
- Cardiovascular: Denies palpitations, angina, new weakness, and dizziness. He has been told he has a slight murmur of no significance.
- Pulmonary: Cough is worse at night, productive for thick green secretions for the past 4 days but his usual secretions are thin and clear. He received a pneumococcal vaccination 5 years ago.
- Gastrointestinal: Denies nausea, vomiting, diarrhea, gastroesophageal reflux disease, and peptic ulcer disease.
- Musculoskeletal: Chronic right arm weakness; denies pain, trauma, or falls.
- Neurological: CVA in 2009 with residual right arm weakness but speech is normal; denies memory loss and seizures.
- Genitourinary: Denies dysuria, frequency, and urgency.
- Endocrine: Denies diabetes, thyroid dysfunction, and hormone therapy.
- Hematological: Denies anemia, human immunodeficiency virus, and cancer.

- Mental health: Grieving wife's death 3 months ago; currently attending grief group that is helpful. He denies suicidal ideation, mania, delusions, or anxiety.

Physical Examination (Completed on Admission to ICU)

- Constitutional: Thin male, appears uncomfortable, but no longer in acute distress.
- Head/eyes/ears/nose/throat: Head is atraumatic with male patterned balding. Pupils are equal, round, reactive to light, 3 mm. Fundus examination findings include silver wiring and cotton wool patches but his optic discs are not elevated. Tympanic membranes are intact with a normal cone of light. Pharynx is pink without exudate; tonsils are absent.
- Pulmonary: The respiratory rate is 24 breaths per minute following the chest tube insertion and his oxygen saturation is 90% on 100% nonrebreather. There are breath sounds in all lobes, with a prolonged expiratory phase and wheezing on expiration.
- Cardiovascular: The cardiac monitor shows sinus tachycardia at 100 beats per minute with occasional premature ventricular beats. The heart sounds have not changed.
- Neurological: He is now more alert with occasional eye contact but is still nonverbal. Protective reflexes, gag, and swallow are intact. He moves all extremities. His neck is supple. The left arm is stronger than his right. He is following some commands and his movements are purposeful. He is no longer attempting to get out of bed.
- Gastrointestinal: Normal bowel sounds in all four quadrants; abdomen is soft without tenderness, bruits, or masses. Liver span is 7 cm.
- Genitourinary: Deferred.
- Integumentary: Skin intact and without lesions.
- Musculoskeletal: Structure and symmetry are within normal limits, right arm 1+ strength and other extremities 2+.
- Lymphatic: No lymphadenopathy.

Results of Diagnostic Testing

Arterial blood gas: On 100% nonrebreather mask

	Results	Normal
pH	7.27	(7.35–7.45)
$PaCO_2$	70 mm Hg	(35–45)
HCO_3	26 mEq/L	(22–26)
PaO_2	60 mm Hg	(>80)
$O_{2\,Sat}$	90%	(>98)

12-Lead ECG: Sinus tachycardia at 100 beats per minute with premature ventricular contractions and short runs of bigeminy. There are nonspecific ST-wave changes.

Portable chest x-ray: Right upper lobe with chest tube in correct position and 15% pneumothorax remaining. Right middle lobe infiltrate consistent with pneumonia, multiple large blebs, and bilateral flat diaphragm consistent with COPD.

? Given the information to this point what elements of the review of systems, physical examination, and diagnostic tests should be added to the list of pertinent positives?

- Ultrasound confirms pneumothorax, chest x-ray shows chest tube is functional, pneumothorax resolved to 15%, and no evidence of hemothorax or pleural effusion.
- X-ray findings consistent with COPD plus pneumonia.
- Respiratory rate 24 breaths per minute and oxygen saturation 90%, showing improvement following needle decompression.
- Improvement in agitation but not at baseline mental status.
- Tachycardia, irregular rhythm, and murmur noted.
- Eye fundus has silver wiring and cotton wool patches (suggests chronic hypertension).
- Residual right arm weakness from the previous CVA—no other deficits.
- Protective reflexes intact.
- Full code status.

? Which items should be added to the list of significant negatives?

- Chest tube insertion without complications
- No blood drainage from chest tube, or bubbles on inspiration in chest drainage system
- Funduscopic examination shows nonelevated disc
- Moves all extremities and neck is supple

? How does this information affect the problem representation?

I restate my problem representation as: "A 65-year-old male hospitalized with pneumonia develops sudden onset of respiratory distress, mental status changes, and agitation, which were partially improved with decompression of a right upper lobe pneumothorax and 100% nonrebreather mask."

Case Analysis

Adequate oxygenation is the priority to prevent end-organ damage, though provision of high levels of supplemental oxygen to patients with COPD requires close monitoring. It is necessary to repeat arterial blood gases periodically to assess his acid-base status as well as oxygenation. With the high level of oxygen that he is receiving he may stop breathing. This is because patients with COPD have a high work of breathing due to the mechanical disadvantage at which they work. Their diaphragm is mechanically forced downward in the chest as the volume of the lung increases (ie, barrel chest). As a result, their ventilatory efficiency decreases and their carbon dioxide rises while the pH decreases. The kidneys compensate by retaining bicarbonate. The result is a higher baseline CO_2 and lower PaO_2. Unfortunately, when provided with high levels of O_2, CO_2 is released from the hemoglobin into the blood, resulting in an increase in $PaCO_2$ and a decrease in pH (the Haldane effect).[1] This may result in apnea. Intubation and mechanical ventilation may be required.

Now that the emergency has been addressed and he is relatively stable, I need to systematically review my differential diagnoses by system. While he did have a pneumothorax, it is essential that I consider other potential causes that may have contributed to his condition.

Pulmonary: The pneumothorax was confirmed by ultrasound and oxygenation improvement with needle decompression and follow-up x-ray. He does not have hemothorax or pleural effusion. A partial pneumothorax persists even with a properly placed functional chest tube. If the pneumothorax is not reduced by tomorrow or if his condition continues to deteriorate, then repositioning of the chest tube or placement of an additional tube may be considered. Resolution of the pneumothorax will be evident on chest x-ray and improved clinical stability.

His pneumonia has not changed in appearance on chest x-ray, which may be a sign of treatment failure, though x-rays often lag behind clinical improvement. He may have aspirated during this acute event, and his low-grade fever may be an indication of early sepsis. I consider escalating his antibiotic therapy as his status is much more serious than when he was admitted. Pulmonary embolus, also on my differential, is still a possibility, though less likely given the absence of lower extremity pain or swelling. The majority of pulmonary emboli emanate from upper and lower extremity deep vein thromboses (DVT), so the absence of these symptoms is reassuring. I can order a lower extremity Doppler ultrasound to be done at the bedside to definitely rule out a DVT. For now it will stay on the differential.

Cardiac: The heart rate decreased after needle decompression, which affirms that his tachycardia was a compensatory response. His ECG did not show cardiac ischemia so myocardial infarction (MI) is unlikely, though he does have tachycardia and premature ventricular contractions, suggesting possible local ischemia due to his acidosis and hypoxemia. A risk of MI remains and cardiac monitoring, serial cardiac enzymes, and repeat ECGs are warranted. The current and past history of heart murmur may represent a chronic cardiac disease such as heart failure or valve disease as he has a history of hypertension and confirmatory physical findings such as cotton wool patches and silver wiring on the funduscopic examination.

Neurological: His acute change in mental state may or may not be due solely to the pneumothorax and subsequent hypoxemia. He is improved now, but has not returned to his baseline. I do not see new focal neurologic deficits such as facial asymmetry that would lead me to consider a new CVA, but I cannot evaluate his speech. His pupils are equal, round, and reactive to light and the discs are normal so a large cranial bleed is less likely. A cerebral anoxic event that is temporary or possibly permanent remains on my differential. A computed tomography (CT) scan of his head is warranted if his mental status does not rapidly improve.

❓ What additional diagnostic testing should be done and in what order?

First I order a repeat arterial blood gas to determine his oxygenation and acid-base status, so that I can provide additional support, mechanical ventilation if needed, or a reduction in his oxygen as he further improves. My goal is an oxygen saturation of 90% without an increase in $PaCO_2$ since hypercapnia may cause respiratory depression. Next I order a repeat 12-lead ECG and serial cardiac enzymes to rule out a myocardial infarction. Blood work including a serum chemistry plus magnesium to evaluate electrolytes, glucose, and acid-base balance, a complete blood count with a differential and a serum lactate will help me determine if he has an electrolyte disturbance or anemia or if he is developing sepsis contributing to his altered mental state. Given his history of CVA and sudden change in neurologic status, I order a computed tomography (CT) scan of the head and will consider consulting neurology if his symptoms do not improve.

CASE INFORMATION

Diagnostics Results

- Chest x-ray: Persistent 15% pneumothorax in the right upper lobe, but the chest tube is in the correct position, otherwise unchanged. I will repeat the chest x-ray in the morning, or sooner if his condition deteriorates, to evaluate the pneumothorax.
- 12-Lead ECG: Sinus rhythm at 96 beats per minute with no ectopy. There are nonspecific ST-wave changes.

Arterial Blood Gas: On 100% Nonrebreather Mask		
	Results	Normal
pH	7.32	(7.35–7.45)
PaCO$_2$	52 mm Hg	(35–45)
HCO$_3$	27 mEq/L	(22–26)
PaO$_2$	88 mm Hg	(>80)
O$_{2\ Sat}$	96%	(>98)

Serum Electrolytes and CBC		
	Patient Value	Reference Range
Serum Chemistry		
Sodium	137	135–145 mEq/L
Potassium	4.0	3.5–5.1 mEq/L
Chloride	99	98–106 mEq/L
Bicarbonate	27	22–26 mEq/L
BUN	22	7–18 mg/dL
Creatinine	0.94	0.67–1.2 mg/dL
Glucose	114	70–115 mg/dL
Magnesium	1.9	1.3–2.1 mEq/L
Lactate	2.4	0.5–2.2 mmol/L
CBC		
WBC	13,000	4,500–11,000 cells/µL
Hemoglobin male	13.7	13.5–17.5 g/dL
Hematocrit male	42	39%–49%
Platelets	300	150–450 × 10^3/µL
RBC male	5.0	4.3–5.7 × 10^6/µL
Bands	12%	0%–10% with rest of differential within normal limits

- Cardiac enzymes: Within normal limits.
- Head CT scan: No mass or bleed. Old lacunar infarct. Unchanged from 2009.
- Chest x-ray the following day: Right upper lobe pneumothorax resolving, now at 10%, with chest tube in correct position. Otherwise unchanged from this admission.

❓ How does the information change your potential list of causes?

There is no evidence of an MI since troponins are normal and no ischemic changes are on the ECG. He still will require the remaining serial enzyme studies to rule out this diagnosis but for now it is low on the differential list. His BUN is elevated likely due to dehydration and will be monitored over time as he is rehydrated.

To further consider sepsis, I measure an anion gap: Anion gap (AG) = $(Na + K) - (Cl + HCO_3)$. A normal AG is 10 to 18 and elevations in the anion gap indicate unmeasured anions such as lactate. His anion gap is 15 so is within normal limits. The lactate level is only slightly elevated so sepsis is lower on my differential list now, particularly since the white blood cell count and bands are only slightly elevated which I attribute to his pneumonia. However, I will continue to evaluate for additional causes of infection over his clinical course.

To further evaluate his persistent hypoxemia, I calculate the alveolar-arterial (A-a) gradient as follows: expected PAO_2 = FIO_2 (barometric pressure: 760 mm Hg – water vapor: 47) – ($PaCO_2$/respiratory quotient: 0.8). His expected PAO_2 calculated by this formula is 648 mm Hg but his actual arterial PaO_2 is only 88 mm Hg, indicating that his A-a gradient is 560. On 100% oxygen, his gradient should be between 50 and 75 or a bit higher due to his age. This abnormal gradient suggests a severe oxygenation problem, which may be due to his persistent pneumonia or a PE. At this point, I will keep the patient in the MICU to closely follow his arterial blood bases, obtain a bedside Doppler ultrasound of his lower extremities, and consult the infectious disease team to address his antibiotic regimen given the severity of his illness.

Diagnosis and Treatment of Pneumothorax

In this case, the pneumothorax was diagnosed by ultrasound, and confirmed by chest x-ray and by the improvement in his condition with chest tube insertion. Pneumothoraces are more common in men (ratio of six men for every woman in the age group 60–89 years.) The majority occur on the right side and in the apices more often than the lower lobes. This patient has a right upper lobe pneumothorax. The patient's emphysematous blebs create a high risk for recurrent pneumothoraces, so carefully educating the patient and family prior to discharge is essential.

Pneumothorax is high on the differential list for any patient with new onset respiratory distress because it is a life-threatening condition.[2] Patients with emphysema, such as the patient in this case, are at increased risk for pneumothorax. Emphysema pathology involves a progressive destruction of the inner walls of the alveolar sacs, resulting in large blebs with a reduced surface area for gas exchange. An emphysema bleb is an enlarged air sac that compresses adjacent parenchyma and these blebs are a frequent site of infections. With increased pressure, such as generated with a cough, the bleb may burst allowing air to flow from the lung into the pleural space, resulting in a pneumothorax. Invading organisms can also erode the parenchyma and cause a pneumothorax.

The treatment of a pneumothorax depends on the extent of lung collapse, the risk for increasing size, and the stability of the patient's condition. For asymptomatic patients observation alone can be considered but if the patient is unstable then immediate intervention is the standard of care. Supplemental oxygenation and a needle decompression to relieve the initial pressure is often a first step until a chest tube to water seal or a one-way valve can be placed. The chest tube is removed when there is no longer air bubbling in the water seal and the chest xray shows full lung expansion. This may take a few days or up to a week or more especially if the patient is on steroids which may delay healing.

If there is recurrence of a pneumothorax, then additional treatment may be considered.[3] If a bleb is large or causes complications, the treatment may be excision by video-assisted thoracoscopic surgery (VATS) or open thoracotomy. Patients with compromised respiratory reserve are surgical risks but generally have improved respiratory status postoperatively. Another treatment is pleurodesis (or sclero-therapy), which involves the insertion of an irritant (talc or minocycline) between the layers of the pleura, causing inflammation and permanent adhesions between the layers, so that air cannot enter the pleural space. This procedure is painful and premedication is warranted.

The patient in this case had a community-acquired pneumonia. Pneumonia may have many causes but in the United States, virus (flu virus is the most common in adults) is the source of one-third of pneumonia cases. However, viral infections do predispose patients to bacterial pneumonias called post-influenza pneumonia. A common bacterial source of pneumonia is *Streptococcus pneumoniae* for which patients can be immunized with a Pneumovax vaccine. This patient did receive this vaccine but other bacteria could have caused his pneumonia, the two most common being *Klebsiella pneumoniae* and *Haemophilus influenzae*. The frequency of pneumonia in the elderly is increased. Patients with HIV who are infected with *Pneumocystis jiroveci* pneumonia (PCP) have a 5% to 10% risk of pneumothorax.[4]

Case Follow-Up

The patient's Doppler ultrasound was negative for DVT, and his oxygenation continued to improve following the change in antibiotics. After another 24 hours of care in the MICU the patient was alert, and weaned from the nonrebreather mask to a nasal cannula. Intubation was averted. His chest tube was removed after 6 days, and his chest x-ray demonstrated improvement in the pneumonia. He was discharged to home with a follow-up appointment with his primary care provider in 3 days.

References

1. West J. *Respiratory Physiology: The Essentials*. 9th ed. New York: Wolters Kluwer/Lippincott Williams and Wilkins; 2012: 81.
2. Cartagenasurgery. Blebs, bullae and spontaneous pneumothorax/thoracic surgery. http://cirugiadetorax.org/2012/02/08/blebs-bullae-and-spontaneous-pneumothorax/. Accessed September 14, 2014.
3. Global strategy for the diagnosis, management and prevention of COPD. Global Initiative for Chronic Obstructive Lung Disease (GOLD). 2011. http://www.goldcopd.org/guidelines-global-strategy-for-diagnosis-management.html. Accessed September 14, 2014.
4. McClellan A, Miller S, Parson P, Cohn D. Pneumothorax with *Pneumocystis carinii* pneumonia in AIDS. Incidence and clinical characteristics. *Chest*. 1991;100(5):1224-1228.

CASE 60

Bonnie Tong

Bonnie Tong works as a cardiology nurse practitioner at Mount Sinai Hospital in New York, NY. Dr Tong is also adjunct faculty for the ACNP Program at New York University.

CASE INFORMATION

Chief Complaint

A 74-year-old woman presents to the emergency room with shortness of breath.

❓ What are the potential causes?

Shortness of breath (SOB) or dyspnea is a subjective symptom that is described by many as difficulty breathing.[1] SOB can be caused by many different etiologies, some of which are life threatening and require rapid diagnosis and treatment. First, I must determine whether the SOB is acute or chronic. The next step is to review the differential diagnoses that can result in dyspnea. One approach is to think of all the physiological processes that can result in dyspnea and identify the associated disease states.

Differential Diagnoses for the Patient With Dyspnea[2]

- Cardiovascular disease: acute coronary syndrome, angina, congestive heart failure, arrhythmias, valvular diseases, congenital heart disease, cardiomyopathy, myocarditis
- Parenchymal lung disease: chronic obstructive pulmonary disease (COPD), pulmonary tumors, infective pneumonitis, noninfective pneumonitis, bronchiectasis, pulmonary contusion, interstitial lung disease, sarcoidosis, pulmonary contusion
- Airway disease: asthma, bronchitis, laryngitis, epiglottitis, obstructive sleep apnea, angioedema, foreign body aspiration, tracheobronchial tumors, diphtheria, vocal cord dysfunction, tracheobronchial tumors
- Pulmonary vascular disease: pulmonary embolus, pulmonary hypertension, pulmonary arteriovenous malformations, hepatopulmonary syndrome
- Pleural disease: pleural effusion, pleural tumors, pneumothorax, pneumomediastinum, mesothelioma, pleuritis, hemothorax

- Hematologic disease: anemia, methemoglobinemia, carbon monoxide poisoning, thrombotic thrombocytopenic purpura, pulmonary leukostasis
- Gastrointestinal disease: gastroesophageal reflux disease (GERD), ascites
- Endocrine disease: thyroid disease, Cushing syndrome, pheochromocytoma
- Musculoskeletal disease: kyphoscoliosis, pectus excavatum
- Allergic/inflammatory disease: shock, anaphylaxis
- Neurologic disease: stroke, botulism, amyotrophic lateral sclerosis, tetanus, polio, acute viral anterior horn infections, Guillain-Barré syndrome, myasthenia gravis, paraneoplastic myasthenic syndrome, respiratory muscle deficiency
- Psychosocial: anxiety, panic attack
- Physiological: aging, deconditioning, obesity

Now that I have compiled a comprehensive list of possible causes for this woman's dyspnea, I will begin to rule in, or rule out, these causes. My next step is to gather more information by performing a general survey of the patient, and obtain the history of this illness as well as her past medical history.

CASE INFORMATION

History of Present Illness

I first perform a general survey of the patient, paying attention to her general state of health, posture, build, motor skills, and any odors from her body or breath: the patient is tachypneic and using her accessory muscles to breath. The patient's eyes are closed, she is leaning forward on her stretcher, and she appears very uncomfortable. Upon asking her how she feels, she reports that she has not had an asthma attack like this before and complains of how warm she feels. She states, "I was at a birthday dinner and all of a sudden felt like I was suffocating. I took my inhalers as I was instructed when I have an asthma attack but it didn't help." She also reports that over the last 3 days she has had worsening swelling in her legs and weakness, to the point where she cannot walk more than 20 steps before having to stop due to shortness of breath. She denies any chest pain, palpitations, or nausea/vomiting. As I speak to the patient, I notice that she is having difficulty speaking without gasping for air.

Before I continue, I conclude that this patient's dyspnea is an acute event and I place a nasal cannula on the patient to deliver 2 L of oxygen. When asked about her medical history she reports having asthma, congestive heart failure (CHF), chronic obstructive pulmonary disease (COPD), and diabetes. Through the review of her medical records, I notice that she also has a history of hypertension, hyperlipidemia, diabetes mellitus type 2, stage III chronic kidney disease, ventricular fibrillation (VF) arrest with an implantable cardioverter-defibrillator (ICD) placed in 2008, an upgrade to a biventricular ICD in 2013, and a ventricular tachycardia (VT) ablation in 2013.

Since initiating the 2 L O_2 by NC she has been placed on pulse oximetry and I note her O_2 saturation is 75%. This is the equivalent of a PaO_2 of approximately 42 mm Hg. I put her on a 100% non-rebreather mask, which immediately brings her oxygen saturation to between 88% and 90%. This will be followed by an arterial blood gas to ensure she is not retaining CO_2 as she has a history of COPD.

? What are the pertinent positives at this time?

- The patient is tachypneic, diaphoretic, and using her accessory muscles.
- The patient's dyspnea occurred suddenly and at rest.
- The patient's sudden shortness of breath was preceded by several days of leg swelling, decreased exercise tolerance to 20 steps, and weakness.
- The patient has a significant history of asthma, CHF, and COPD.
- The patient has a history of HTN, hyperlipidemia, and CKD stage III.
- The patient was at a birthday dinner prior to arriving to the hospital.
- The dyspnea occurred abruptly at a birthday dinner.

? What are the pertinent negatives at this time?

- The patient denies chest pain and palpitations.
- The shortness of breath is different from her asthma attacks and the patient had no relief with the use of inhalers.

? Does the information gathered so far give you an insight into the possible causes of her dyspnea and what other information would be helpful?

Summing up the information gathered so far will help highlight the pertinent information. The summation may look like this:

"A 74-year-old woman with a medical history of hypertension, hyperlipidemia, DM type 2, CKD stage III, VF arrest with an ICD placed in 2008, an upgrade to a biventricular ICD in 2013, and a VT ablation in 2013 presents with acute shortness of breath at rest."

Case Analysis

The patient's acute shortness of breath can be caused by an exacerbation of her COPD or her CHF, or an asthma attack. Although, I note that her current symptom is different from her prior asthma attacks and this differential is lower on my list, because of its severity and the possibility of a life-threatening untreated asthma attack, asthma must be ruled out. In addition, her history of hypertension, age, CHF, and hyperlipidemia increases her chances of having coronary artery disease (CAD). I must rule out a myocardial infarction as well. Although the patient denies any chest pain or nausea/vomiting, I keep in mind that women and people with diabetes often manifest CAD in atypical ways. The patient has a history of VT and VF, and due to her history of HTN, CHF, and hyperlipidemia, there is an increased risk of developing an arrhythmia. Another differential diagnosis I must keep in mind is a pulmonary embolus (PE) due to its high mortality and the sudden onset of her shortness of breath is consistent with this diagnosis.[3] Most pulmonary emboli begin as a lower extremity deep vein thrombus so the associated symptom of leg swelling raises my concern for this diagnosis. Her leg swelling also raises concern for a CHF exacerbation but ruling out MI, asthma attack, and PE is a higher priority at this time.

My next step is to begin obtaining the information I need to rule out the high priority diagnoses. I order blood work including brain natriuretic peptide (BNP), cardiac markers to rule out MI, and a D-dimer, as well as standard labs that include complete blood count with differential, a comprehensive metabolic panel, and thyroid function tests. An elevated BNP will increase the likelihood of acute on chronic CHF as the cause of dyspnea and a positive D-dimer increases the likelihood of a PE. I also order an ECG, a stat chest x-ray, and a transthoracic echo (TTE). In addition, an interrogation of her ICD is warranted to look for any recent arrhythmias and to assess the functioning of her device. The results of these tests will determine the cause of the patient's dyspnea, but will be performed after I have confirmed that the patient is stable and completed a history and physical. In the meantime, I order an albuterol nebulizer treatment. Her O_2 saturation is now 90%, she is still short of breath but she is able to speak and is alert.

CASE INFORMATION

Prior to Admission Medications

Metolazone 5 mg PO three times a week
Furosemide 80 mg daily
Carvedilol 6.25 mg PO twice a day
Amiodarone 200 mg twice a day
Albuterol 90 µg/actuation aerosol, one puff by mouth every 6 hours as needed

Ipratropium bromide 0.02% solution, inhale via nebulizer every 6 hours as needed

Aspirin 81 mg PO daily

Fluticasone propionate 220 µg/actuation aerosol, inhale one puff by mouth twice a day

Insulin glargine 100 units/mL (3 mL) pen: Inject 10 units SQ daily

Review of Systems

The patient is a good historian.

- Constitutional: reports feeling lousy and has not been able to do as much usual over the last 3 days, states she takes her medications as prescribed, endorses weight increase of approximately 15 lb in 2 weeks
- Head/eyes/ears/nose/throat: denies sinus drainage, or sore throat
- Cardiovascular: denies chest pain or palpitations, positive bilateral lower extremity edema, positive paroxysmal nocturnal dyspnea (PND), and sleeps on three pillows
- Pulmonary: positive shortness of breath, denies wheezing, denies cough
- Gastrointestinal: denies any changes in bowel movements, last bowel movement was yesterday evening. Denies nausea/vomiting. Denies any bloating, cramping, or epigastric pain
- Genitourinary: endorses decreased urination, denies urgency, frequency, or painful urination
- Musculoskeletal: denies any joint pain
- Neurological: denies stroke, transient ischemic attacks
- Endocrine: denies any heat/cold intolerance,
- Psychiatric: denies depressed mood, anxiety at this time

Physical Examination

- Vitals: blood pressure 196/87 mmHg, heart rate 60 beats per minutes, respiratory rate 35 breaths per minute, temperature 36.1°C, oxygen saturation on 100% O_2 via non-rebreather is 90%
- Constitutional: ill appearing, appears stated age, and in respiratory distress
- Cardiovascular: regular rate and rhythm, +II/VI systolic murmur, jugular venous distension at 10 cm sitting up, 3+ bilateral pitting edema up to thighs, upper and lower extremities cool to touch, nail beds are pale, brisk capillary refill
- Pulmonary: tachypneic, + use of accessory muscles, lungs with crackles bilaterally ¾ way up, no wheezing noted
- Gastrointestinal: normoactive bowel sounds, tympanic on percussion, abdomen soft, no tenderness
- Neurologic: alert and oriented to name, place, and time, no focal neurologic deficits.

Diagnostic and Laboratory Testing

ECG: (biventricular pacing deactivated) underlying rhythm is NSR 60, LVH, no ST changes noted, no significant changes from prior ECG

Chest x-ray: cardiomegaly, pulmonary vascular congestion (hilar engorgement), bilateral diffuse interstitial and alveolar filling throughout both lung fields

Transthoracic Echocardiogram: severe left ventricular dilatation, overall severe decreased left ventricular systolic function (diffuse), severe decreased right ventricular dilatation; ejection fraction = 18%

Device interrogation:

Parameters: DDD 60-110

Tachycardia parameters: VT 166 beats per minute

Events: None

Conclusion: Appropriate device function

Laboratory values:

ABG on 100% O_2: pH 7. 32, $PaCO_2$ 32 mm Hg, PaO_2 54 mm Hg.

Brain natriuretic peptide: 1145.

D-dimer: Negative.

Comprehensive metabolic panel reveals a BUN/creatinine of 81/2.84, CO_2 23.1. The patient does have a history of CKD, but I notice from her chart that her baseline creatinine is around 1.5 to 2.

CBC reveals WBC 7, Hgb/Hct 11.9/37.7.

Troponin ×1: 0.0.

LFTs: Within normal limits.

TSH: 0.5 μU/mL.

Case Analysis

The next step in this process is to sort the differential diagnoses and classify the dyspnea.

❓ What are the pertinent positives from the review of systems, physical examination, and diagnostic and laboratory testing?

- The patient reports paroxysmal nocturnal dyspnea with three-pillow orthopnea, bilateral lower extremity swelling, and increased weight gain.
- The patient is hypertensive, hypoxemic, has elevated neck veins, +II/VI systolic murmur, 3+ bilateral pitting edema up to thighs, lungs with crackles bilaterally ¾ way up, decreased urination, bilateral upper and lower extremities cool to touch, and her nail beds are pale.

- The transthoracic echocardiogram reveals severe left ventricular dilatation, overall severe decreased left ventricular systolic function (diffuse), severe decreased right ventricular dilatation; ejection fraction = 18%.
- The chest x-ray reveals cardiomegaly and congestion.
- The patient's ECG revealed left ventricular hypertrophy (LVH).
- The patient has an elevated BNP and increased creatinine.

❓ What are the pertinent negatives from the review of system, physical examination, and diagnostic and laboratory testing?

- The patient denies chest pain and palpitations.
- The patient is not wheezing.
- The patient's ECG revealed no new changes and her troponin level is negative.
- The CBC is at baseline and D-dimer is negative.

❓ Does the new information gathered increase your insight into the possible causes of her dyspnea?

I feel comfortable ruling out an infectious process and anemia as the cause of her dyspnea given her normal complete blood count. An acute myocardial infarction is less likely due to negative troponin levels and baseline ECG. In addition, PE is unlikely given the normal D-dimer, and I am less concerned about lower extremity deep vein thrombosis (DVT) now that I see that her swelling is equal in both legs. Bilateral DVT is very unlikely, so unilateral swelling would be much more concerning. Based on my examination, I am less concerned that this is an asthma attack; the patient has no wheezing, and did not respond to stat nebulizer treatment.

Now I have gathered enough information to believe that heart failure is the cause of her dyspnea. The patient's increased BNP, increased neck veins, bilateral crackles on auscultation, and lower extremity edema suggest fluid overload. Her chest x-ray is descriptive of an enlarged heart (cardiomegaly), hilar engorgement, and bilateral interstitial and alveolar filling pattern consistent with pulmonary edema. All these findings suggest acute on chronic systolic heart failure. In addition, the patient's increased creatinine level is most likely due to decreased perfusion. Due to the acuity of her dyspnea, these findings, and her hypoxemia, I conclude that the patient is having flash pulmonary edema. What differentiates an acute exacerbation of chronic heart failure from flash pulmonary edema is the speed in which the severe dyspnea develops. In this case, her condition was likely exacerbated by the food she had at the birthday dinner.

My summation of the problem can now be: "A 74-year-old ill-appearing female with a medical history of hypertension, hyperlipidemia, DM type 2, CKD stage III, VF arrest with an ICD placed in 2008, an upgrade to a biventricular ICD in 2013, and a VT ablation in 2013 presents with rapidly developing dyspnea due to acute onset pulmonary edema."

❓ What diagnostic tests should be done?

At this time, prompt treatment of the patient is essential as she is in respiratory distress. Diagnostic testing such as those listed above should be performed only after the patient is stabilized.

Flash Pulmonary Edema: Diagnosis and Management

Flash pulmonary edema is a dramatic form of fluid accumulation in the interstitial and alveolar spaces in the lung that results from an imbalance in the pulmonary fluid homeostasis, in this case, the birthday dinner, which worsened her acute decompensated heart failure.[4] Other triggers include myocardial infarction, malignant hypertension, and volume overload due to chronic kidney disease. Flash pulmonary edema is largely a clinical diagnosis with patients complaining of dyspnea, tachypnea, pulmonary rales/crackles on auscultation, increased jugular venous pressure, and peripheral edema.

Accepted treatments for flash pulmonary edema related to decompensated heart failure include loop diuretics, which not only relieve the volume overload in acute decompensated heart failure but also have a vasodilatory effect.[5] Vasodilators are also utilized to relieve pulmonary congestion. In patients refractory to diuretics, inotropes may be necessary.

As noted this patient was rapidly transitioned to a 100% nonrebreather as her oxygen saturation was only 75% on 2 L of oxygen via nasal cannula. She was then given furosemide 80 mg intravenously and placed on a nitroglycerin drip. Her oxygen saturation slowly improved to 95% and her blood pressure started to normalize. She was eventually weaned off the 100% nonrebreather and was admitted to the hospital with the continuation of intravenous furosemide to treat her decompensated systolic heart failure.

References

1. Peters SP. When the chief complaint is (or should be) dyspnea in adults. *J Allergy Clin Immunol Pract.* 2013;1:129-136. http://dx.doi.org/10.1016/j.aip.2013.01.004.
2. Kamal AH, Maguire JM, Wheeler JL, Currow DC, Abernathy AP. Dyspnea review for the palliative care professional: assessment, burdens, and etiologies. *J Palliat Care.* 2011;14:1167-1172. doi: 10.1089/jpm.2011.0109.
3. Moua T, Wood K. COPD and PE: a clinical dilemma. *Int J Chron Obstruct Pulmon Dis.* 2008;3:277-284.
4. Rimoldi SF, Yuzefpolskaya M, Allemann Y, Messerli F. Flash pulmonary edema. *Prog Cardiovasc Dis.* 2009;52:249-259. doi: 10.1016/j.pcad.2009.10.002.
5. Evaluation of dyspnea. Epocrates Web site. https://online.epocrates.com/u/2912862/Evaluation+of+dyspnea/Differential/Etiology. Published 2014. Accessed August 6, 2014.

CASE 61

Carol K. Thompson

Carol is a Professor in the AG-ACNP Program at the University of Kentucky. Dr Thompson was one of the first 100 to be certified as an ACNP and currently is a member of an all NP intensivist team at the University Hospital, Lexington, KY. She was the first ACNP to be President of the Society of Critical Care Medicine and continues to lead internationally.

CASE INFORMATION

Chief Complaint

A 35-year-old African American female comes to the emergency room complaining of bilateral leg swelling and left leg redness.

❓ What is the potential cause?

There are many etiologies of leg swelling and redness and each of these symptoms may have a separate cause. However, I start with a comprehensive differential that is inclusive of both symptoms since it is likely they are related. Some conditions that result in leg swelling and redness are serious and I will focus on ruling them out first so that appropriate treatment is provided quickly.

Comprehensive Differential Diagnoses for Acute Unilateral or Bilateral Leg Swelling and Redness

Unilateral
Deep vein thrombosis, cellulitis, burn, bone or muscle trauma, and other musculoskeletal causes such as sprain, strain, tear, tendon rupture, fracture

Bilateral
- Cardiac: heart failure from cardiomyopathy, pericarditis, arrhythmias
- Renal: nephrotic syndrome, renal insufficiency/failure
- Vascular: stenosis, venous insufficiency, mass/tumor/lesion impeding flow
- Infection: sepsis
- Gastrointestinal: cirrhosis, liver failure
- Hormonal: pregnancy, hormone therapy
- Lymphatic: lymphedema

CASE INFORMATION

General Survey and History of Present Illness

My first priority is to assess how the patient is tolerating her condition. Thus I quickly assess her airway, breathing, and circulation—does she look distressed? She is sitting up in the bed with her forearms resting on pillows at her side, tachypneic at 26 breaths per minute, but has no accessory muscle use. Her face is pink and there is no diaphoresis or asymmetry. Her speech is clear and she greets me with "hello." No one has accompanied her to the emergency department so any information that I obtain will depend on her ability to provide it. For now she appears to be in slight respiratory distress but appears to be tolerating her condition. She is well developed, well nourished, obese, and is wearing worn, wrinkled, but unsoiled clothing.

When asked why she came to the emergency room, she responds, "Both legs have been swelling but this morning the left one started turning red." She noticed that over the past 2 days her ankles have become swollen and the swelling has increased from the ankles up to her knee and thigh. She denies pain, lesions, insect bites, trauma, recent surgery, or being out of any of her medications. Nothing seems to decrease the swelling, "they just keep getting larger." She has never had leg swelling before. Prior to the onset of the swelling, she was ill with a subjective fever, runny nose, nonproductive cough, and sore throat, and this led her to spend most of 3 days in bed. Her nephew had the same symptoms when he visited a few days before she got sick. She has not been seen at this facility before and no records are available for review. Upon initial triage her vital signs are temperature 99°F, blood pressure is 146/92 mm Hg, heart rate 107 beats per minute, respiratory rate 26 breaths per minute, pulse oximetry 92% on room air.

Past Medical and Surgical History

She denies any history of heart disease, lung disease, liver problems, or cancer. She also reports she does not have diabetes, and has never been pregnant. She is not aware of any allergies to any medications.

Social History

Divorced, lives with male partner, employed as computer programmer sitting most of the day, smokes 2 packs per day for the past 20 years, occasional wine, denies liquor or illicit drug use.

Family Medical History

Both parents died in an auto accident 10 years ago, but no chronic illnesses. Sister has diabetes and hypertension. She denies family history of myocardial infarction, stroke, cancer, anemia, clotting disorders, congenital defects.

Medications

Her medications include over-the-counter daily vitamins, calcium citrate, green tea extract; azithromycin two refills for when she gets sinusitis. She says she started a course of azithromycin on day 3 of her illness.

? What are the pertinent positives from the information given so far?

- Patient is alert and able to give history
- Bilateral leg swelling
- Left leg redness
- Bedridden for 3 days prior to leg swelling
- Recent upper respiratory illness with possible low-grade fever
- Tachypnea (26 breaths per minute) and sitting upright
- Tachycardia (107 beats per minute)
- Pulse oximetry: 92% on room air

? What are the significant negatives from the information given so far?

- No apparent distress
- No prior leg swelling, trauma, recent surgery
- No pain in legs

? What is the problem representation?

I state the problem as: "A 35-year-old female with bilateral leg swelling for 2 days with left leg redness noted today with respiratory compromise. Recently bedridden with upper respiratory infection (URI)."

? How does this information affect the list of possible causes and what do you need to do now?

The patient does not seem critical but she is stressed. She has been ill for the past 5 days and is now seeking medical treatment. I am concerned that this is a serious condition as it is newly acquired and associated with a sedentary state due to a recent illness. Her leg edema appears to be getting worse and now one leg has redness. She also is tachypneic and has signs of respiratory compromise as well. A saturation of 92% is a PaO_2 of 70 mm Hg or less. I immediately put her on 100% nonrebreather mask, order continuous cardiac and pulse oximetry monitoring and a peripheral IV with a "keep open infusion rate" of 0.9% NS.

I order a stat formal ECG, arterial blood gas, and portable chest x-ray, which are standard tests when a patient presents with signs of respiratory compromise. The ECG will evaluate for cardiac ischemia and infarction, which requires prompt treatment, and the arterial blood gas will confirm her hypoxemia and demonstrate her acid-base balance. The portable chest x-ray is diagnostic for a number of pulmonary disorders, including pneumothorax, pneumonia, congestive heart failure, and pleural effusion. In addition, I can estimate her heart size on the chest x-ray, which is helpful when cardiomyopathy is on my differential.

While I must consider all the potential causes in my differential the ones that have the most serious potential outcomes include deep vein thrombosis (DVT) with migration of a clot to the lungs (ie, pulmonary embolus [PE]), sepsis from a cellulitis of her leg or other source such as an abscess, and a cardiac cause. While DVTs are most commonly unilateral, I keep this diagnosis high on my differential due to the seriousness of a PE. The patient's age, the fact that she has not experienced similar symptoms in the past, and her medication list suggest this is not an exacerbation of a previously diagnosed chronic condition such as heart failure. However, given the preceding URI, cardiomyopathy from a viral source is a possibility so new onset heart failure is also high on my differential. A comprehensive history and physical are warranted.

CASE INFORMATION

Review of Systems

- Constitutional: Bedridden with URI 3 days and states she did not have an appetite and did not get out of bed often to get fluids or food. She denies chills but states she thought she had a low-grade fever.
- Head/eyes/ears/nose/throat: Winter sinusitis × 4 years, treated with azithromycin. Started this medication on day 3 of recent URI symptoms, which included runny nose (clear secretions), nonproductive cough, and sore throat. Denies pain or discomfort in ears, endorses sore throat with recent illness but this is now improving.
- Cardiovascular: Denies chest pain, palpitations, and irregular heartbeats, endorses bilateral leg edema.
- Pulmonary: Denies orthopnea or shortness of breath until today, but today she states she feels better sitting up.
- Gastrointestinal: Denies nausea, vomiting, diarrhea, abdominal pain, unusual flatus, belching. Last bowel movement was yesterday, soft, brown, and without obvious blood.

- Neurological: Denies syncope, dizziness, weakness, numbness, paresthesias, slurred speech, sleepiness, seizures, memory loss
- Genitourinary: Urinary tract infection (UTI) 6 months ago treated with cranberry juice, irregular menstrual cycles, sexually active single partner without protection, denies prior pregnancies or sexually transmitted diseases. Currently denies dysuria, vaginal discharge. Last menstrual period "a while ago—not sure when."
- Musculoskeletal: Denies leg pain, recent trauma, or lesions. Denies numbness in extremities.
- Skin: Notes recent left leg redness from ankle to knee, denies recent bug bites, rashes, or trauma or abnormal bruising.
- Endocrine: Denies diabetes, thyroid disorder, hormone therapy.
- Hematological: Denies blood clotting abnormalities, infections, cancer. HIV negative single test after divorce 3 years ago.
- Mental health: Denies ever having suicidal ideation, mania, depression, hallucinations, delusions. Describes work as "usual stress." Manages stress with daily meditation and journaling. Satisfied with current male partner relationship.

Physical Examination

- Vital signs: Temperature 99°F oral, heart rate 107 beats per minute, respiratory rate 26 breaths per minute, blood pressure 146/92 mm Hg, weight 250 lb, and body mass index is 44.3.
- Bedside monitor: Pulse oximeter 96% on 100% nonrebreather, cardiac monitor—sinus tachycardia (107 beats per minute) without ectopy or ST-segment changes.
- General: 35-Year-old African American female, well developed, obese, hair matted, clothing worn, communicates with few sentences, occasionally making eye contact, in moderate distress. Appears more stressed now than during initial survey.
- Head/eyes/ears/nose/throat: Pupils equal, round, reactive to light and accommodation, 3 mm. Sclera clear without lid crusting. Maxillary sinus dullness and tender to palpation and percussion. Nasal membranes pale. Tympanic membranes clear bilaterally, no fluid noted, normal color, no exudates. Posterior pharynx without erythema or exudate.
- Cardiovascular: Point of maximal impulse fifth intercostal space midclavicular line, without gallops, murmur, rub, or click. S2 split with pulmonic increased loudness. Jugular venous distension (JVD) 9 cm at 45° head of bed elevation.
- Extremities: Nonpitting edema right leg 2+ at ankles and 1+ at knee without erythema, hyperthermia, lesions. Nonpitting edema left leg 3+ ankles to mid-thigh, erythema from ankle to knee, hyperthermia, without lesions.

Upper extremities without edema, erythema, movement impairment, pain, or lesions.

- Pulmonary: Symmetric breathing pattern with slight sternocleidomastoid muscle use. Using short answers/sentences. Percussion reveals bilateral dullness in lower bases. Breath sounds bilaterally diminished, technically difficult examination due to body habitus.

- Gastrointestinal: Bowel sounds present in all four quadrants. Liver span unable to assess due to body habitus. Negative abdominal tenderness, masses or nodes, bruits.

- Integumentary: Good skin turgor, intact, without lesions. Left leg redness is uniform without rash or streaking from ankle to knee. No stasis dermatitis or other abnormal vascular patterns.

- Musculoskeletal: Symmetrical, well developed with full range of motion of upper extremities and lower extremity range of motion limited by edema. No effusion, crepitus, or movement tenderness. Straight legs raise 70° bilaterally before pain limits movement.

- Neurological: Alert and oriented ×3, cranial nerves II-XII intact. Deep tendon reflexes 2+ bilaterally upper extremities but unable to elicit in lower extremities bilaterally. Upper and lower extremity sensory intact bilaterally. Logical thought process but somewhat sluggish in response to questions. Flat affect.

- Lymphatic: No lymphadenopathy appreciated but limited by body habitus.

Her stat diagnostics have been completed and yield the following:
- Chest x-ray: No fluid, infiltrates or pneumothorax noted. Difficult interpretation due to body habitus.
- ECG: Sinus tachycardia, no arrhythmias or ischemic changes. No cardiomegaly
- ABG: pH 7.27, PCO_2 32 mm Hg, PaO_2 78 mm Hg Bicarbonate 19 on 100% non-rebreathing mask.

? Given the information to this point what elements of the review of systems and the physical examination should be added to the list of pertinent positives?

- Oxygen saturation of 96% on 100% nonrebreather
- Respiratory rate 26 breaths per minute with slight sternocleidomastoid use and reports moderate shortness of breath today
- Speaking in short sentences
- Bilateral pulmonary basilar dullness and diminished breath sounds
- Cardiac examination reveals P_2 heart sound accentuation, JVD to 9 cm

- Both legs swollen from ankles to knee on the right and mid-thigh on the left but redness and hyperthermia of left leg only
- Absent lower extremity reflexes but present in upper extremities
- Evidence of maxillary sinus congestion with dullness and tenderness, clear secretions
- Irregular menstrual cycle in sexually active female, with unknown last menses
- Chest x-ray-normal, ECG essentially normal except tachycardia
- Arterial blood gas: partially compensated metabolic acidosis with hypoxemia

---

❓ Which items should be added to the list of significant negatives?

- No leg lesions
- Full range of motion with only edema limitation
- No sensory deficits in legs or feet
- No pain
- Nonproductive cough
- No lymph node engorgement or tympanic membrane abnormalities

---

❓ How does this information affect the list of possible causes?

The review of systems helps narrow down the primary systems involved. I am very concerned about the pulmonary system because she is tachypneic, has distant breath sounds (perhaps due to shallow breathing, atelectasis, or obesity), JVD 9 cm at 45° head of bed elevation, and P_2 increased loudness. Both enhanced P_2 and JVD are consistent with pulmonary hypertension and potentially a pulmonary embolism. Her x-ray, along with physical findings, suggests there is no cardiomyopathy or heart failure, pneumothorax, or pneumonia but technically it was somewhat limited due to her obesity.

The fact that she is only speaking in short sentences and that initial oxygen saturation was 92% on room air and now is 96% on 100% nonrebreather mask (this is the equivalent of a PaO_2 of about 70–75 mm Hg) tells me she is severely compromised. Her ABG reflects a partially compensated metabolic acidosis, which may be a result of hypoxemia and the development of lactic acid. I must quickly evaluate her and take action to ensure she does not have a cardiopulmonary arrest. On percussion I noted some dullness in her bases, which is abnormal but again, her examination is somewhat difficult due to her size. Regardless, it is possible she has some atelectasis or small pleural effusions that I cannot yet detect. I also know that PEs are more prevalent in the lower lobes and can cause local infarctions and atelectasis. I will need to explore these findings with other diagnostics.

Her ECG is normal except for tachycardia, which may be compensatory for hypoxemia. There is an absence of chest pain, diaphoresis, and nausea so cardiac ischemia is less likely the primary cause of her condition. Heart failure is also lower on my differential but I will need additional diagnostics before I rule this out. I move DVT higher on my differential now based on my examination of her lower extremities. I think cellulitis is less likely in the absence of any open sores, and the patient has no history, such as diabetes, which would predispose her to this diagnosis.[1] Musculoskeletal conditions have moved lower on the list since range of motion is only limited by the edema and her movement is pain free.

Given her condition, which is quite serious, I consider DVT with PE highest on my list until I rule them out definitively. Using the Wells criteria for pulmonary embolism, I calculate her risk score as a 9, indicating that she is at high risk of having a PE.[2] Her positive Wells score includes clinical signs and symptoms of DVT, heart rate >100 beats per minute, and immobilization for more 3 days or more. Other potential causes of leg swelling and redness are much lower on my differential and will be explored after I rule out PE which is life threatening.

While the reason for development of a DVT is as yet unclear, a plausible explanation is that her recent illness increased her sedentary lifestyle and resulted in poor fluid intake, both of which may have potentiated the formation of DVTs. But other causes that may result in DVT such as pregnancy or a clotting disorder must be considered as part of Virchow triad (stasis, hypercoagulability acquired with pregnancy, congenital etiology, or injury induced.)[3]

While the chief complaint of the patient upon admission to the ED was leg swelling and redness, her acid-base status and progressive respiratory compromise suggest impending emergency. Further stat diagnostic testing is necessary at this point to evaluate for PE.

❓ What diagnostic testing should be done and in what order?

Spiral computed tomography (CT) with contrast or CT pulmonary angiogram (CTPA) provides visualization of the pulmonary vessels and so is the goal standard for diagnosing a pulmonary embolism. Because I am suspicious that she has bilateral DVTs but unsure if she is pregnant or not, I order a stat human chorionic gonadotropin (hCG) test and a stat bedside Doppler ultrasound of her legs to evaluate for clots. If the hCG is positive, I basically have two choices. I can notify the radiology department of the pregnancy and they may be able to modify the radiation dose somewhat. However, the alternative to CTPA, a ventilation/perfusion (V/Q) scan, poses a greater risk to the fetus, so CTPA would still be my choice of tests. Or I could make the diagnosis of PE based on my index of suspicion (which is very high), and begin treatment, especially if the Doppler study is positive for clot. At this point I order a stat CTPA and will provide the hCG results to radiology. Some institutions also complete a leg CT to evaluate for the presence of thrombi at the same time as the CTPA is done. Other stat labs include repeat arterial blood gas, complete metabolic profile, CBC, coagulation times, and type and cross.

CASE INFORMATION

Diagnostic Testing Results

- hCG: negative
- ABG on FiO_2 1.0 nonrebreather mask

	Results	Normal
pH	7.30	(7.35–7.45)
$PaCO_2$	30 mm Hg	(35–45)
HCO_3	18 mEq/L	(22–26)
PaO_2	75 mm Hg	(>80)
O_{2Sat}	96%	(>98)

- Complete metabolic profile: normal with the exception of a serum carbon dioxide of 18
- CBC with differential: normal, no anemia, white blood cell count and bands within normal limits
- Coagulation times: normal

Imaging studies

- Doppler ultrasound: left femoral vein thrombus, right leg ultrasound negative for thrombus
- CTPA: shows bilateral scattered small pulmonary emboli in both the main pulmonary arteries and the segmental branches

Case Analysis

Her CTPA confirms the diagnosis in this case. While the Doppler study did not show a clot in her right leg, it is possible that the large left femoral clot partially obstructed the right femoral vein, causing edema. It is also possible that a smaller clot was not detected due to technical or mechanical issues related to the difficulty in performing bedside studies in obese patients. I admit the patient to the medical intensive care unit to initiate anticoagulation, provide pulmonary and cardiac support, fluids, and monitor for complications.

Diagnosis and Treatment: Deep Vein Thrombosis and Pulmonary Emboli

According to American College of Chest Physicians (ACCP) guidelines, for antithrombotic and thrombolytic therapy, thrombolytic therapy is recommended if a PE is associated with hypotension. In this case, the patient is not hypotensive, and has no evidence of serious cardiac dysfunction. These findings are associated with a relatively low risk of mortality from PE.[4,5] If the patient is not hypotensive, then low-molecular-weight heparin and cardiac support would be the dominant treatments. Thrombolytics such as tissue plasminogen activator (abbreviated tPA or PLAT) may be necessary if hemodynamic instability ensues. However, the use of thrombolytic agents requires careful risk/benefit analysis because it can lead to uncontrolled bleeding, particularly intracranial bleeding, which is more likely to be fatal than the pulmonary embolism.

In the case of this patient, her DVT is proximal rather than distal and antico-agulants are the standard of care for at least 3 months, assuming bleeding risk is low. For the first few days enoxaparin, dalteparin, tinzaparin, or fondaparinux with rapid onset of anticoagulant action may be given in the acute care setting as the transition to oral warfarin is accomplished. Warfarin's onset of action is 24 hours but does not peak for 72 to 96 hours. Because anticoagulant therapy with warfarin is given for months, home management is appropriate after stabilization. The risk of recurrent PE is significant[6] so prevention education is an essential part of the plan of care.

The patient in this case has both a DVT and a PE, which most likely seeded from her DVT, but DVTs and PEs can also occur independent of each other. DVTs are divided into categories of distal (calf) or proximal (popliteal, femoral, or iliac veins) with proximal associated with highest mortality. Proximal DVTs are more likely to migrate than distal clots. The classic symptoms of DVT include pain, swell-ing, warmth, and discoloration in the affected leg. But these are not always reliably present, and these symptoms do not always predict DVT. In one study, only 17% to 32% of patients with these signs and symptoms had DVTs[4] so further diagnos-tic testing is generally indicated to make the diagnosis. Contrast venography has higher accuracy but greater risk, since the contrast used can actually potentiate the development of a DVT, so noninvasive testing such as ultrasound is preferred. D-dimer is a degradation product of cross-linked fibrin obtained from a blood sam-ple and is sensitive but not specific for DVT so is generally only useful if negative. If the suspicion of DVT is low a D-dimer may be helpful.

DVT formation is attributed to a specific set of conditions occurring simulta-neously and referred to as Virchow triad. The three conditions are venous stasis, hypercoagulability (acquired or congenital), and vessel wall injury.[3] In this case, 3 days of immobility contribute to her venous stasis and this was probably exac-erbated by dehydration. Another potential cause to be considered since her clot occurred in the left leg is May-Thurner syndrome, which is compression of the left common iliac vein by the overlying right common iliac artery. This abnormality is present in 20% of individuals and the risk of recurrent thrombi is high so stenting is warranted after the first DVT.[7]

Conditions that often predispose patients to DVT include pregnancy and cancer. Vascular injury from trauma or invasive procedures should also be consid-ered when taking the health history. However, if a clear source or reason for DVT formation such as pregnancy or cancer is not elucidated, additional coagulation studies and a hematology consultation may be considered to evaluate for a hyper-coagulable state.

Over 90% of acute PEs are from DVTs in the proximal veins of the lower extremities.[8] Air and amniotic fluid are less common causes of PE. Symptoms may be abrupt or progress over time. The classic presentation of PE is pleural chest pain, shortness of breath, and hypoxemia. This patient has both shortness of breath and hypoxemia. Dyspnea is present in only 60% of those who die of PE. However, there are many atypical presentations that are nonspecific. Some examples include hemoptysis, new onset wheezing, chest pain, new cardiac arrhythmias, chest wall tenderness, back pain, shoulder pain, upper abdominal pain, and syncope. Determining pretest probability of PE with the modified Wells scoring system or revised Geneva scoring system before proceeding to diagnostic testing is an evidence-based tool for use in practice.[2] Spiral (helical) CT scan is currently the standard of care. Ventilation perfusion scans are useful if CT is unavailable or contraindicated. Treatment options include anticoagulants, thrombolytics, and, in the most severe and life-threatening cases, embolectomy.

Case Conclusion

The patient in this case had risk factors and symptoms of DVT and PE as well as confirmatory diagnostic tests. Narrowing the differential systematically helped guide the prioritization of diagnostics. Once the diagnosis was confirmed and treatment was initiated, other diagnoses on my patient's differential were quickly eliminated. The patient was started on warfarin following initial use of low-molecular-weight heparin. Once she achieved a therapeutic level, as evidenced by a rise in her international normalized ratio (INR), the patient was discharged home on day 5 with instructions to continue warfarin for 6 months. She was given educational materials, a warfarin prescription, and a follow-up appointment with her primary care provider to have her INR retested in 1 week.

References

1. Keller E, Tomecki KJ, Chadi Iraies M. Distinguishing cellulitis from its mimics. *Cleve Clin J Med.* 2012;79(8):547-552.
2. Well's criteria for pulmonary embolism. MDCalc Web site. http://www.mdcalc.com/wells-criteria-for-pulmonary-embolism-pe/. Accessed December 4, 2014.
3. Fauci AS, Kasper DL. Coagulation disorders. In: Longo DL, Fauci AS, KasperDL, Hauser SL, Jameson JL, Loscanzo J., eds. *Harrison's Principles of Internal Medicine.* 18th ed. New York, NY: McGraw-Hill Co, Inc; 2012:chap 116.
4. Konstantinides S, Torbicki A, Agnelli G, et al. 2014 ESC guidelines on the diagnosis and management of acute pulmonary embolism. *Eur Heart J.* 2014;35(43):3033-3080.
5. Guyatt GH, Akl EA, Crowther M, et al. Executive summary: antithrombotic therapy and prevention of thrombosis, 9th ed: American College of Chest Physicians evidence-based clinical practice guidelines. *Chest.* 2014;141(2 suppl):7s-47s.
6. Barker RC, Marval P. Venous thromboembolism: risks and prevention. *Contin Educ Anaesth Crit Care Pain.* 2011;11(1):18-23.
7. O'Sullivan GJ, Ujiki M, Goodwin AL, Eskandari M, Yao J, Matsumura J. Endovascular management of iliac vein compression (May-Thurner) syndrome. *J Vasc Interv Radiol.* 2000;11(7):823-836.
8. Browse NL, Thomas ML. Sources of non-lethal pulmonary emboli. *Lancet.* 1974;1:258.

CASE 62

Jie Chen

Jie works for the abdominal solid organ transplant service at the University of Virginia Medical Center. She has been working with the abdominal organ transplant patient population since 2006 first as a bedside nurse and then as an NP.

CASE INFORMATION

Chief Complaint

A 65-year-old female who is 2 weeks status post deceased donor liver transplant due to nonalcoholic steatohepatitis (NASH) cirrhosis is transferred to the emergency room (ER) from an acute rehabilitation center for new onset tachycardia and worsening pedal edema. Transplant surgery has been called to evaluate the patient due to her recent transplant history.

❓ What is the potential cause?

Tachycardia is a nonspecific symptom, which can be caused by many underlying conditions. The patient recently had major surgery and thus I immediately consider the potential that her symptoms are related. Some of the etiologies can be life threatening, such as pulmonary embolism (PE), sepsis, bleeding, or myocardial infarction (MI). Meanwhile, others can be quite benign as tachycardia is a normal response to exercise and any conditions in which catecholamine release is physiologically increased. I need to prioritize the list of potential etiologies and quickly determine what interventions are needed. This list will direct me to collect pertinent data in order to sort the potential etiologies efficiently.

Differential Diagnoses for New Onset Tachycardia

- Pulmonary embolism
- Hypotension caused by bleeding or volume depletion
- Sepsis
- Acute coronary syndrome (ACS) or MI
- Medications
- Heart failure
- Anemia
- Anxiety
- Hyperthyroidism

CASE INFORMATION

General Survey and History of Present Illness

When I walk in the patient's room I note she is lying in the bed without apparent distress. She immediately recognizes me as I took care of her for a few days post-liver transplant surgery and I remember her. Her surgery went well without complications. The liver graft function improved as expected. However, she was quite deconditioned at the time of the transplant due to her chronic illness. Once medically stable, postoperatively she was discharged to an acute rehabilitation center in town.

I ask her how she is feeling. She becomes tearful, and says that she felt that she was getting stronger with intensive physical therapy at the rehab center, but then she was told that her heart rate was too fast. She says she did not feel her heart racing at all. She states that she is sad and frustrated that she has to come back to the hospital. She denies fever, chills, palpitations, cough, or chest pain. She endorses slight shortness of breath with exertion but thinks it is because she is still not strong enough. She does notice that both her legs have been swollen and that the swelling has increased but she denies any pain in her calves. When I ask about her operative incision site, she says that the pain is getting better and the incision is healing well.

Review of the medical chart shows her hemoglobin was trending downward from 11.3 to 9.5 g/dL in the days she spent at the rehab center. Her most recent hemoglobin is 8.9 g/dL (normal range 12–15 g/dL). Her heart rate has been ranging between 110 and 130 beats per minute (bpm) since yesterday. Her blood pressure is stable at 110–120/50–60 mmHg and oxygen saturation is 94% to 96% on room air. A bilateral lower extremity ultrasound obtained in the emergency room to rule out DVT is negative. Her last echocardiogram was done prior to the transplant as part of the evaluation was normal with ejection fraction 55% to 60%.

Past Medical History

She denies any heart or lung diseases, denies diabetes. She had echocardiogram done as part of her transplant evaluation and it showed a normal ejection fraction of 55% to 60%.

She reports having blood clots in her left leg when she was in her 40s that were attributed to taking birth control pills.

Medication List

The patient has no known medication allergies. She is on a complicated regimen of oral medications to suppress her immune system and prevent organ rejection. The risk of this therapy is that she will develop opportunistic infection so she takes additional medications as a preventive measure. Her regimen is as follows:

- Immunosuppressant medications include tacrolimus, mycophenolate, and prednisone.
- Anti-infective medications include valganciclovir, trimethoprim/sulfamethoxazole, and nystatin suspension.
- Aspirin 81 mg once a day for prophylaxis.
- Sennosides for constipation.
- Multivitamin as well as calcium with vitamin D and iron, which she took prior to transplant.
- Omeprazole, which she took prior to transplant as well, to prevent gastro-intestinal bleeding.

? What are the pertinent positives from the information given so far?

- Emotional: sad and frustrated
- Liver transplant surgery 2 weeks ago
- Deconditioned with limited mobility
- Slight shortness of breath with exertion
- Bilateral leg swelling without pain
- History of deep vein thrombosis (DVT) 25 years ago while on birth control pills
- Hemoglobin downtrending at the rehab center
- Oxygen saturation of 92% on room air

? What are the significant negatives from the information given so far?

- No apparent distress
- Denies fever, chills, palpitation, cough, or chest pain
- Denies heart or lung diseases
- Normal lower extremity ultrasound on this admission
- Normal echocardiogram prior to transplant
- Stable blood pressure, absence of fever or tachypnea, normal temperature and respiratory rate

❓ Can the information gathered so far be restated in a single sentence highlighting the pieces that narrow down the cause?

The problem representation: a 65-year-old female status post-liver transplant 2 weeks ago with history of DVT who presents with a 2-day history of asymptomatic tachycardia, lower extremity edema, and decreased oxygen saturation levels without evidence of lower extremity DVTs.

❓ How does this information affect the list of potential etiologies?

The absence of chest pain or tachypnea, negative Doppler ultrasound, and relatively stable blood pressure make me think that PE is less likely but it cannot be excluded yet because of her decreased oxygen saturation level. A computed tomography (CT) arteriogram with contrast will be required to definitively rule out PE, if she does not have renal dysfunction. Similarly acute rejection cannot be definitely ruled out without a biopsy. I will alert the transplant surgery team as we may need to progress to this step but first I should gather more data with less invasive means. The patient is asymptomatic with her tachycardia, and she denies chest pain, but she could have an arrhythmia such as atrial fibrillation. In addition, acute coronary syndrome or MI can be silent in women and in the elderly. So I will order a stat ECG, a noninvasive test that will help me prioritize my differential.

In light of her drop in hematocrit, bleeding is a potential cause of tachycardia and remains high on my list. Surgical bleeding is unlikely as the surgery was 2 weeks ago, but gastrointestinal bleeding is a possibility especially as she did resume her daily aspirin. I need more information to confirm or refute that potential cause; I will order serial blood, ask pertinent questions on the review of systems, and check for signs of bleeding on examination.

The absence of fever does not exclude sepsis and transplant patients are at high risk for infection, especially during the early post-transplant period. This is because of immunosuppressant induction therapy, surgery, and hospitalization. Bacterial and candidal wound infections, urinary tract infections, catheter-related infections, bacterial pneumonias, and *Clostridium difficile* colitis are common infections during this period.[1] In addition, transplant patients do not always present with typical signs and symptoms of infection. So infection remains high on my list right now; I will gather more information on the review of systems and physical examination to determine a possible site of infection.

I recognize that the patient is deconditioned due to her chronic illness and recent major surgery, and she may be correct in assuming this is the reason for her dyspnea on exertion. However, fluid balance following liver transplant is also a consideration. Fluid retention and recurrent ascites are common post-liver transplantation particularly in patients who had ascites and edema prior to transplant.[1] While the liver transplant resolves portal hypertension immediately, the rest of the patient's circulatory status takes weeks to equilibrate and normalize. Preoperative circulation in these patients is generally hyper-dynamic, characterized by an increased cardiac output and heart rate and decreased systemic vascular resistance with a resultant low arterial blood pressure. In addition, patients with liver failure are often malnourished. Because of these patients' low albumin stores (related to their nonfunctioning presurgical liver), the intravascular oncotic pressure is decreased. Postsurgical blood volume is often increased causing elevation in the hydrostatic pressure, which moves fluid into the tissues causing "third spacing." Intravascular volume can be low while extravascular fluid is increased and manifested by edema formation especially in dependent parts of the body such as the legs. I need more information to evaluate my patient's fluid balance.

There is no new medication that has been added since discharge. Therefore, the patient's tachycardia is unlikely to be caused by medications. She does take an iron supplement as one of her home medications, but chronic anemia is unlikely the etiology for the new onset tachycardia. The patient appears to be concerned with her readmission and overall health. However, anxiety is unlikely to be the sole responsible underlying condition. In addition, she reports that her pain has improved so I do not believe this is contributing to her high heart rate.

CASE INFORMATION

Review of Systems

- Constitutional: Endorses malaise and fatigue. Denies fever, chills, weight loss, or diaphoresis.
- Cardiovascular: Endorses leg swelling. Denies chest pain, palpitation, orthopnea, or paroxysmal nocturnal dyspnea.
- Pulmonary: Endorses slight shortness of breath on exertion. Denies cough or wheezing.
- Gastrointestinal: Denies nausea, vomiting, abdominal pain, diarrhea, constipation, melena, or bright red blood in stool.
- Genitourinary: Endorses frequency. Denies dysuria, denies hematuria.
- Musculoskeletal: Not pertinent.
- Neurological: Endorses generalized weakness. Denies dizziness, tremor, or headache.
- Endocrine: Denies heat or cold intolerance.

Physical Examination

- Vital signs upon arrival to ER are: Temperature 36.7°C, pulse 110 bpm and regular, blood pressure 114/60 mmHg, respiratory rate 15 breaths per minute, and oxygen saturation 92% on room air.

- General: Well developed. No apparent distress. Tearful.
- Head/eyes/ears/nose/throat: Normocephalic and atraumatic, pupils equal, round, reactive to light, buccal mucosa and oropharynx moist, sclera icterus. Neck supple with normal range of motion. No jugular venous distension present. No thyromegaly present.
- Cardiovascular: Tachycardic with regular rhythm, no murmur, gallops, or rubs, cardiac apex 4/5 intercostal space, midclavicular line, 2+ nonpitting edema to bilateral lower extremities, pulses intact throughout.
- Pulmonary: Respiratory rate and rhythm are normal, no use of accessory muscles, lungs diminished at bases to auscultation, no crackles or wheezes.
- Gastrointestinal: Abdomen distended, firm, normoactive bowel sounds. No tenderness, guarding, or rebound. Recent surgical incision to abdomen intact with staples, healing well. No erythema or drainage noted.
- Skin: No lesions, skin is warm and dry.
- Neurological: No focal neurologic deficits, face symmetric, alert, oriented to person, time, and place, answers questions and follows commands appropriately, moves all extremities.

The ECG shows normal sinus tachycardia, and there is no change when compared to the ECG from pre-transplant surgery 2 weeks ago other than the increase in heart rate.

? **What elements of the review of systems and the physical examination should be added to the list of pertinent positives? Which items should be added to the list of significant negatives?**

Pertinent Positives

- Malaise and fatigue
- Generalized weakness
- Scleral icterus
- Lungs sounds diminished at bases to auscultation
- Lower extremity edema
- Abdomen distended and firm
- Urinary frequency

Significant Negatives

- Afebrile with stable blood pressure
- No orthopnea or paroxysmal nocturnal dyspnea

- No jugular venous distension present
- Regular heart rhythm
- Normal point of maximal impulse
- ECG shows sinus tachycardia and is negative for signs of ischemia
- No crackles or wheezes
- No nausea, vomiting, abdominal pain, diarrhea, constipation, melena, or bright red blood in stool
- No dysuria
- No dizziness, tremor, or headache
- No heat or cold intolerance
- No thyromegaly present
- No signs of infection at the incision site

❓ How does this information affect the list of possible causes?

Given the absence of cardiac symptoms, normal ECG, and normal cardiac examination, heart failure and acute coronary syndrome are less likely to be underlying etiologies for her tachycardia. The patient denies nausea, vomiting, tarry stools, or blood in stools, which makes gastrointestinal bleeding unlikely as the cause of hypovolemia contributing to tachycardia. Sepsis is still on my mind even though her incision is intact and there is no obvious source on her examination. But, as mentioned earlier, the signs and symptoms of infection for transplant patients can be very subtle. While the absence of diarrhea makes *Clostridium difficile* colitis very unlikely, pneumonia, peritonitis, or urinary tract infection are all still possible.

❓ What diagnostic testing should be done and in what order?

I order a complete blood count with differential, basic metabolic panel, hepatic panel, prothrombin time with international normalized ratio (PT/INR), troponin, and thyroid function tests. Two sets of blood cultures drawn percutaneously and urinalysis with reflex culture are also obtained. Chest x-ray is not the most sensitive imaging test for pneumonia but it is part of the initial infection workup, and it will provide additional information about potential pulmonary edema and/or pleural effusions that may be affecting her oxygenation. To evaluate the patient's abdominal distension and hepatic vasculature following transplant, I also order a hepatic Doppler ultrasound. If her distension is due to significant ascites, I may need to proceed with paracentesis to determine if she has peritonitis.

CASE INFORMATION

Results of Diagnostics

CBC With Differential		
White blood cells	12.38	4.0–11.0K/µL
Neutrophils percent	83	40%–60%
Neutrophils absolute	10.27	
Lymphocytes percent	0.0	20%–40%
Lymphocytes absolute	0.00	
Red blood cells	3.04	4.20–5.20M/µL
Hemoglobin	9.4	12.0–16.0g/dL
Hematocrit	29.5	35.0–47.0%
Platelet	141	150–450K/µL
Comprehensive Metabolic Panel		
Na	139	136–145mmol/L
K	4.8	3.4–4.8mmol/L
Cl	105	98–107mmol/L
CO_2	23	22–29mmol/L
BUN	14	9.8–20.1mg/dL
Cr	0.8	0.6–1.1mg/dL
Glucose	94	74–99mg/dL
Glomerular filtration rate	>60	
Total bilirubin	2.0	0.3–1.2mg/dL
Alkaline phosphatase	200	40–150U/L
AST	31	<35U/L
ALT	141	< 55U/L
Protime	10.8	9.8–12.6 seconds
Protime INR	1.0	0.9–1.2
TSH	5.11	0.45–4.5mIU/L
T3 free	1.5	2.3–4.2pg/mL
T3 total	50	58–159ng/dL
T4 free	0.97	0.7–1.5ng/dL
T4 total	4.9	4.9–11.7µg/dL
Troponin	<0.02	<0.02

The chest x-ray (compared to previous post-transplantation x-rays) shows a persistently low lung volume and right basilar discoid atelectasis; improving partial left lower lobe collapse; and pleural spaces within normal limits. Atelectasis is not the cause of her presenting symptoms but I will manage this with an incentive spirometer.

The hepatic Doppler ultrasound shows: postsurgical changes associated with liver transplantation and a new moderate volume ascites. The hepatic Doppler suggests a stenosis at the hepatic transplant arterial anastomosis. This is probably not causing her tachycardia and dyspnea but it does need to be addressed. I consult interventional radiology to perform a hepatic arteriogram to confirm this diagnosis and to determine appropriate treatment. The hepatic arteriogram confirms hepatic artery stenosis, and a stent is placed.

❓ How do the results of the diagnostics affect your list of potential causes?

Her white blood cell count and neutrophils are elevated, which is an indication of infection and her zero lymphocyte count is the result of recent immunosuppression induction therapy. Her hemoglobin is low but stable compared to prior values, so I do not believe she is bleeding and she does not require blood transfusion at this time. Her platelet count is acceptable in the setting of a post-liver transplant. Her mildly elevated thyroid stimulating hormone rules out hyperthyroidism as the cause of her high heart rate. Her serum potassium level is slightly elevated but with normal kidney function as demonstrated by normal blood urea nitrogen (BUN) and creatinine levels, her hyperkalemia is not worrisome at this level and is likely caused by medications such as tacrolimus.

Reviewing the patient's liver function, I find a concerning trend. While her total bilirubin and liver enzymes were trending downward following her transplantation, her bilirubin has now increased to 2.0 from the last value of 1.5. Her urinalysis also shows the presence of bilirubin. In addition, her alkaline phosphatase of 200 is elevated compared to 117 at last check. AST level is normal and ALT is elevated, but down to 141 compared to the last check at 154. The rising total bilirubin and alkaline phosphatase could be due to the hepatic arterial stenosis seen on ultrasound but rejection and bile leak are also important considerations with these lab results. Rejection is less likely in the setting of adequate immunosuppressive therapy; however, I cannot completely rule this out without a liver biopsy. Early bile leaks (4 weeks from transplant) may be caused by ischemia and technique issues[2] and require immediate intervention to prevent progression to sepsis.

Because the patient has a moderate amount of ascites on ultrasound, I order a paracentesis so I can further test for a bile leak as well as infection and decide further treatment. The paracentesis yields 6360 mL of tea-colored fluid and I send samples for bilirubin and culture. Ascites fluid bilirubin is 31.3, which is much higher than the serum level, and her fluid culture Gram stain is negative with culture pending.

Diagnosis and Treatment: Sepsis due to Bile Leak

At this point, the diagnosis of sepsis due to bile leak as a source of infection is confirmed by the presence of ascites fluid with a bilirubin of 31.3, tachycardia, leukocytosis, and low oxygen saturation level. According to the American Association for the Study of Liver Diseases Cirrhosis Management Guidelines, 50 g (6–8 g/L) 25% albumin needs to be given to replete the amount of ascites fluid removed in order to prevent acute kidney injury due to volume loss.[3] Additional volume will also be necessary. Normal saline or 5% albumin is generally used with albumin specifically selected if third spacing is an issue. Broad-spectrum antibiotics are initiated immediately.[4] Piperacillin-tazobactam is a common choice of antibiotic for intra-abdominal or biliary tract infections if the patient does not have allergy to penicillin. If allergic to the β-lactams, the combination of cefepime and metronidazole can be used. Bile leak can be treated with endoscopic retrograde cholangiopancreatography (ERCP) with biliary stenting.[1,5]

The patient undergoes ERCP with a stent placed at the biliary anastomosis where the leak occurred. She completes a 7-day course of piperacillin-tazobactam and her final ascites fluid culture was negative. Her tachycardia resolved as did her leg edema, and she was discharged back to the rehab center.

References

1. Eghtesad B, Miller CM, Fung JJ. Post-liver transplant management. Cleveland Clinic Center for Continue Education. http://www.clevelandclinicmeded.com/medicalpubs/diseasemanagement/hepatology/post-liver-transplantation-management/. Published August 1, 2012. Accessed November 6, 2014.
2. Ayoub WS, Esquivel CO, Martin P. Biliary complications following liver transplant. *Dig Dis Sci.* 2010;55:1540-1546. doi: 10.1007/s10620-010-1217-2.
3. Runyon BA. Management of adult patients with ascites due to cirrhosis: update 2012. AASLD practice Guideline. doi: 10.1002/hep.00000.
4. Azar R, Jonnalagadda SS. Severe and complicated biliary tract disease. In: Irwin RS, Rippe JM, eds. *Irwin and Rippe's Intensive Care Medicine*. Philadelphia, PA: Lippincott Williams & Wilkins; 2008.
5. Ostroff JW. Management of biliary complications in the liver transplant patient. *Gastroenterol Hepatol*. April 2010;6(4):264-272.

CASE 63

Steven W. Branham and Tara C. Hilliard

Steve Branham is an Assistant Professor in the ACNP Program at Texas Tech University and serves as adjunct faculty at Texas Woman's University. Dr Branham maintains an active clinical practice focused on critical and emergency care. Tara C. Hilliard is an Assistant Professor at Texas Tech University Health Sciences Center School of Nursing.

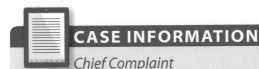

CASE INFORMATION

Chief Complaint

MW is a 55-year-old female who is admitted to the emergency room after "passing out for about 6 minutes."

❓ What is the potential cause?

In a case such as this with life-threating implications, I need to act promptly. Because her loss of consciousness may represent a life-threatening condition, I must quickly evaluate the patient while simultaneously providing initial stabilization and resuscitation measures as necessary. I start by developing a system-focused differential for syncope, defined as "a transient loss of consciousness and postural tone, characterized by a rapid onset, lasting for a short duration, and with a spontaneous recovery."[1]

Differential Diagnoses for Syncope[1]

Neurologic
- Intracerebral bleed
- Vertebrobasilar stroke
- Migraine
- Seizure

Pulmonary
- Severe pneumonia
- Pneumothorax
- Pulmonary embolism

Cardiovascular
- Myocardial infarction
- Aneurysm rupture, both thoracic and abdominal
- Ventricular arrhythmia
- Sinus node dysfunction
- Long QT syndrome
- Atrioventricular block

- Cardiac tamponade
- Volume depletion
- Aortic stenosis
- Mitral stenosis
- Cardiogenic shock
- Orthostatic hypotension

Gastrointestinal
- Acute abdominal pathology or bowel perforation
- Gastrointestinal bleeding

Genitourinary
- Urosepsis

Metabolic dysfunction states
- Diabetic ketoacidosis (DKA)
- Hyperglycemic hyperosmolar nonketotic coma (HHNC)
- Hypoglycemia
- Distributive shock states such as sepsis

Iatrogenic or self-inflicted causes
- Excessive blood pressure medication dosing or accidental overdose
- Drug overdose

Armed with a list of "most common and likely causes" I need to narrow the list and establish evaluation and treatment priorities. Some diagnoses on the differential list such as cerebral bleed and myocardial infarction are potentially life threatening and require evaluation before I move to less critical diagnoses. To that end, my initial steps include a rapid survey of the patient in the emergency room, including vital signs, history of this illness and any associated symptoms, and a focused physical examination. Based on these findings I will be able to move quickly through my differential list to isolate the etiology of the patient's symptoms and consider initial treatment, prioritize diagnostic testing, and review treatment options.

CASE INFORMATION

History of Present Illness

MW is a professor at a local community college and during her early morning class, her students reported that she "passed out" and they could not awaken her for about 6 minutes. A nursing student in the class detected a weak pulse and said that MW's breathing was "rapid and shallow." She awakened slowly but was lethargic and too weak to get up. Emergency medical service was called, an ECG in the field showed sinus tachycardia, and the rest of her vital signs revealed mild hypotension and tachypnea. They brought her to the local emergency department for further evaluation and treatment. In transit, oxygen was started and a peripheral intravenous access was established.

I arrive at the patient's bedside in the emergency room and she is awake but drowsy, able to speak clearly, with symmetric facial expressions. She is in mild respiratory distress and complains of pain in her right buttock that has been present for approximately 5 days. She rates the pain in her right buttock as an "8" on a scale of 0 to 10. Three days prior to her syncopal episode she reports having fever, chills, and sweats. The following day, she awoke with rigors. She thought she might have the flu. Additional symptoms included a general malaise, loss of appetite, nausea, and "dry heaves." She tells me "today I feel so bad, I think I am going to die." The ED nurse has already obtained a set of vital signs for me to review.

Vital Signs

- BP 90/50 mm Hg supine and 80/40 mm Hg with head of bed at 45°
- Pulse 125 beats per minute, RR 28/min, and labored with four- to five-word dyspnea
- Temperature 102.6°F orally
- Height: 5 ft 3 in
- Weight 226 lb, BMI 39.5
- Pulse oximetry: 90% on 100% nonrebreather mask

Case Analysis

I see that MW is febrile, hypotensive, and tachycardic, and that she has an extremely painful right buttock. At this point, the most likely cause of her presentation with syncope is an infectious process. While I need more information to rule out the other diagnoses, including the cardiovascular and pulmonary disorders that can cause syncope, I also know that these are less common conditions. Her rapid recovery to normal neurological status makes it very unlikely that her syncope is due to a stroke and her ECG findings make cardiac arrhythmia, such as prolonged QT, less likely. I need to gather more history to exclude some of the other diagnoses such as DKA and drug overdose. Based on her vital signs alone, however, I can diagnose systemic inflammatory response syndrome, which, when occurring in conjunction with a source of infection, supports the diagnosis of sepsis[2] (see Table 63-1). When evaluating a patient with signs of sepsis, the focus of the history and physical is to determine likely sources of infection. Given the report of pain in her right buttock, I am thinking that this is the source and will investigate this further in my history and physical examination.

Table 63-1   Sepsis Markers

General Variables	Organ Dysfunction Variables	Inflammatory Variables	Tissue Perfusion Variables	Hemodynamic Variables
Fever (>38.3°C)	Arterial hypoxemia (PaO_2/FiO_2 <300)	Leukocytosis (WBC count >12,000 cells/μL)	Hyperlactatemia (>1 mmol/L)	Arterial hypotension (SBP <90 mm Hg, MAP <70 mm Hg, or an SBP decrease >40 mm Hg in adults or less than two SD below normal for age)
Hypothermia (core temperature <36°C)	Acute oliguria (urine output <0.5 mL/kg/h for at least 2 h despite adequate fluid resuscitation)	Leukopenia (WBC count <4000 cells/μL)	Decreased capillary refill or mottling	
Heart rate >90/beats/min[1] or more than two SD above the normal value for age	Creatinine increase >0.5 mg/dL or 44.2 μmol/L	Normal WBC count with greater than 10% immature forms		
Tachypnea	Coagulation abnormalities (INR >1.5 or aPTT >60 s)	Plasma C-reactive protein more than two standard deviations above the normal value		
Altered mental status	Ileus (absent bowel sounds)	Plasma procalcitonin more than two standard deviations above the normal value		
Significant edema or positive fluid balance (>20 mL/kg over 24 h)	Thrombocytopenia (platelet count <100,000 cells/μL)			

General Variables	Organ Dysfunction Variables	Inflammatory Variables	Tissue Perfusion Variables	Hemodynamic Variables
Hyperglycemia (plasma glucose >140 mg/dL or 7.7 mmol/L) in the absence of diabetes	Hyperbilirubinemia (plasma total bilirubin >4 mg/dL or 70 μmol/L)			

Severe sepsis definition = sepsis-induced tissue hypoperfusion or organ dysfunction (any of the following thought to be due to the infection):
  Sepsis-induced hypotension
  Lactate above upper limits of laboratory normal
  Urine output <0.5 mL/kg/h for more than 2 hours despite adequate fluid resuscitation
  Acute lung injury with PaO_2/FiO_2 <250 in the absence of pneumonia as infection source
  Acute lung injury with PaO_2/FiO_2 <200 in the presence of pneumonia as infection source
  Creatinine >2.0 mg/dL (176.8 μmol/L)
  Bilirubin >2 mg/dL (34.2 μmol/L)
  Platelet count <100,000 cells/μL
  Coagulopathy (international normalized ratio >1.5)
Data from Dellinger RP, Levy MM, Rhodes A, et al. Surviving sepsis campaign: international guidelines for management of severe sepsis and septic shock: 2012. *Crit Care Med.* 2013;41(2):580–637.

CASE INFORMATION

History and Physical Examination

Appears generally ill, disoriented to date. Because the patient is groggy, her husband, who is at her bedside, provides most data. Additional history is obtained from the electronic health record.

Past Medical History

- Hypertension
- Type 2 diabetes mellitus
- Dyslipidemia
- Obesity
- Seasonal allergies
- History of pancreatitis when taking eventide (Byetta) (this is a protein that is injected to help the pancreas release insulin)
- DKA in the past year which required a 24-hour intensive care unit and 2-day hospital stay
- In the past year she was twice treated for cutaneous abscesses, which cultured positive for methicillin-resistant *Staphylococcus aureus* (MRSA)

Immunizations

- Tetanus current
- Flu shot current, no pneumonia vaccine

Past Surgical History
- Noncontributory

Social History
- Married for 27 years, two children in good health
- Tobacco: current smoker, smokes 1 pack per day × 45 years
- Alcohol: states she and her husband usually have wine each night
- Drug use: negative illicit drug use

Family History
- Father died at age 68 of myocardial infarction.
- Mother is alive and resides in a nursing home and has advanced Alzheimer disease and breast cancer.
- Brother age 53 has bipolar disorder and type 2 diabetes mellitus.
- Sisters age 48 and 51 are both in good health.
- No known drug allergies.

Current Medications
- Metformin 1000 mg twice a day
- Lisinopril 5 mg once a day
- Metoprolol, extended release 50 mg once a day
- Fenofibrate 145 mg once a day
- Hydrochlorothiazide 50 mg once a day
- Pioglitazone 30 mg once a day
- Insulin glargine 10 units SQ twice a day
- Loratadine/pseudoephedrine one once a day
- Azelastine two puffs each nostril at bedtime
- Acetaminophen as needed for pain

Review of Systems
- Constitutional: Fever, chills, sweats, weakness, fatigue × 3 days and has had no recent sick contacts or travel.
- Head/eyes/ears/nose/throat: Denies vision or hearing loss, earaches, tooth aches, recent sinus conditions, or thrush.
- Cardiovascular: Denies chest pain, positive recent syncope but denies previous similar episodes. No history of myocardial infarction or heart failure.
- Pulmonary: Positive for shortness of breath, and denies history of respiratory infections, denies snoring, daytime somnolence, or morning headaches (ie, signs of sleep apnea).

- Gastrointestinal: Nausea for the past 3 days with vomiting, twice in the last 6 hours, now with dry heaves.
- Genitourinary: Has only urinated once in past 24 hours, denies burning, denies hematuria.
- Musculoskeletal: Increasing pain to right buttock area, cannot lie on affected area
- Endocrine: No appetite.
- Neurologic: Recent mental status changes, groggy, disoriented to date, no seizures or recent reported headaches.
- Psychiatric: No history of suicidal ideations or depression.
- Lymphatics: Denies any nodes.

Physical Examination

- Vital signs and constitutional (as previously described).
- Head/eyes/ears/nose/throat: Oral mucosa dry. Tongue furrowed. Lips cracked. Pupils are 3 mm with brisk response to light, ear examination shows tympanic membranes with distinct light reflex, no erythema. Neck is supple and there are no noted masses or swelling on palpation.
- Cardiovascular: Tachycardia, S1, S2 without noted murmur, rub, or gallop.
- Pulmonary: Noted tachypnea, increased work of breathing, on auscultation crackles throughout all lung fields, no wheezing.
- Gastrointestinal: Obese, hypoactive bowel sounds in all quadrants. On palpation, nontender, no masses or organ enlargement. Rectal examination diffusely tender and painful so entire digital vault examination could not be performed.
- Genitourinary: External examination grossly normal and total pelvic examination deferred due to the patient's condition.
- Musculoskeletal. No gross deformity or extremity edema. Pulses in feet are +1. Limb strength is grossly 5/5.
- Integumentary: 5 cm area of severe erythema with edema and fluctuance in right buttock area. Streaking noted extending to rectum 6 cm in length. The area is warm and tender to touch.
- Neurological: Lethargic, responsive to verbal stimulation, oriented to person, place, and time. Cranial nerves II-XII grossly intact.
- Lymphatics: Unable to appreciate nodes due to body habitus with the exception of bilateral femoral node tenderness.

Case Analysis

The history and physical both support a diagnosis of sepsis. When evaluating these findings it is important to determine the relationship of abnormal organ system findings to the diagnosis of sepsis. Finding the source of the sepsis is essential. Many of the potential diagnoses on my initial list seem less likely as the case for sepsis seems more compelling. A brief review of the further positive and negative findings will guide the next stage of evaluation, the ordering of diagnostic tests.

❓ What are the pertinent positives and significant negatives obtained in the information collected so far?

Pertinent Positives

At this point, MW has a toxic appearance with fever and chills.

- Her history of diabetes and recent admission for DKA indicate that her blood sugar is not well controlled predisposing her to infection.

- The recent history of MRSA infections is also an ominous indicator of potential risk as well as a suspected pathogen.

- Her tachypnea and hypoxia reflect respiratory system compromise, suggesting that if her pulmonary system is not the primary source of her sepsis, it is definitely suffering secondary damage.

- Her furrowed tongue most like indicates volume system compromise.

- The noted neurologic dysfunction, abdominal pain, and decreased urine output could be a sign of primary site of infection or a site of secondary insult related to sepsis.

- The most important finding is the abscess area on her right buttock, indicating a focal source of infection, which could seed systemically, leading to sepsis.

Significant Negatives

- Neurologic dysfunction that seems to be improving makes intracerebral pathology a less likely cause of the current events but cannot be fully excluded without further evaluation.

- Cardiac indicators of tachycardia may simply be an indication of systemic compensatory mechanisms and not the true source of the problem.

- A relatively normal abdominal examination serves as a strong indicator that abdominal pathology is probably not the primary source of her infection.

- Her relatively normal physiological profile helps further narrow down suspicions.

The next stage is to progress to testing which will further hone the potential causes of this patient's syncope and systemic inflammatory response syndrome.

❓ What diagnostic tests are needed and in what order?

The patient's positive history and physical findings suggest a serious infection in her buttock, and her vital signs demonstrate hypotension and orthostasis. These key findings support the diagnosis of severe sepsis. However, other causes must stay on my differential for now. I order the following diagnostics to determine the status of her critical illness, other potential sources of infection, and so that I can initiate essential therapies to prevent organ failure and death.

These include stat: complete blood count (CBC) with differential, metabolic panel, serum osmolality, and cardiac enzymes. I also order a PT and PTT, D-dimer, lactic acid, arterial blood gas, urinalysis, urine drug screen, and blood cultures. These tests will help determine the gravity of her infection and evaluate the potential secondary effect of sepsis on her end organs.[3]

Other diagnostics: Chest x-ray, ECG, and a stat computed tomography (CT) of the head without contrast to rule out cerebral bleed.[2]

Simultaneous to ordering these diagnostics I start intravenous fluids (0.9% NS) at 200 mL/hour.

CASE INFORMATION

Results of Diagnostics

- ECG: Sinus tachycardia 128 without ST elevation or depression. Axis is normal.
- Chest x-ray: Patchy confluent alveolar infiltrates bilaterally with slight elevation of the right hemidiaphragm consistent with volume loss.
- Head CT: Negative for intracranial bleed or gross pathology

Labs

CBC		
	Result	Reference range
White blood cell count	25.3	(4.5–11.0 cells/µL)
Red blood cell count	5.43	(4.40–6.00 cells/µL)
Hemoglobin	14.5	(14.0–18.0 g/dL)
Hematocrit	44.3	(41.0%–51.0%)
MCV	85.2	(82.0–100.0 fL)
MCH	29.3	(27.0–34.0 pg)
MCHC	33.1	(31.0–37.0 g/dL)
Platelets	375	(150–400 K/µL)
Bands	28	(0%–8%)
Neutrophils	92	(44%–88%)
Lymphocytes	34	(12%–43%)
Monocytes	2	(2%–11%)

Complete Metabolic Panel		
	Result	Reference range
Sodium	125	(135–145 mEq/L)
Potassium	5.5	(3.5–5.0 mEq/L)
Chloride	89	(99–109 mEq/L)
CO_2	22	(24–31 mEq/L)
BUN	55	(8–24 mg/dL)
Creatinine	1.5	(0.5–1.5 mg/dL)
Glucose	340	(65–110 mg/dL)
Protein	7.5	(6.3–8.2 g/dL)
Albumin	3.0	(3.5–5.0 g/dL)
Total bilirubin	0.7	(0.2–1.2 mg/dL)
Alk phosphatase	112	(30–115 U/L)
AST (SGOT)	15	(15–46 U/L)
ALT (SGPT)	27	(10–55 U/L)
Serum osmolality	305	(280–300)
Lactic acid	10.4	(≥4 mmol/L)
PT/PTT		Normal limits
Cardiac enzymes		Normal limits
D-dimer	2.2	<5
ABG Drawn on 100% Nonrebreather Mask		
	Result	Reference range
pH	7.28	pH 7.35–7.45
$PaCO_2$	32	$PaCO_2$ 35–45 mmHg
PaO_2	55	HCO_3 22–26 mEq/L
HCO_3	29	PaO_2 >80 mmHg
Oxygen saturation	88%	O_{2Sat} 96% (>98)
BE	−4	
Urinalysis		
Specific gravity	1.030	
Glucose	Trace	
Ketones	Negative	
RBCs	1	
WBCs	0	
Leukoesterase	Negative	
Urine drug screen	Negative	

Case Analysis

The patient's lab results further confirm my diagnosis of infection and probable sepsis. The complete blood count shows an elevated white blood cell count, with 25.3 total white blood cells, and a left shift, which refers to the elevated percent of white blood cells that are bands, or immature white blood cells, released too early in response to overwhelming infection. With a suspected site of infection, leukocytosis with bandemia confirms a bacterial cause of sepsis. Given the history of two MRSA infections in the last year, I am concerned about MRSA as the possible causative organism. While her lab work confirms my findings on examination that the patient has sepsis, I cannot rule out diabetic ketoacidosis (DKA) because DKA frequently presents concurrently in diabetic patients with sepsis and her serum glucose is very high.

Based on the results of diagnostic testing, I can quickly rule out many of the other differential diagnoses on my list. With a normal CT scan I am comfortable ruling out intracerebral bleed as a cause of her syncopal episode. A thrombotic stroke is still possible but seems less likely as her neurologic status is improving and other examination findings do not support a stroke.

Her chest x-ray does not show pneumonia or pneumothorax although it does show evidence of patchy bilateral alveolar filling infiltrates that are seriously affecting her oxygenation. Her negative D-dimer, for now, puts pulmonary embolism as the cause of her hypoxia very low on the differential. At this point I am comfortable ruling out thoracic aneurysm rupture as there is no sign of "widening mediastinum" or severe chest pain which would have supported that diagnosis. There is no history of chest pain and her cardiac enzymes and ECG do not show any sign of ischemia, so myocardial infarction is excluded. Her abdominal examination was unremarkable and coupled with the fact that she has no complaints of abdominal pain, perforation and abdominal aneurysm are unlikely. Her serum glucose of 340 and negative urine ketones suggest she does not have DKA; instead, the high glucose may be due to dehydration. It is not high enough to suggest hyperosmolar hyperglycemic state (HHS), as this typically occurs with glucose levels closer to 1000. Her urinalysis is negative for white blood cells and leukoesterase and this rules out sepsis of urinary origin. Coupled with a no history of suicidal ideations and negative drug screen, drug overdose is no longer a concern. Iatrogenic overdose on blood pressure medications is simply ruled out as overwhelming evidence supports a more likely etiology of her critical illness.

At this point I am comfortable with the following diagnoses:

I. Severe sepsis with distributive shock secondary to gluteal abscess, which may have perirectal tunneling, based on the examination. I highly suspect it is due to MRSA given her treatment in the past year for two confirmed MRSA infections. Her history of diabetes further predisposes her to infections. Her case is compelling for severe sepsis as she has hypotension, elevated lactate level (10.4), acute lung injury, and decreased urine output as she has voided only once in 24 hours. Each one of these factors alone raises the level of sepsis to severe sepsis.[2]

Table 63-2   Berlin Criteria of ARDS

Presentation	PaO$_2$/FiO$_2$ Ratio	Classification
Lung injury/acute onset, within 1 week of clinical insult and with progression of respiratory symptoms	201–300 mm Hg (≤39.9 kPa)	Mild
Bilateral opacities on chest imaging not explained by other pulmonary pathology	101–200 mm Hg (≤26.6 kPa)	Moderate
Respiratory failure not explained by volume overload or heart failure	≤100 mm Hg (≤13.3 kPa)	Severe

Data from Ferguson ND, Fan E, Camporota L, et al. The Berlin definition of ARDS: an expanded rationale, justification, and supplementary material. *Intensive Care Med.* 2012;38(10):1573-1582.

II. Hypoxic respiratory failure related to severe sepsis. The acute onset of respiratory failure without a known pulmonary cause and refractory hypoxemia of a PaO$_2$ of 55 on 100% oxygen correlates with a P/F ratio of 55. She has adult respiratory distress syndrome (ARDS) and based on the Berlin criterion, this PF ratio stratifies the severity of the ARDS to "severe ARDS"[3,4] (see Table 63-2).

III. Metabolic acidosis due to severe sepsis. This is confirmed both by the arterial blood gas, which show acidosis (pH of 7.28), PaCO$_2$ of 32, which indicates partial respiratory compensation, and a base deficit of −4 indicating that she has a metabolic acidosis and that all hydrogen ions present in the blood are not offset by available bicarbonate. The elevated lactate level further confirms a metabolic acidosis.

IV. Hyperglycemia with a history of type 2 diabetes. This may be secondary to dehydration and may respond simply to fluid resuscitation.

V. Stage II chronic kidney disease (CKD) based on borderline creatinine elevations. Given her long history of diabetes this is highly likely and as noted may be an acute on chronic insult from dehydration. This will need to be assessed closely as volume status is restored.

VI. Electrolyte derangement due to severe sepsis and distributive shock,

(a) Her serum sodium is measured 125 mmol/L, which, when corrected for her glucose of 340, gives her sodium level 129 mmol/L, indicating hyponatremia. This is an unusual finding as normally in hypovolemic states the sodium level is high. It may be that her low sodium represents renal sodium loss from early acute tubular necrosis (ATN), which is also suggested by her high BUN and high/normal creatinine. The sodium level may also be affected by her medications. Specifically, angiotensin-converting enzyme inhibitors, such as lisinopril, can cause a low sodium. But having only one set of labs to evaluate, I cannot determine if the low sodium is chronic in nature or an acute on chronic insult. Further evaluation is needed once volume status is fully restored and urine output further evaluated.

(b) Hyperkalemia related to severe sepsis and volume contraction (serum K^+ of 5.5). I feel that this is not a true increase in total body potassium and should be rechecked once volume status is restored.

Management of Sepsis and Severe Sepsis

Initial management of sepsis includes aggressive fluid resuscitation, blood cultures (prior to antibiotics), serum lactate level, placement of a central line to assess volume status, and urinary catheter to assess urine output. Fluid resuscitation is accomplished with crystalloids such as normal saline, via a peripheral IV until a central line in placed. Once a central line is in place, additional information about the patient's volume status can be obtained by transducing a central venous pressure (CVP). Once CVP monitoring is established, fluids are administered with a target CVP of 8 to 12 mm Hg. Empiric antibiotic coverage is initiated within an hour of drawing blood cultures. Given the patient's recent history of MRSA infections, targeted antibiotic therapy will include vancomycin 1 g every 8 hours, with further dosing based on levels and the patient's renal function. Given that the suspected source of infection is a gluteal abscess with possible perirectal extension, additional coverage for gram-negative organisms including pseudomonas is appropriate. Dual coverage includes a β-lactam and an aminoglycoside or pseudomonal active fluroquinolone.[2]

The patient's respiratory failure due to ARDS secondary to sepsis requires aggressive management. Prompt measures to reduce hypoxia include positive end expiratory pressure to increase alveolar recruitment. This can be accomplished with continuous positive airway pressure (CPAP) for noninvasive ventilation or positive end-expiratory pressure (PEEP) when intubated and placed on mechanical ventilation. A brief trial of BiPAP may be tried, but given this patient's critical condition, I think intubation and mechanical ventilation is the preferred and most prudent strategy until she is stabilized. Intubation and mechanical ventilation offer the added benefit of significantly reducing the work of breathing that is contributing to the patient's underlying catabolic state, a hallmark of sepsis.

In addition to the initial treatment for sepsis, prompt surgical consult is needed to evaluate the abscess area for surgical drainage and debridement and to determine the need for additional imaging studies. The patient is transferred to the ICU for close monitoring, including continuous cardiac and pulse oximetry monitoring, frequent vital signs, and repeat arterial blood gases, blood counts, and comprehensive metabolic panels to evaluate her response to interventions. Her home medications will be held until she is more stable. She will be started on intravenous insulin with blood glucose checks done hourly and the infusion titrated to maintain blood glucose below 160.[5]

Case Follow-Up

MW had a rocky hospital course. She was taken to the operating room a total of three times for surgical debridement. During her ICU stay she required vasopressors, mechanical ventilation, and enteral feedings. A tracheostomy was placed after 10 days as she was not weaning from the ventilator as anticipated. A month later she was transferred to a long-term acute hospital for ventilator weaning, ongoing antibiotics, and aggressive physical therapy and rehabilitation. Three months after her initial admission to the acute care hospital, she was discharged to home. Her total recovery took about 9 months at which point she was able to return to work and normal activity.

References

1. Syncope evaluation. Epocrates Web site. https://online.epocrates.com/noFrame/showPage?method=diseases&MonographId=248&ActiveSectionId=11. Updated July 4, 2014. Accessed December 5, 2014.
2. Dellinger RP, Levy MM, Rhodes A, et al. Surviving sepsis campaign: international guidelines for management of severe sepsis and septic shock: 2012. *Crit Care Med*. 2013;41(2):580-637. doi: 10.1097/CCM.0b013e31827e83af.
3. Dries DJ. *Fundamental Critical Care Support*. 5th ed. Mount Prospect, IL: Society of Critical Care Medicine; 2012.
4. Ferguson ND, Fan E, Camporota L, et al. The Berlin definition of ARDS: an expanded rationale, justification, and supplementary material. *Intensive Care Med*. 2012;38(10):1573-1582.
5. Gielen M, Vlasselaers D, Van den Berghe G. Glucose in the ICU—evidence, guidelines, and outcomes. *N Engl J Med*. September 27, 2012;367(13):1208-1219, 1259-1260. *N Engl J Med*. 2012;367(25):2451. doi: 10.1056/NEJMc12129.

CASE 64

Sarah A. Delgado

Sarah A. Delgado is an acute nurse practitioner, currently working for the American Association of Critical-Care Nurses as a clinical practice specialist. She has over 10 years experience in advanced nursing practice, focusing on the management of adults with chronic diseases. In the past, she taught acute care graduate and undergraduate nursing students at the University of Virginia, and developed a chronic disease management program at an integrated delivery system in Whittier, California.

CASE INFORMATION

Chief Complaint

A 70-year-old-male comes to a follow-up appointment in a chronic disease management clinic with a complaint of severe left wrist pain that kept him up all night.

? What is the potential cause?

Pain in a single joint immediately brings to mind trauma, so some of the first questions I ask will be about recent activity and any falls. There are other causes to consider, however, and I will need to keep these in mind as I proceed in gathering more information from my patient.

Comprehensive Differential Diagnoses for Patient With Left Wrist Pain

- Trauma causing fracture or sprain
- Septic arthritis
- Gout or pseudogout
- Tenosynovitis
- Osteoarthritis
- Psoriatic arthritis
- Rheumatoid arthritis
- Hemarthrosis
- Renal osteodystrophy
- Calcific periarthritis
- Overuse injury

CASE INFORMATION

History of Present Illness

The patient who has chronic kidney disease (CKD) and congestive heart failure (CHF) came to clinic with his son but he prefers to come into the examination room alone and he is able to give his own history. He reports his left wrist started hurting 3 days ago; he first noticed it while reaching to take dishes out of a cabinet. It gradually worsened and yesterday he noticed redness and swelling on the front of his wrist extending to the area distal to his thumb. He holds his wrist out to demonstrate the area of concern. When I touch it lightly he winces and I notice that the red skin is also very warm.

He denies any falls, trauma, or change in activity. He has mostly been taking it easy since his recent hospital stay (described later) and is not even sitting at his computer much. Because the pain is exacerbated by any activity, he has avoided using his left hand. He is not aware of ever having symptoms like this before in his wrist or any other joint, and he has no pain anywhere else other than his usual back pain, which he has "learned to ignore."

Last night the pain was so bad that he took a hydrocodone-acetaminophen tablet from an old prescription prior to going to bed. In spite of this, he woke up twice in the night because of the pain and ended up taking two more pills, without noticing much improvement. He was surprised this did not help because in the past, hydrocodone-acetaminophen made him really groggy so he thought it was a strong medication. He was really frightened this morning by the severity of his pain and considered going to the emergency room but then he saw on his calendar that he had this appointment scheduled.

This is the patient's second appointment in the chronic disease clinic; his initial appointment was 2 weeks ago, and occurred 3 days after discharge from the hospital. He was admitted for small bowel obstruction but his hospital stay was complicated by CHF exacerbation, treated with diuresis leading to worsening renal function. He then developed nosocomial pneumonia, which required 14 days of intravenous (IV) antibiotics. At his insistence, the hospital team arranged for the last 4 days of IV antibiotics to be given at home with a home health service through a midline catheter. His total length of stay, because of the complications, was 21 days. He stated on his initial visit to this clinic that if "I never go to the hospital again, it will be too soon."

Past Medical History (From Hospital Record and From His Initial Visit to This Clinic)

- Systolic heart failure, echocardiogram on recent admission showed ejection fraction of 35%
- Chronic kidney disease, stage 3, his baseline creatinine is 1.7 mg/dL, with a glomerular filtration rate of 40 mL/min/1.73 m^2
- Coronary artery disease, underwent angioplasty 8 years ago
- Chronic low back pain with degenerative joint disease of lumbar spine
- Protein calorie malnutrition worsening in the last month
- Anemia of chronic disease

- Osteoarthritis
- Small bowel obstruction: managed conservatively on recent hospital stay
- Nosocomial pneumonia treated with 14 days of IV cefepime
- Denies any history of diabetes, cancer, gout, rheumatoid arthritis, psoriasis, or other autoimmune disorders

Past Surgical History

- Right total knee arthroplasty 10 years ago for osteoarthritis
- Partial colectomy for recurrent diverticulitis 7 years ago
- Hernia repair 6 years ago
- Cataract removal 1 year ago

Family and Social History

- His father died of myocardial infarction in his 70s and his mother died at age 92, "she didn't need a reason." Not aware of any family history of rheumatoid arthritis or other autoimmune disorders.
- Used to drink two to three glasses of wine a day but he gave this up after his colectomy 7 years ago.
- Smoked a couple of cigarettes a day for a few years as a teenager but "it didn't really stick with me."
- He lives alone, but his son lives only a few minutes away and helps him with errands and rides to doctor appointments. Otherwise, he cares for himself independently.

CASE INFORMATION

Medications

- Aspirin 81 mg oral tablet once daily
- Calcitrol 0.5 µg oral tablet once a day
- Centrum silver oral tablet once a day
- Ferrous sulfate 324 mg once a day
- Metamucil one packet mixed with 8 ounces of water once a day
- Ondansetron 4 mg every 8 hours as needed for nausea
- Hydrocodone-acetaminophen 7.5/325 mg one tablet three times a day as needed for back pain

Allergies

The patient has no known drug allergies but was told not to take any over-the-counter medications other than acetaminophen (Tylenol) because of his kidney function, and his nephrologist discontinued his angiotensin-converting enzyme inhibitor because of hyperkalemia.

❓ What are the pertinent positives from the information given so far?

- Severe left wrist pain for 3 days that interfered with sleeping
- Pain had a sudden onset and is worsened by movement
- Redness and swelling of left wrist for the past 24 hours
- History of osteoarthritis
- Recent complicated hospital admission
- Recent intravenous antibiotics
- Chronic kidney disease, stage 3
- Systolic congestive heart failure
- Malnutrition

❓ What are the significant negatives from the information given so far?

- No falls or trauma, no change in activity
- No history of gout, psoriasis, rheumatoid arthritis, or other autoimmune disease

---

❓ Can the information gathered so far be restated in a single sentence highlighting the pieces that narrow down the cause?

The problem representation in this case might be: "a 70-year-old male with CHF and CKD stage 3 presents with acute onset of severe left wrist pain, redness, and swelling."

❓ How does this information affect the list of possible causes?

I can immediately cross trauma and overuse injury off my differential list as the history of this illness is not consistent with these causes. In evaluating a painful joint, it is often useful to determine the response to rest and movement. Inflammatory disorders cause pain with motion and at rest while noninflammatory disorders, such as degenerative joint disease, cause pain that is worse with motion and improves with rest.[1] This patient's pain is worse with motion but also woke him from sleep so it is more likely an inflammatory process. The triad of redness, swelling, and warmth also supports an inflammatory disorder. This makes the noninflammatory disorders on my list, osteoarthritis and renal osteodystrophy less likely.

While the location of the pain, in his wrist, makes me consider rheumatoid arthritis (RA), I put this low on my list because RA usually has a more insidious onset, and is usually symmetric, not unilateral. Psoriatic arthritis is unlikely since he does not have a history of psoriasis. I need to examine the joint carefully but there is no history of repetitive lifting, which would place the patient at risk for tenosynovitis. He has anemia and he is on low-dose aspirin but has no other risk factors for hemarthrosis and this, in and of itself, is less common and therefore less likely.

Clearly the triad of redness, swelling, and warmth along with the severity of his pain, which does not improve with rest, suggests an acute inflammatory process, most likely gout or septic arthritis. Gout usually involves the great toe or knee but it can occur in the wrist. The patient has several risk factors for gout including CKD, HF, use of diuretics, and male gender. In addition, patients with gout often complain of difficulty sleeping, as this patient does, because any slight stimulation such as the sheet overlying the affected joint exacerbates acute gout pain. The patient's age and the absence of a history of gout, however, make this diagnosis less likely; usually the first attack of gout occurs between 40 and 60 years of age.[1]

Risk factors for septic arthritis include the presence of a joint prosthesis, recent joint surgery or intra-articular injection, skin infection, diabetes, rheumatoid arthritis, intravenous drug use, alcoholism, and age over 80 years.[2] The patient actually has none of these risk factors; his joint surgery was long ago and his symptoms are not even in that joint. I recognize though that while he has not used illicit injectable drugs, he recently had an intravenous access for antibiotics, which could have been a portal for bacterial infection.

At this point, even before examining the patient, I know I am going to need some help. Differentiating gout and septic arthritis on the basis of clinical presentation alone is challenging at best, and the imperative of treating this condition quickly, both for the patient's comfort and to ensure he maintains function in the joint, requires efficient diagnosis. I suspect he will require joint aspiration as part of his diagnostic workup. Before proceeding with the review of systems and physical examination, I step out of the examination room and ask the licensed vocational nurse (LVN) assisting me to call the rheumatology office and see if any urgent appointments are available that day.

CASE INFORMATION

Review of Systems

- Constitutional: Denies fever or chills, denies body aches. Endorses fatigue and poor appetite since discharge. He generally sleeps well at night but could not sleep last night.
- Head/eyes/ears/nose/ throat: Noncontributory.
- Cardiovascular: Denies chest pain, leg swelling, or difficulty breathing when lying down.
- Pulmonary: Denies shortness of breath or cough.
- Gastrointestinal: Denies nausea, vomiting, constipation, or diarrhea.
- Genitourinary: Denies any changes in urination.
- Integumentary: Denies rash, denies itching, denies any wound.
- Musculoskeletal: Endorses left wrist pain as described above. Has chronic low back pain that is worse when he stands up for a prolonged period and worse since his hospitalization. Reports knee surgery 10 years ago was uncomplicated and improved his functional status.
- Neurological: No headaches, no dizziness, no numbness or tingling.
- Endocrine: Denies increased hunger, thirst, or urination.

Physical Examination

- Vital signs: Pulse is 74 beats per minute, blood pressure is 144/80 mm Hg on this visit, 100/60 on last visit, and never over 120 during recent hospital admission. His respiratory rate is 16 breaths per minute, and temperature is 98.5°F axillary, oxygen saturation by pulse oximeter is 95% on room air. He weighs 136 lb, which is 2 lb less than he weighed 2 weeks ago.
- Constitutional: Appears older than stated age, underweight, and uncomfortable on this examination, holding his left arm with his right hand away from his body.
- Head/eyes/ears/nose/throat: Deferred.
- Cardiovascular: Heart rate and rhythm regular, no murmurs, no gallops, nail beds are pale, cool to touch, brisk capillary refill, no peripheral edema.
- Pulmonary: Respiratory rate and rhythm are normal, without use of accessory muscles, lungs clear to auscultation.
- Gastrointestinal: No nausea, vomiting, diarrhea, or constipation.
- Neurological: No focal neurologic deficits, face symmetric, speech is clear, gait is steady.
- Integumentary: Scattered old bruises on both forearms. There is a small round black scab in the left antecubital space where the midline catheter was placed. There is no redness, warmth, or tenderness at that site.

- Musculoskeletal: Left wrist is red, warm, and swollen from the ulnar process around to the dorsal surface just proximal to the thumb; the inflamed area ends just below the metacarpophalangeal joints. It is exquisitely tender and he is unable to demonstrate range of motion due to pain with adducting or abducting the wrist. He is able to flex and extend his left fingers without discomfort but movement of his thumb is very painful. Demonstrates full range of motion in all other joints, no redness, swelling, or warmth in his feet, knees, elbows, or shoulders.
- Endocrine: Noncontributory.

? What elements of the review of systems and the physical examination should be added to the list of pertinent positives? Which items should be added to the list of significant negatives?

Pertinent Positives

- Left wrist range of motion limited by pain.
- Blood pressure above his baseline, likely due to discomfort.

Significant Negatives

- Normal review of systems and examination other than left wrist.
- He is afebrile; the insertion site of the midline catheter shows no sign of infection.
- The area of inflammation is confined to the wrist joint, and does not appear to involve the metacarpophalangeal joints.

? How does this information affect the list of possible causes?

Based on the patient's stable weight, clear breath sounds, and absence of lower extremity edema, I am able to confirm that his HF is compensated, which was really the condition I planned to address on this visit. However, this is no longer the priority for this patient.

Unfortunately, gout and septic arthritis can appear very similar on examination. In addition, gout and infection can occur simultaneously in the same joint. While it is tempting to check a radiograph and do blood work, such as a uric acid level, C-reactive protein, and white blood cell count, I recognize that none of these tests will definitively determine the underlying pathology. Serum uric acid is not a sensitive or specific test for gout; patients can have a high level and no gout, or acute gout and a normal level.[2] C- reactive protein and white blood cell count indicate that infection is present but this patient could have gout in his wrist and an infectious process elsewhere. In addition, if I believe this could be septic arthritis, I need to culture the synovial fluid before I start antibiotics to ensure that the regimen I select adequately covers the infecting organism.

Joint aspiration is the gold standard for differentiating gout and septic arthritis. If a patient has uric acid crystals in the joint aspirate, then gout is present. The absence of crystals makes gout less likely but does not definitely rule it out, since the sample may have been inadequate. Similarly, the presence of bacteria on aspiration definitely rules in septic joint. Bacteria can be detected by Gram stain and by culture, or inferred based on the appearance of the synovial fluid and a high level of white blood cells. The LVN assisting me tells me the rheumatologist will see the patient as an urgent case, if I call and discuss the case with her first. After calling and explaining my findings to her, I ask the patient to go to her office, located in the building next door, for joint aspiration.

CASE INFORMATION

Diagnostic Testing

Prior to leaving my office, the patient reminds me that he does not want to end up back in the hospital. I explain that I will try my best but that at this point, my first priority is to alleviate his extreme discomfort and he concurs with that priority. I recognize that if this is indeed an infectious process, he will require intravenous antibiotics, and possibly drainage of the joint and this would need to be done in an inpatient setting.

Two hours later, the rheumatologist calls me to request that I arrange for the patient to be directly admitted to the hospital for septic arthritis. She was able to aspirate a sample of synovial fluid, which was opaque, cream colored, and presumably purulent; normal synovial fluid is transparent and clear to pale yellow.[3] No uric acid crystals are seen. A Gram stain, cell count, and culture are pending, but based on the appearance of the fluid, she advises initiating intravenous antibiotic therapy and consulting orthopedics for arthroscopic drainage.

Management of Septic Arthritis

A suspicion for septic arthritis requires urgent evaluation because untreated infection can lead to joint destruction and loss of the distal limb. Gout is a self-limiting disease process but is often treated with corticosteroids, either oral or injectable, or nonsteroidal anti-inflammatory medications due to the extreme discomfort it causes. Empiric treatment for gout without ruling out an infectious process can have deleterious consequences as the immunosuppressive effects of corticosteroids can promote spread of the infection. In addition, giving antibiotics when the source of infection is unclear can contribute to the growing issue of antibiotic resistance.

Septic arthritis is usually caused by hematogenous spread of bacteria though it is not always associated with positive blood cultures. It may be that the infecting organism was only briefly present in the blood stream before seeding in the joint.

Gout, rheumatoid arthritis, and osteoarthritis can predispose a particular joint to infection, though the mechanism by which a particular joint is affected is not clearly understood. The acute inflammatory cellular response within the synovial membrane includes cytokines and proteases that cause cartilage destruction and inhibit cartilage synthesis. The joint may also be affected by necrosis due to pressure from large-volume synovial effusions.[3]

Staphylococcus aureus is the most common causative organism in septic arthritis. Streptococci, including *Streptococcus pneumoniae* are also commonly implicated. Gram-negative organisms usually occur only in the setting of trauma, intravenous drug use, or immunosuppressed states. It is unusual for septic arthritis to occur from polymicrobial infection unless trauma leads to direct exposure of the joint or in the case of septic arthritis of the hip due to seeding from a bowel perforation.[3]

The treatment of choice is vancomycin, particularly when a Gram stain confirms a gram-positive infection. Gram-negative infections are usually treated with a third-generation cephalosporin. In situations where pseudomonal infection is suspected, dual antibiotic therapy is warranted with either ceftazidime or ciprofloxacin and an aminoglycoside. If the Gram stain does not show any bacteria but there are other signs indicating septic arthritis, such as altered appearance of synovial fluid and a cell count showing 50 to 150 white blood cells, primarily neutrophils, the recommendation is to treat with vancomycin while awaiting culture results.[3]

Drainage of the joint is also a key element in the management of septic arthritis.[3] This can be achieved through needle aspiration, arthroscopy, or surgical drainage. If the involved joint is prosthetic, or if the infection is in a large joint such as the hip or shoulder, surgical drainage is often the treatment of choice. With smaller joints, such as this patient's wrist, arthroscopy is the preferred approach. Any patient who does not demonstrate clinical improvement with less invasive drainage should be evaluated for surgical intervention.

Case Follow-Up

The following day, I round at the hospital and see my patient. He is much more comfortable, on as needed doses of intravenous narcotics, and following 24 hours of intravenous vancomycin. I acknowledge that we have not met our original goal, established during his first visit, to avoid hospital admission. On his initial clinic visit, I assessed fluid imbalance would be the most likely cause of readmission based on the issues during his hospital stay with HF and acute renal failure following diuresis. I believed with close follow-up and careful titration of diuretic medications that preventing readmission for his HF was feasible. I did not anticipate this complication! While I wish that I had been successful in managing the patient without hospital admission, I feel confident that reaching out to the rheumatologist for assistance was the right course of action.

The patient asks how quickly he might be discharged. I discuss the case with the adult hospitalist and he agrees to place a midline catheter for home antibiotics, and as long as his symptoms continue to improve, he can be discharged after 72 hours of inpatient therapy. We schedule a follow-up appointment in the chronic care clinic to resume management of his chronic health issues.

References

1. Baer AN, Patel V, McCormack R. The approach the painful joint. Medscape Web site. http://emedi cine.medscape.com/article/336054-overview#showall. Updated January 23, 2014. Accessed May 3, 2015.
2. Rothschild BM, Miller AV, Francis ML. Gout and pseudogout. Medscape Web site. http://emedicine. medscape.com/article/329958-overview. Updated March 16, 2015. Accessed May 3, 2015.
3. Goldenberg DL, Sexton DJ. Septic arthritis in adults. UptoDate Web site. Topic 7666. Version 17.0. http://www.uptodate.com/contents/septic-arthritis-in-adults?topicKey=ID%F7666. Updated April 2, 2015. Accessed April 17, 2015.

CASE 65

Karen L. Kopan

Karen Kopan is an NP with the critical care consult team in the Surgical Intensive Care Unit at NorthShore University HealthSystem, Evanston Hospital. Dr Kopan is also an Assistant Professor in the Department of Adult Health and Gerontological Nursing at Rush University College of Nursing.

CASE INFORMATION

Chief Complaint

A 63-year-old female was brought to the emergency room of an outside hospital with complaints of headache and elbow laceration after a fall while walking her dog.

History of Present Illness

Because of her headache an initial head CT was done at approximately 7:00 PM and revealed a 9 × 10 mm rounded density within the left occipital lobe. Her mental status quickly declined in the emergency room and a repeat head CT at approximately 8:15 PM showed an interval increase in the left occipital lesion compatible with acute occipital parenchymal hemorrhage, measuring 10.4 × 13.6 mm. She was intubated and ventilated for airway protection and impending acute respiratory failure and transferred by the neurosurgery team to the intensive care unit at this hospital. A third head CT obtained at approximately 10:00 PM showed further increase in the size of the hemorrhage, measuring 3.3 × 3 cm with increased vasogenic edema. The patient remained intubated overnight on light sedation with propofol infusion. She received Keppra for seizure prophylaxis and platelet transfusion for a prolonged platelet function assay (PFA). Cardiology was consulted for elevated cardiac markers and recommended β-blocker and statin therapy. A nicardipine hydrochloride infusion was initiated for hypertension. Old records were requested from the outside hospital and urinalysis, blood cultures, and chest x-ray were obtained. The patient was started on stress ulcer prophylaxis and a sequential compression device was applied for deep vein thrombosis prophylaxis. At 4:00 AM a repeat head CT showed significant increase in the hemorrhage, a new moderate right frontal subarachnoid hemorrhage, and small right temporal subarachnoid hemorrhage. The neurosurgery team evaluated her and concluded that she could not be taken to surgery for evacuation as her neurological status was still evolving. In addition the head CTs showed no midline shift or downward pressure and the cisterns were open. She is sent to the surgical ICU.

During sign out at 6:00 AM, the patient becomes hypotensive to the 80s systolic. Her nicardipine infusion is off, having been weaned as of 2:00 AM and the propofol was discontinued at 4:00 AM. She is given a 500 mL intravenous (IV) fluid bolus of 0.9% normal saline over 30 minutes to address the hypotension, but this has little effect. The patient is now in my care and my job is to stabilize the patient.

After the bolus, the patient's blood pressure is 76/54 mm Hg, pulse rate 83 beats per minute, respiratory rate 30/min, and temperature is 103.1°F.

❓ What is the potential cause?

Hypotension is common in the intensive care unit, especially the surgical intensive care unit. My initial thought at seeing hypotension with a fever is the diagnosis of severe sepsis. Severe sepsis is defined as sepsis-induced tissue hypoperfusion or organ dysfunction due to infection.[1] Criteria for severe sepsis include sepsis-induced hypotension, lactate above upper limits of laboratory normal, urine output less than 0.5 mL/kg/hour for more than 2 consecutive hours despite fluid resuscitation, acute lung injury in the absence of pneumonia, creatinine greater than 2.0 mg/dL, bilirubin greater than 2 mg/dL, platelet count less than 100,000 µL, or coagulopathy with international normalized ratio (INR) greater than 1.5. I am comfortable giving another 500 to 1000 mL IV fluid bolus of 0.9% normal saline as I think through the reasons for severe sepsis in a patient who presented with a fall and intraparenchymal bleeding who also has subarachnoid hemorrhage.

I quickly assess the ABCs: airway, breathing, and circulation. Her airway is secured because she is intubated, though I will confirm placement of the tube myself by physical examination and by viewing the morning's chest x-ray. To assess breathing and adequate ventilation, I will check an arterial blood gas to rule out an acidemia. To assess circulation, I systematically think my way through the approach to hypotension or shock: heart rate, preload, afterload, and contractility. The heart rate is normal and the rhythm is regular so I wonder if the hypotension is caused by decreased circulating blood volume, decreased systemic vascular resistance, or decreased contractility. From my experience with managing very sick patients, I know to request placement of an arterial line and central line in order to stay ahead of the game. I anticipate that I will be spending many intensive hours managing this complex patient and these lines will allow minute-to-minute assessments of her response to my interventions. I keep my comprehensive differential in mind as I further assess and care for this patient.

Comprehensive Differential Diagnoses for a Patient With Hypotension[2]

Hypovolemia or Decreased Venous Return

Hypovolemia due to losses from: hemorrhage, GI tract, kidneys, third spaced fluids, diabetes insipidus Decreased venous return: increased intrathoracic or intraabdominal pressure, cardiac (pericardial) tamponade, profound venous dilation

Low afterload

Anaphylaxis, sepsis, spinal shock, drug effects from anesthesia or drug overdose

Contractility

Myocardial causes: infarction, sepsis with myocardial depression Mechanical problems: acute valvular regurgitation or rupture of the mitral valve associated with myocardial infarction, left ventricular outflow obstruction

With the differential list complete, I begin to gather more detailed information from the patient's history, physical examination, chart review, diagnostics including labs, radiographs, electrocardiograms, and microbiology data, and refine my treatment plan accordingly.[3] Severe hypotension with intraparenchymal and subarachnoid hemorrhages in a patient who was just out walking her dog does not add up to a clear diagnosis so I need to step back and consider what else is happening. Has she had an acute myocardial infarction? She is not responding to the IV fluid boluses; could she have severe sepsis along with intracerebral/subarachnoid bleeds? Does she have loss of autoregulation of her blood pressure from increased intracranial hypertension?

CASE INFORMATION
Medical history from the chart

This 63-year-old female has a past medical history that is significant for hypertension, an ascending aortic aneurysm repair with a mechanical aortic valve replacement in 2010, and an epidural steroid injection in the lumbar spine for degenerative disc disease in 2013. She takes aspirin daily along with a thiazide diuretic, statin, and calcium channel blocker. She has no allergies and no significant family history. She is divorced with two adult children and the family reports heavy alcohol use.

I then review the diagnostic testing done on admission to the outside emergency room. The electrocardiogram (ECG) is normal though cardiac markers are elevated. The patient did not complain of chest pain or pressure initially in the emergency room and has no prior history of coronary artery disease. The white blood cell count was normal and the oral temperature was 101.0°F on admission. No bands or schistocytes were present on the differential. The serum sodium was 130 mEq/L and the serum bicarbonate was 17 mEq/L. The creatinine was 2.0 mg/dL with a glomerular filtration rate (GFR) of 33.7 mL/min/1.73 m² (the normal value for females is approximately 120 mL/min/1.73 m²).[4] The arterial blood gas was pH = 7.58/$PaCO_2$ = 19 mm Hg, PaO_2 = 79 mm Hg on room air prior to intubation with a respiratory rate of 40 to 50. Her chest x-ray showed mild pulmonary edema on admission. Transaminases were mildly elevated and prothrombin time was normal.

❓ What are the pertinent positives from the information given so far?

- The patient fell and has intraparenchymal and subarachnoid hemorrhages with vasogenic edema.
- The patient is hemodynamically unstable with hypotension, elevated cardiac markers and has a history of ascending aortic aneurysm repair with a mechanical aortic valve replacement and mild pulmonary edema on chest x-ray.
- The patient had respiratory alkalosis with fever and tachypnea prior to intubation.
- The patient has a decreased serum bicarbonate level, an elevated creatinine, and a decreased glomerular filtration rate on admission.
- Transaminases are mildly elevated and the patient has a history of family-reported heavy alcohol use.

❓ What are the pertinent negatives from the information so far?

- The patient has no history of coronary artery disease.
- There is no evidence of gastrointestinal losses, renal losses, pancreatitis, burns, or recent abdominal surgery.
- There is no anaphylaxis or cervical spinal cord injury.
- There is no diffuse erythroderma or transfusion reaction.
- There is no arrhythmia.

❓ Can the information gathered so far be restated in a single sentence highlighting the pieces that narrow down the cause?

The problem representation in this case might be: "a 63-year-old female with hypertension, lumbar stenosis, daily alcohol use, and an ascending aortic aneurysm s/p repair with mechanical aortic valve replacement who presents with new intraparenchymal and subarachnoid hemorrhages with development of shock state."

Initially the case presents as a fall and an intraparenchymal lesion that quickly changes to an evolving hemorrhagic stroke with subarachnoid hemorrhages. The patient was intubated and ventilated for airway protection and impending respiratory failure. Initially vital signs were unstable, in fact requiring a nicardipine hydrochloride infusion for hypertension and propofol for sedation, and in early morning she became hypotensive with fever.

Case Analysis

Now the various shock states need to be considered. I consider hypovolemic shock. The patient did fall and may have sustained an internal abdominal or splenic injury or retroperitoneal bleeding. And she has a history of an aortic aneurysm repair, so a leak or dissection of her aorta is also possible. To further evaluate, I will need a CT scan of the chest and abdomen to look for any signs of hemorrhage. Dehydration is also possible. I can rule out neurogenic diabetes insipidus as the cause of hypovolemia because her urine output is low, and I can further confirm this by sending urine and serum osmolalities, particularly if she continues to have abnormal sodium levels.

Cardiogenic shock is another possibility, due to myocardial infarction, underlying/undiagnosed heart failure, or valvular disease. To evaluate for this, I will need an echocardiogram, starting with a transthoracic echo but moving to a transesophageal to examine the valves for vegetation and the integrity of the aortic valve and ascending aorta if necessary. I will also continue to follow her cardiac markers, though these can be elevated due to acute brain injury.

Obstructive shock, though low on the differential list, must also be ruled out. A repeat chest x-ray is ordered to rule out a tension pneumothorax. It is possible that a rib fracture occurred with the fall, causing a small pneumothorax that is now under pressure with positive pressure ventilation (ie, a tension pneumothorax). The echocardiogram will rule out cardiac tamponade from a pericardial effusion. To rule out auto-PEEP I will check the ventilator waveforms for pressure and flow. A pulmonary artery computed tomography scan (CT-PA) will rule out pulmonary embolism.

The most likely cause of shock, based on the information I have so far, is distributive shock due to sepsis. Respiratory alkalosis, tachypnea, and fever are the harbingers of severe sepsis. Her temperature has risen from 101.1°F to 103.1°F. To evaluate the patient for this type of shock, I will send another set of blood cultures and follow up on previous blood and urine cultures. Source control is a priority in the management of sepsis. I will review her antibiotic regimen and ensure she is receiving broad-spectrum coverage. There is no history of recent immunosuppression so for now I will not add antibiotic coverage for atypical organisms. I will check her amylase and lipase to rule out pancreatitis, and I will check another differential on the next complete blood count to look for bands and elevated neutrophils, which suggest a bacterial infection. Even though the chest x-ray was negative for an infiltrate, I will send a sputum culture. Anaphylaxis is low on the differential list but I will send a toxicology screen if it was not sent already. Of course my physical examination will also provide data on possible sources of infection.

CASE INFORMATION

Review of Systems

I am unable to complete review of systems due to decreased mental status.

Physical Examination

- Vital signs: Pulse is 83 beats per minute and normal sinus rhythm, blood pressure is 76/54 mm Hg, respiratory rate is 16 breaths per minute, and temperature is 103.1°F oral. Oxygen saturation is 96%.
- Constitutional: Unresponsive, ventilated.
- Head/eyes/ears/nose/throat: Scalp laceration dressing intact, orally intubated, no scleral icterus, ears unremarkable, no carotid bruits, no jugular venous distension at 30°, no nuchal rigidity.
- Cardiovascular: Heart sounds normal S1, S2, no murmur, rub, or gallop, valve click noted, normal sinus rhythm.
- Vascular: No clubbing, +dusky fingers, pale feet, weak thready pulses throughout extremities, no peripheral edema.
- Pulmonary: Symmetrical expansion, lung sounds with rhonchi in left upper lobe, diminished lower lung fields bilaterally, breathing over the preset ventilator rate, stable oxygen saturation.
- Gastrointestinal: Abdomen soft, rounded, without distension, active bowel sounds, no hepatomegaly.
- Genitourinary: Catheter in place, otherwise normal.
- Integumentary: No petechiae, Osler nodes, or splinter hemorrhages. No rashes, lesions, or erythema noted. Skin mottled; integrity intact with exception of scalp laceration.
- Neurological: Pupils are equally reactive, sluggish, at 3 mm, no spontaneous motor movement, no commands, no withdrawal to pain, +corneal, +cough, and +gag reflexes.

Laboratory Test Results

Repeat complete blood count, coagulation studies, chemistry panel, cardiac markers, arterial blood gas and mixed venous oxygen saturation ScVO$_2$ are sent stat. The repeat blood count shows normal hemoglobin and hematocrit values. Repeat coagulation studies are normal. The white blood cell count is normal, but there is an increased number of neutrophils and bands of 16%, which indicates a "left shift" suggesting an infection. Her platelet count is low at 99,000/µL and may signify increased platelet destruction from infection or sepsis. The complete metabolic profile is significant for a low serum bicarbonate (ie, serum CO_2) of 12 mEq/L, indicating a severe metabolic acidosis. She also has a high creatinine level of 2.6 mg/dL, indicating acute kidney injury likely due to shock, dehydration, or acute heart failure, and elevated transaminases, likely related to her history of alcohol use in the setting of decreased perfusion to the liver with shock. Her arterial blood gas also demonstrates a severe metabolic acidosis with partial respiratory compensation: pH = 7.14, $PaCO_2$ = 25 mm Hg, PaO_2 = 131 mm Hg, and bicarbonate = 10 mEq/L. Her anion gap is 19 (Normal = 10–14 mmol). Correcting for a low albumin level, the anion gap is 23.5! I attribute the anion gap to lactic acidosis and severe sepsis. The lactic acid level is very high at 11.9 (due to anaerobic metabolism-shock state) and the $ScVO_2$ is low at 56.7% (consistent with sepsis). Cardiac markers continue to rise with a troponin level of greater than 95 µg/L, myoglobin greater than 4000 ng/mL, and a total creatine kinase (CK) of 8499 µ/L, revealing massive myocardial injury and acute kidney injury. The ECG shows normal sinus rhythm with first-degree atrioventricular block but is otherwise normal. The toxicology screen is negative for drugs and alcohol. Urinalysis is negative, urine culture is negative. Repeat chest x-ray shows the endotracheal tube in correct position 3 cm above the carina, no pneumothorax, but there is left basilar atelectasis.

❓ What elements of the physical examination and diagnostic testing results should be added to the list of pertinent positives? Which items should be added to the list of significant negatives?

- **Pertinent positives:** hypotension, fever, rhonchi left upper lobe, diminished sounds lower lung fields bilaterally, dusky fingers, thready pulses, mottled skin, sluggish pupillary reaction, no spontaneous movement off sedation and no response to pain, bandemia, thrombocytopenia, acute kidney injury, anion gap metabolic acidosis, elevated cardiac markers, and decreased $ScVO_2$.

- **Significant negatives:** no icterus, no jugular venous distension at 30°, no nuchal rigidity, normal heart sounds with appropriate valve click, no arrhythmia, breathing over the preset ventilator rate, stable oxygen saturation, abdominal examination benign, no peripheral edema, no petechiae, Osler nodes, or splinter hemorrhages, no skin rashes or erythema, +corneal, +cough, +gag reflexes. Normal hemoglobin, hematocrit, and coagulation panel. Normal ECG, urinalysis, and toxicology screen.

❓ How does this information affect the list of possible causes?

Hypovolemic shock is unlikely without hemorrhage or volume losses; her hemoglobin is normal and there is no sign of acute volume loss. Furthermore, the patient did not present with compensatory signs of hemorrhage such as tachycardia, thirst, and hypotension. Obstructive shock due to cardiac tamponade, pulmonary embolism, or a tension pneumothorax is also unlikely. She does not have jugular venous distension, muffled heart tones, or a scenario consistent with pericardial effusion or tamponade. Her initial chest x-ray showed only mild pulmonary edema, no pneumothorax, and no central line was attempted that might have caused a pneumothorax following that x-ray. In addition, the patient did not report chest trauma prior to her mental status decline.

Cardiogenic shock may be present and the echo will help establish this. She does not have signs of heart failure such as exertional dyspnea, crackles, S3, cardiomegaly, peripheral edema, or arrhythmias. She does have decreased renal function, mild pulmonary edema on initial chest x-ray, history of heavy alcohol use, and previous aortic valve surgery. So I cannot rule out cardiogenic shock without more information.

Distributive septic shock is still the most likely source of this patient's shock state. She may be harboring an infectious source in her mechanical valve that threw emboli to her brain, causing small embolic insults that converted to a hemorrhagic stroke. It is also possible that she has an undiagnosed urinary tract infection or a pneumonia that did not show up on the initial chest film. And it may be that she had an infection prior to her fall and that the infection contributed to her being weak and off balance, thus contributing to her fall and serious head injury.

I appreciate that hemorrhagic intraparenchymal and subarachnoid strokes in combination with distributive septic shock state are life threatening for this patient. There are advanced directives in the chart and the patient is currently a full code. As I move forward establishing a medical plan of care, I need to discuss the severity of this case with the primary neurosurgical team, attending critical care physician, bedside nurse, social worker, chaplain, and most importantly, family members.

❓ What diagnostic testing should be done and in what order?

I order a stat transthoracic echo to rule out cardiogenic shock and a stat chest, abdomen and pelvis CT scan (whichever can be done first) to evaluate for a source of infection and rule out additional trauma.

CASE INFORMATION
Diagnostic Testing Results

Blood cultures drawn on admission grow gram-positive cocci in clusters, positive in two peripheral venous samples. The transthoracic echo preliminary report shows an ejection fraction of 35%, globally depressed myocardial function, no valvular dysfunction, and no signs of dissection in the thoracic aorta. The stat chest/abdomen/pelvis CT scan reveals fatty liver, changes to the kidneys consistent with acute tubular necrosis, and possible pyelonephritis. Arterial and central lines are placed and the initial central venous pressure (CVP) is 15 mm Hg.

Diagnosis and Management of Gram-Positive Bacteremia with Septic Shock

The diagnosis of septic shock is defined as sepsis-induced hypotension (systolic blood pressure [SBP] less than 90 mm Hg or mean arterial pressure [MAP] less than 70 mm Hg or an SBP decrease greater than 40 mm Hg or less than two standard deviations below normal for age in the absence of other causes of hypotension) that persists despite adequate fluid resuscitation.[1] Sepsis-induced tissue hypoperfusion is defined as infection-induced hypotension, elevated lactate, or oliguria.[1] It is recommended that appropriate cultures are obtained before antimicrobial therapy is initiated provided doing so does not cause significant delays in the administration of antimicrobial agents. Imaging studies should be performed promptly to confirm or rule out potential sources of infection.

The initial management of severe sepsis, within the first 3 hours, is fluid resuscitation with 30 mL/kg crystalloid to treat for hypotension or a lactate level greater than or equal to 4 mmol/L. The goals of fluid resuscitation include a central venous pressure (CVP) 8 to 12 mm Hg, MAP greater than or equal to 65 mm Hg, urine output greater than 0.5 mL/kg/h and a central venous oxygen saturation of at least 70%.[3] After obtaining cultures and completing imaging studies to identify the source of infection, broad-spectrum antimicrobial therapy is administered, ideally within the first hour of recognizing septic shock. Within 6 hours, vasopressors are added if hypotension does not respond to initial fluid resuscitation. A specific anatomical source of infection should be considered or excluded within the first 12 hours and selective oral and digestive tract decontamination should be introduced to reduce incidence of ventilator-associated pneumonia.[3]

Case Follow-Up

The patient receives 3 liters of crystalloid therapy followed by norepinephrine, vasopressin, and phenylephrine drips at maximum doses to maintain MAP greater than 65 mm Hg. Inotropic therapy for cardiogenic shock is considered though not initiated after consultation with the cardiology team. To manage the patient's profound acidosis, ventilator settings are adjusted to increase removal of carbon dioxide, and a bicarbonate drip is initiated. Nephrology is consulted to place a line and start continuous renal replacement therapy to address her acute kidney injury. A dextrose infusion is started after several episodes of hypoglycemia and stress dose steroids are given to empirically address adrenal insufficiency. She is started on antibiotic therapy including vancomycin and piperacillin/tazobactam.

In between the acute management of the patient, I ascertain that the patient's ex-husband was not a consistent supportive figure for the patient or their college-aged children, and is not involved in the medical decision making for the patient. Advanced directives in the chart indicate that the patient does not want her life prolonged in the event that there is little hope of recovery. The patient's children mention a plan to leave the hospital and come back the next day. I take this opportunity to slow down and spend some time discussing the situation with the children. I ask them what they understand of the situation with their Mom and realize they do not have the whole picture. I explain that her situation is very critical; she may not survive to the next day. I assure them we are doing everything possible to save her life. I pause to let this information sink in before I continue. I then explain that her critical condition means she could pass away during the night, which they need to know before they make the decision to leave the hospital. I ask if their Mom has other family members who might want to know about this critical illness and offer them support at this time. They decide to call additional family and not to leave the hospital. Social work and chaplain services are consulted. Later in the evening the family decides on a DNR status to honor her wishes and when her systolic blood pressure drops acutely into the 40s followed by pulseless electrical activity (PEA) arrest, no CPR is performed. Her family is in the room with her when she dies.

References

1. Dellinger RP, Levy MM, Rhodes A, Annane D, Gerlach H, Opal SM, et al. Surviving sepsis campaign: international guidelines for management of severe sepsis and septic shock. *Crit Care Med.* 2013;41(2):580-637.
2. Lanken PN, Manaker S, Kohl BA, Hanson CW III. *The Intensive Care Unit Manual.* Philadelphia, PA: Elsevier Saunders; 2014.
3. Society of Critical Care Medicine. *Fundamental Critical Care Support.* 5th ed. Mount Prospect, IL: Society of Critical Care Medicine; 2012.
4. Stevens LA, Coresh J, Greene T, Levey AS. Assessing Kidney Function – Measured and Estimated Glomerular Filtration Rate. *N Engl J Med.* 2006;354:2473-2483. doi: 10.1056/NEJMra054415.

CASE 66

Carolyn Brady

Carolyn Brady works in the Heart Failure Nurse Practitioner Clinic at the University of Virginia Medical Center.

CASE INFORMATION

Chief Complaint

A 55-year-old man presents to the outpatient heart failure nurse practitioner clinic with a new complaint of night sweats.

❓ What is the potential cause?

Night sweats are a common complaint with many possible etiologies. The first step is to develop a precise definition of night sweats and differentiate it from other benign symptoms such as hot flashes, flushing, or sweating from being in an overheated room, wearing too many layers of clothing, or using too many blankets. Night sweats is defined as drenching sweats at night that require a person to change their bed sheets or clothing. Once this is confirmed, then I can create a list of all the possible causes.

Comprehensive Differential Diagnoses for a Patient With Night Sweats[1]

- Malignancy: lymphoma (Hodgkin lymphoma and non-Hodgkin lymphoma), solid tumors (germ cell tumors, medullary carcinoma of the thyroid, prostate cancer, renal cell carcinoma), leukemia
- Infections: mycobacterium (tuberculosis, atypical mycobacterium), bacterial (brucellosis, abscess, endocarditis, osteomyelitis), fungal, viral (human immunodeficiency virus [HIV] infection, chronic hepatitis C)
- Medications: antidepressants (bupropion, selective serotonin reuptake inhibitors, tricyclic antidepressants, norepinephrine reuptake inhibitors), antimigraine drugs ("triptans," serotonin 5-HT [1B/1D] agonists), antipyretics (acetaminophen, NSAIDs, ASA), cholinergic agonists (bethanechol, pilocarpine), hormonal agents (gonadorelin, goserelin, histrelin, leuprolide, nafarelin, anastrazole, exemestane, letrozole, flutamide, raloxifene, tamoxifen), hypoglycemic agents (insulin, sulfonylureas, thiazolidinediones), sympathomimetic agents (β-agonists, phenylephrine), alcohol, β-blockers, bromocriptine, calcium channel blockers, clozapine, cyclosporine, donepezil, fluvoxamine, hydralazine, imatinib, infliximab, interferon α-2b, morphine, niacin, nitroglycerin,

omeprazole, opioids, protease inhibitors, rituximab, ropinirole, sildenafil, theophylline, tramadol
- Endocrine disorders: pheochromocytoma, carcinoid syndrome, hyperthyroidism, hypoglycemia, diabetes insipidus, and postorchiectomy
- Neurological disorders: autonomic neuropathy, autonomic dysreflexia, stroke, posttraumatic syringomyelia
- Miscellaneous: menopause, anxiety/panic disorder, chronic fatigue syndrome, common blushing, food additives, gastroesophageal reflux, mastocytosis, rosacea, temporal arteritis, sleep disorders/sleep apnea, and idiopathic hyperhidrosis
- Substance withdrawal: alcohol, cocaine, opioids[1]

Now that I have a list of all the possible etiologies, I begin to gather data. As I gather data, I review the differential diagnosis list and begin to rule out some possible causes while making note of other causes as possible diagnoses.

CASE INFORMATION

History of Previous Illness

While observing the patient, I am able to gather helpful information. The patient presents alone to clinic and is sitting on the examination table in no apparent distress. He appears his stated age, well-nourished, well-developed, and is appropriately groomed. His face is symmetrical and he is able to move all extremities. He smiles when greeted by the provider, answers questions appropriately, and is oriented to person, place, and time. The provider asks the patient how he has been feeling and the patient replies, "I feel great since they got all that fluid off my legs in the hospital last week. The only thing that is bothering me now is I keep waking up at night soaked in sweat and have to change my clothes." He goes on to report that his wife has complained for many years that he snores loudly and is scared when he stops breathing while sleeping. He denies any recent illnesses or fever. He has resumed his daily walk through his neighborhood and is able to walk 1 mile in 20 minutes without stopping to rest.

I ask the patient about his past medical history and he replies, "I have a heart problem. My heart is weak and sometimes I get fluid on my legs. I was just in the hospital last week for fluid buildup in my legs and they did a really good job getting all that fluid off. I lost over 15 lb and now I feel much better." I then ask the patient what medications he takes regularly, including over-the-counter and prescription medications. The patient responds, "I take four pills every day: two heart pills, a baby aspirin, and a fluid pill." The patient denies any prior history of malignancy, infections, substance abuse, intravenous (IV) drug use, blood transfusions, stroke, gastroesoph-ageal reflux disease, fatigue, neurological problems, diabetes, thyroid disorders, anxiety/panic disorder, recent invasive procedures, any surgery, travel outside the United States, working with animals or animal products, eating raw or unpasteurized foods. He mentions, "I had a bad cold that lasted 4 months. I never really felt great after that but didn't go to my doctor until I had trouble breathing and couldn't finish my usual walk in the neighbor-hood. He gave me some antibiotics and I felt better for a while but then got worse again. He also wanted me to be checked out for sleep apnea last year but I never got an appointment."

In review of the patient's electronic medical record, I discover that he had an admission last week for a heart failure exacerbation. A review of daily prog-ress notes shows no fevers, a blood pressure range of 90–110/50–62 mmHg, and a heart rate range of 55 to 82 beats per minute (bpm). During that admission, he was diuresed for a total of 9 liters. He had a posterior-anterior (PA) and lateral chest x-ray (CXR), which showed no acute focal airspace dis-ease, pneumothorax, malignancy, or effusion and stable, mild cardiomegaly, likely left atrial enlargement. He had a transthoracic echocardiogram (TTE), which revealed normal left ventricular wall thickness and the left ventricular cavity was moderately dilated. The left ventricular ejection fraction (EF) was 25% to 30%. Left ventricular systolic global function was severely decreased and there was severe diastolic dysfunction. This was compared to his prior TTE from 3 months ago and was unchanged. Lab work, including a com-plete blood count (CBC) with differential and comprehensive metabolic panel (CMP), was normal. Troponin I initially was 0.03 (Normal = <0.01 ng/mL), then was rechecked 8 hours later and was 0.02, suggesting that he may have heart disease but not an acute myocardial infarction. On admission, his B-type natriuretic peptide (BNP) was 1070 (Normal = 100 pg/mL). Thyroid-stimulating hormone with reflexive T4 were both normal. Twelve-lead electrocardio-gram (ECG) showed normal sinus rhythm at 72 bpm. His past medical history includes a former 15-year chewing tobacco history and he quit 7 years ago.

He had one other hospital admission 3 months ago for shortness of breath and after an extensive workup; he was diagnosed with nonischemic cardiomyopathy of unclear etiology. His workup during that admission included a D-dimer = 268 ng/mL (normal = <231 ng/mL), chest-computed tomography (CT) scan showed stable multiple small pulmonary nodules consistent with benign etiology but no acute cardiopulmonary abnormal-ity. Computed tomography pulmonary angiography (CTPA) chest showed no evidence of pulmonary embolism to the subsegmental level. He had a TTE, as described above. He declined cardiac catheterization and thus underwent a cardiac magnetic resonance imaging (MRI), which showed left ventricular enlargement with severely reduced systolic function (EF = 25%). Normal-sized right ventricle with mildly reduced systolic function (EF = 39%). No evidence of myocardial ischemia or late gadolinium enhancement.

Mild mitral regurgitation. He was started on lisinopril 10 mg daily, metoprolol succinate 25 mg daily, aspirin 81 mg daily, and furosemide 40 mg daily.

In review of the outpatient office notes, I note that his primary care MD prescribed a z-pack 4 months ago for the patient's bronchitis. He also made a sleep clinic referral but the patient did not attend that appointment. However, the patient did recently begin to work with his primary cardiologist to optimize his heart failure medications. Standard medications for patients with heart failure with reduced ejection fraction (HFrEF), defined as left ventricular (LV) dysfunction with EF <40%, are used to reduce morbidity and mortality and include an angiotensin-converting enzyme inhibitor (ACE-I) (or angiotensin II receptor blocker if ACE-I not tolerated) and a β-blocker (one of the following three β-blockers: carvedilol, metoprolol succinate, or bisoprolol), unless contraindicated.[2] For patients with EF ≤35% and NYHA class II-VI (NYHA class II patients should also have a history of prior cardiovascular hospitalization or elevated plasma BNP), an aldosterone agonist (spironolactone or eplerenone) is also indicated, if tolerated. Tolerance is defined as a serum creatinine of ≤2.5 mg/dL in men, or ≤2.0 mg/dL in women, and a serum potassium <5.0 mEq/L (or estimated glomerular filtration rate >30 mL/min/1.73 m²).[2] Aldosterone antagonists require frequent lab monitoring to detect renal insufficiency and hyperkalemia.[2,3] Loop diuretics are used in patients who are volume overloaded (bumetanide, furosemide, and torsemide).[2] Goals of therapy are to increase the heart failure medication doses to the maximum tolerated dose.[2,3] Unfortunately this patient's low blood pressure has prevented any medication dose adjustments and he remains on lisinopril 10 mg daily and metoprolol succinate 25 mg daily. He previously took spironolactone 25 mg daily for 3 weeks but that was discontinued due to hyperkalemia (serum potassium [K$^+$] = 5.6 mmol/L).

❓ What are the pertinent positives gathered from the information gathered thus far?

- The patient has a known heart failure diagnosis, with systolic and diastolic dysfunction evident on echocardiogram.
- The patient has a history of snoring with witnessed apneas by his wife.
- The patient is taking two medications that are known to potentially cause night sweats: aspirin and metoprolol succinate.
- The patient was previously referred to sleep clinic for evaluation of sleep-disordered breathing.

• The patient is currently well, having resumed physical activity with daily walking and reporting that he feels better than he did prior to his recent hospital stay.

❓ What are the significant negatives from the information gathered thus far?

• CTPA chest and chest CT show no evidence of malignancy, infectious process, or acute cardiopulmonary disease. In review of the patient electronic medical record, he has had recent lab work with normal, or unrevealing, results including CBC, CMP, and troponin.

• The patient denies history of, and review of the patient's electronic medical record shows no evidence of, malignancy, infection, endocrine disorders, neurologic disorders, chronic fatigue syndrome, gastroesophageal reflux disease, mastocytosis, panic disorder/anxiety, rosacea, temporal arteritis, hyperhidrosis, substance abuse, chronic opioid use.

❓ Can the information gathered so far be restated in a single sentence highlighting the pieces that narrow down the cause?

The problem representation in this case might be: "A 54-year-old man with known heart failure presents to the outpatient heart failure nurse practitioner clinic with a new complaint of night sweats."

Case Analysis

The patient has had an extensive diagnostic workup over the past 3 months without evidence of malignancy or infectious process. In addition, he has resumed his usual activities of daily living, daily exercise regimen of walking 1 mile in 20 minutes without stopping to rest, and is feeling better since he was discharged from the hospital, making infection and malignancy less of a concern. These conditions can be moved down on the list of potential etiologies for night sweats. Evaluating for these conditions is a high priority because they require additional testing and referral to other health care specialists for treatment. Review of the patients electronic medical record shows he was diagnosed with nonischemic cardiomyopathy and that he is on the appropriate evidence-based medications including lisinopril 10 mg daily (ACE-I), metoprolol succinate 25 mg daily (β-blocker), aspirin 81 mg daily, and furosemide 40 mg daily. Beta-blockers and aspirin can potentially cause flushing and/or night sweats. However, the patient has been on stable doses of these for 3 months and only recently developed night sweats, so these are less likely to be the cause of his symptoms and may be moved down the list. Patients with heart failure often have sleep-disordered breathing and sleep apnea. This patient has a history of loud snoring and his wife has witnessed apnea during his sleep. This information is important and will make sleep apnea move up higher on my differential as a possible etiology of night sweats.

CASE INFORMATION

Review of Systems

- Constitutional: The patient denies fever, chills, fatigue, appetite changes, unplanned weight changes, dental pain, vision changes, recent falls or injuries. He does endorse night sweats for the past week described as sweating over his entire head and upper body bilaterally and soaking his clothes. He recently lost over 15 lb while hospitalized for heart failure secondary to diuresis.
- Cardiovascular: The patient denies chest pain, palpitations, waking up at night short of breath, difficulty breathing when lying flat, leg swelling, loss of consciousness, or feeling as if he may lose consciousness.
- Pulmonary: The patient denies shortness of breath at rest or with activity, cough, or wheezing. He does endorse snoring that will occasionally wake him up at night. He reports his wife has complained that he snores loudly and "she gets upset when I stop breathing and starts shaking me to wake me up." He reports walking 1 mile daily in 20 minutes through his neighborhood and has not needed to stop and rest. He reports being able to climb two flights of stairs without stopping to rest.
- Gastrointestinal: The patient denies abdominal bloating, early satiety, nausea, vomiting, reflux, appetite changes, bowel changes, constipation, diarrhea, black stools, or blood in stools.
- Genitourinary: The patient denies blood in urine, pain with urination, change in urine color or odor, urinary hesitancy, urinary urgency (except after taking diuretic), incomplete bladder emptying, urinary incontinence. The patient does endorse frequent urination after taking diuretics and he reports waking up once nightly to urinate.
- Musculoskeletal: The patient denies muscle, joint pain, or any pain. The patient denies muscle weakness, falls, spinal cord or recent injuries.
- Neurological: The patient denies dizziness, falls, unsteady gait, numbness, tingling, weakness, or change in speech. The patient endorses occasional morning headaches.
- Endocrine: The patient denies changes in adjusting to cold or hot temperatures, increased thirst, hunger, or urination.
- Lymphatic: Denies nodes.

Physical Examination

- Vital signs: Height 5 ft 6 in, weight 273 lb, BMI 44.1 kg/m², pulse 72 bpm, blood pressure 102/54 mm Hg, respiratory rate 16, temperature 98.4°F oral, oxygen saturation 99 % on room air.
- Constitutional: Obese, well appearing and in no distress, sitting on the examination table. Appears his stated age.

- Head/eyes/ears/nose/throat: Pupils are equal, round, and reactive to light. Atraumatic, normocephalic, extraocular movements intact. No scleral icterus. Neck is thick, supple, trachea midline. Neck circumference = 44 cm. Oropharynx is moist with narrowing of lateral walls and enlarged tonsils bilaterally. Jugular venous distension difficult to appreciate given thick neck and body habitus.
- Cardiovascular: Heart rate and rhythm regular, no murmurs, no rubs, or gallops. Normal S1 and S2. No edema. Brisk capillary refill. Distal pulses, DP and PT, 1+ bilaterally.
- Pulmonary: Respiratory rate and rhythm are regular. Lungs are clear to auscultation bilaterally throughout. No accessory muscle use.
- Gastrointestinal: Obese, abdomen soft, nontender, nondistended without rebound or guarding. Normoactive bowel sounds. No ascites appreciated. No hepatomegaly or splenomegaly appreciated. Abdominal examination difficult given body habitus.
- Genitourinary: Normal examination.
- Neurological: No focal neurological deficits. Face is symmetrical, clear speech, moves bilateral upper and lower extremities spontaneously with 5/5 strength. Oriented to person, place, and time. Cranial nerves (CN) 2–12 intact.
- Skin: Intact without rashes, lacerations, excoriations, lesions, or ecchymoses. Normal skin turgor. No peripheral edema.
- Lymphatic : No lymphadenopathy although difficult to appreciate given body habitus.

? **What elements of the review of systems and physical examination should be added to the list of pertinent positives? Which items should be added to the list of significant negatives?**

- **Pertinent positives:** the patient endorses night sweats, occasional morning headaches, snoring, witnessed apneas, large neck circumference, enlarged tonsils, and patient is morbidly obese. The patient did recently lose 15 lb but that was secondary to diuresis while hospitalized for heart failure.

- **Significant negatives:** the patient denies fever, fatigue, unplanned weight changes, cough, hemoptysis, recent medication changes, hypertension, diarrhea, wheezing, heat or cold intolerance, spinal cord or other injuries. The patient's physical examination shows no fever, rashes, or lesions (present in mastocytosis), joint pain, lymphadenopathy, splenomegaly, abscess.

? How does this information affect the differential diagnosis list?

In reviewing the differential diagnosis list, it is most important to initially evaluate for malignancy or infection, as these will both require additional testing and possible referral to other health care specialists.[1] His admission records show no documentation of fever and all lab work, CXR, chest CT, and chest CTPA show no evidence of infection or malignancy. The patient denies any fever, fatigue, unplanned weight changes. His physical examination is unremarkable for lymphadenopathy or splenomegaly. I can now rule out lymphoma or other malignancies as a cause for night sweats in this patient. The patient denies travel outside the United States, cough, fever, fatigue, and hemoptysis. Diagnostic studies show no evidence of infectious processes so tuberculosis can be ruled out. The patient denies working with animals or animal products, eating raw or unpasteurized foods, or joint pain so brucellosis is not likely the cause and can also be ruled out as the cause for night sweats.[1] The patient has no known risk factors for HIV, including intravenous (IV) drug use or blood transfusion, so I can rule this out as a potential cause for night sweats.

The patient had normal TSH and T4 while hospitalized last week, which rules out hyperthyroidism as the cause of his night sweats. The patient has no known history of hypertension or tachycardia. Hospital records show blood pressure has ranged on the lower side and ECG documents normal sinus rhythm so pheochromocytoma is unlikely the cause of night sweats and can be ruled out. The patient denies flushing, which is a classic symptom in carcinoid syndrome. He also denies diarrhea or wheezing, thus carcinoid syndrome can be excluded as a cause.[1] He has not had any injuries. Medical records show no evidence of a neurological event and his physical examination was nonfocal so neurological disorders (autonomic dysreflexia, autonomic neuropathy, post-traumatic syringomyelia) can be excluded as the etiology for night sweats in this patient. The patient is male, so menopause is not the cause for night sweats. The patient has no known history of idiopathic hyperhidrosis, gastro-esophageal reflux, or diabetes, so those can be moved lower on the differential list. The patient has no evidence of rashes or lesions, nausea or vomiting, diarrhea, fatigue, infections, bone or muscle pain, anaphylaxis so mastocytosis can be ruled out as a potential cause for night sweats.[1] He has not had temporal pain, vision changes, jaw pain, scalp tenderness, fever or unplanned weight loss so temporal arteritis can now be excluded as a cause as well.[1] The patient has not had recent diet changes or a history of anxiety so those may also be excluded as the cause for night sweats.

At this point, I need to reexamine the data. The problem representation now is: "A 54-year-old morbidly obese man with a known history of heart failure, snoring, and witnessed apnea presents to the outpatient heart failure nurse practitioner clinic with a new onset of 'night sweats'." I have safely ruled out many of the causes on the differential diagnosis list and am now ready to order some further diagnostic testing.

❓ What diagnostic testing should be done and in what order?

The remaining diagnoses on the differential diagnosis list that have not been ruled out are stroke, infection, substance abuse with withdrawal, idiopathic hyperhidrosis, gastroesophageal reflux, diabetes, and sleep disorders. The patient shows no evidence of altered mental status and his physical examination shows he has no focal deficits so stroke is unlikely and I will not order a head CT scan at this time. The patient's history, physical examination, and review of medical records lack evidence for substance abuse or withdrawal. I review his information in the physician prescription monitoring program and find no history of any opioid prescriptions filled by the patient. For these reasons, I will not order a toxicology screen and rule out substance abuse and withdrawal as possible causes for night sweats. The patient denies any history of sweating or gastroesophageal disease so these can now be ruled out as the cause.

I order lab work including CBC with differential, comprehensive metabolic panel, B-type natriuretic peptide, urinalysis with culture, and two sets of blood cultures because infection was still a concern given the recent hospital stay. All results are normal and blood and urine cultures show no growth at 48 hours. The patient's white blood cell count (WBC) and urinalysis results are normal, he is afebrile, blood and urine cultures show no infection, and all recent diagnostic testing and physical examination show no evidence of an infectious processes. Infection can now be ruled out as the cause of night sweats in this patient.

The remaining diagnosis is sleep-disordered breathing. The patient endorses snoring that wakes him up at night and his wife has witnessed apneas while he is sleeping. His physical examination shows an obese body habitus, thick neck, enlarged tonsils, which all are common findings in patients with sleep-disordered breathing or sleep apnea. He has a history of heart failure and sleep-disordered breathing is known to be common in patients with heart failure. Ordinarily, sleep apnea is also associated with poorly controlled hypertension, which is absent in this case. However, given that there is strong evidence in favor of this diagnosis and the patient's PCP suspected sleep apnea on a prior examination, I conclude that sleep-disordered breathing is the most likely primary diagnosis in this patient with a complaint of night sweats. I refer the patient to the sleep clinic for in-laboratory overnight polysomnography. Results show the patient has severe obstructive sleep apnea.

Sleep-Disordered Breathing: Diagnosis and Treatment

Patients with heart failure, regardless of ejection fraction, have a high incidence of sleep-disordered breathing and it is thought to be underdiagnosed.[4] The reason sleep apnea is very prevalent in patients with heart failure is unclear; regardless diagnosing sleep-disordered breathing is important in these patients because when untreated, it is associated with adverse cardiovascular outcomes and a higher mortality.[4] Treatment of sleep-disordered breathing in patients with heart failure is associated with improved outcomes, increased left ventricular ejection fraction, improved functional status, and improved quality of life.[4] The most common types of sleep-disordered breathing found in patients with heart failure are obstructive sleep apnea and central sleep apnea with Cheyne-Stokes breathing.[4] Obstructive sleep apnea is defined as reduction or cessation of airflow during sleep due to upper airway closure, regardless of respiratory efforts.[4] During REM sleep, there is a generalized hypotonia of the muscles and with spontaneous breathing (negative pressure breathing) the airways collapse causing obstruction. Cheyne-Stokes breathing is defined as cyclical crescendo-decrescendo inspiration and expiration while the patient is awake or asleep and is without obstruction.[4] When apnea accompanies decrescendo breathing, central sleep apnea syndrome is generally the diagnosis.[4] The gold standard testing for sleep-disordered breathing is an overnight polysomnogram.[4] This can be done in a sleep clinic laboratory or by in-home portable monitoring, though in-home portable overnight polysomnogram has not been well studied and is not recommended for patients with heart failure due to the complexity of sleep-disordered breathing commonly found in this patient population.[4]

2013 Guidelines for the Treatment of Sleep-Disordered Breathing[2-6]

The 2013 American College of Cardiology Foundation/American Heart Association guidelines recommend treating sleep-disordered breathing in patients with heart failure. Goals of treatment are improved functional capacity and increasing left ventricular ejection fraction.[2] The primary treatment of sleep-disordered breathing is accomplished with the provision of continuous positive airway pressure (CPAP) during sleep. CPAP provides a pneumatic splint to the upper airways continuously throughout the respiratory cycle, which prevents obstruction and subsequent apneas. If apnea is not due to airway obstruction, Bi-PAP (two levels of positive pressure: pressure support [inspiratory pressure] and PEEP [positive end-expiratory pressure]) can be used with a backup respiratory rate to prevent apneic episodes.

In a large randomized controlled trial with 258 patients, aged 53 to 73 years old, with a diagnosis of heart failure with ejection fraction ranging 16.8% to 32.3%, and on optimal medical therapy for heart failure, patients were randomly assigned to receive CPAP or no CPAP and were followed for 2 years. Results suggested that the use of CPAP for obstructive sleep apnea effectively decreased the apnea-hypopnea index, improved nocturnal oxygenation, increased LVEF, lowered norepinephrine levels, and increased the distance walked in 6 minutes. These benefits were sustained for up to 2 years.[2]

Estimates related to adherence to the use of CPAP indicate that 83% of patients do not adhere.[5] Adherence may be defined as wearing CPAP for at least, or more than, 4 hours during sleeping.[6] Some potential predictors of CPAP adherence include adherence with CPAP the first week of therapy, higher self-reported daytime sleepiness with moderate to severe OSA, higher severity of oxyhemoglobin desaturation while sleeping, lower nasal volume, the patient is not claustrophobic, the patient has positive problem-solving skills and is optimistic about the benefit of CPAP therapy, the patient has self-efficacy or confidence to engage in healthy behaviors, and the patient sought medical attention.[6] Interventions that have been shown to be helpful in improving CPAP adherence are the management of the side effects of CPAP therapy and behavioral therapy.[6] Examples of managing CPAP side effects are: including the patient in the choice of mask type and fit, humidification, and discussing ways to cope with the potential interference of intimacy or sexual activity.[6] Behavioral therapy interventions include regular patient follow-up, support, and education.[6]

Obstructive sleep apnea can have serious comorbidities and adherence to CPAP is challenging despite its importance. However, improvement of the patient's status is possible if the provider works with the patient to manage side effects of CPAP, educates the patient, and provides close follow-up.[6] In this case, the patient was prescribed nasal CPAP at 11 cm H_2O and he reported using CPAP while sleeping for a minimum of 5 hours each night. After 3 months, the patient returned for a follow-up visit and reported he felt much better and that prior to using his CPAP, he was not aware how fatigued he had become. The patient has continued to walk daily but recently increased walking up to 1.5 miles in 25 minutes. He also planted a new vegetable garden in his yard. He was planning to go on a family vacation and had already contacted his home supply company to look into how to travel with his CPAP, as now he reports not being able to sleep without it.

References

1. Smetana G. Approach to the patient with night sweats. UptoDate Web site. http://www.uptodate.com/contents/approach-to-the-patient-with-night-sweats. Accessed July 22, 2014.
2. Yancy CW, Jessup M, Bozkurt B, et al. 2013 ACCF/AHA guideline for the management of heart failure: a report of the American College of Cardiology Foundation/American Heart Association Task Force on Practice Guidelines. *J Am Coll Cardiol*. 2013;62(16):e147-e239. doi: 10.1016/j.jacc.2013.05.
3. Lindenfeld J, Albert NM, Boehmer JP, et al. Executive summary: HFSA 2010 comprehensive heart failure practice guideline. *J Card Fail*. 2010;16(6):475-539. doi: 10.1016/j.cardfail.2010.04.
4. Malhotra A, Fang JC. Sleep disordered breathing in heart failure. UptoDate Web site. http://www.uptodate.com/contents/sleep-disordered-breathing-in-heart-failure. Accessed August 6, 2014.
5. Bradley TD, Alexander GL, Kimoff RJ, et al. Continuous positive airway pressure for central sleep apnea and heart failure. *N Engl J Med*. 2005;353(19):2025-2033.
6. Weaver TE, Grunstein RR. Adherence to continuous positive airway pressure: the challenge to effective treatment. *Proc Am Thorac Soc*. 2008;8:173-178. doi: 10.1513/pats.200708-119MG.

Susan Yeager and April J. Kastner

Susan is the Lead NP in the Neurocritical Care Unit at The Ohio State University Wexner Medical Center and serves as Clinical Instructor at The Ohio State University College of Nursing in Columbus. April works as an NP in the Neurocritical Care Unit at The Ohio State University Wexner Medical Center in Columbus.

CASE INFORMATION

Chief Complaint

A 65-year-old male was brought by the rescue squad to the emergency room after being found comatose on the floor of his garage at the bottom of a 15-ft ladder. He was intubated at the scene for airway protection and remains unresponsive. Past medical history is unknown as a neighbor found the patient; however, the neighbor notes alcohol intake of unknown frequency or quantity. Computed tomography scan (CT scan) imaging of his cervical spine was negative but brain imaging showed diffuse, traumatic subarachnoid hemorrhage; small right-sided epidural hematoma (EDH); and large holohemispheric left subdural hematoma (SDH) with subsequent tentorial herniation. The left-sided SDH was evacuated and a hemicraniectomy was performed to minimize the mass effect of the cerebral edema. The patient was admitted to the neurocritical care unit (NCCU) for ongoing management and treatment. The patient initially regained some movement in the left upper and the left lower extremities postoperatively. However, we are now called by the bedside nurse on postoperative day 1 because of an acute loss of his left-sided motor function, new right eye deviation, and coma.

❓ What is the potential cause?

Acute neurologic changes in this patient warrant immediate attention with rapid prioritization of potential causes. Organic and neurologic sources are both possibilities and can be ruled out with both bedside and diagnostic evaluations. System-specific potential etiologies are listed below.

> **Focused Differential Diagnoses for Acute Neurologic Changes Resulting in Coma in a Postoperative, Traumatic Brain Injured Patient**
>
> • Neurologic: seizure or nonconvulsive status epilepticus, postictal state, reaccumulation of left-sided SDH, right EDH expansion, herniation from expanding cerebral edema or hematoma, diffuse axonal injury,

anoxic injury, acute hemorrhagic or ischemic stroke, tension pneumocephalus, elevated intracranial pressure (ICP), or acute spinal compression

- Metabolic: hyper- or hypoglycemia, hyper- or hyponatremia
- Psychiatric: supratherapeutic sedation, slow metabolism of analgesics
- Infection: meningitis, encephalitis, brain abscess, urinary tract infection, aspiration pneumonia
- Toxicology: alcohol withdrawal

 CASE INFORMATION

While the above list of potential etiologies is lengthy, the advantage of experience and previous knowledge of this patient's history enables us to quickly scan the patient and data to rapidly prioritize our list of diagnoses. The initial approach to this patient is to review the vital signs, including the intracranial pressure (ICP), and complete a thorough neurologic and total body examination.

His vital signs are as follows: temperature 97.6°F, heart rate 105 beats per minute; systolic blood pressure 148 mm Hg; mean arterial pressure 80 mm Hg; oxygen saturation 98% on 40% oxygen; respiratory rate is 18 breaths per minute with a set ventilator rate of 12 breaths/minute. His intracranial pressure is 18 mm Hg with a cerebral perfusion pressure of 70 mm Hg. The intraventricular catheter is leveled at 10 mm Hg and is actively draining clear cerebral spinal fluid. A normal intracranial pressure waveform is noted. The patient is currently on 5 mg/hour of nicardipine by intravenous (IV) infusion along with maintenance IV normal saline at 75 mL/hour. Per the bedside nurse, the propofol infusion has been off for approximately 30 minutes and the patient's last dose of bolus, as needed, fentanyl was 6 hours ago. Laboratory findings are: sodium 142 mEq/L, blood urea nitrogen 8 mg/dL, creatinine 0.7 mg/dL, glucose 105 mmol/L, white blood cell count 11,000 cells/mL, hemoglobin 11 g/dL, platelets 205,000/µL, international ratio 1.1, and admission urinalysis and toxicology screen are both negative.

? What are the pertinent positives from the information given so far?

- Neurological: A high normal ICP is noted in a patient with a hemicraniectomy.
- Cardiopulmonary: The patient is tachycardic with blood pressure elevation requiring continuous infusion of nicardipine.
- Psychiatric: The patient has the potential history of recent alcohol consumption of an unknown amount, frequency, or last date of consumption.

❓ What are the significant negatives from the information given so far?

- Neurological: Ventriculostomy is draining without blood or abnormal waveform or cerebral perfusion pressure (CPP) findings. He is breathing over the ventilator. Fentanyl has not been given in 6 hours and the propofol has been off for at least 30 minutes.
- Cardiopulmonary: The patient is without hypoxemia.
- Laboratory: No abnormalities are noted with the patient's chemistry, hematology, coagulopathy, toxicology, or urinalysis results.

❓ What is the problem representation at this point?

The problem representation in this case might be: "a 65-year-old male postoperative day 1 from left-sided hemicraniectomy with SDH evacuation now with declining neurologic examination."

Case Analysis

Given the information obtained so far we quickly consider the findings and begin to sort our differential. We note that the normal laboratory findings and normothermia rule out infectious (meningitis, encephalitis, sepsis, abscess, urinary tract infection, or aspiration pneumonia) or metabolic causes (hypo/hyperglycemia or hypo/hypernatremia). Given the negative toxicology screen, and the fact that alcohol withdrawal does not cause lateralizing findings, the likelihood that alcohol withdrawal is the cause of the patient's changes is low. High normal ICPs in a patient with a partial skull removal, and the report of new left-sided weakness, are concerning because there may be a new space-occupying lesion such as worsening brain edema or bleeding. New onset seizure or acute stroke can also cause heart rate, blood pressure, and intracranial reading elevation. Pain and agitation, or a sympathetic surge following his trauma and operation, can also be associated with these vital sign findings but are not associated with the loss of motor function. While diffuse axonal injury and/or anoxic brain may be present, these pathologies do not generally cause acute localized findings. Therefore, pain, agitation, sympathetic surge, anoxic brain, or diffuse axonal injury are no longer in our immediate list of potential causes of the acute neurologic changes. We will need additional information and thus proceed with a full evaluation of the patient.

CASE INFORMATION

Review of Systems

Unable to obtain due to coma.

Physical Examination

- Constitutional: The patient is intubated without diaphoresis or abnormal breathing.

- Cardiovascular: His bedside ECG shows sinus tachycardia without ischemic changes. Heart sounds demonstrate a normal S1, S2 without a murmur, rub, gallop, or click. An arterial line is present in his left radial artery with a normal waveform. 2+ pulses are noted throughout.
- Pulmonary: The patient is breathing over the 12 ventilator-assisted breaths with a total respiratory rate of 18 respirations per minute without accessory muscle use. Lungs are clear to auscultation but diminished in the bases bilaterally. Previously obtained chest radiography is negative for acute pulmonary processes.
- Gastrointestinal: His abdomen is soft, obese, and with hypoactive bowel sounds. Nasogastric intact with green gastric drainage.
- Genitourinary: Foley catheter in place with clear yellow urine. Urinary output is within normal range.
- Integumentary: With the exception of his sutured forehead laceration and postoperative site, his skin is intact, without rashes, lesions, or sores. Normal skin turgor.
- Neurological: Positive cough, corneal, gag reflexes; conjugate gaze with right eye deviation; equal, round, and reactive pupils at 3 mm, new left-sided hemiplegia and baseline right-sided hemiplegia despite noxious stimulation. He is not following commands but this finding is unchanged from his postoperative baseline. No facial asymmetry or ptosis but these are difficult to assess given the presence of life support devices and his unresponsiveness. No tonic clonic or twitching motor findings are evident. His Miami J collar is intact and is appropriately sized and placed. His neck is midline and no step-offs or deformities of his spine are palpated. His left hemicraniectomy incision is open to air without drainage. His brain is palpable beneath skin over the hemicraniectomy site and is slightly firm.

❓ What elements of the review of systems and the physical examination should be added to the list of pertinent positives?

- Neurological: New findings include right eye deviation, and left-sided plegia. He has no response to noxious stimulation. His hemicraniectomy site is slightly firm.

❓ What elements of the review of systems and the physical examination should be added to the list of significant negatives?

- Neurological: The spine is without step-off or deformity. As stated earlier (and in case 70, Part A of this case), the CT scan of his cervical spine did not demonstrate fractures or obvious spinal cord injury. The Miami J collar is appropriately fitted; therefore, no cervical venous compression is likely. Pupils are symmetric and his gaze is not disconjugate. Cough, gag, and corneal reflexes are intact. Facial asymmetry does not appear to be present though difficult to ascertain. No visible signs of seizure are noted.

- Cardiovascular: No murmurs, rubs, or gallops are noted. No arrhythmias or abnormalities are appreciated on bedside telemetry. Pulses and arterial line waveforms are within normal limits. No diaphoresis noted.

- Pulmonary: No ventilator asynchrony, abnormal x-ray findings, or hypoxia are noted. The patient is breathing above the ventilator.

- Gastrointestinal, genitourinary, integumentary systems are all without abnormal findings.

❓ How does this information affect the list of possible causes?

The addition of the right eye deviation increases the likelihood of new onset subclinical seizures, expanding right epidural hematoma, acute stroke, or acute intraparenchymal hemorrhage. Generally, if a patient is having seizures, the eyes will deviate away from the seizure ictus. In the event of intracranial bleeding, the patient's eyes will deviate toward the source of bleeding or intracranial abnormality. His left-sided subdural hematoma and brain injury can cause brain inflammation, which causes brain irritation and puts him at higher risk for seizure. As no outward signs of seizure are appreciated, we need to consider subclinical seizure activity. The term "subclinical seizures" means that despite the lack of physical motor signs, abnormal electrical brain activity (ie, intermittent seizure or status epilepticus) is a possibility.[1] An EEG to record electrical brain activity will determine if the patient is having subclinical seizures. Once in place, the EEG can be left in place for continuous monitoring for seizure activity.

Other possible explanations of his acute left-sided hemiplegia with right eye deviation include the expansion of the known right-sided epidural hematoma, the development of new hemorrhagic or ischemic stroke, or the evolution of brain contusion. Acute ischemic stroke can occur when increased intracranial pressure and acute herniation cause vascular and tissue compression. For example, small vessel compression from brain edema and acute subdural hematoma can result in a lack of blood flow with subsequent ischemic changes. Additionally, the rapid reexpansion of the brain following hematoma evacuation can lead to blood vessel shearing, which may result in new brain hemorrhage or epidural expansion. Brain contusions can be microscopic upon patient admission and can blossom to larger space-occupying lesions despite small or limited presence on the initial CT head.

❓ What diagnostic testing should be done and in what order?

Immediate radiographic, diagnostic testing should begin with a noncontrast CT scan of his head. This will quickly rule out new or expanding brain bleeding. We would not obtain an MRI in this patient at this point for several reasons. First, in all TBI patients, brain monitoring system compatibility with the MRI magnet needs to be considered. While this patient's intraventricular device is compatible with MRI, this diagnostic is not necessary for treatment at this point in his evaluation. The reason for this is that the results will not change our course of management. If he did suffer a stroke, his recent surgery and brain bleeding are both contraindications for thrombolytic therapy, such as tissue plasminogen activator (TPA). Additionally, the source of this patient's ischemia would not be amenable to thrombolytic therapy. This is because the likely source of ischemia, if it has occurred, is brain compression from acute herniation syndrome. For this patient, the compression syndrome has already been minimized with the evacuation of his subdural hematoma and his hemicraniectomy. Ischemic stroke in a trauma patient may also be related to carotid artery dissection. While this is a possibility, it is less likely in this patient given the absence of cervical vertebral fracture. If carotid dissection were to occur, antiplatelet therapy would be the treatment strategy. Given his fresh intracranial bleeding, this treatment would not be started at this point in his recovery.

CASE INFORMATION

Diagnostic Testing Results

CT scan imaging on this patient rules out a new or an expanding bleed. Therefore, seizure should be considered the most likely differential diagnosis for his acute neurologic changes. To evaluate the presence of nonconvulsive seizures, a stat continuous EEG is ordered. With application of the EEG device, the patient is noted to have nonconvulsive status epilepticus (NCSE).[1]

Nonconvulsive Status Epilepticus: Diagnosis and Treatment

As with any patient situation, treatment should begin by ensuring that the patient has a stable airway, is breathing effectively, has circulatory access, and is hemodynamically stable. This patient already has an endotracheal tube with ventilator support that is effective based on stable oxygen saturations and synchronous breathing. He has central venous access and his vital signs are stable, indicating adequate circulation. An additional consideration in a neurologic patient is that even though vital signs are within an appropriate range, augmentation of a patient's blood pressure with vasoactive agents may be required to maintain adequate cerebral perfusion pressures (CPP). In traumatic brain injured patients, the CPP goal is 70 mm Hg.[2] His CPP is above this goal. Therefore, the priority goal of treatment is to emergently stop electrographic seizure activity. Lorazepam is the preferred intravenous agent but if access is limited, midazolam can be administered intramuscularly and diazepam can be administered rectally. This patient is given 4 mg of lorazepam intravenous bolus and loaded with 20 mg/kg of fosphenytoin followed by a maintenance dose of 100 mg every 8 hours. Administration of all antiepileptic agents should always be followed by the administration of a maintenance dose. The approved agents used to control NCSE are fosphenytoin/phenytoin and valproate sodium, phenobarbital, levetiracetam, or continuous infusions of midazolam, propofol, or ketamine. A combination with escalation of these medications may be necessary to maintain a seizure-free situation. The favored agent in most patients is fosphenytoin; however, in those with a history of primary generalized epilepsy, valproate sodium is the choice agent. Continuous EEG monitoring even when the initial seizure activity has ceased is needed as there is a risk of reoccurrence.[1]

Case Follow-Up

After several days without seizure on the cEEG, the patient remains comatose with a very poor examination. Because of this, the decision is made to obtain an MRI. The results show severe diffuse axonal injury (DAI) as well as holohemispheric stroke to the left side of his brain. Diffuse axonal injury occurs when there is sheer force to the brain that causes stretching with nonreversible damage to the neuronal axons.[3] In the majority of patients, the left brain hemisphere controls language expression and comprehension. Given the severity of the DAI and language effects of the left brain injury, prognosis and goals of care were discussed with the family. Palliative medicine is involved in this discussion and ultimately the collaborative decision is made for terminal withdrawal of life support.

References

1. Brophy GM, Bell R, Claassen J, et al. Guidelines for the evaluation and management of status epilepticus. *Neurocrit Care*. August 2012;17(1):3-23. doi: 10.1007/s12028-012-9695-z.
2. Brain Trauma Foundation. Guidelines for the management of severe traumatic brain injury. *J Trauma*. 2007;24(1):1-116.
3. Craniocerebral trauma. In: Hickey JV, ed. *The Clinical Practice of Neurological and Neurosurgical Nursing*. 8th ed. Lippincott Williams & Wilkins; 2014:382-385.

CASE 68

Nicolle L. Schraeder

Nicolle Schraeder works as an Acute Care NP with Neuroscience Department at Littleton Adventist Hospital. Nicolle follows all neurosurgery patients in the acute care setting from ED to discharge. Nicolle also leads education efforts for nursing staff regarding neurological injuries and disorders.

CASE INFORMATION

Chief Complaint

A 50-year-old female is admitted to the emergency department with headache, dysarthria, and left-sided weakness.

❓ What is the potential cause?

A change in neurological status with focal deficits and left-sided weakness is likely related to some disruption within the brain or spine. However, my differential must be comprehensive and broad so the correct diagnosis is determined and treated. In addition, life-threatening causes must be immediately identified and treated emergently.

> ### Comprehensive Differential Diagnoses for Patients With Acute Headache[1]
>
> - Neurologic: Elevated intracranial pressure, benign intracranial hypertension, brain tumor, hypertension encephalopathy, eclampsia, acute hydrocephalus, ischemic versus hemorrhagic acute stroke, venous sinus thrombus, epidural hematoma, subarachnoid hemorrhage, subdural hematoma, traumatic brain injury, seizure, multiple sclerosis, migraines.
> - Cardiovascular: Hypertensive encephalopathy.
> - Musculoskeletal: Spinal cord stenosis, spinal cord injury, tension headaches, temporomandibular joint syndrome (TMJ).
> - Trauma: Unwitnessed fall with possible trauma.
> - Infectious: Meningitis, brain abscess, acute sinusitis.
> - Facial: Trigeminal neuralgia.
> - Other: Acute mountain sickness/hypoxia, cluster headaches, acute angle-closure glaucoma.

I begin my evaluation with the history of present illness. This includes determining the duration and severity of symptoms as well as any related sequelae that may indicate whether this is slowly presenting presentation or an acute or life-threatening presentation. If the condition is life threatening, immediate action is required.

CASE INFORMATION

History of Present Illness

This 50-year-old female has not seen a doctor in a number of years and reports headaches over the past 2 weeks, which she treated at home with ibuprofen. The night of admission, she went to bed but woke around midnight to get some water and ibuprofen, and fell. Her husband heard her fall and when he arrived at her side he noted she was not moving her left side and was confused and disoriented. She also had garbled speech and was complaining of headache by holding her head and moaning. The husband called 911 and EMS arrived approximately 5 to 10 minutes after the fall. The paramedics stated that she vomited en route to the hospital and again in the emergency department (ED). Her blood pressure en route was 208 over palpable, she was in sinus rhythm, and her blood sugar was 91. The EMS assessment also noted confusion, garbled speech, and absence of movement on her left side to painful stimuli. EMS called the ED en route to initiate a "stroke alert." The estimated time elapsed from the fall to the patient's arrival in the ED is 15 to 20 minutes.

General Survey

I arrive at the patient's bedside as she is being admitted to the ED and I note the patient's altered and nonverbal status. Her speech is garbled and she is confused and unaware of where she is. I obtain some information from the patient's husband. He states that she has not been diagnosed with chronic medical problems such as diabetes, hypertension, heart disease, cancer, and he is not aware of her ever having a seizure or stroke. To his knowledge, she has no recent history of fevers, chills, nausea, vomiting, dyspnea, cough, pain in the chest, abdomen, or back. She has not complained of numbness, tingling, paresthesias, or edema of the extremities. Her mood and affect were normal with the exception of having recurrent headaches.

? **What are the pertinent positives from the information given so far?**

- The patient has had headaches for 2 weeks that were mildly relieved with ibuprofen.
- The patient fell with noted left-sided weakness, mental status changes, dysarthria, and vomiting.
- The patient has significantly elevated blood pressure in the ambulance and in the ED.

> **?** **What are the significant negatives from the information given so far?**

- The patient has not had any recent fevers, chills, vomiting (prior to her fall), dyspnea, and cough, pain in the chest, abdomen, or back.
- No history of prior falls.
- No medical history of chronic disorders such as seizures or stroke.
- No trauma prior to episode such as blow to the head.

> **?** **Can the information gathered so far be stated in a single statement—a problem representation?**

The problem representation at this time might be: "A 50-year-old female with unknown prior medical history presents with new onset mental status changes, dysarthria, left-hemiparesis, headaches, vomiting, and elevated blood pressure."

> **?** **How does this information affect the list of possible causes?**

I first consider life-threatening causes of my patient's neurologic symptoms. Given what I know so far about the patient, I am mostly concerned that the patient's mental status changes may be due to a neurologic event. As the patient presents with a focal neurological deficit, left-sided weakness, it is possible that she may have sustained an ischemic or hemorrhagic stroke. A cardiac cause of her neurologic status is unlikely as she is in normal sinus rhythm and has no noted history of chest pain or rhythm disturbances such as atrial fibrillation. But I cannot rule out stroke from an embolus as a result of atrial fibrillation. Although she is in sinus rhythm now it is possible that she has experienced intermittent atrial fibrillation with clot formation and subsequent embolization to her brain. Ischemic and hemorrhagic strokes are treated differently but in both, time is of essence.

I recognize that the focal weakness as noted in the patient may help me rule out many differential diagnoses that present with more generalized or isolated symptoms. As I continue to think through my differential, I keep this in mind. To that end, I quickly and efficiently evaluate her further for stroke while also continuing to consider other specific diagnostic possibilities.

Per the husband's account, the patient's overall well state of health and the absence of fever or chills prior to the event make an acute infection less likely; however, encephalitis or meningitis is not ruled out at this point. Endocrine disorders such as adrenal insufficiency, diabetic coma, and thyrotoxicosis are unlikely since they tend not to present with focal changes but rather general changes such as weakness and confusion. This is also the case with severe electrolyte disturbances. For now they are much lower on my differential but cannot yet be ruled out. Further testing will be necessary.

Benign intracranial hypertension rarely presents with focal one-sided weakness, nor does hypertensive encephalopathy unless it results in hemorrhage. Acute hydrocephalus presents with generalized deficits not with one-sided weakness. And, acute hydrocephalus is rarely seen in isolation without other medical causes.

The patient's medical history obtained from her husband does not include pregnancy and this is unlikely given her age so eclampsia is quickly ruled out. The patient does have headaches and dysarthria, which makes a spinal diagnosis unlikely as well, but not completely ruled out. This is especially true if the defect is in the cervical spinal region such as with cervical injury. Vertebral dissection at this level may cause decreased blood flow to the brain. Trigeminal neuralgia does not present with left-sided weakness. I quickly eliminate acute mountain sickness and acute glaucoma from the differential as she is not at an elevated altitude and acute glaucoma presents with vision changes and not left-sided weakness.

Migraines can cause focal neurological changes and stroke; however, the patient is deteriorating quickly and this is unusual in the case of severe status migraines. Cluster headaches are also a less likely cause because they present with unilateral, orbital, supraorbital, and/or temporal area pain. These headaches predominately affect men and are not associated with cranial nerve deficits or confusion and altered mental status as I see in my patient. For now migraines and cluster headaches are much lower on my differential.

While I am considering all of the possible causes for my patient's condition I place stroke highest on my differential and proceed to complete a rapid and comprehensive history and physical. I also order a stat ECG to rule out an acute cardiac event or arrhythmia that may put her at risk for stroke, and a stat non-contrast computed tomography (CT) scan of her head.[2]

CASE INFORMATION

Physical Examination

- Vital signs on arrival: Temperature 36.0°C oral, heart rate 79 beats per minute, respiratory rate 20 breaths per minute, blood pressure 251/136 with a mean arterial pressure of 174 mm Hg, oxygen saturation 96% on 3L nasal cannula, ECG at bedside: sinus rhythm with rate of 79 beats per minute.
- General appearance: Decreased mental status, she opens eyes to verbal and tactile stimuli and is able to follow commands, yet with dense left hemiparesis (meaning no movement at all even to painful stimuli).
- Head/eyes/ears/nose/throat: Normocephalic, atraumatic. Pupils equal and round, reactive to light. The patient does have disconjugate gaze. Normal extraocular movements with the right eye, left eye is unable to look laterally. Mucous membranes moist, throat without erythema. Able to stick out her tongue to command without noted deviation.

- Cardiovascular: Regular rate and rhythm, no murmur, rubs, or gallops, 2+ bilateral radial and dorsalis pedis pulses.
- Pulmonary: No accessory muscle use or labored breathing, retractions, lungs are clear bilaterally to auscultation, without wheezes, crackles, or rhonchi.
- Gastrointestinal: Normal bowel sounds, abdomen is soft and nontender, no masses
- Neurological: Initially opens eyes to verbal stimuli and follows commands with right side 5/5 strength and slight movement to left side 1/5 strength. However, within 5 minutes of arrival, and before the head CT scan, her mental status rapidly deteriorates and she is unable to protect her airway or follow commands. A positive left Babinski is noted (which presents with upward flaring of the great toe). She is unable to follow commands with her legs upon arrival, but on my examination, both her left arm and left leg are flaccid with no movement at all-even to painful stimuli. The patient initially had good grip strength with her right hand but this deteriorates rapidly during my assessment. The p atient's initial National Institutes of Health Stroke Scale (NIHSS) score is 28, but after her rapid decline the second NIHSS score is unobtainable due to her unresponsiveness (see Table 68-1 and Box 68-1).
- Skin: Warm and dry, no rashes.
- Musculoskeletal: Neck is supple, no cervical tenderness or palpable deformity. Extremities are symmetrical and no lower extremity edema.
- Psychiatric: Noncontributory.

Table 68-1   NIH Stroke Scale

Instructions	Scale Definition	Score
1a. Level of consciousness	0 = Alert; keenly responsive.	
	1 = Not alert; but arousable by minor stimulation to obey, answer, or respond.	
	2 = Not alert; requires repeated stimulation to attend, or is obtunded and requires strong or painful stimulation to make movements (not stereotyped).	_____
	3 = Responds only with reflex motor or autonomic effects or totally unresponsive, flaccid, and areflexic.	
1b. LOC questions	0 = Answers both questions correctly.	
	1 = Answers one question correctly.	_____
	2 = Answers neither question correctly.	

(continued)

Table 68-1 **NIH Stroke Scale** (Continued)

Instructions	Scale Definition	Score
1c. LOC commands	0 = Performs both tasks correctly.	
	1 = Performs one task correctly.	
	2 = Performs neither task correctly.	_____
2. Best gaze	0 = Normal.	
	1 = Partial gaze palsy; gaze is abnormal in one or both eyes, but forced deviation or total gaze paresis is not present.	_____
	2 = Forced deviation, or total gaze paresis not overcome by the oculocephalic maneuver.	
3. Visual	0 = No visual loss.	
	1 = Partial hemianopia.	
	2 = Complete hemianopia.	_____
	3 = Bilateral hemianopia (blind including cortical blindness).	
4. Facial palsy	0 = Normal symmetrical movements.	
	1 = Minor paralysis (flattened nasolabial fold, asymmetry on smiling).	
	2 = Partial paralysis (total or near-total paralysis of lower face).	_____
	3 = Complete paralysis of one or both sides (absence of facial movement in the upper and lower face).	
5. Motor arm	0 = No drift; limb holds 90° (or 45°) for full 10 seconds.	
	1 = Drift; limb holds 90° (or 45°), but drifts down before full 10 seconds; does not hit bed or other support.	
	2 = Some effort against gravity; limb cannot get to or maintain (if cued) 90° (or 45°), drifts down to bed, but has some effort against gravity.	
	3 = No effort against gravity; limb falls.	
	4 = No movement.	
	UN = Amputation or joint fusion, explain: _____	
	5a. Left arm	_____
	5b. Right arm	_____
6. Motor leg	0 = No drift; leg holds 30° position for full 5 seconds.	
	1 = Drift; leg falls by the end of the 5-second period but does not hit bed.	
	2 = Some effort against gravity; leg falls to bed by 5 seconds, but has some effort against gravity.	
	3 = No effort against gravity; leg falls to bed immediately.	
	4 = No movement.	
	UN = Amputation or joint fusion, explain: _____	
	6a. Left leg	_____
	6b. Right leg	

Table 68-1   NIH Stroke Scale (Continued)

Instructions	Scale Definition	Score
7. Limb ataxia	0 = Absent.	
	1 = Present in one limb.	_____
	2 = Present in two limbs.	
	UN = Amputation or joint fusion, explain: _____	
8. Sensory	0 = Normal; no sensory loss.	
	1 = Mild to moderate sensory loss; the patient feels pinprick is less sharp or is dull on the affected side; or there is a loss of superficial pain with pinprick, but patient is aware of being touched.	_____
	2 = Severe to total sensory loss; patient is not aware of being touched in the face, arm, and leg.	
9. Best language	0 = No aphasia; normal.	
	1 = Mild to moderate aphasia; some obvious loss of fluency or facility or comprehension, without significant limitation on ideas expressed or form of expression. Reduction of speech and/or comprehension, however, makes conversation about provided materials difficult or impossible. For example, in conversation about provided materials, examiner can identify picture or naming card content from patient's response.	_____
	2 = Severe aphasia; all communication is through fragmentary expression; great need for inference, questioning, and guessing by the listener. Range of information that can be exchanged is limited; listener carries burden of communication. The examiner cannot identify materials provided from patient response.	
	3 = Mute, global aphasia; no usable speech or auditory comprehension.	
10. Dysarthria	0 = Normal.	
	1 = Mild to moderate dysarthria; patient slurs at least some word and, at worst, can be understood with some difficulty.	_____
	2 = Severe dysarthria; patient's speech is so slurred as to be unintelligible in the absence of or out of proportion to any dysphasia, or is mute/anarthric.	
	UN = Intubated or other physical barrier, explain:_____	
11. Extinction and Inattention (formerly neglect)	0 = No abnormality.	
	1 = Visual, tactile, auditory, spatial, or personal inattention or extinction to bilateral simultaneous stimulation in one of the sensory modalities.	_____
	2 = Profound hemi-inattention or extinction to more than one modality; does not recognize own hand or orients to only one side of space.	

Reproduced from National Institute of Neurological Disorders and Stroke. National Institutes of Health (NIH). Retrieved June 11, 2015. http://www.ninds.nih.gov/disorders/stroke/strokescales.htm. Updated June 2, 2008.

> **BOX 68-1** NIHSS Score and Use of tPA
>
> The NIHSS score is initially completed with any patient presenting with stroke symptoms. The greater the score, the more severe the stroke or neurological deficit. This score guides practice related to the use of thrombolytic agents. For example, a very high score of 21 may preclude the use of tissue plasminogen activator (tPA) or other thrombolytic therapy while a score of less than 4 indicates a minor stroke and risks of tPA may outweigh the benefits, thus tPA may not be given.[2] When the score is between 4 and 21, that is when tPA is most often given. Giving tPA with high or low scores warrants risk-benefit discussion among the team and the patient and family. Generally, the score is recalculated after treatment with thrombolytic or interventional treatment and at the time of discharge. But because the scale serves as a useful measure of progression of recovery, some hospitals use it throughout the hospital stay.[2]

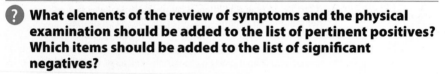

? What elements of the review of symptoms and the physical examination should be added to the list of pertinent positives? Which items should be added to the list of significant negatives?

Pertinent Positives

- Elevated blood pressure
- Rapidly deteriorating neurological examination
- Disconjugate gaze
- Unable to protect airway
- Left hemiparesis
- Positive left Babinski
- The patient able to follow commands on arrival but rapidly declined to unresponsive.

Significant Negatives

- No neck or back pain on palpation,
- no noted visual trauma to head or bruising indicating significant traumatic event,
- no noted muscle twitching or noticeable seizure like movements on examination.
- Normal cardiovascular and pulmonary examinations.

? How does this information affect the list of possible causes?

My differential is rapidly evolving and I revisit and re-sort the diagnoses given confirmatory and/or negative evidence as noted in my examination. A cardiac event is very unlikely due to the focal neurological deficits noted and because her cardiac exam is normal and her ECG shows normal sinus rhythm. However, because she has neurological deficits that can potentially be related to an ischemic event, paroxysmal atrial fibrillation cannot be ruled out yet. As noted earlier, hypertensive encephalopathy is less likely with focal neurological deficits. Encephalopathy and meningitis without brain injury present with generalized confusion, decreased level of consciousness, and general neurological deficits versus focal deficits. There has been no blunt trauma to her head and there are no notable assessment findings that suggest that a blow to the head might be responsible for her neurological deficits. The patient has hemiparesis on her left side along with cranial nerve deficits, which rules out a spinal stenosis or trauma. In spinal stenosis the patient would not have cranial nerve deficits such as the disconjugate gaze, thus spinal cord involvement is less likely.

At this point I think a cranial process is the most likely cause of the patient's symptoms. It is important to identify symptoms that need to be treated urgently, such as the patient's ability to protect her airway and emergency treatment options. Cranial processes that need urgent treatment include ischemic and hemorrhagic strokes.

❓ What diagnostic tests should be done at this time?

CT scan of the head is the highest priority diagnostic test. Many facilities have a CT protocol that takes a patient directly from the ambulance to radiology for a CT scan if they have stroke-like symptoms. Once the CT scan of the head

CASE INFORMATION

Diagnostic Testing Results

The patient's CT scan shows a large 6-cm right-sided intraparenchymal hemorrhage with a 16-mm leftward midline shift (Figure 68-1). While the patient was in the CT scanner, CT angiography was completed to assist with identifying the source of the bleed. Results did not identify an aneurysm.

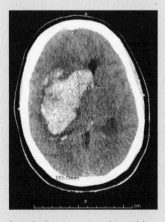

Figure 68-1   6-cm right-sided intraparenchymal hemorrhage with a 16-mm leftward midline shift.

is completed this will guide further tests and treatments related to cranial processes. With a CT scan of the head, brain masses can usually be identified as well as intracranial bleeds and large vessel emboli. CT angiography also assists with identifying aneurysms and perfusion mismatch to help identify ischemic strokes.

Diagnosis and Management of Acute Strokes

Appropriate management of ischemic and hemorrhagic strokes in the immediate presentation stage is essential to the patient's recovery. Quick decision making is needed for both types of strokes because the window for providing thrombolytic therapy is 3 to 4.5 hours from the onset of symptoms,[2] and the sooner a hemorrhagic stroke is diagnosed and treated, the greater the chance of recovering functional status. To that end, it is essential to gather data and act quickly, particularly when the NIHSS score and the timeframe are considered since symptom onset indicates eligibility for tPA.

Establishing the timeframe from symptom onset is sometimes challenging, as it is in this case. It is unclear whether this patient's stroke symptoms are 2 weeks old, beginning with the onset of her headaches, or if the related symptoms occurred just prior to her getting out of bed to get ibuprofen. When the time frame is uncertain, careful discussion with the team and with the patient's family about the risks and benefits of tPA is warranted. Of course a stat head CT scan needs to be completed prior to considering tPA, both to confirm the presence of ischemic stroke and to ensure that the patient does not have a brain hemorrhage as thrombolytic therapy in the presence of hemorrhage would be devastating. The CT images will guide other diagnostic and treatment options as well.

A key difference in the management of ischemic stroke compared to hemorrhagic stroke is blood pressure control. With ischemic strokes, blood pressure is not aggressively corrected though the systolic blood pressure must be lower than 185 for treatment with tPA.[2] Because the vasculature is blocked with an ischemic stroke, perfusion to the brain beyond the area of injury must be maximized. In hemorrhagic stroke, the goal is to reduce systolic blood pressure to less than 140 mm Hg, as higher blood pressures can lead to more extensive bleeding and devastating clinical outcomes. A systolic blood pressure greater than 140 to 150 mm Hg more than doubles the risk of death and dependency.[3] In some cases a vasodilator may also be necessary to decrease the BP.

Due to the rapid decline of this patient's neurological status, and before obtaining the head CT, the patient was intubated in the ED. Her blood pressure was severely elevated on admission to the ED so intravenous hydralazine was administered. Because the patient's head CT scan shows a large bleed with rapidly declining neurological status, she is rushed to the operating room for an emergent right craniotomy and hemorrhagic clot removal.[3] She was then admitted to the ICU for further monitoring and care.

This patient stayed in the ICU for 2½ weeks recovering from her stroke. Her hemorrhagic stroke was attributed to a prehospital elevated blood pressure. Supportive care required placement of a tracheostomy and a feeding tube. She regained consciousness, was following commands, answering questions by nodding and eating small amounts of food prior to discharge to a long-term acute care facility. To date she continues to have little function of her left side but has regained function on her right side. Her recovery will be a long process and she will require long-term rehabilitation. Return to her prestroke life status and function is limited by her left-sided deficit, which makes her dependent on a caregiver for her activities of daily living (ADLs). Long-term stroke prevention management for her includes close monitoring of her blood pressure and limiting other risk factors such as hyperlipidemia and weight management.

While this case presents decision making as a stepwise process, the reality is that in the case of possible stroke, many of the described tests and assessments are completed rapidly and often simultaneously. For example, a stat CT scan of the head and initiation of blood pressure management are accomplished at the same time as interviewing the family to gather data and conducting a physical examination of the patient. "Time is brain!"

References

1. Epocrates [online]. San Mateo, CA: Epocrates, Inc; 2014. http://www.epocrates.com. Updated continuously. Accessed September14, 2014.
2. Jauch EC, Saver JL, Adams HP Jr, et al. Guidelines for the early management of patients with acute ischemic stroke. *Stroke.* 2013;44(3):870-947. doi: 10.1161/STR.0b013e318284056a. http://stroke.ahajournals.org/lookup/doi/10.1161/STR.0b013e318284056a.
3. Morgenstern LB, Hemphill JC 3rd, Anderson C, et al. Guidelines for the management of spontaneous intracerebral hemorrhage: a guideline for healthcare professionals from the American Heart Association/American Stroke Association. *Stroke.* 2010;41:2108-2129. Originally published online July 22, 2010. http://stroke.ahajournals.org/content/41/9/2108.full.pdf.

CASE 69

Angela Nelson

Angela Nelson works as an NP for the Department of Neurosurgery at New York University Langone Medical Center.

CASE INFORMATION

Chief Complaint

A 53-year-old black male presents with severe headache (10/10) to an out-side hospital where a computed tomography (CT) scan of his head identi-fied a subarachnoid hemorrhage. He was immediately transferred to a large academic medical center for further evaluation and treatment.

? What is potential cause?

Subarachnoid hemorrhage (SAH) is bleeding into the subarachnoid space. SAH must always be considered when a patient presents with complaints of severe, sudden onset headache. The most common cause of an SAH is intracra-nial aneurysmal rupture. This blood acts as an irritant to the brain, potentially causing vasospasm, which can lead to severe neurological damage. The initial goal is to quickly determine the cause of the bleed and control the blood pres-sure to prevent further bleeding.

Comprehensive Differential Diagnoses for Patient With Subarachnoid Hemorrhage[1]

- Neurologic: perimesencephalic nonaneurysmal SAH, vascular mal-formation, spinal vascular malformation, cerebral venous thrombo-sis, cerebral amyloid angiopathy or brain or cervical tumor, migraine headache
- Cardiovascular: hypertensive bleed
- Pulmonary: none
- Gastrointestinal: none
- Genitourinary: none
- Musculoskeletal: traumatic SAH
- Endocrine: pituitary apoplexy
- Psychiatric disorder: none
- Metabolic: none
- Hematologic: sickle cell disease and bleeding disorders
- Exogenous: cocaine abuse and anticoagulant therapy

With an awareness of the potentially devastating effects of cerebral vasospasm, my first priority is to control the blood pressure to prevent any further bleeding and to monitor the patient very closely for neurological changes. Nicardipine is a short-acting drug, which is easy to titrate as an intravenous infusion. It effectively controls blood pressure in this patient population. The patient was admitted to the neurosurgical intensive care unit to closely monitor blood pressure and perform frequent neurologic examinations. An additional essential goal is to manage the patient's headaches so that they do not contribute to hypertension. At this point my goal is to obtain a cerebral angiogram within 24 hours or sooner to determine the cause of the SAH.

CASE INFORMATION

General Survey and History of Present Illness

A general survey of the patient reveals a black male, thin and fit looking, appearing younger than stated age. He reports severe headache and neck stiffness, which began within 1 hour prior to admission to the outside hospital. He prefers to keep his eyes closed but responds appropriately. He denies any photophobia, nausea, or vomiting at this time. He states that he was at work talking to his supervisor when the headache suddenly started. He reports it as a 10/10. He was taken to an outside hospital where he was treated with ibuprofen and morphine for the headaches and a noncontrast head CT was done revealing the SAH. He was then transferred to our hospital for further evaluation and treatment.

Upon arrival to our hospital another noncontrast head CT is done to make sure that he did not have any further bleeding during the transfer. The head CT reveals diffuse acute subarachnoid hemorrhage and a small amount of intraventricular hemorrhage with mild communicating hydrocephalus. A review of the labs obtained initially reveals a normal metabolic panel with sodium of 138 (normal = 135–147 mEq/L) on admission. Coagulation studies are borderline abnormal with an INR of 1.1 (normal = 0.8–1.2). The alkaline phosphatase is borderline elevated at 120 IU/L (normal = 40–120 IU/L). The complete blood count reveals a normal white blood cell count at 8.3 cells/µL (normal = 4500–10,000 cells/µL); however, the differential shows a shift to the left with neutrophils of 91% (normal = 54%–62%). His drug screen is negative. His ECG on admission has some T-wave inversion but he remains in a normal sinus rhythm. He was started on levetiracetam (Keppra), an antiepileptic, for seizure prophylaxis and nimodipine, a calcium channel blocker that helps reduce brain damage caused by bleeding in the brain from a burst blood vessel. His drug screen is negative.

Past Medical History

This patient has no known past medical history. He denies any history of hypertension or any recent smoking history that may be a risk factor for the development of aneurysms.

Family and Social History

The patient arrives to the hospital alone stating he is married but separated at present. He denies any drug use or trauma or falls. He denies any family history of aneurysms.

Medications

He takes no medications on a regular basis.

? What are the pertinent positives from the information given so far?

- 10/10 headache with sudden onset
- Neck stiffness
- Noncontrast head CT with subarachnoid hemorrhage
- ECG with T-wave abnormalities thought to be secondary to acute hypertension or SAH (SAH can result in the release of catecholamines, resulting in various cardiac arrhythmias and ECG changes).

? What are the significant negatives from the information given so far?

- Intact neurological examination on initial survey
- No history of smoking, hypertension, recent trauma, or drug use
- No family history of aneurysms
- Negative drug screen

? Can the information gathered so far be restated in a single sentence highlighting the pieces that narrow down the cause?

Putting information obtained so far in a single statement—a problem representation—sets the stage for gathering more information and determining the cause. The problem representation at this point is: The patient is a 53-year-old male with no past medical history presenting with a sudden onset of severe headache and neck stiffness with head CT scan revealing a subarachnoid hemorrhage.

? How does this information affect the list of possible causes?

The patient reports no medical history or hospitalizations. He denies any recent trauma as a cause for the SAH. The most common differential diagnosis would be an aneurysm rupture, despite his lack of risk factors. The lab work obtained so far is essentially normal with incidental findings of a mildly elevated INR at 1.1 excluding any bleeding disorders as a cause for the rupture. His drug screen is also negative.

CASE INFORMATION

Review of Systems

- Constitutional: Denies any recent weight loss, fever, night sweats, or weakness. The patient is alert and oriented although prefers to keep his eyes closed but answering all questions.
- Head/eyes/ears/nose/throat: Reports 10/10 headache. Denies nasal discharge, sore throat, difficulty swallowing or hearing or ringing in ears, discharge from ears or visual changes.
- Cardiovascular: Denies chest pain, palpitations, orthopnea, or peripheral edema.
- Pulmonary: Denies dyspnea or cough.
- Gastrointestinal: Denies nausea, vomiting, blood in stools, or heartburn. Reports bowel movements every couple of days.
- Genitourinary: Denies frequency, urgency, dysuria, or blood in urine.
- Musculoskeletal: Denies joint pain or swelling.
- Neurological: Denies any history of migraines. Reports current headache was abrupt in onset and severe and unlike any other headache he has ever had. Also reports neck stiffness. Denies seizures, weakness, or coordination problems. Denies any drug or alcohol problems.
- Lymphatic: Denies nodes.
- Endocrine: Denies cold or hot intolerance, diabetes, thyroid conditions.

Physical Examination

- Vital signs: Pulse is 64 beats per minute, blood pressure is 135/74 mm Hg, respiratory rate is 14 breaths per minute, and temperature is 98.3°F orally, oxygen saturation (O_2 sat) by pulse oximetry is 99% on room air, and a fingerstick blood glucose is 93 (normal = 60–110 mg/dL).
- Constitutional: Appears healthy in no apparent distress except that he is lying in bed preferring not to open his eyes but denying photophobia.
- Head/eyes/ears/nose/throat: Normocephalic, atraumatic. Pupils equal, round, reactive to light and accommodation. Uvula midline. Buccal mucosa moist.
- Cardiovascular: Heart rate and rhythm regular. No murmurs or gallops. No jugular venous distension. S1, S2 normal. Skin warm to touch. No edema. + pedal pulses. Capillary refill 2+.

- Pulmonary: Clear to auscultation bilaterally. No use of accessory muscles.
- Gastrointestinal: Bowel sounds all four quadrants. Soft nontender.
- Genitourinary: Normal genitalia, urine clear yellow.
- Integumentary: Intact, no lesions, rash, or open areas. Skin turgor normal.
- Neurological: Awake, alert, and oriented ×3. Moving all extremities with full strength. No drift. No dysmetria. Pupils equal, round, reactive to light. Extraocular movements intact. V1-V3 facial sensation intact. Cranial nerves II-VII grossly intact. Deep tendon reflexes nonpathologic. Tongue midline. Toes bilaterally downgoing. Negative Hoffman. Negative clonus. Joint position sense intact. Sensation to light touch and proprioception intact. No extinction to double simultaneous stimuli. Speech fluent. Follows complex commands without difficulty.

? What elements of the review of systems and physical examination should be added to the list of pertinent positives? Which items should be added to the list of significant negatives?

Pertinent Positives

- Worst headache he has ever had
- Headache had abrupt onset
- Blood pressure elevated

Significant Negatives

- Review of systems shows no symptoms of other acute or chronic disease
- Physical examination is normal except for neck stiffness
- No trauma
- No history of high blood pressure

? How does this information affect the list of possible causes?

Given the information obtained so far I think the most likely cause of his SAH is a ruptured aneurysm. This accounts for the majority of SAHs and is even more likely in this case as he has no known risk factors such as hypertension, bleeding disorders, tobacco, alcohol or drug use, or any recent trauma. Though this is high on my differential I recognize that his history is incomplete. Regardless of the etiology of SAH, blood pressure management remains the same. The single most important task at this stage is to maintain his systolic BP <130 mm Hg with the use of nicardipine. Close neurological monitoring is an important focus in order to rapidly recognize deterioration and treat promptly.

CASE INFORMATION

He is emergently taken for a cerebral angiogram and diagnosed with a ruptured right anterior communicating berry aneurysm. The following day, he
is taken to the operating room for clipping of the aneurysm and the placement of a ventricular drain. His initial cerebrospinal fluid (CSF) values are as
follows: glucose 80 mg/dL (normal = 40–80 mg/dL), protein 19 mg/dL (normal = 15–45 mg/dL), red blood cells 67,000 cells/μL (normal = 0), and white
blood cells 90 cells/μL (normal = 3). These results are expected given the
blood in the ventricles.

Diagnosis and Treatment: SAH

As in the case of this patient, an emergent CT of the head should be done in any
patient presenting with symptoms of SAH. The evidence-based guidelines recommend that patients with SAH be transferred, if possible, to an institution where a
large volume of patients with SAH are treated as the best outcomes are typically
achieved at these centers.[2] If a SAH is suspected and the CT is negative, then a
lumbar puncture should be done. Lab tests include serum chemistries, coagulation
studies, complete blood count, toxicology screen, and ECG. The goal after diagnosis is to control blood pressure and the current recommendation is to do so with
nicardipine.

The most common test to diagnose aneurysm as the cause of a SAH is
cerebral angiography. Computed tomography angiography can sometimes be
obtained more quickly, depending on the center, but it has imperfect sensitivity
in detecting aneurysms. Aneurysmal rupture is not detected in 24% of patients
with an initial cerebral angiographic study but instead on subsequent scans.
Patients with ruptured aneurysms typically present with a sudden onset of a
severe headache and stiff neck, brief loss of consciousness, or focal neurological
deficits like cranial nerve palsies. The current guidelines state that there is large
risk of a recently ruptured aneurysm rebleeding and thus prompt and accurate
diagnosis is essential.[2] Once diagnosed, the patient should be graded using one
of the generally accepted grading systems, as this can be important in planning
future care (see Tables 69-1 and 69-2). The higher grades typically have worse
outcomes.

Once the diagnosis of a ruptured cerebral aneurysm is established, blood pressure control is the main priority until the patient undergoes a procedure, either clipping or coiling to prevent rebleeding. Coiling is an endovascular procedure, while
clipping is a surgical procedure. The decision to do either is based on the expertise
of the provider, location and size of the aneurysm, grade when first presented, age,
and comorbidities of the patient.

Postoperatively, the most critical complication is cerebral vasospasm. The risk
of vasospasm is highest between day 5 and 14 following the initial bleed. Early

Table 69-1   Hunt and Hess Scale[3]

Classification of patients with intracranial aneurysms according to surgical risk:

Grade I—Asymptomatic or minimal headache and slight nuchal rigidity

Grade II—Moderate to severe headache, nuchal rigidity, no neurological deficit other than cranial nerve palsy

Grade III—Drowsiness, confusion, or mild focal deficit

Grade IV—Stupor, moderate to severe hemiparesis, possibly early decerebrate rigidity, and vegetative disturbances

Grade V—Deep coma, decerebrate rigidity, and moribund appearance.

Table 69-2   World Federation of Neurosurgeons SAH Grading Scale[4]

Glasgow Coma Scale	Motor Deficits	Grade
15	Absent	1
13-14	Absent	2
13-14	Present	3
7-12	Present or absent	4
3-6	Present or absent	5

Data from Teasdale GM, Drake CG, Hunt WE, et al. A universal subarachnoid hemorrhage scale: report of a committee of the World Federation of Neurosurgical Societies. *J Neurol Neurosurg Psychiatry.* November 1988;51(1):1457.

treatment of the aneurysm, and the use of nimodipine can help prevent vasospasm. Other care measures include bedrest and treatment with fibrinolytic therapy short-term perioperatively. In the past, a common practice for managing cerebral vasospasm was "triple H" therapy, which included hypervolemia, hypertension, and hemodilution.[2] New guidelines by the Neurocritical Care Society suggest that hypervolemia is associated with some undesirable outcomes, including permanent neurological injury. As a result, they recommend euvolemia as the goal.[5] Transcranial Doppler can be used to detect vasospasm as flow velocity increases with vasospasm. Regular serial measurements are a useful monitoring strategy. Lastly, if vasospasm occurs, it may potentially be managed with cerebral angioplasty or with the use of selective intraarterial vasodilator therapy.

Hydrocephalus is also a complication frequently seen with SAH patients. This is managed with the use of external ventricular drains for CSF diversion; often long-term diversion with the use of internal shunts is necessary. Hyponatremia occurs in 10% to 30% of these patients. The recommendation for management of low serum sodium is to reduce fluid administration and use isotonic rather than hypotonic fluids. There is some evidence that the use of fludrocortisone may also be useful in concentrating serum sodium.[2] Recent recommendations suggest that the use of 3% hypertonic IV infusions may be warranted.5 Routine use of prophylactic seizure medications during the immediate post-hemorrhagic period is considered but not recommended long term unless the patient has a history of seizures, infarction, or middle cerebral artery aneurysm.

Case Follow-Up

The patient in this case was found to have a ruptured berry anterior communicating artery aneurysm and was taken to the OR for clipping of that aneurysm. His post-op course was complicated by persistent fevers, *serratia marcescens* meningitis treated with cefepime (fourth generation cephalosporin, resistant to β-lactamases) and vancomycin (glycopeptide antibiotic); acute bilateral lower extremity deep vein thromboses in the soleal veins with subsequent inferior vena cava filter placement; obstructed ventricular drains requiring the administration of tissue plasminogen activator; and multiple replacements of ventricular external drains (at one point he required bilateral drains), cerebral vasospasms of the right anterior cerebral artery segments, hyponatremia, and persistent obstructive hydrocephalus requiring the placement of a ventriculoperitoneal shunt (delayed due to the meningitis). His hospital course was greater than 30 days and although he developed many complications he remained neurologically stable and was eventually sent to a rehab facility and then home.

The management of patients with SAH due to ruptured aneurysm is quite complex and evolving. In 2009, the American Heart Association and American Stroke Association developed guidelines for the diagnosis and management of aneurysmal SAH.[2] Twenty-five percent of patients with aneurysmal SAH die, and of those who survive, 50% are left with persistent neurological deficits. Appropriate management is crucial to preventing these devastating complications. Risk factors for SAH include smoking, hypertension, alcohol and drug use particularly sympathomimetic drugs such as cocaine. Any patient who presents with an acute onset of a severe headache should be evaluated for these risk factors. The initial clinical severity should be assessed using one of the validated scales such as the Hunt and Hess Scale or the World Federation of Neurosurgeons Scale (Tables 69-1 and 69-2). These scales are useful in stratifying severity of the insult and linking them to potential outcomes. My patient's Hunt and Hess grade was level II; he had severe headaches and nuchal rigidity, but no neurological deficits. If using the WFN SAH scale, his score would have been a grade I.

References

1. Singer RJ, Ogilvy CS, Rordorf G, et al. Clinical manifestations and diagnosis of aneurysmal subarachnoid hemorrhage. 2015 UpToDate Web site. www.uptodate.com. Updated September 26, 2013. Accessed March 3, 2015.
2. Bederson JB, Connolly SE, Batjer HH, et al. Guidelines for the management of aneurysmal subarachnoid hemorrhage. *Stroke.* 2009;40(3):994-1025. 10.1161/STROKEAHA.108.191395. Epub 2009 Jan 22.
3. Hunt WE, Hess RM. Surgical risk as related to time of intervention in the repair of intracranial aneurysms. *J Neurosurg.* January 1968;28(1):14-20.
4. Teasdale GM, Drake CG, Hunt WE, et al. A universal subarachnoid hemorrhage scale: report of a committee of the World Federation of Neurosurgical Societies. *J Neurol Neurosurg Psychiatry.* November 1988;51(1):1457.
5. Diringer MN, Bleck TP, Claude Hemphill J III, et al. Critical care management of patients following aneurysmal subarachnoid hemorrhage: recommendation from the Neurocritical Care Society's Multidisciplinary Consensus Conference. *Neurocrit Care.* October 2011;15(2):211-240.

CASE 70

Susan Yeager and April J. Kastner

Susan works as the Lead Nurse Practitioner in the Neurocritical Care Unit at The Ohio State University Wexner Medical Center and as an Acute Care Nurse Practitioner Clinical Instructor at The Ohio State University College of Nursing in Columbus. April works in the Neurocritical Care Unit at The Ohio State University Wexner Medical Center in Columbus.

CASE INFORMATION

Chief Complaint

A 65-year-old male was brought into the emergency room by the rescue squad after being found by a neighbor comatose on the floor of his garage at the bottom of a 15-ft ladder. He was breathing but was intubated at the scene for airway protection and remains unresponsive, with a Glasgow coma scale of 6 according to emergency responders. The neighbor is unable to provide the patient's medical history except for confirming alcohol intake; he is unsure of the frequency or amount.

❓ What is the potential cause?

Coma as a presenting symptom is associated with a large list of differential diagnoses. In this scenario, the fact that he was found at the bottom of a ladder means that traumatic injuries need to be ruled out. His Glasgow coma score (GCS) was 6, indicating severe brain injury. Brain or spine trauma is high on the list, but given the height of the ladder, internal trauma is also possible. While trauma seems likely, it is possible that a cardiovascular event, metabolic alteration, or drug/toxin exposure caused the patient to fall. Because the fall was not witnessed, it is unclear whether he fell from a standing position or from a significant height. The patient's unresponsive state precludes gathering additional medical history to focus the workup during this initial evaluation. Therefore, a quick but comprehensive evaluation of all body systems is essential, with the priority of determining if the patient has a life-threatening condition. This workup begins in the trauma bay with primary and tertiary examinations focused first on the stabilization of airway, breathing, and circulation, and then neurological and systemic examination.

Comprehensive Differential Diagnoses for Patient With Coma

- Neurologic: cerebral contusions, subdural hemorrhage, epidural hemorrhage, traumatic versus aneurysmal subarachnoid hemorrhage, diffuse axonal injury, anoxia, acute hemorrhagic or ischemic stroke, seizure or nonconvulsive status epilepticus, brain tumor, encephalitis, meningitis, brain abscess, spinal bone fracture or dislocation, spinal cord injury, or ligamentous injury

- Cardiovascular: myocardial infarction, cardiac arrhythmia, hypotension, aortic trauma
- Pulmonary: hypoxia, carbon monoxide poisoning, pulmonary embolism, pneumonia, COPD exacerbation, rib fractures, pulmonary contusion, pneumothorax, or hemothorax
- Gastrointestinal: gastrointestinal bleeding, spleen or liver trauma with subsequent hypovolemic shock
- Genitourinary: urosepsis from urinary tract infection
- Musculoskeletal: fracture, mechanical fall
- Endocrine: hypo- or hyperglycemia, diabetic ketoacidosis
- Psychiatric: suicide attempt
- Metabolic: dehydration, electrolyte imbalance, hypernatremia, hyponatremia, hepatic encephalopathy, uremia, profound nutritional deficiency, septicemia
- Intoxications: alcohol withdrawal or intake, illicit drug usage, drug overdose

CASE INFORMATION

By calling a trauma alert, a total body examination can be done quickly by a multidisciplinary team of experts. The primary examination consists of an evaluation of the patient's airway integrity, breathing effectiveness and pattern, and circulatory stability (ABCs).[1] The patient was intubated in the field and maintained on 100% oxygen, and then moved several times throughout the patient's transport to the hospital. Therefore, the first items to evaluate are those related to his airway placement and patency, oxygenation, and ventilation, including to check his end-tidal carbon dioxide ($ETCO_2$), pulse oximetry, and the presence of bilateral breath sounds. From this evaluation, we confirm that the airway is intact, oxygenation on the pulse oximetry is 98% with manual resuscitation bag (MRB) ventilation, and cervical spine immobilization is present. The patient was paralyzed and sedated for intubation. While the effects of the paralytic are wearing off, it is necessary to support the patient's breathing with MRB until mechanical ventilation is initiated. The paralytic used was of short duration and he begins breathing spontaneously just minutes after his arrival. No asynchrony in breathing is noted and his oxygen saturation readings remain at 98% with MRB ventilation so we move on to evaluate circulation. Two 18-gauge intravenous catheters were placed by the prehospital providers and appear functional. Normal saline is infusing. Upon arrival he was originally hypertensive but quickly became hypotensive. Fluid boluses were initiated with an immediate increase in blood pressure to 120/82 mm Hg.

After addressing the ABCs, a quick neurologic examination reveals the following: no eye opening or attempts to follow commands, his left pupil is 4 mm and the response to light is sluggish, the right pupil is 3 mm and brisk, gaze is conjugate but without tracking, minimal corneal, cough, and gag reflexes, but he localizes to painful stimulation with his left upper and lower extremity and withdraws slightly with his right upper and lower extremity. There is no step-off (misalignment of the spine that might indicate a fracture or dislocation) or deformity of the cervical, thoracic, or lumbar spine. He has intact rectal tone. Facial symmetry is unable to be determined due to the presence of the endotracheal tube (ETT). The patient is becoming increasingly more agitated.

A quick secondary examination notes a left forehead laceration with no active bleeding but otherwise his examination is negative for thoracic, abdominal, or musculoskeletal findings. Vital signs are fluctuating with the heart rate ranging from 55 to 115 beats per minute, blood pressure from a systolic pressure of 90 to 220 mm Hg and diastolic pressure from 70 to 110 mm Hg, and a respiratory rate from 18 to 30 breaths per minute. The patient is given Fentanyl 50 µg intravenously to treat pain, which may be the cause of his agitation and fluctuating vital signs.

❓ What are the pertinent positives from the information given so far?

- Neurological: The patient is agitated, does not follow commands, has asymmetrical pupils and asymmetrical motor response.
- Cardiopulmonary: The patient's vital signs are intermittently rising and decreasing
- Dermatologic: He has a forehead laceration.
- Psychiatric: He has a history of alcohol consumption although it is unclear the amount or frequency of intake.
- Possible fall from height.

❓ What are the significant negatives from the information given so far?

- Neurological: No visible seizures are noted. The entire spine is without step-off or deformity. Rectal tone is intact.
- Thoracic/gastrointestinal/genitourinary/musculoskeletal systems are without acute external findings.

❓ Can the information gathered so far be summarized in a single statement or problem representation?

The problem representation in this case might be: "a 65-year-old male with possible alcohol use presents following a presumed fall from a 15-ft ladder onto a cement floor with possible acute brain trauma and impending herniation."

Case Analysis

The presence of a head laceration suggests that a traumatic injury to the head occurred. Whether it was a fall from a height or from a standing position may never be determined without a witness to the event. In this situation, a fall from a height is the working diagnosis so we do not miss other injuries that might surround that mechanism of injury. Unequal pupillary responses can occur as the patient is recovering from the effects of the paralytic agents given during the intubation process. While we consider this information, we are concerned that the patient has motor changes consistent with contralateral pupillary changes. These findings lead us to prioritize our evaluation of brain etiologies, and interventions to prevent herniation. Vital sign variability may be part of arousal from the paralytic agent or may be the emergence of the Cushing triad where increased brain pressure causes irregular breathing, hypertension, and bradycardia.[2] While evaluation and treatment for brain trauma are a priority, we must continue to consider potential reasons the patient may have lost consciousness and/or the reason for the fall. A mechanical fall (in which he slipped, tripped, or lost his balance) is possible but other cardiopulmonary and metabolic causes may be responsible.

Because of the urgency of this patient's evolving neurological status we order a stat blood glucose and urine dipstick for ketones, leukoesterase and toxicology, a stat ECG, and an arterial blood gases (ABG) at the bedside.

CASE INFORMATION

Review of Systems

Unable to obtain due to coma and unaccompanied by family.

Physical Examination

- Vital signs: Sinus tachycardia with a heart rate of 117 beats per minute, blood pressure is 185/110 mm Hg, respiratory rate is 28, and temperature is 97.5°F, oxygen saturation by pulse oximeter is 97% on the following ventilator settings: mode-synchronized intermittent mechanical ventilation (SIMV) plus pressure support ventilation (PSV), tidal volume of 550 mL, respiratory rate of 12 breaths per minute, positive end-expiratory pressure of 5 cm H_2O pressure support of 10 cm H_2O, and an FiO_2 of 100%.
- Constitutional: Lying in bed, intubated, breathing is rapid but otherwise does not appear to be in distress, with no facial grimacing, although heart rate and blood pressure remain elevated. No distinct odors are noted.
- Cardiovascular: Heart rate and rhythm are regular but fluctuating between tachycardia and bradycardia, hypertensive blood pressure readings are fluctuating with bradycardia, both heart rate and blood pressure are unresponsive to pain medication or fluids, no murmurs, no gallops, no visible

edema, 2+ pulses throughout. No jugular venous distension with head of bed elevated at 30°. Nail beds pink, <3 second capillary refill.

- Pulmonary: Synchronous with ventilator, without use of accessory muscles, tachypneic with a total rate of 26 breaths per minute (set ventilator rate is 12). Lungs clear to auscultation but diminished at bases bilaterally.
- Gastrointestinal: Normoactive bowel sounds, abdomen soft, no visual cues indicating tenderness over entire abdomen including liver and spleen areas but this is difficult to assess due to unresponsiveness, rotund abdomen, no liver or spleen enlargement, no flank or abdominal ecchymosis noted.
- Genitourinary: Urine clear yellow.
- Integumentary: Intact except 4 in, linear, left forehead laceration that is approximately 4 mm in depth, otherwise no rashes, lesions, or sores, normal skin turgor.
- Neurological: Does not open eyes to stimulation, weak cough, gag, and corneal reflexes. Unable to test extraocular movements due to coma. Left pupillary response is 4 and minimally responsive, right pupil 3 and sluggish. Gaze is conjugate. Left upper extremity with minimal movement, left lower extremity has slight withdrawal to pain. Right upper extremity and right lower extremity without response.

Diagnostic Testing

- His blood glucose by fingerstick is 101 mg/dL.
- Urine dipstick results: No ketones, leukocyte esterase, or nitrates and toxicology negative.
- ECG shows a sinus tachycardia with no signs of ischemia.
- Arterial blood gas results are: pH 7.42, CO_2 32 mm Hg, bicarbonate 22 mmol/L with a base deficit of -1, and PaO_2 119 mm Hg.

❓ What elements of the review of systems and physical examination should be added to the list of pertinent positives?

- Neurological: Worsening neurologic examination. Does not open eyes to stimulation, weak cough, gag, and corneal. Left upper extremity now with minimal movement, left lower extremity only slight withdrawal to pain and right upper and lower extremity no longer moving even to painful stimuli, pupillary signs with minimal response on left and sluggish response on the right.
- Cardiovascular: Fluctuating heart rate and blood pressure unchanged after pain medication and intravenous fluid.

❓ What elements of the review of systems and physical examination should be added to the list of significant negatives?

- Electrocardiogram is negative for arrhythmia or sign of ischemia.
- Chest/abdomen/extremities without ecchymosis or signs of trauma.
- Afebrile, lung sounds clear, urine without signs of infection.
- Glucometer with normal glucose and urine check negative for ketones.
- No distinct odors and spot urine toxicology negative.
- Normal arterial blood case on mechanical ventilation.

❓ How does this information affect the list of possible causes?

A cerebral neurological cause is most likely given the abnormal, worsening neurological examination. Spinal irregularities cannot be fully identified with a clinical examination on an unconscious patient and therefore require further study. The fluctuating heart rate, respiratory rate, and blood pressure can be multifactorial including Cushing reflex, sepsis, pain, or exposure to toxins. Herniation syndromes remain at the top of the differential list for these findings given his worsening neurologic examination. There is no obvious source of infection and he has a normal base excess so infection is lower on the differential. Pain does not seem to be contributing to his altered vital signs as administration of pain medication has no impact. The normal spot toxicology screen makes alcohol intoxication unlikely as the cause of his unresponsiveness, but other toxins or illicit drug exposures require further exploration.

His normal cardiac examination, lack of acute ischemic changes on the cardiac monitor and ECG, and sinus bradycardia and tachycardia via continuous telemetry lessen, but do not rule out, a cardiac cause of unresponsiveness. The lack of hypoxia noted on the arterial blood gas (PaO$_2$ of 119 mm Hg) and essentially normal breath sounds make a respiratory cause unlikely but may not reflect prehospital events given that these readings were taken while the patient was intubated. However, continued hypertension and tachycardia after intubation and with a normal arterial blood gas, and clear lung sounds do not suggest an exacerbation of a chronic condition such as chronic obstructive pulmonary disease (COPD), congestive heart failure (CHF), or status asthmaticus. Pulmonary embolism is unlikely, but still on the differential until it can be ruled out. Pneumothorax or hemothorax remain on the list. Anoxic injury remains a diagnosis to consider as prehospital respiratory status is unknown. Hypoglycemia and hyperglycemia are ruled out given the normal blood glucose reading. The patient's abdomen is soft but the presence of abdominal pain is indeterminate given the patient's unresponsiveness, so intraabdominal trauma cannot be ruled out.

❓ What diagnostic testing should be done and in what order?

Considering the above information, we will begin to prioritize additional diagnostic and imaging studies. Portable chest and pelvic imaging are automatically and simultaneously obtained with the secondary examination in the trauma bay as part of the multidisciplinary evaluation. The team also does a focused abdominal sonographic test (FAST) at the bedside while other evaluations continue. The FAST examination is a rapid bedside ultrasound examination that specifically screens for blood around the heart, or abdominal organs. These tests quickly rule out the presence of pneumothorax, hemothorax, pulmonary consolidation, widened mediastinum, pelvic fracture pathology, pericardial effusion, and intra-abdominal free fluid. We also send blood at this time to evaluate the patient's electrolytes, troponin, complete blood count with differential, prothrombin (PT), international normalized ratio (INR) and partial thromboplastin time (PTT), liver function tests, and drug toxicology to screen for alcohol, amphetamines, barbiturates, benzodiazepine, cocaine, methadone, opiates, and cannabinoids.[3] As there are multiple practitioners assisting with the trauma examination, blood work can be obtained without interrupting the physical examination or treatment measures. However, further care and evaluation is not to be delayed to obtain or wait for the results.

Given the patient's signs and symptoms of Cushing reflex, rapid imaging of the head needs to be done. Chest and abdominal computed tomography (CT) scans are generally done at the same time as a part of the rapid trauma pan scan.[3] Given that he is unconscious, it is unknown whether he struck his chest or abdomen if he did fall. The addition of these studies rapidly rules out intrathoracic or intraabdominal pathology not seen on plain films. While no signs of external trauma are noted, ecchymosis may not be apparent immediately and rib fractures are not always picked up with plain films given the curved nature of the bones. In a fall from a height, the ligament of arteriosum that attaches the aorta may be stretched, causing a tear, which can progress to full aortic rupture. While the plain chest x-ray did not reflect a widened mediastinum, chest CT scan will definitively rule out dissection.[3] Abdominal injury is less likely given the lack of abdominal or flank ecchymosis, negative FAST examination, and mechanism of injury. Cervical, thoracic, and lumbar sacral spinal images can be reconstructed from the CT scan imaging. Spinal imaging will rule out obvious bony fractures, spinal dislocation, or obvious spinal cord injury. Given the suspected fall from a height and the forehead laceration, cervical flexion or extension injury or spinal compression injuries are suspected.

Electrographic cardiogram (ECG) and ongoing telemetry with troponin trending are recommended for the basic cardiac workup to evaluate the source of the slight troponin elevation. Echocardiogram should also be ordered to identify cardiac structural problems that might have caused a cardiac dysrhythmia and a subsequent fall. Ongoing cerebral edema management may continue with either 3% hypertonic saline or mannitol with frequent monitoring of serum sodium and osmolality to guide treatment changes.

CASE INFORMATION

Results of Diagnostics

Findings reveal normal complete blood count, coagulation studies, sodium, potassium, magnesium, creatinine, blood urea nitrogen, glucose, liver function, portable chest x-ray, pelvic x-ray, FAST, CT chest/abdomen/pelvis, and total spine imaging. The initial troponin was slightly elevated at 0.3 ng/mL.

The CT of the head reveals an acute large holohemispheric left-sided subdural hematoma (SDH), extensive, diffuse subarachnoid hemorrhage (SAH), as well as a small right-sided epidural hematoma (EDH) overlying the right temporal lobe with overlying comminuted left temporal bone fracture. These findings were associated with a midline shift of 3 cm with signs of tentorial herniation.

Traumatic Brain Injury With Malignant Intracranial Hypertension With Pending Tentorial Herniation Diagnosis and Treatment

Our evaluation confirms that our patient had extensive intracranial bleeding with signs of tentorial herniation, a life-threatening neurological injury that presented with coma. The presentation of coma warrants a multipronged approach to evaluation. The EMS report for this patient focused on likely trauma as the most pressing source of the coma with the inciting event being unknown.

Traumatic brain injury is a neurological emergency that requires immediate attention, diagnosis, and treatment.[1] Early and rapid treatment is essential to prevent or limit life-changing deficits. Diagnostic evaluation begins with the neurologic examination and head CT imaging without contrast as the initial standard of care for suspected brain trauma. Immediate medical treatment starts with the stabilization of the patient's airway, breathing, and circulation. Intubation, ventilator support, and intravenous fluids, 0.9% normal saline through two large bore IVs, are the interventions applied to achieve stabilization. Neurologic evaluation follows ABC management.

This patient demonstrated signs and symptoms of cerebral malignant hypertension with impending herniation. In this situation, trauma guidelines recommend the use of short-term hyperventilation and pharmacologic intervention with mannitol or hypertonic saline to decrease brain swelling and maintain a systolic blood pressure greater than 90 mm Hg. In this situation, 0.5 to 1 g/kg of mannitol with or without 23.4% saline may be given. The medication we initially choose is mannitol as it can be given through peripheral access. Hypertonic saline at 23.4% requires central access. Maintaining a systolic blood pressure greater than 90 mm Hg and pulse oximetry readings of greater than 90 percent are shown to improve outcomes.[1] Hyperventilation is only used as a temporizing measure to transition the patient to surgical intervention. If no surgical lesion is noted and medical management is the plan of care, $PaCO_2$ readings should be maintained between 35 and 40 mm Hg. As carbon dioxide is a potent vasodilator, $PaCO_2$ levels higher than this can dilate the blood vessels, causing the blood volume within the skull to increase. As the blood volume increases, the intracranial pressure increases, which can result in brain compression and possibly herniation. Therefore, hyperventilation is an effective temporary measure to minimize venous dilation. In this case, the subdural hematoma and associated edema are pushing against normal brain structures. Hyperventilation should be temporary because the ensuing decrease in arterial blood flow from hypocarbia can actually result in cerebral cell ischemia if maintained over time. With this patient's intracranial findings, a neurosurgical consult should occur as soon as an intracranial process is identified. Our patient's subdural hematoma was associated with a large midline shift and such a finding should prompt an immediate transfer to the operative suite. Placement of an intracranial pressure monitor is a standard intervention in patients with a Glasgow coma scale less than 8.[1] If used, the neurosurgical team is asked to assist with the placement of the monitoring device. In this patient, an external intraventricular device was placed when the patient underwent immediate surgical evacuation of his subdural hematoma and hemicraniectomy. The hemicraniectomy consisted of the removal of the left side of his skull and dura to minimize brain compression. Implementation of antiepileptic medications without the presence of seizures is a topic of debate. But given the coup subdural hematoma and contrecoupe[4] epidural lesions found in this patient, prophylactic medications were given.

After the emergency operative intervention described above, the patient was admitted to the neurologic critical care unit for ongoing evaluation and management (Follow up on this patient can be found in Case 67.)

References

1. Brain Trauma Foundation. Guidelines for the management of severe traumatic brain injury. *J Trauma.* 2007;24(1):1-116.
2. Hickey JV and Bettina CP. Craniocerebral injuries. In: Hickey JV, ed. *The Clinical Practice of Neurological and Neurosurgical Nursing.* Philadelphia, PA: Lippincott Williams & Wilkins; 2014:380.
3. American College of Surgeons Committee on Trauma. *Thoracic Trauma in the Advanced Trauma Life Support for Doctors Student Course Manual.* 8th ed. Chicago, IL: American College of Surgeons; 2008:85-103.
4. Brophy GM, Bell R, Claassen J, et al. Guidelines for the evaluation and management of status epilepticus. *Neurocrit Care.* August 2012;17(1):3-23. doi: 10.1007/s12028-012-9695-z.

CASE 71

Sarah A. Delgado

Sarah A. Delgado is an acute nurse practitioner, currently working for the American Association of Critical Care Nurses as a clinical practice specialist. She has over 10 years experience in advanced nursing practice, focusing on the management of adults with chronic diseases. In the past, she taught acute care graduate and undergraduate nursing students at the University of Virginia, and developed a chronic disease management program at an integrated delivery system in Whittier, California.

CASE INFORMATION

Chief Complaint

An 80-year-old female comes to the emergency room (ER) with her son, due to a complaint of new onset confusion.

? What is the potential cause?

Confusion, particularly in an older adult, is a nonspecific symptom and the list of potential etiologies is long. One approach to generating a complete list of possible causes is to go through each system in the body and consider the pathologies that can cause confusion. While some conditions are more likely to cause a given symptom, others are more essential to discover and treat quickly because they are life threatening or threatening to the patient's functional status. For instance, in the case of this patient, I need to quickly determine if her confusion might be caused by a cerebrovascular accident or myocardial infarction, which are both unlikely causes but require immediate intervention to ensure a successful outcome.

Comprehensive Differential Diagnoses for Patient With Altered Mental State[1]

- Neurologic: acute stroke (embolic or hemorrhagic), traumatic head injury, seizure with postictal state, seizure, brain tumor, meningitis
- Cardiovascular: myocardial infarction, cardiac arrhythmia, congestive heart failure (CHF) exacerbation, hypertensive encephalopathy
- Pulmonary: hypoxia, carbon monoxide poisoning, pulmonary embolism, pneumonia, chronic obstructive pulmonary disease (COPD) exacerbation
- Gastrointestinal: ischemic bowel, cholecystitis, appendicitis, diverticulitis, constipation, gastritis, colitis
- Genitourinary: urinary tract infection, urinary retention or obstruction
- Musculoskeletal: fracture
- Endocrine: adrenal insufficiency, myxedema, thyrotoxicosis

- Psychiatric disorder: depression, new onset or exacerbation of bipolar disorder, psychosis
- Metabolic: dehydration, electrolyte imbalance, hyperglycemia, hypoglycemia, hypernatremia, hyponatremia, hepatic encephalopathy
- Exogenous: medication side effect or interaction or withdrawal, drug overdose, alcohol withdrawal

With the list of all possible causes in mind, my next step is to begin gathering data, which when applied to the case will rule out some of the possible causes and make other choices more likely. One advantage of experience is the ability to prioritize the patient assessment so that the differential diagnosis is sorted efficiently and effectively.

CASE INFORMATION

General Survey and History of Present Illness

In this case I begin with a general survey of the patient: she is a well-nourished well-developed appropriately groomed female in no distress, her face is symmetric, and she is able to move all extremities. She is fidgeting with her sheets and does not make eye contact when spoken to. I ask the patient what happened and she loudly states, "I'm not really ready to talk about it right now" and continues fussing with the sheet. The patient's son, Robert, quickly steps in, "I brought my mom to the ER because she was acting really strange when I got home from work. She has been kind of forgetting things the last few months, that's why I moved in to help her out, but today she was trying to make a phone call using the TV remote, and when I told her that it wasn't the phone, she got kind of upset." The patient looks at her son and says clearly, "I'm not sure what you are talking about" then goes back to pulling the sheets through her hands. The patient's son goes on to state that he called her today, as he usually does at the end of his lunch break, and she sounded fine but said she was going to lie down for a while. This is not her normal routine; she usually stays up all day doing her word puzzles or sewing. The patient's son also states that until today "she seemed fine," no recent illness, no fevers, no falls, no new complaints though she probably ate less than usual this morning and last night. Otherwise she seemed in her usual state of health until he came home from work.

Past Medical History

When asked about her past medical history the patient gives a puzzled look and the son again intervenes to help her. "She's really pretty healthy. I think they told us once that she might be starting to get diabetes but she doesn't use insulin or anything, she just has to be careful about eating sweets. She has pills she takes; one is orange for her blood pressure. She takes a blue pill also—that one is for her nerves. I think that's all there is." The patient shakes her head no when asked about any history of cancer, heart disease, stroke, or seizure; son confirms that, as far he knows, this is true.

When I review the hospital's electronic medical record I learn that the patient was seen once in the emergency room for a complaint of palpitations about a year ago. She was observed for 24 hours in the observation unit, and remained in normal sinus rhythm on telemetry. Additional workup during that visit was benign. The discharge summary from lists hypertension and mild cognitive impairment but does not mention diabetes, and her blood sugar on that visit was normal. The patient also had a knee replacement for osteoarthritis 6 years ago. The family confirms that they do not go to any other hospital; their home is only six blocks away. The medical record from the primary care provider's office is unavailable at this time.

Family and Social History

The patient and son deny any relevant family history. The son reports that the patient has never smoked cigarettes, and does not use alcohol other than a glass of wine once a week at the most if she goes out to dinner.

❓ What are the pertinent positives from the information given so far?

- The patient was more tired than usual and eating less in the 24 hours before the confusion started.
- The patient seems to have mild cognitive impairment or dementia.
- The patient has a history of hypertension, has osteoarthritis, and has either prediabetes or diet-controlled diabetes.
- She has a recent history of palpitations but no confirmed diagnosis of cardiac arrhythmia.
- The patient is on two prescription medications although they have not been identified yet.

❓ What are the significant negatives from the information given so far?

- The patient is in no distress.
- No facial droop, no slurred speech, moving both hands equally.
- There is an absence of chronic health problems such as CHF, COPD, cancer, and she is in good health generally and able to care for her own basic needs.
- No history of seizures or prior stroke.
- No falls.

❓ Can the information gathered so far be restated in a single sentence highlighting the pieces that narrow down the cause?

Putting the information obtained so far in a single statement—a problem representation—sets the stage for gathering more information and determining the cause. The problem representation in this case might be: "an 80-year-old female with hypertension and mild cognitive deficits who presents with new onset altered mental state."

❓ How does this information affect the list of possible causes?

The patient's overall good health makes an acute exacerbation of a chronic disease such as CHF or COPD less likely to be the cause of her acute confusion. In addition, the general survey finding that the patient is well appearing and in no apparent distress makes ischemic bowel, pulmonary embolism, sepsis, myocardial infarction, and acute stroke very unlikely. The history of diabetes or prediabetes raises concern for a metabolic cause of her confusion. In addition, the history of palpitations and the patient's age raise concern for cardiac arrhythmia, particularly atrial fibrillation, which can lead to transient ischemic attack. However, the story of her illness makes this less likely; the symptoms of transient ischemic attack usually resolve, and this patient is still altered from her baseline mental state. Medication side effect or overdose cannot be ruled out until more is known about which medications she takes and how she takes them.

More information needs to be collected, but at this point a metabolic cause, dehydration, constipation, urinary tract infection, or an adverse reaction to medication seems most likely. I will order an ECG because the idea of cardiac arrhythmia based on the past visit to the ER is still on my mind, and she does have cardiac risk factors (age, diabetes, hypertension). Along with the ECG a troponin is drawn, as there is the possibility of infarction that does not cause ECG changes (non-ST-elevation myocardial infarction). I will ask the ER nurse to initiate bedside telemetry monitoring. Routine blood work including a complete blood count, comprehensive metabolic panel, and urinalysis are also ordered but I will not have these results immediately. A blood glucose by fingerstick, on the other hand, will immediately determine if hypoglycemia or hyperglycemia are contributing to her symptoms.

CASE INFORMATION

Medications

The ER nurse calls the patient's pharmacy and learns that she is prescribed sertraline (Zoloft) 50 mg once a day, and hydrochlorothiazide 25 mg once a day. The son and the pharmacist are both unaware of any medication allergies or adverse reactions.

Review of Systems

- The patient is a poor historian and is assisted by her son.
- Constitutional: Denies fever, her appetite is normally good but did not eat well at breakfast the morning of this event, no recent falls, no trauma.
- Head/eyes/ears/nose/throat: Denies headache and vision changes. Ate with her son this morning, had no difficulty chewing or swallowing food. Denies recent cold or upper respiratory tract infection systems.
- Cardiovascular: Denies chest pain, leg swelling, or difficulty breathing when lying down
- Pulmonary: Denies shortness of breath or cough.
- Gastrointestinal: Denies nausea/vomiting, reports she had a bowel movement this morning (son cannot confirm this), denies blood in stools.
- Genitourinary: Denies blood in her urine, change in urine smell, frequency, or amount. Endorses occasional "leaking" for which she wears a sanitary napkin in her underwear.
- Musculoskeletal: Endorses occasional knee pain she attributes to osteoarthritis. Takes ibuprofen once in a while with relief.
- Neurological: Denies headache, falls, history of seizure disorder or stroke, numbness, tingling, or extremity weakness, change in speech. Son has not noted any facial changes.
- Endocrine: Denies increased hunger, thirst, or urination, states, "I'm always cold."

Physical Examination

- Vital signs: Pulse is 80 beats per minute, blood pressure is 154/78 mm Hg, respiratory rate is 16 breaths per minute, and temperature is 98.5°F axillary, oxygen saturation by pulse oximeter is 97% on room air, and a fingerstick blood glucose is 108 mg/dL.
- Constitutional: Well appearing, appears stated age, but anxious/fidgety, cannot hold her hands still, poor eye contact during interview, looks tired.
- Head/eyes/ears/nose/throat: Pupils are equal, round, reactive to light, extraocular movements intact, buccal mucosa moist, oropharynx is moist and rises symmetrically, dentures in place upper and lower.
- Cardiovascular: Heart rate and rhythm regular, no murmurs, no gallops, trace edema in both ankles, nail beds are pale, fingers are cool to touch, brisk capillary refill. Her ECG shows normal sinus rhythm, and there is no change when compared to the ECG from a year ago. On bedside telemetry she remains in normal sinus rhythm.
- Pulmonary: Respiratory rate and rhythm are normal, without use of accessory muscles, lungs clear to auscultation and resonant to percussion.
- Gastrointestinal: Normoactive bowel sounds, tympanic on percussion, abdomen soft with mild tenderness over left lower quadrant on deep palpation.

- Neurological: No focal neurologic deficits, face symmetric, speech is clear, upper and lower extremity strength 5/5 throughout, oriented to person but not to place or time, shakes her head or nods to questions, occasionally looks to son to answer for her. Cranial nerves 2–12 intact.
- Integumentary: Intact, no rashes, lesions, or sores, normal skin turgor.
- Endocrine: Normal hair distribution, no involuntary movements, thyroid palpable without nodules. Her blood glucose by fingerstick is 108 mg/dL.

❓ What elements of the review of systems and physical examination should be added to the list of pertinent positives? Which items should be added to the list of significant negatives?

- **Pertinent positives:** Cold intolerance, high blood pressure, mild left lower quadrant abdominal tenderness, fidgety behavior consistent with son's sense that his mother is altered.

- **Significant negatives:** The review of systems and the physical examination are both negative for focal neurological deficits. Her blood glucose by fingerstick is normal. In addition, the ECG is negative for arrhythmia or sign of ischemia. The review of systems reveals no localizing complaints such as pain in a specific area or pulmonary symptoms such as cough or shortness of breath. The physical examination is essentially normal with the few exceptions noted above.

❓ How does this information affect the list of possible causes?

A neurological cause, such as acute stroke, is very unlikely given the normal neurological examination. In addition, the patient's normal cardiac examination and ECG make arrhythmia less likely to be a cause, though paroxysmal atrial fibrillation cannot be ruled out based on a single ECG. The possibility of the patient having an acute exacerbation of CHF or COPD is ruled out based on the absence of any sign or symptom of these diseases and her benign pulmonary and cardiovascular examinations. Her normal blood glucose rules out hypoglycemia and complications of diabetes, such as diabetic ketoacidosis. The absence of a fall or any sign of injury makes fracture or head injury unlikely. A gastrointestinal process is also less likely as the patient's abdominal examination is normal. While left lower quadrant tenderness might indicate constipation, the patient denies this on review of systems. It is possible though that confusion makes her an unreliable historian.

Urinary tract infection is still a possibility as elderly adults often present with confusion and do not present with fever, abdominal pain, or burning on urination and other classic symptoms. In addition, hyponatremia is a potential cause as this is a side effect of both of the medications she is on and may not be revealed on physical examination. With a moist oropharynx and normal skin turgor, dehydration moves lower on the list. The information gathered to date does not rule out a psychiatric process, drug or alcohol withdrawal, or hepatic encephalopathy, however the patient's benign medical and social history make these disorders less likely.

At this point, I reexamine the problem representation. The new problem representation reads: "an 80-year-old female, generally in good health, with hypertension and mild cognitive deficits who presents with mild confusion." I now believe there is something acutely wrong, but it is unlikely that there is something terribly wrong with the patient. Most likely, she has an electrolyte imbalance or a urinary tract infection, both of which cause nonfocal, reversible neurological changes. I am able to reassure the patient's son, and consider additional diagnostic testing.

CASE INFORMATION

Review of Diagnostic Testing

Computed tomography (CT) scan of the head should be considered in any patient who presents with possible stroke. Early treatment is essential to limit deficits and therefore warrants rapid assessment. In this patient, stroke is very unlikely given the information gathered so far and I have other test results to review. Troponin drawn in conjunction with the ECG comes back as 0.024 ng/mL, inconsistent with acute coronary syndrome. A comprehensive metabolic panel shows mildly elevated blood urea nitrogen at 25 mg/dL, normal creatinine, normal blood glucose, and normal electrolytes, ruling out hyponatremia. A normal bilirubin, liver function tests, and normal albumin definitively rule out hepatic encephalopathy. A complete blood count shows mild anemia with a normal white count and normal platelet count. The urinalysis with microscopy shows positive leukocyte esterase, positive nitrates, greater than 10 white blood cells per milliliter, and confirms the presence of bacteria; a culture is pending. With this result, I defer ordering a CT scan. At this point I am ready to list urinary tract infection (UTI) as my primary diagnosis.

Urinary Tract Infection: Diagnosis and Treatment

A diagnosis of urinary tract infection can be made with the presence of symptoms and pyuria, or white blood cells in the urine on microscopic examination. When only a dipstick is available the presence of leukocyte esterase suggests pyuria and urinary tract infection. The presence of nitrates on urine dipstick is highly specific for urinary tract infection but not highly sensitive. In other words, if nitrates are present the person has a urinary tract infection but the absence of nitrates does not rule out urinary tract infection.[2] While guidelines state that a culture is not needed to confirm the diagnosis, it is helpful in guiding treatment, particularly if there is reason to suspect antimicrobial resistance. The need to treat a symptomatic patient prior to having culture data means that a urinary tract infection is often treated empirically, based on the most likely organisms to cause the infection. Uncomplicated urinary tract infection (UTI), defined as UTI in the absence of a urinary catheter or recent procedure, is usually caused by *Escherichia coli* (*E Coli*), which accounts for at least three-fourths of all UTIs. Less often UTI is caused by *Staphylococcus*, *Proteus mirabilis*, *Klebsiella*, enterococci, group B streptococci, or *Pseudomonas*.[3]

Antibiotic choice is guided by patient allergies, interactions with other medications, renal function, and local patterns of antibiotic resistance.[2] It is also wise to consider the number of daily doses needed as adherence to medications dramatically falls when patients are required to take a medication more than twice a day. Side effects that a particular individual may find more troubling should also be considered. For instance, prescribing an antibiotic that causes photosensitivity to a person who spends most of their day outdoors is unwise.

Current guidelines advise a 3-day course of antimicrobial therapy for uncomplicated urinary tract infection, which is any urinary tract infection that is not associated with urinary catheterization or a genitourinary procedure. This recommendation holds true regardless of the patient's age.[4] Specific agents recommended by the guidelines are: trimethoprim-sulfamethoxazole, ciprofloxacin, levofloxacin, norfloxacin, gatifloxacin, nitrofurantoin macrocrystals and nitrofurantoin monohydrate macrocrystals, fosfomycin tromethamine. Some authors advise reserving the fluoroquinolones for complicated UTIs due to increasing microbial resistance.[2]

Additional interventions to consider in the management of a patient who presents with UTI include education about hygiene to prevent further UTI, and the use of cranberry juice or cranberry pills to prevent recurrent infection. For this patient in particular, hygiene should be reviewed with the patient and her son as the patient is unlikely to retain this information in her current state. I also reassure the son, who was clearly frightened by this episode, that UTIs frequently cause acute confusion in older adults.

Case Follow-Up

The patient is given her first dose of trimethoprim-sulfamethoxazole in the emergency room and admitted to the observation unit overnight on telemetry. She remains in normal sinus rhythm and a second troponin level is normal. Early the next morning, her mental status is better. I advise the patient and her son to follow up with her primary care provider (PCP) in the next 2 weeks and I dictate a note to be sent to her PCP's office. The nurse on the observation unit reviews written information about urinary tract infection prevention with the patient and her son and she is discharged home with a prescription for 3 days of trimethoprim-sulfamethoxazole.

References

1. Blanchard G, Dosa D. Evaluation of altered mental status. Epocrates Web site. https://online.epocrates.com/u/2911843/Evaluation+of+altered+mental+status. Accessed March 31, 2015. Updated December 12, 2014.

2. Brusch JL, Bavaro MF, Cunha BA, Tessier JM. Cystitis in females: work up. Medscape Web site. http://emedicine.medscape.com/article/233101-workup#aw2aab6b5b1aa. Accessed June 7, 2014. Updated April 7, 2014.

3. Patel BN, Lee UJ, Goldman HB. Urinary tract infections in women. Epocrates Web site. https://online.epocrates.com/u/291177/Urinary+tract+infections+in+women. Accessed March 31, 2015. Updated September 5, 2014.

4. Treatment of urinary tract infections in non-pregnant women. American College of Obstetricians and Gynecologists Practice Bulletin; number 91. Agency for Healthcare Research and Quality Web site. http://www.guideline.gov/content.aspx?id=12628&search=uti. Published March 2008 and reviewed 2012. Accessed June 7, 2014.

INDEX